SOLVE
IT WITH
SUPPLEMENTS

SOLVE
IT WITH
SUPPLEMENTS

The Best Herbal and Nutritional Supplements to Prevent and Heal More Than 100 Common Health Problems

Robert A. Schulman, MD

Physiatrist and Medical Acupuncturist

with Carolyn Dean, MD, ND, Medical Advisor

RODALE

© 2007 by Rodale Inc.

Rodale books may be purchased for business or promotional use or for special sales. For information, please write to: Special Markets Department, Rodale Inc., 733 Third Avenue, New York, NY 10017

Printed in the United States of America
Rodale Inc. makes every effort to use acid-free ♾, recycled paper ♻.

(*Front cover images*) Jim Ballard /Getty Images *(left)*; Getty Images *(center and spine)*; Mark Bolton/Corbis *(right)*

Library of Congress Cataloging-in-Publication Data

Schulman, Robert A.
Solve it with supplements : the best herbal and nutritional supplements to help prevent and heal more than 100 common health problems / Robert A. Schulman, with Carolyn Dean.
p.   cm.
Includes index.
ISBN–13 978–1–57954–942–8 paperback
ISBN–10 1–57954–942–X paperback
1. Dietary supplements—Popular works.   I. Dean, Carolyn.   II. Title.
RM258.5.S38   2006
613.2'8–dc22   2004015154

Distributed to the book trade by Holtzbrinck Publishers
4   6   8   10   9   7   5   3   paperback

RODALE
LIVE YOUR WHOLE LIFE™

We inspire and enable people to improve their lives and the world around them
For more of our products visit **rodalestore.com** or call 800-848-4735

CONTENTS

ABOUT THIS BOOK

WHETHER YOU ARE SURFING THE INTERNET, shopping at your local health food store, or simply talking to a friend who swears that her memory has improved after taking a particular herb, it is nearly impossible to escape the various health claims made about dietary supplements. While there is certainly no lack of information about supplements, finding information that is reliable or that suits your particular needs can be an extremely time-consuming and sometimes fruitless endeavor. To make matters worse, the media's coverage of vitamins, minerals, and herbs vacillates between scaring consumers and creating an exaggerated hype around a particular supplement. As a result, information tends to be distorted and consumers are left in a steadily growing mire of supplemental confusion.

In 2002, the Council for Responsible Nutrition (CRN) published a report stating that the consistent use of multivitamins and other key supplements can promote good health and help prevent disease. While few people would dispute the benefits of dietary supplements for particular populations—such as pregnant women and seniors—many people are confused about the health benefits they can attain from dietary supplements for disease prevention and treatment.

Solve It with Supplements brings you the most up-to-date information on vitamins, minerals, and herbs and helps you understand the various conditions they may prevent and treat. You will no longer have to scratch your head while trying to decipher exactly what the information on a supplement label means. Our writers, author, and medical advisor have sifted through a variety of media—including scientific studies, news articles, supplement databases, and Web sites—in order to assemble a comprehensive reference book that does not require a medical degree to read. Our author also ensured the content's accuracy and included his own experience with supplements in his clinical practice.

Use *Solve It with Supplements* as a tool to help you get the most health benefits from various vitamins, minerals, and herbs and to determine which supplements are appropriate for your health needs. Be sure to speak to you doctor about whether a particular supplement is right for you and always disclose any supplements you are taking to your healthcare provider.

Solve It with Supplements will ensure that you reap the greatest rewards from nutritional supplements, when using them alone or as a successful complement to your traditional medical care in order to achieve optimum health and wellness.

HOW TO USE THIS BOOK

SOLVE IT WITH SUPPLEMENTS HAS BEEN CAREFULLY arranged to provide instant and easy access to the information you seek. Part One: "What Supplements Can Do for You" is a thorough introduction to supplements that will give you a solid base of knowledge about vitamins, minerals, and herbs and why they are so important. Reading this introduction will also teach you to become an educated consumer so that you can go to the health food store or pharmacy armed with the knowledge you need to purchase the product you want.

In Part Two: "A Guide to Supplements" you can look for a particular supplement to learn more about its characteristics, including:

What It Is	Is the supplement a vitamin, mineral, herb, enzyme, or amino acid?
What It Does	The role that the supplement plays in health and the various conditions it treats
How It Works	The mechanism of action of the supplement
How to Take It	General dosage guidelines for the supplement
Look Out for This!	Safety risks for certain populations (for example, seniors)
What to Avoid	Interactions that the supplement may have with other supplements, herbs, or prescription medications

All material is cross-referenced so that you may easily search Part Three: "Using Supplements to Manage Health" for detailed information about specific conditions and ailments.

Part Three: "Using Supplements to Manage Health" allows you to look up information about particular health conditions and the supplements that may help treat them. For instance—you return from your annual physical only to discover that your cholesterol is high. You can look up "High Cholesterol" and read about the various supplements that are recommended for this condition. Furthermore, you can call your doctor and ask his or her opinion about taking a particular supplement in conjunction with the cholesterol-lowering medication the doctor just prescribed. It's that simple. Each profile in this section will provide a general overview of an ailment or condition, a list of the best supplements recommended to help treat, prevent, or alleviate it, and the specific dosages for each supplement. The sections in each profile include:

What Is It?	A general overview of the condition
What Should I Take?	A list of supplements recommended for the condition and information about why they are believed to be effective
My Supplement List	Dosage information about recommended supplements

PART ONE

....

*What Supplements
Can Do for You*

THE BENEFITS
OF SUPPLEMENTS

LOOKING FOR WAYS TO IMPROVE YOUR OWN and your family's health and well-being? The quality of your diet is one very important place to start. Nutrition has an enormous impact on your health, affecting how you feel, how well you function, how well your body can fight infection . . . even how long you live. It can also play a role in preventing many diseases and certain birth defects.

There's no question that a balanced diet (along with regular exercise) is critical to health maintenance and disease prevention (see "Food Packs a Punch," page 13). However, some researchers believe that certain nutrients are deficient in soil, and that as a result, the food we consume—even if it's the correct food—may be lacking in some nutrients. Since plants cannot manufacture minerals, and soil that was once enriched with minerals may be depleted, supplements can help make up for a deficiency of minerals in the foods we eat, as well as give us an additional health boost.

A growing body of evidence suggests that dietary supplements play an important part in health maintenance. Studies show that both men and women fail to meet the Recommended Daily Allowances (RDAs; see page 7) for a variety of important nutrients, including calcium, vitamin E, vitamin B_6, magnesium, copper, and zinc. It's no wonder that people are turning to supplements to get the important nutrients they require and to treat specific ailments—as many as 50 percent of Americans use dietary supplements. And in 2000 alone, they spent an estimated $15.7 billion on more than 29,000 different products—from vitamins and minerals to herbal supplements and other specialty products.

THE ABCs OF SUPPLEMENTS
A Definition

Before 1994, the term "dietary supplements" referred only to products made from one or more of the essential nutrients (such as vitamins, minerals, and proteins). In 1994, the U.S. Congress passed the Dietary Supplement Health and Education Act (DSHEA). This act created a new framework for labeling and assuring the safety of dietary supplements. It also redefined a dietary supplement as a product that is:

- Meant to supplement the diet
- Made up of one or more of the following:
  - Vitamins
  - Minerals
  - Herbs or substances derived from plants (except tobacco)
  - Amino acids (the building blocks that make up proteins)
  - Other substances that increase the total dietary intake (such as enzymes or organ tissue)
  - Concentrates, metabolites, constituents, or extracts of all the substances named above

■ Taken by mouth in the form of tablets, capsules, softgels, gelcaps, liquids, or powders*
■ Labeled as a dietary supplement

*Note: Dietary supplements are available in other forms as well (for example, snack bars).

The Benefits

The range of dietary supplements now available to you and your family is vast. And so are the benefits they may provide. From your heart and mind to your joints and bones, there are dietary supplements purporting to help you from head to toe. Many benefits of supplements are supported by sound scientific evidence; others are not. This is mainly because supplement research is still in its infancy. Knowing the difference is essential for responsible supplement use (see "Becoming a Wise Consumer," page 15, for tips on buying and using supplements).

Supplements are often placed into broad categories that describe their action and claimed and/or potential benefits. For example:

■ Antioxidants (such as vitamins C and E) are substances that slow oxidative processes in the body, protecting the body from damage caused by the cell-damaging molecules called "free radicals." They reduce the transformation of low-density lipoprotein (LDL) cholesterol ("bad" cholesterol) into damaging substances and may reduce the risk of heart disease, prevent cancer, and protect the body from the effects of aging.
■ Anti-inflammatory supplements (such as glucosamine) are thought to suppress tissue irritation, therefore reducing associated pain (see "Glucosamine," page 144).

Who Needs Supplements?

In general, all adults, and all teenagers and children with poor appetites or irregular eating habits, can benefit from a multivitamin with minerals, since it provides extra insurance of obtaining the nutrients needed for good health.

Other supplements that may be necessary, depending upon a person's age, gender, and eating habits, are:

■ Calcium—For people who don't regularly eat dairy products or other calcium-rich foods and for postmenopausal women at risk for osteoporosis.
■ Folic acid (folate)—For women planning to become pregnant. Since many pregnancies are unplanned, it is recommended that all women of childbearing age (who might become pregnant) receive additional folic acid.
■ Iron—For pregnant women and people with anemia.
■ Magnesium—For people who don't eat vegetables, nuts, seeds, and whole grains.
■ Vitamin B_{12}—For vegetarians (adults, teenagers, and children) who do not eat animal products, or for adults over age 50 who are deficient in this vitamin.
■ Vitamin D—For older adults and people who are rarely in sunlight.

You may also consider using other key supplements (such as vitamins C or E), herbal products (such as St. John's wort or ginkgo biloba), or specialty supplements (such as glucosamine) for specific conditions. Remember, it's never too late to begin reaping the rewards of dietary supplements. You too can enjoy greater health with a few simple steps.

MICRONUTRIENTS: ESSENTIALS FOR GOOD HEALTH

Proper nutrition is made up of six types of nutrients that must come from your diet—carbohydrates, fats, proteins, vitamins, minerals, and water. Carbohydrates, fats, and proteins are called macronutrients because they are needed in large amounts to produce energy for your body. Vitamins and minerals are called micronutrients because they are needed in small amounts. These micronutrients don't produce energy, but are needed for all parts of the body to function properly.

Vitamins

So far, researchers have identified 13 essential vitamins, which are divided into two categories: water-soluble vitamins and fat-soluble vitamins.

Water-Soluble Vitamins
- Need water to be absorbed
- Leave the body in the urine
- Include vitamin C and the eight B vitamins (biotin, folate, niacin, pantothenic acid, riboflavin, thiamine, and vitamins B_6 and B_{12})

Fat-Soluble Vitamins
- Need fat to be absorbed
- Are stored in fat tissue
- Include vitamins A, D, E, and K

Each of the vitamins plays at least one major important role in your body—for example, vitamin A protects your eyesight, vitamin D helps you absorb calcium (thereby promoting healthy bones and teeth), and vitamin K is essential for blood clotting.

Minerals

Sixteen essential minerals are separated into two categories: major or macrominerals, and trace or microminerals.

Major or Macrominerals
- Are needed by the body in large amounts (more than 100 milligrams/day).
- Include calcium, chloride, magnesium, phosophorus, potassium, sodium, and sulfur.

Trace or Microminerals
- Are needed in much smaller (or trace) amounts than macrominerals.
- Include chromium, copper, fluoride, iodine, iron, manganese, molybdenum, selenium, and zinc.

Like vitamins, minerals are vital for good health—for example, calcium, phosophorus, and magnesium help develop and maintain healthy bones and teeth. Sodium, potassium, and chloride maintain the right balance of water and electrolytes in your body, which aids metabolism. Many sports drinks include sodium and/or potassium to help maintain the balance after exercise.

When Micronutrients Are Missing

When essential micronutrients are missing from your diet or are taken in amounts less than those recommended (see "How Much You Need" on next page), the body cannot perform at its best, and serious health problems can develop. Vitamins and minerals act as essential cofactors in all the metabolic processes of the body; if they are not present, the body cannot function properly. Pregnant women and young children are among the groups most vulnerable to this problem, since a lack of micronutrients can interfere with the development of basic functions (such as intellect) during periods of rapid growth. The elderly are also vulnerable because they are more susceptible to illness and disease.

The Pyramid Controversy

The USDA Food Guide Pyramid was introduced in 1992 to help promote healthy nutrition. Its intent was to help consumers choose the proper foods for maintaining a healthy diet by providing a visual image of dietary concepts. The pyramid aimed to promote a diet that incorporated adequate amounts of protein, vitamins, minerals, and dietary fiber while eliminating excessive amounts of fat, saturated fat, cholesterol, sodium, added sugars, and calories. The pyramid highlights many different types of foods in order to illustrate that a diversity of foods should be consumed from within various food groups.

However, the Food Guide Pyramid came under attack because of its emphasis on carbohydrates, whereas current trends focus on a diet that includes more fat and fewer carbohydrates. Furthermore, the Food Guide Pyramid became a subject of consternation for many people because of the growing number of people diagnosed with diabetes and obesity, possibly because of a high carbohydrate and fat intake. As a result, the USDA released a revised version of the Food Pyramid called My Pyramid.

Many alternative pyramids have been developed, designed for particular populations, each taking into consideration cultural and/or nutritional eating habits.

The Mayo Clinic Healthy Weight Pyramid—Emphasizes foods that are low in calories but can be consumed in large amounts (such as fruits, vegetables, legumes, poultry, fish, and whole grains).

The Asian Diet Pyramid—Emphasizes grains such as rice and noodles and contains limited dairy products.

The Latin Diet Pyramid—Emphasizes maize (corn) and potatoes and includes daily meal options (including fish, shellfish, plant oils, dairy products, and poultry) and weekly meal options (including red meat, sweets, and eggs).

The Mediterranean Diet Pyramid—Emphasizes fresh fruits and vegetables, grains, and legumes and uses olive oil in the place of other fats and oils.

The Vegetarian Diet Pyramid—Emphasizes grains, legumes, fruits, vegetables, nuts, and seeds and includes egg whites, soy milk, dairy products, and plant oils in moderation.

How Much You Need

Fortunately, there are many resources in the United States (such as the U.S. Department of Agriculture [USDA] Food Guide Pyramid; see previous page) that can offer guidelines to help you plan a healthy diet and, when necessary, use dietary supplements to avoid micronutrient deficiencies and their consequences.

Percent daily values, which appear on food labels (see "Read Labels Wisely," page 18), provide a simple way to plan your supplement use to meet recommended intakes of various nutrients. These values are based on a diet of 2,000 calories per day (for adults and children over 4 years of age), and they indicate the percent of the recommended daily amount of a nutrient that is supplied by one serving of a supplement.

By using the percent daily value for a particular nutrient, you can tell whether the amount you're taking is too high (over 100 percent) or too low (less than 100 percent). For example, if the label on your multivitamin bottle says that your multivitamin provides 20 percent of the daily value for calcium, you'll need another 80 percent from other sources to meet the recommended goal.

Daily values meet or exceed the recommended micronutrient needs for most people, so you can rely on them as an accurate guide to your own recommended daily use of supplements.

The U.S. Recommended Dietary Allowance (RDA)

How Much is Enough?

The RDA—created by the Food and Nutrition Board of the U.S. National Academy of Sciences' Institute of Medicine—was established to provide nutritional guidelines to the general public and health professionals. The RDA number was developed to reflect the intake of essential nutrients that were judged to be adequate to meet the known needs of practically all healthy people. For many years, the RDAs for these nutrients served as the "gold standard" against which people could measure the nutritional adequacy of their own diets.

Although the RDA system has undergone various updates, many people in the nutrition community feel that the current RDAs are too low and are calling for major revisions. The basis of this argument was discussed in a symposium that was published under the title of "Future Directions for the Recommended Daily Allowances Under Discussion by the Food and Nutrition Board" in 1994. This report may be viewed online at no cost at http://books.nap.edu/books /NX004037/html/17.html#pagetop.

Many members of the nutritional community desire a revision of RDAs because:

■ New knowledge has accumulated for various nutrients that should be taken into consideration.

■ The formulation of new RDAs should include the reductions they will provide in the risks of developing various chronic diseases when there is sufficient information about the safety and efficacy of those nutrients.

In order to keep the RDAs for various nutrients up to date, the 1994 Food and Nutrition Board Symposium also discussed a new format for future RDAs, which includes more detail about how these recommendations are derived, their flexibility to address multiple uses of nutrients, information on interactions between different nutrients, information about the principles and scientific evidence underlying RDAs, and dietary patterns for specific age groups and physiological states.

However, considering the ill health of a large part of the population, many doctors recommend doses of vitamins and minerals above the Recommended Dietary Allowance (RDA) and daily intake values to try to prevent and treat chronic disease.

Want to Know More about Intake?

While percent daily values are a simple, at-a-glance guide for planning your supplement use, you may be interested in more detailed information about recommended nutrient intake. "Daily values" is an umbrella term that includes Dietary Reference Intakes (DRIs). These DRIs are based on at least three reference values:

- Estimated average requirement (EAR)—The usual average intake of a particular nutrient that can meet the needs of half the healthy people in a particular age and gender group.
- Recommended dietary allowance (RDA)—The average daily intake of a nutrient that meets the requirement of nearly all healthy people in a particular age and gender group.
- Adequate intake (AI)—If there is not enough information to set the EAR, the AI is suggested, rather than the RDA.
- Upper limit (UL)—The highest level of a nutrient that is unlikely to pose risks to almost all people in a particular age and gender group. In other words, this is the safe upper limit.

When it comes to micronutrients, your goal should be to meet the RDA (or the AI if no RDA is established) and not to exceed the UL. However, your doctor may recommend higher amounts of particular vitamins or nutrients for your specific condition. Some people aim to meet the UL, because the RDAs for various supplements are now often considered to be inadequate and are constantly changing.

Since 1995, several expert committees in the United States and Canada have been establishing DRIs for each nutrient. The reports on these DRIs have so far been completed and published and are available from the Food and Nutrition Board of the Institute of Medicine of the National Academy of Sciences. The reports can either be purchased online or viewed online at no cost at http://www.iom.edu/project.asp?id=4574.

Alternatively, you can contact the National Academies Press:

Tel: (800) 624-8373 or (202) 334-3313
Fax: (202) 334-2451
Mail: National Academies Press
       500 Fifth Street, NW
       Washington, DC 20055

Where to Get Your Micronutrients

Finding the right balance of vitamins and minerals is important to your health. How can you achieve that balance? A multi-pronged approach is best.

Healthy food choices, especially fruits, vegetables, seeds, nuts, whole grains, and fresh herbs should definitely be part of your overall plan (see "Food Packs a Punch," page 13). Sometimes, fortified foods (see "Facts on Fortified Foods," below) can be beneficial as well. And for many people, a basic multivitamin with minerals makes good sense.

What You Need to Know About Multivitamins

Thousands of multivitamins (with and without minerals) are available on the market. What's more, they're not all "created equal." So when choosing a multivitamin, there are several tips to keep in mind. A good-quality supplement:

- *Should* provide 100 percent of the daily value for
  - Vitamins: A, B_1 (thiamine), B_2 (riboflavin), B_3 (niacin), B_6, B_{12}, D, and folic acid.
  - Minerals: calcium,* copper, zinc, magnesium, iron, iodine, selenium, and chromium.
- *Should not* exceed 100 percent of the daily value for each vitamin and mineral (unless your doctor advises otherwise).
- *Should not* provide megadoses of one or more nutrients (for example, 300 percent of the daily value), unless recommended by your doctor. Megadoses of some vitamins and minerals can be dangerous.

*Most multivitamins don't contain 100 percent of the daily value for calcium. If they did, the supplement tablet or capsule would be far too large to take. A separate calcium supplement needs to be taken to achieve the recommended intake of this mineral.

Make sure to check that the expiration date of a supplement has not passed. This date should be listed on the label (see "Read Labels Wisely," page 18). If it isn't there, don't buy the product.

Facts on Fortified Food

When food is fortified, nutrients are added to the food that weren't originally there. (This is a separate process from enriching foods, in which nutrients that were lost during processing are added back.)

A quick look at the food's nutrition facts (listed on the label) will tell you if it's been fortified, which nutrients have been added, and the percent daily value for each nutrient. However, all of the added vitamins in fortified foods are synthetic and don't come close to replacing what's lost in food refining.

The U.S. government sets the standards for the fortification of certain foods by specifying the amount of certain micronutrients they must contain, such as:

- Vitamins A and D in milk
- Folic acid* and iron in grain products
- Iodine in salt

*Note: For women of childbearing age, eating foods fortified with folic acid is not enough to meet the new recommendations for this supplement (400 micrograms/day). Additional supplementation is necessary.

A Word of Caution

Many food producers voluntarily enhance their products with micronutrients (for example, calcium-fortified orange juice and iron-enriched breakfast cereals). On the one hand, this expands your choice of beneficial foods. But on the other hand, it can put you at risk of getting too much of a micronutrient, since there is no limitation on the amount that can be added. This can be a problem for people with chronic health conditions. For instance, the excess iron in fortified foods can be a serious hazard to the health of people who have conditions in which the body stores or absorbs too much iron.

There is no doubt that fortified foods can give a needed boost of a particular vitamin or mineral for people with poor dietary habits. However, keep in mind that while these foods may help to reverse the symptoms that come from a lack of a particular nutrient, they do not treat the problem itself, which stems from poor dietary habits. Nothing, not even fortified foods, can replace a wholesome, well-balanced diet.

HERBAL ALTERNATIVES

Herbal medicine has a long history of use in various cultures around the world, including North America. When the first edition of the *United States Pharmacopeia* was published in 1820, 67% of the total number of entries were botanical substances. It was not until the 1920s that herbs began to lose popularity, when they were replaced with prescription drugs that could offer more dramatic results at a more economical price. In the 1990s, however, sales of herbal products dramatically increased, and herbs continue to be an important element in many people's health regimens.

Herbal supplements contain active ingredients from various plant parts, including the roots, berries, seeds, leaves, stems, bark, and flowers. Many have been used for millennia to prevent and treat illness. In fact, a multitude of our best-known pharmaceutical medicines are derived from plants. Aspirin, for example, originally came from white willow bark and meadowsweet. Taxol, derived from the yew tree, is used to treat breast and ovarian cancer. Quinine, which comes from the bark of the Peruvian cinchona tree, was once a common treatment for malaria. Lanoxin, originally derived from the foxglove plant, is used to treat certain heart conditions. And colchine, which is prescribed as an anti-inflammatory medicine, comes from the autumn crocus plant.

An enormous range of herbal supplements are available on the market. Many, such as garlic and ginseng, are well known; others, like kava root and saw palmetto, may be less familiar. Turn to "A Guide to Supplements," starting on page 25, for a detailed explanation of individual herbal and botanical supplements.

While you may take vitamin and mineral supplements to get nutrients that your diet doesn't provide, most people take herbs to treat specific symptoms, such as joint pain or a depressed mood. Some herbal supplements have been proven safe and effective by scientific research (St. John's wort is a good example); the effectiveness of others remains unknown. The best way to tell the difference is to do your own research.

Types and Forms of Herbal Supplements

Herbs are divided into the two main categories of specific herbs and tonics.*

Specific Herbs
- Target a specific symptom
- Usually are taken for brief periods

An example of a specific herb is echinacea for the common cold.

Tonics
- Are meant to enhance the health of an organ or body system
- Usually are taken over a long term (sometimes with short breaks)

An example of a tonic is ginkgo (ginkgo biloba) to increase blood flow to the brain (potentially improving memory and other functions of the brain).

Note: Some herbs can fall into both categories.

Herbal supplements are available in many forms—fresh from the plant, capsules, tablets, standardized extracts, teas, infusions and decoctions, tinctures and glycerites, infused and essential oils, and sprays. Some herbal supplements are sold as capsules because they are convenient, easy to take, and portable, but some ailments require another form such as topical. Herbal supplements do, however, have some drawbacks:

- Herbs that are dried and ground may lose potency more quickly when this is done. Whole-herb capsules (as opposed to a concentrated extract) need to be taken in larger amounts to get enough of the herb.
- The form you use can depend on the herb you are taking. For example, enteric-coated peppermint capsules are often useful for treating irritable bowel syndrome. If you are suffering from sunburn, aloe vera gel is often applied topically. And if you feel queasy, a cup of ginger tea, made from fresh ginger, may be just what the doctor ordered. Many herbs do come in different forms, to be used depending on the condition being treated.

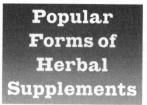

Popular Forms of Herbal Supplements

Standardized Extracts—Extracts are concentrated products obtained by treating an herb with a solvent such as water or alcohol; standardized extracts contain the same amount of active ingredient(s) in all batches made by the manufacturer.

Capsules and Tablets—Contain the herb or extract in an easy-to-swallow form.

Teas—Require steeping the herb in water.

Decoctions—Ingredients extracted from the herb in boiling water. A decoction is the strongest of the water-based preparations of an herb.

Tinctures—Alcohol-based preparations of an herb and usually more potent than water-based preparations.

Glycerites—Made by extracting an herb with glycerine instead of alcohol.

Infused and Essential Oils—Oils extracted from an herb by distilling it. Essential oils contain many, if not most, of the medicinal properties of an herb and are highly concentrated. Infused oils are produced by soaking the plant material in warm oil over a period of time and are less concentrated.

Sprays—Used topically or for aromatherapy.

How to Use Herbs

Compared to drugs, most herbal supplements have fewer and milder side effects. But like drugs and other supplements, herbs can be harmful if used improperly. "Becoming a Wise Consumer" on page 15 provides strategies for smart supplement use that apply equally to herbs. However, there are some specific tips to keep in mind when using herbs:

- Start slowly. Dosages of herbs are often given in ranges. Always start at the low end, and if you don't feel any relief, gradually increase the dose. If you reach the top of the recommended range and still haven't experienced any benefit, consult your doctor or herbal practitioner (see "When You Need Help," below).
- Most herbs are best taken on an empty stomach, half an hour before or two hours after meals, to achieve maximum absorption.
- If you ever feel any unusual symptoms after taking an herbal supplement, stop taking it immediately and consult your doctor or herbal practitioner.
- Single-herb products indicate how much of the herb is in each dose. Some products contain a mixture of herbs (called "formulas" or "combination products") that may have inadequate doses of each of the constituent herbs but may work synergistically. They may also contain herbs that are not well researched and may not seem suitable for the condition being treated. However, trained herbalists understand the synergism of herbs and often prescribe an herbal formula, which is a traditional way of giving herbal prescriptions.
- Never give herbal supplements to children younger than two years old (unless approved by a doctor).

When You Need Help

With all of the herbal supplements available on the market and the seemingly endless array of the benefits they offer, it's not surprising that you might want and need assistance in choosing

Standardized Products

The standardization of herbal products was a process designed to guarantee that they included a certain amount of an active ingredient. Since the types and contents of chemicals in an herb can vary greatly, depending on a host of conditions—including growing conditions, environment, harvest times, handling, storage, age, and extraction techniques—a process was needed to ensure that consumers could expect the same quality and consistency in the herbal products they purchase. Standardization allows manufacturers to have greater consistency from one batch to another of the herbs they use in making an herbal product. The process of standardization is extremely complex and requires manufacturers to adhere to various codes of ethics, in addition to stringent documenting processes and standards, throughout all stages of herb production.

However, it is important to keep in mind that standardizing a product does not guarantee its potency. In many cases the medicinal activity of an herb is not due to one ingredient, but rather to a mixture of many ingredients working together, some of which may not even be identified. Still, standardization helps both consumers and manufacturers attain a more consistent product.

those that are best for you. You might get this assistance from your primary care doctor (since more and more doctors in the United States are knowledgeable in this field). There are also people trained specifically in herbal medicine who can help you. Look for the following designations after their names:

- *ND (naturopathic doctor)*—A person trained for four years at a certified naturopathic medical school (not all states recognize this degree).
- *MNIMH* or *FNIMH*—A person trained at the National Institute for Medical Herbalism (NIMH) in England.
- *AHG*—A certification given by the American Herbalists Guild to people who have either attended a three- to four-year program or who have a similar depth of training or experience obtained from elsewhere.
- *LAc*—A licensed acupuncturist. Some of these specialists may have received additional training and certification in herbal medicine as well.
- *NCCAOM*—The National Certification Commission provides certification for Acupuncture and Oriental Medicine to qualified practitioners of acupuncture and oriental medicine.

FOOD PACKS A PUNCH

Last but far from least in your health is food. Your daily diet has a powerful influence on your health and is often the best and most complete way to ensure a proper intake of vitamins and minerals. Dietary supplements can be an important partner in achieving this goal, but they should never replace eating right every day.

The good news is that studies indicate that dietary supplement users do not appear to take supplements as a "substitute" for a healthy diet. Instead, they use supplements as part of an overall nutritional strategy that includes sensible and varied food choices. Along with regular exercise, this should also be your guiding principle.

The Benefits of Healthy Eating

- Whole foods contain a wide variety of nutrients needed by your body. For example, an orange contains not only vitamin C, but also contains beta carotene, calcium, and other nutrients integral to good health.
- Whole foods provide dietary fiber, which you need for proper digestion. Fiber also appears to reduce the risk of developing heart disease, diabetes, diverticular disease, and constipation.
- Other substances in whole foods may protect you from disease. There are many compounds in foods (other than the essential nutrients) that can provide an abundance of health benefits. Fruits and vegetables have compounds called phytochemicals that may prevent diseases such as cancer, diabetes, osteoporosis, and heart disease. And foods may contain many other, as-yet-unidentified compounds that provide important health benefits. Eating a wide variety of foods is the best way to boost your chances of obtaining healthy nutrients, especially ones that are organic, free range, or grown by local farmers.

Getting the Most Nutrients

Specific foods can provide "the best buck" for certain nutrients. These nutrients and the foods that best provide them are:

Calcium
- Yogurt, milk, and natural cheeses (for example, cheddar)
- Dark green, leafy vegetables
- Nuts (for example, almonds and Brazil nuts)
- Seeds (for example, sunflower and sesame)
- Sardines (with bones)
- Blackberries and cherries
- Beans (for example, pinto and soybeans)

Iron
- Eggs
- Shellfish (for example, shrimp or clams), sardines
- Lean meats (particularly beef) and beef liver
- Spinach
- Cooked dry beans (for example, kidney beans), peas, and lentils
- Pumpkin seeds
- Wheat bran

Vitamin A
- Orange fruit (for example, mango, cantaloupe, and papaya) and vegetables (for example, carrots and sweet potatoes)
- Dark green, leafy vegetables (for example, spinach and kale)
- Yellow butter
- Organ meats (consider organically fed organ meats)
- Cod liver oil

Vitamin C
- Citrus fruits, kiwi fruit, strawberries, and cantaloupe
- Broccoli, peppers, tomatoes, potatoes, and sauerkraut
- Leafy greens (for example, romaine lettuce and spinach)

Folate
- Oranges, orange juice, bananas, pineapple, and berries
- Dark green, leafy vegetables (for example, spinach and brussels sprouts)
- Green peas

Potassium
- Baked potatoes (white or sweet); green, leafy vegetables (for example, spinach); and winter (orange) squash
- Bananas and dried fruit (for example, apricots and prunes)
- Cooked dry beans and lentils

- Avocados
- Seeds and nuts
- Fish (for example, salmon, cod, flounder, and sardines)

SUPPLEMENT SAVVY:
BECOMING A WISE CONSUMER

Some dietary supplements can be a boon to your health and well-being. Others can create unexpected risks or unnecessary expenses. How can you become a smart supplement user and tell the good from the bad? It's not always easy, particularly since the Food and Drug Administration (FDA) has only limited control over the quality and safety of the herbal supplements that are available on today's market.

In 1993, there was a movement by the FDA to tighten the regulation of dietary supplements. The goal was to require manufacturers to prove that their supplements actually did what they claimed, by subjecting them to extensive scientific studies. While this was sound in theory (and is the same process required for all drugs sold in the United States), it would have required supplement manufacturers to make a huge investment—one from which they might never have recovered economically, since many supplements would be difficult to patent and make profitable. In response, supplement manufacturers garnered public support and fought back with a grassroots writing campaign that stopped the FDA proposal in its tracks.

What resulted was the Dietary Supplement Health and Education Act (DSHEA), which became law in 1994. This act limits the FDA's power to ensure the safety and effectiveness of herbal supplements. While organizations selling supplements can make limited health claims without FDA approval (see "Read Labels Wisely," page 18), the FDA can order removal of a product from the market if it is thought to be dangerous. Furthermore, the DSHEA prevents supplement makers from saying that a particular product can "cure" or "treat" a particular health condition. Ultimately, the DSHEA gives you greater freedom—and greater responsibility—in deciding which supplements may benefit you and your family.

In contrast to the DSHEA, a more rigorous and restrictive approach to supplements has been adopted outside the United States (see "Germany Takes a Different Track," page 16). And it appears that a tighter rein on supplements is now being advocated in the United States as well. In March 2003, the FDA proposed a rule that would establish new standards for the manufacturing and labeling of dietary supplements. According to the FDA, "the proposed rule would not limit consumers' access to dietary standards." If adopted as proposed, the rule "would give consumers greater confidence that the dietary supplement they use will have the identity, purity, quality, strength, and composition that is claimed on the label." The rule would still not, however, address the product's safety or effectiveness. Many consumers see this more restrictive approach as limiting their freedom of choice.

Until the proposed FDA rule is formally enacted by the FDA (if, indeed, it is), the onus is on you to assess the safety and effectiveness of the supplements you use. Although this may seem a daunting task, some practical strategies can help you to avoid the pitfalls of supplement misuse and take full advantage of the many benefits supplements can offer.

Practical Strategies for Smart Supplement Use

Consult Your Doctor

Before you or your family use a dietary supplement, it's wise to consult your doctor. A frank discussion of your plans to take any supplement is vital, especially if you are taking a prescription medication, are pregnant or nursing a baby, or have a chronic medical condition such as diabetes, heart disease, glaucoma, depression, kidney failure, or high blood pressure. Consulting your doctor is also important if you are experiencing specific symptoms. While many supplements can relieve certain symptoms, a proper medical diagnosis of any symptoms is essential.

Be sure to tell your doctor and pharmacist about all the supplements you are planning to take or are currently taking.

- Some supplements may interact with other medicines—both over-the- counter (OTC) and prescription medicines—and produce serious, and sometimes life-threatening reactions. Be on the lookout for advisories (see "FDA MedWatch," page 22) that warn of these interactions.
- Some supplements may interact with medications used during surgery, causing changes in heart rate, blood pressure, and increased bleeding (for example, ginseng can increase blood pressure that's already high, while garlic, ginger, and feverfew can increase the risk of bleeding). Your doctor may ask you to stop taking supplements at least two to three weeks before a surgical procedure in order to avoid these serious complications.

Germany Takes a Different Track

In contrast to the United States, Germany requires that herbal supplements undergo the same process that is required for the approval of new drugs. In 1978, the German government formed an expert scientific committee that it called Commission E, to evaluate the safety and efficacy of all herbal supplements released after that date. A "Traditional Medicine" status was granted to old herbal products already on the market and which could not meet the Commission E standards. These products must also pass a review by a special committee established in 1996. Based on these ongoing evaluations, Commission E then approves the sale of certain herbs or combinations of herbs.

The German Commission E has published the evaluations of more than 300 herbs in the form of official monographs containing approved uses, contraindications, side effects, dosage, drug interactions, and other vital information about these herbs. Both approved and unapproved herbs were included in these monographs.

All Commission E monographs have been translated and compiled into one text that is available at most major bookstores, *The Complete German Commission E Monographs: Therapeutic Guide to Herbal Medicines,* edited by Mark Blumenthal and others and published in 1998.

And remember, *never* discontinue any medication and substitute a dietary supplement for it without your doctor's knowledge and consent.

Be Informed

Take the time to be a well-informed consumer. Reading all you can about supplements before taking them is critical. This book is an excellent place to start. Talk to your doctor as well. An increasing number of doctors are taking an interest in therapies that are used alternatively to or together with conventional medical treatment—and which are therefore grouped together under the heading of complementary and alternative medicine (CAM)—and many are knowledgeable about the benefits and risks of dietary supplements.

SEARCHING THE WEB

An enormous amount of information on dietary supplements is available on the internet. The challenge is to differentiate credible, reliable information from misleading, outdated, or potentially harmful material.

- Avoid "blind" searches with a search engine. Go instead to directory sites of respected organizations.
- Identify the organization that runs the Web site. Your best choices are sites operated by the government, a university, or a reputable medical, holistic, or health organization, such as the National Institutes of Health or the American Holistic Medical Association.
- Determine if the information is current—look for the date when the material was posted or updated on the Web site. The most reliable Web sites are updated on a frequent basis.
- Ascertain if the information is supported by sound evidence (see "The Scientific Approach," below) from reputable sources, such as well-known medical journals or scientific organizations. Ideally, a site should back up its information with a list of references containing details about where you can find specific studies (so that you can check them out yourself).

The Scientific Approach

Not all scientific evidence is sound. In general, the best way to judge the quality of the evidence provided by a scientific study is to look at a study's design. In general, if a study of a supplement is conducted as a prospective, double-blind, placebo, randomized controlled trial (RCT), you can be more confident that the results it provides are accurate. It is also important to look at who is conducting the study, how the study was designed, how the treatment groups for the study were selected, and most importantly, how the data produced by the study were analyzed and the study's conclusions were reached. An RCT is a sure way to know if a treatment is effective and works better than a placebo (a "fake" treatment such as a sugar pill). A well-designed RCT has the following characteristics:

- A large group of people take part in the study to ensure that the results are not due to a coincidence or error.
- The study occurs over a reasonable length of time (such as 6 months or more).

- Participants are randomly selected and assigned ("randomized") to one of two or more treatment groups (see below), so that results of the study are not biased.
- One group of participants is treated with the supplement, and another group—called the control group—is given the placebo instead.
- Both the participants in the study and the scientists conducting the study are "kept in the dark" about who receives the supplement and who receives the placebo (a procedure called "double-blinding").

Ultimately, good recommendations about health-related products and procedures generally rely on a body of evidence, not on one single study. Therefore, if a study's results are confirmed by at least one other study, you can be more confident about the results.

However, it is important to note that studying nutrients and supplements may not be the same as studying prescription medications, which traditionally use RCTs. There is growing debate about studying nutrients and supplements individually, as many work synergistically in the body. While RCTs may be the most accepted method used currently, scientists still are unclear about how to best measure supplement benefits.

Regarding dietary nutrients, look for studies that review whole populations eating a good diet, such as the Loma Linda University studies about vegetarian lifestyles, or studies of cultures prior to the introduction of refined foods. From such studies one can conclude that a balanced, organic diet and supplementation with supplements from natural sources can be your best bet toward getting and remaining healthy.

Read Labels Wisely

Making sense of dietary supplement labels can be tricky if you're not familiar with the system they use. However, being able to decipher the label's information is a quick way to find the best product to suit your needs. Understanding labels will help you make smart choices and steer you clear of supplements that may be hazardous or ineffective.

In 1999, the FDA changed the labeling system for dietary supplements. The goal was to present a list of useful information, much like that found on all commercial food labels, to help you make more informed choices when buying dietary supplements. The new labeling

The Future of Testing

Many researchers are trying to devise new methods of testing natural products in a way that would increase the efficiency, accuracy, and cost-effectiveness of such testing. In early 2003, researchers at Purdue University discovered a faster, less expensive method of testing the quality and purity of 14 dietary supplement oils (including flaxseed, borage seed, and grape seed oil) as well as five common food oils (including canola, corn, and peanut oil). Through the use of infrared spectroscopy (a tool that uses different wavelengths of light to determine the chemical structure of a substance), the Purdue researchers were able to identify compounds present in natural products with a great deal of accuracy. Since many food and pharmaceutical companies already own the equipment used for infrared spectroscopy, this new method of purity testing may be an important step forward in supplement testing.

system includes a standardized information panel that, by law, must appear on all supplement containers.

The main elements of the new labeling requirements for supplement-product containers include:

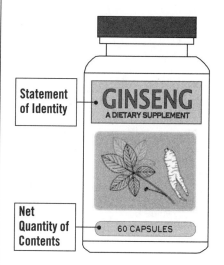

- *Statement of Identity* —The name of the product. The name must indicate the type of the product, such as "dietary," "herbal," or "vitamin" supplement.
- *Net Quantity of Contents*—How much of a supplement is contained in the supplement bottle or other container (for example, "60 capsules").
- *Structure-Function Claim and Statement*—Statements made by the manufacturer that describe how the product affects the structure or function of the body (for example, "When you need to perform your best, take supplement X"). FDA regulations make it illegal for supplement manufacturers to make any disease claims (stating that a supplement can prevent, treat, cure, or diagnose a disease) without this first being reviewed and approved by the FDA.

Since the FDA does not use scientific testing to evaluate structure-function claims, such claims must be followed by a statement that reads: "This statement has not been evaluated by the FDA. This product is not intended to diagnose, treat, cure, or prevent any disease." It is up to the supplement manufacturer to ensure that claims made for a supplement are truthful and not misleading, although an independent commission on dietary supplements does monitor these claims.

The new requirements for supplement products also require that their labels contain the following:

- *Directions*—How to take the supplement (for example, "Take one capsule daily").

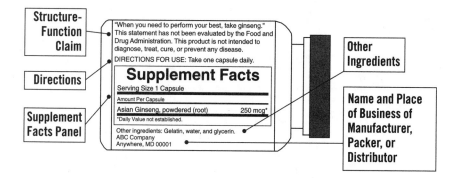

- *Supplement Facts Panel*—A list of the serving size, amount, and active ingredients of the supplement (see "How to Read the Supplement Facts Panel," page 21).
- *Other Ingredients*—A listing of other added ingredients in the supplement product in descending order according to their amounts and by their common names.
- *Name and Place of Business of the Supplement Manufacturer, Packer, or Distributor*—The address where consumers may write for additional product information about the supplement.

In some cases, the manufacturer of a supplement product may choose to include additional information on its label, such as

- *Warnings and Cautions*—Restrictions and cautions about the use of the product. The absence of a warning/cautionary statement does not mean that the product has no adverse effects.
- *Interactions and Side Effects*—A list of potential reactions that might arise from combining

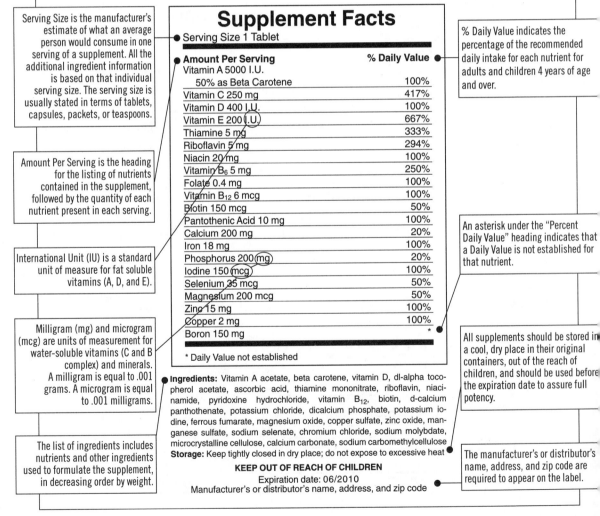

Serving Size is the manufacturer's estimate of what an average person would consume in one serving of a supplement. All the additional ingredient information is based on that individual serving size. The serving size is usually stated in terms of tablets, capsules, packets, or teaspoons.

Amount Per Serving is the heading for the listing of nutrients contained in the supplement, followed by the quantity of each nutrient present in each serving.

International Unit (IU) is a standard unit of measure for fat soluble vitamins (A, D, and E).

Milligram (mg) and microgram (mcg) are units of measurement for water-soluble vitamins (C and B complex) and minerals. A milligram is equal to .001 grams. A microgram is equal to .001 milligrams.

The list of ingredients includes nutrients and other ingredients used to formulate the supplement, in decreasing order by weight.

% Daily Value indicates the percentage of the recommended daily intake for each nutrient for adults and children 4 years of age and over.

An asterisk under the "Percent Daily Value" heading indicates that a Daily Value is not established for that nutrient.

All supplements should be stored in a cool, dry place in their original containers, out of the reach of children, and should be used before the expiration date to assure full potency.

The manufacturer's or distributor's name, address, and zip code are required to appear on the label.

Supplement Facts

Serving Size 1 Tablet

Amount Per Serving	% Daily Value
Vitamin A 5000 I.U.	
50% as Beta Carotene	100%
Vitamin C 250 mg	417%
Vitamin D 400 I.U.	100%
Vitamin E 200 I.U.	667%
Thiamine 5 mg	333%
Riboflavin 5 mg	294%
Niacin 20 mg	100%
Vitamin B₆ 5 mg	250%
Folate 0.4 mg	100%
Vitamin B₁₂ 6 mcg	100%
Biotin 150 mcg	50%
Pantothenic Acid 10 mg	100%
Calcium 200 mg	20%
Iron 18 mg	100%
Phosphorus 200 mg	20%
Iodine 150 mcg	100%
Selenium 35 mcg	50%
Magnesium 200 mcg	50%
Zinc 15 mg	100%
Copper 2 mg	100%
Boron 150 mg	*

* Daily Value not established

Ingredients: Vitamin A acetate, beta carotene, vitamin D, dl-alpha tocopherol acetate, ascorbic acid, thiamine mononitrate, riboflavin, niacinamide, pyridoxine hydrochloride, vitamin B₁₂, biotin, d-calcium panthothenate, potassium chloride, dicalcium phosphate, potassium iodine, ferrous fumarate, magnesium oxide, copper sulfate, zinc oxide, manganese sulfate, sodium selenate, chromium chloride, sodium molybdate, microcrystalline cellulose, calcium carbonate, sodium carbomethylcellulose

Storage: Keep tightly closed in dry place; do not expose to excessive heat

KEEP OUT OF REACH OF CHILDREN

Expiration date: 06/2010

Manufacturer's or distributor's name, address, and zip code

the supplement with prescription and over-the-counter medicines, as well as with foods or other supplements.

■ *Expiration Date*—The date after which the product should not be used.

How to Read the Supplement Facts Panel

Learning to decipher the supplement facts panel is an important part of becoming supplement savvy. Read on for information on how to properly read supplement labels:

Carefully Assess Claims

A good rule of thumb when assessing claims made by supplement manufacturers is the saying, "If it sounds too good to be true, it probably is." In particular, exercise a healthy skepticism about:

■ Products promoted as "quick-fix remedies" or "miraculous" or "magical" cures.

■ Claims that the product has only benefits and no side effects.

■ Personal testimonials and information from people who have no formal training in nutrition or supplements.

■ Claims that the product can treat or cure a wide range of diseases that are unrelated to one another.

■ Promises of a "no-risk, money-back guarantee."

Challenge Old Assumptions

You may have many long-standing assumptions about dietary supplements. So take the time to check them against reality.

If It's Natural, It Must Be Safe

Never assume that a product is entirely safe just because it's natural. Some supplements (whether natural or synthetic) can have side effects if taken incorrectly, or they may interact in dangerous ways with prescription drugs, over-the-counter medications, or other supplements.

If a Little Is Good, a Lot Is Better

It is simply not true that if a little of anything is good, a lot must be better. Just like drugs, some supplements can be dangerous if taken in large doses. Use supplements in moderation

---

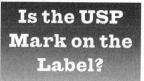

Is the USP Mark on the Label?

In 2001, the United States Pharmacopeia (USP), a nongovernmental medical research group, introduced a program that aims to inform and safeguard supplement users. The USP "Dietary Supplement Verified" mark on the label of a supplement means that it:

• Contains the ingredients that are listed on the label.
• Contains the stated amount and strength of each ingredient.

• Will easily break down in the stomach, so that your body can absorb the supplement's nutrients.
• Has been tested for harmful substances (such as heavy metals or pesticides).
• Has been made in a safe, clean, and controlled environment.

Be aware that the USP program is voluntary for supplement manufacturers. Furthermore, the USP mark does not guarantee a product's safety or that the supplement works as claimed. However, the USP mark is definitely something to look out for.

and follow your doctor's instructions about appropriate dosage. However, keep in mind that although certain supplements (such as vitamin A) can cause serious health problems when taken at very high doses, on the whole, people rarely die from supplement overdoses compared to many from prescription medication overdoses.

A Supplement Is Safe If There Are No Warnings on the Label

While some manufacturers do place appropriate warnings and cautionary statements on their products, there is no obligation for them to do so (see "Read Labels Wisely," page 18). If in doubt, contact the manufacturer directly about the safety of a specific supplement.

Consider the Manufacturer

Most supplement manufacturers operate responsibly and carefully. However, less restrictive regulations in the United States create the potential for poor manufacturing practices. New FDA standards for the labeling and manufacturing of dietary supplements may soon be in place. But until then, consider the following steps to protect yourself.

- Choose supplements made by a well-known, reputable manufacturer that produces other food or drug products. This type of organization will already adhere to high-quality standards called "Good Manufacturing Practices" (GMPs) set for its other products. Those manufacturers that do adhere to GMPs for making a supplement will often mention it on their labels or in promotional material.
- Choose a supplement that has a USP mark on its label (see "Is the USP Mark on the Label?" page 21). However, keep in mind that many brand-name supplements do not have the USP mark, often because the manufacturer chooses to rely on its name, rather than an outside authority, to guarantee the product.
- Write to the manufacturer for more information. For example, you might ask about
  - Test results on the safety and efficacy of the product
  - Quality control systems used in making the product
  - Information to substantiate the manufacturer's claims
  - Reports of adverse effects from the product
  - Requesting an independent, third-party assay (analysis) of the product

Contact information for the manufacturer of a supplement can be found on the supplement's label (see "Read Labels Wisely," page 18).

- If you want to avoid pesticide and herbicide residues, make sure to choose a certified organic source of herbs.

Report Harmful Effects

If you or your family ever suffer a serious adverse reaction to a supplement, or encounter a problem with product quality, stop taking the supplement immediately and report the problem to FDA MedWatch. This program, set up originally to monitor drug use, enables health-care professionals and consumers to voluntarily report serious problems related to supplement use as well. Such reporting can be done as follows:

- Online: www.fda.gov/medwatch/
- By phone: (800) FDA-1088 [(800) 322-1088]
- By submitting the MedWatch 3500 form (available online) by mail or fax to:
  U.S. Food and Drug Administration
  MedWatch Office
  5600 Fishers Lane, HFD-410
  Rockville, MD 20857
  Fax: (301) 827-7241

The FDA encourages you to ask your doctor to complete and submit the reporting form, since he or she can provide pertinent information, based on your medical record, that will help the FDA accurately evaluate your report. However, you may also complete the form yourself. Once that is done, there is no need for follow-up. The FDA will acknowledge receipt of your report and will contact you only if more information is needed.

Also be sure to report any problems with a drug or supplement product to the manufacturer or distributor, as well as to the store or pharmacy where you purchased the product.

PART TWO

....

A Guide to Supplements

ALOE VERA

WHETHER YOU REFER TO IT AS A "miracle plant" or simply by its "last name"—*vera*, meaning "truth" in Latin—the semi-tropical aloe vera plant *(Aloe vera, Aloe barbadensis)* has been deemed a treatment for every ailment under the sun, from blisters and burns to indigestion and cancer. Aloe vera has a time-honored and romantic history: Its medical properties were first described over two thousand years ago. In ancient Egypt, aloe was used for embalming. It was a plant literally fit for a queen—Cleopatra used aloe vera to beautify her complexion. Today, aloe vera is one of the most widely used natural ingredients in skincare products. Many people keep an aloe vera plant at home from which they can break off the tip of a leaf and use the gel to treat minor burns and skin irritations.

WHAT IT DOES

The clear gel from the leaves of the aloe vera plant is used to treat cuts, wounds, infections, burns, rashes, and other skin conditions. While some of the claims for moisturizing and penetrating properties of the gel have held up, other claims, such as its healing and pain-killing properties, are less clear. Some studies suggest that aloe may be useful in the treatment of skin rashes, psoriasis, and genital herpes, although the evidence is not definitive. Taken orally, aloe latex is a potent laxative. While its use as a laxative has been recognized for centuries, at present this use is not recommended because it is too potent and is contraindicated in many serious health conditions. Animal studies suggest that aloe juice may help in regulating blood sugar levels in diabetes, though human studies have not yet been performed. One study found aloe gel to be useful for ulcerative colitis, but more research is needed before this can be recommended.

For additional information on specific health conditions and how you can treat them with supplements, see Part 3 of this book, beginning on page 309.

HOW IT WORKS

When the leaf of an aloe vera plant is cut, an orange-yellow sap, or latex, called aloin, is released. Because it is an irritant, this bitter sap stimulates the colon, producing a strong laxative effect, so strong that it is no longer recommended for internal use. Note: This is not the same as the aloe juice or gel and has very different properties.

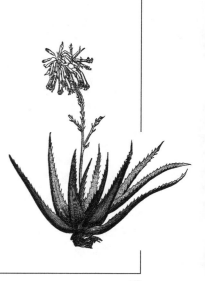

Removing the tough, green skin of the leaf exposes a transparent, mucus-like substance that contains a colorless, semisolid gel. Known as aloe vera gel, it has healing properties for skin irritations and also reduces inflammation and pain. Aloe vera gel is believed to work because of its ability to penetrate deep into the skin, to the level where cells grow and multiply, helping to feed and repair damaged skin cells.

HOW TO USE IT

Aloe gel may be used in a variety of forms. It may be applied topically, as a gel, or in an ointment that often includes other ingredients such as mineral oil or castor oil. Topical aloe creams should contain 0.5 percent aloe and may be used as needed. Aloe gel may also be applied directly from an aloe plant by breaking off an aloe leaf and applying the gel directly onto skin.

Except in rare cases in which a person has an allergy to aloe, the topical application of aloe is generally safe. Anyone allergic to garlic, onions, tulips, or other plants of the *Liliaceae* family—of which aloe is a member—may have a reaction to aloe. It is also possible to develop an allergic reaction, such as hives or a rash, after using aloe gel for an extended period of time.

In 2002, the U.S. Food and Drug Administration issued a final rule stating that aloe products are not generally recognized as safe

Grow This!

Aloe is a useful plant to have around the house or in the garden (in a frost-free area) for topical use on the skin. Keep in mind that aloe gel—which is the sap of the plant—should be used immediately because its medicinal properties deteriorate when it is stored in a container.

Do not ingest any part of the aloe plant before consulting your doctor, since it is hard to control the dosage of material taken directly from the plant.

- **Light:** Bright filtered light (as in a sunny windowsill) or light shade.
- **Temperature:** Room temperature.
- **Water:** Aloe should be watered every 1 to 2 weeks from March through September (its growing season). Allow soil to become dry between waterings. From October through February (its resting period), aloe should be watered every 2 to 3 weeks.
- **Repotting:** The key to potting aloe is making sure the soil is well drained. Aloe will grow in poor soil and during drought in a garden as long as the soil is draining well. In containers, use regular potting soil or a special cactus mix. A low, wide planter is ideal for aloe, since the roots grow in a shallow, spread-out pattern. Use a planter with one or more drainage holes. Feed aloe plants monthly during their active growing period with compost tea or liquid seaweed. Aloe may be propagated by removing the offsets from mature plants and potting them in individual containers.

and effective and banned the use of aloe (and cascara sagrada) as laxative ingredients in over-the-counter drug products. Bitter aloe (the latex form) should not be taken orally since it may cause nausea, vomiting, and diarrhea. Children and pregnant or nursing women should avoid using aloe as a laxative. The latex form, called bitter aloe (often yellow in color and sold in capsule form), should never by anyone with appendicitis or inflammatory intestinal diseases such as Crohn's disease or ulcerative colitis without the supervision of a doctor.

WHAT TO AVOID

Medication: Aloe gel or juice, when taken orally, should be used with caution by people taking laxative drugs, loop diuretics, zidovudine (AZT), or medications for blood-sugar reduction or heart-rhythm disturbances.

Herbs and Dietary Supplements: Aloe, when taken orally, should be used with caution by people taking licorice root, other laxative herbs, and blood-sugar-lowering herbs or supplements.

Food: Taking aloe orally for long periods of time may interfere with the body's ability to absorb nutrients in the intestine.

ALPHA LIPOIC ACID

ALPHA LIPOIC ACID (ALA) is a fatty acid that contains sulfur and is essential to the body's production of energy. What makes ALA different from many other antioxidants is that it can function in both water and fat, which gives ALA an increased range of action.

Although ALA can be found in foods such as meat, liver, yeast, spinach, and broccoli, the human body manufactures its own ALA, so healthy people don't usually need to take ALA as a supplement. However, supplements are necessary for people who want to obtain therapeutic dosages of ALA.

WHAT IT DOES

ALA may be helpful in treating complications associated with diabetes, especially when taken in conjunction with other antioxidants (such as vitamin E). In Germany and Russia, ALA is used to treat symptoms of diabetic peripheral neuropathy—a complication of diabetes in which nerves are damaged—by reducing the pain, burning, itching, tingling, and numbness associated with this condition. Studies also suggest that ALA when given intravenously may decrease insulin resistance in people with diabetes.

ALA may prevent or treat a variety of other conditions, including cataracts, glaucoma, heart disease, human immunodeficiency virus (HIV) infection and acquired immune deficiency syndrome (AIDS), and Parkinson's disease. Creams containing ALA may also protect the skin from sun damage.

Preliminary animal research suggests that ALA may reduce the effects of aging and, in particular, may slow aging of the brain and increase long-term memory, although more research is needed to test its efficacy in these areas.

For additional information on specific health conditions and how you can treat them with supplements, see Part 3 of this book, beginning on page 309.

HOW IT WORKS

ALA has two major roles in the body—to help cells produce energy and to act as an antioxidant. ALA can be found in the mitochondria, the parts of cells that generate energy. ALA is essential to the metabolic functioning that transforms glucose into the energy we need to stay alive.

As an antioxidant, ALA not only neutralizes the cell- and tissue-damaging free radical molecules but also appears to help recycle or regenerate other antioxidants, such as vitamins C and E and glutathione (an antioxidant produced directly by the body), when they become depleted.

HOW TO TAKE IT

ALA is commercially available in capsule and tablet form. As a general antioxidant, ALA is usually recommended at a dosage of 50 to 100 milligrams per day. However, ALA appears to be safe when taken in dosages as high as 1,800 milligrams daily.

LOOK OUT FOR THIS!

ALA is generally considered safe, with few side effects, even when taken in high doses.

If you have diabetes and take insulin or other diabetes medication, consult your doctor before taking ALA, since it may decrease your blood sugar even further than these drugs do, and your doctor may therefore need to adjust the dosages of your diabetes medication.

The safety of ALA has not been established in pregnant or nursing women, children, and people with liver or kidney disease. Anyone in these groups should consult a doctor before taking ALA.

WHAT TO AVOID

There are no known interactions of ALA with other drugs, herbs, or supplements.

ARGININE

ARGININE, ALSO KNOWN AS L-ARGININE, is an amino acid that plays a key role in numerous body processes including the healing of wounds, the removal of ammonia from the body, the functioning of the immune system, and the secretion of important hormones. Until recently, it was thought that if the diet lacked arginine, the body would produce the amount of arginine that it needed in order to keep levels of this amino acid within an adequate range. However, new studies suggest that the body's rate of arginine synthesis may be insufficient, in which case supplementation may be necessary.

WHAT IT DOES

For individuals at risk for coronary artery disease, arginine may improve circulation to the heart and other blood vessels, slow the progression of atherosclerosis, and reduce blood pressure. However, l-arginine may be harmful after a heart attack. Arginine may also

Arginine Shows Promising Results for Hospitalized Patients

Did You Know?

In hospitals, some nutritional products contain arginine. These products are designed to aid recovery after major surgery, illness, or injury. These products are usually administered enterally (through a tube in the stomach).

An analysis of 15 studies comparing hospital patients who received standard enteral—or orally ingested—nutrition to patients who received enteral nutrition that was enhanced with arginine and other amino acids found that the arginine-enhanced products sped up recovery as well as improving the degree of recovery. The report found that arginine-enhanced hospital diets appear to help reduce episodes of infection, length of hospital stay, and the time during which the patients require a ventilator for breathing assistance.

improve sexual dysfunction in men with impotence, without causing the adverse side effects often associated with prescription medications. Some studies indicate that arginine may help treat infertility in both men and women.

Many bodybuilders take arginine in the belief that it causes the body to produce growth hormones, thus increasing muscle mass. However, research indicates that arginine is not effective for this purpose.

Preliminary research suggests that arginine may work to boost the immune system of hospitalized and severely ill people (see Did You Know, page 31). Recent studies also suggest that arginine may decrease insulin resistance in people with type 2 diabetes, as well as help in treating ulcers and esophageal reflux and improving cognition. More research is needed to support these findings.

For additional information on specific health conditions and how you can treat them with supplements, see Part 3 of this book, beginning on page 309.

HOW IT WORKS

One of the main roles of arginine is to help the body produce nitric oxide, a substance that dilates blood vessels and relaxes them to allow blood to flow more freely throughout the body. Arginine is absorbed by the small intestine and is transported to the liver, where it enters into various metabolic pathways.

The exact way in which arginine works is unknown.

HOW TO TAKE IT

People with heart disease should consult their doctor before taking arginine supplements. Do not try to self-treat with supplements if you have a heart condition.

Arginine is commercially available in the form of L-arginine (the L stands for "levo," which is the form in which arginine occurs naturally) and arginine-derived nitric oxide (also known as "AD-NO"). It is available in tablets, capsules, and even as an ingredient in heart-healthy candy bars. Typical dosages of arginine range from 6 to 9 grams daily, although dosages vary for different health conditions.

LOOK OUT FOR THIS!

Arginine is generally considered safe, with few side effects. At high doses, it may cause diarrhea, nausea, and dizziness.

Arginine may reactivate latent herpes virus infections, and individuals with genital herpes and cold sores may therefore want to avoid taking it, particularly if they are taking lysine to treat herpes, since arginine can counteract the benefits of lysine. (For more on lysine and herpes, see page 200.)

People with diabetes should consult their doctor before taking arginine.

Pregnant and nursing women should not take arginine.

WHAT TO AVOID

Medication: Consult your doctor before taking arginine with medications that dilate the blood vessels, such as nitroglycerin, erectile dysfunction drugs (such as Viagra), diuretics, and angiotensin converting enzyme (ACE) inhibitors for high blood pressure. Individuals taking drugs that have effects on the stomach, including nonsteroidal anti-inflammatory drugs (NSAIDs) such as ibuprofen, and medications that may alter the balance of potassium in the body should consult their doctor before taking arginine.

A R N I C A

DERIVED FROM THE DRIED FLOWERS and roots of the plant *Arnica montana*—a member of the daisy family—arnica has a long tradition as a folk remedy for easing muscle aches and pains and treating a variety of external injuries. In highly diluted form it is a well-known homeopathic remedy, and there is a high demand for arnica-based products in Europe; more than 300 varieties of arnica products are available in Germany.

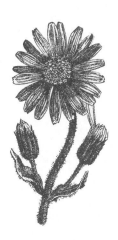

WHAT IT DOES

Topical applications of arnica have been claimed to soothe sore muscles and joints and have been used to treat swelling and pain caused by injuries such as dislocations, fractures, and the bruising injuries known as contusions. The German Commission E (see page 16) has approved these uses of arnica, as well as its topical

SUPPLEMENTAL TRIVIA

Derivatives of arnica were part of Native American medicinal potions used to treat wounds, sprains, and bruises. The Native Americans called arnica by the name of mountain tobacco and leopard's bane, and it is even today known in some places as wolf's bane.

use for treating inflammation caused by insect bites and minor vein inflammation. Arnica has also been recommended to treat inflammation in the mouth and throat, but the internal use of undiluted arnica is extremely dangerous as it contains poisons that can be harmful if ingested.

Increasing numbers of studies are beginning to show that arnica does have anti-inflammatory properties. Preliminary studies suggest that arnica may have promise in reducing pain after carpal tunnel surgery and in mild osteoarthritis of the knee. Homeopathic arnica may diminish bruising after plastic surgery and reduce postpartum blood loss. Other studies suggest that arnica may kill various types of bacteria that inhabit the mouth and can cause gum problems. However, the results of many studies are conflicting, and more research is needed to confirm arnica's benefits.

For additional information on specific health conditions and how you can treat them with supplements, see Part 3 of this book, beginning on page 309.

HOW IT WORKS

Some studies have found that components in arnica have anti-inflammatory, antiseptic, and pain-killing properties when applied topically. This may come from an active component of arnica called sesquiterpene lactone. Other studies indicate that the sesquiterpenes in arnica may also work as antibacterial, fever-reducing, and stimulant agents when taken internally. However, more research is needed to determine the safety and effectiveness of undiluted arnica for internal use.

HOW TO TAKE IT

Because of the danger of poisoning—as indicated above—undiluted arnica should never be taken internally. However, homeopathic preparations of arnica, in which it is highly diluted, have no reported toxic effects and are usually quite effective.

Practitioners who recommend arnica for oral inflammation suggest mouth rinses with dilute solutions prepared from this herb. But here too it is necessary to be very careful, since ingesting arnica can cause severe and even potentially fatal side effects.

External preparations of arnica include tinctures, oils, and ointments in which arnica is highly diluted, usually by as much as

10 parts of liquid to 1 part of arnica. Arnica oil contains 5 parts of fatty oil for every 1 part of arnica.

LOOK OUT FOR THIS!

The U.S. Food and Drug Administration (FDA) lists arnica as an unsafe herb. If ingested, arnica can cause nausea and vomiting, abdominal pain and diarrhea, and potentially life-threatening cardiac arrhythmias or irregular heartbeats, as well as coma and death.

External applications of arnica can cause side effects that include contact dermatitis accompanied by swelling. The long-term use of arnica may cause eczema and more serious toxic skin reactions. Arnica should never be applied to open wounds or broken skin and is best used on a short-term basis.

WHAT TO AVOID

When used topically, arnica has no known interactions with other drugs, herbs, or supplements.

ASTRAGALUS

IN TRADITIONAL CHINESE MEDICINE, the root of the astragalus plant *(Astragalus membranaceus)* is known for supporting the "Qi" (pronounced "chi"), a Chinese word meaning life force. It is often combined with other herbs to treat a variety of conditions including colds, flu, fatigue, and heart disease.

WHAT IT DOES

Astragalus is often combined with other herbs (such as echinacea) for the treatment of common respiratory infections such as colds, flu, and bronchitis by boosting the immune system. One clinical trial found that by curtailing infections, astragalus helped boost the immune system in people undergoing kidney dialysis. A clinical trial conducted in the United States suggested that in combination with chemotherapy, astragalus might be able to boost the immune system in cancer patients, raising the number of cancer-fighting cells known as T cells.

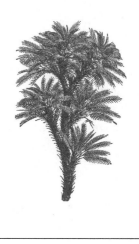

Among the most fascinating effects of astragalus is its ability to improve the functioning of the heart after a heart attack. Evidence indicates that astragalus helps the left side of the heart, which pumps

RESTORATIVE RECIPES

HERBAL CHICKEN SOUP

Chicken soup is a staple when it comes to treating coughs, colds, and other respiratory infections. Next time you're sick, try making an herbal chicken soup, packed with immune-boosting ingredients that will help put you back on your feet naturally.

Ingredients

1 small to medium-size chicken
1 bay leaf
2 teaspoons sea salt
2 to 3 teaspoons dried astragalus
1/2 inch chopped ginger
5 to 7 chopped garlic cloves
1 thinly sliced green onion
3 small, chopped chili peppers

Directions: Rinse the chicken thoroughly and remove all of the excess skin and fat. Place the chicken in a covered pot and fill the pot so that the water is 2 inches above the chicken. Add the bay leaf and sea salt to the mixture and bring the water to a boil. Once the water is boiling, lower to a gentle boil and add astragalus, ginger, and garlic. Cook for 2 hours or until the chicken is thoroughly cooked. Once the soup is complete, garnish it with green onions, chili peppers, and salt to taste.

out blood to most of the body, to work better after a heart attack, as well as helping to ease chest discomfort and shortness of breath in people with heart failure.

Although most of these benefits suggest that astragalus enhances the immune system, there's also preliminary evidence that astragalus may help control a malfunctioning immune system in people with lupus; a Chinese clinical trial found that astragalus suppressed the immune response in lupus patients, helping combat the disease. Preliminary research also suggests that astragalus may be useful in the treatment of diabetes and also inhibit the herpes simplex virus. More research is needed to confirm these uses of astragalus.

For additional information on specific health conditions and how you can treat them with supplements, see Part 3 of this book, beginning on page 309.

HOW IT WORKS

As with many other herbal therapies, the exact way in which astragalus works is unknown. Studies indicate that it boosts the activity of several types of cells of the immune system, including phagocytes, macrophages, and antibodies, and increases the number of T cells.

Astragalus contains a number of active components, including flavonoids, amino acids, and trace minerals. It also apparently has antioxidant effects, which may in part explain its ability to strengthen the heart. One study indicated that chemical compounds present in astragalus suppress the replication of the coxsackie virus, which causes a condition called myocarditis, a dangerous swelling of the heart muscle.

HOW TO TAKE IT

Dried astragalus root is traditionally made into a tea by steeping it in hot or boiling water for 15 to 30 minutes. Some practitioners recommend using from 9 to 15 grams of the dried root daily. Astragalus is also available in extract form. Dosage recommendations vary; some practitioners suggest taking 500 milligrams a day, divided into two equal doses, to stimulate the immune system, while others suggest taking two 250 or 500 milligram capsules three times a day.

Astragalus may be found in combination with ginseng or echinacea in supplement products for preventing common respiratory infections and easing the effects of stress.

LOOK OUT FOR THIS!

Although astragalus is recommended to fight colds and the flu, Chinese medicine practitioners believe it is best taken *before* the first sign of infection because it can bring colds to "a head" if it is taken after symptoms have already developed. Consult a doctor or herbalist for more information about astragalus.

Few side effects have been reported with astragalus, but these may include mild gastrointestinal upset and diarrhea when the herb is taken at very high doses. Because of the potential effects of astragalus on the immune system, patients receiving immunosuppressive therapy or who have an autoimmune disease should consult their doctor before taking astragalus.

No safe dosage levels have been established for astragalus for young children, pregnant and nursing women, or people with severe kidney or liver disease.

WHAT TO AVOID

Medication: Using astragalus with anticoagulant medications (such as warfarin) may increase the risk of bleeding.

BEE POLLEN

BEE POLLEN IS ABOUT AS NATURAL a supplement as you're likely to find, and for some people that's apparently enough to justify its use. But what does bee pollen contain that gives it its reputed beneficial effects? The answer remains unknown. The composition of bee pollen is literally as diverse as the flowers,

Bee Pollen Leads to Advances in Alternative Medicine Research

Did You Know?

Several years ago, Iowa senator Tom Harkin, who had been convinced to try bee pollen pills for his allergies, announced that they'd worked and he was cured. Not long afterward, the manufacturer of the pills was fined $200,000 for false advertising, claiming that his product cured allergies, helped consumers lose weight, and even reversed the aging process.

No one knows what led to Harkin's "cure," but in some cases, allergies may simply disappear with the passage of time. Harkin was so encouraged by the apparent effectiveness of the non-medical remedy that had seemingly cured his allergies that he began working with the National Institutes of Health Office of Alternative Medicine, which has been instrumental in providing reliable information on complementary and alternative medicine.

trees, and plants from which bees collect it. And while bee pollen contains vitamins, minerals, carbohydrates, and amino acids, their precise percentages vary from one batch to another. That's one part of the reason why scientists hesitate to ascribe any specific benefits to bee pollen supplements.

WHAT IT DOES

Bee pollen was first purported to have beneficial effects in the 1970s, when several athletes claimed that it improved their performance; they called it a natural "energy food," stating that it increased their endurance. But the evidence for this was purely anecdotal. In 1975 and again in 1976, clinical trials of the effect of a bee-pollen supplement versus a placebo on a university swim team and on long-distance runners found no significant difference between the two.

I have heard that some products produced by bees have health benefits. Is this true?

A number of bee-derived products are purported to have health benefits. The "glue" that bees use to hold their hives together, and the resin that they collect from coniferous trees and poplars, called *propolis*, may have antibacterial and anti-inflammatory properties. In fact, propolis apparently helps keep beehives germ-free! Studies show that propolis may help fight influenza ("flu") and herpes viruses, as well as the gum inflammation known as gingivitis. Propolis has been a part of folk medicine for generations and is an ingredient in some cold lozenges, cough syrups, and mouth rinses.

Another possibly health-beneficial product derived from bees is royal jelly, which is loaded with vitamins and proteins. Royal jelly is a bee food produced by worker bees. Preliminary studies suggest that it may lower blood pressure and cholesterol levels. A study of mice that were fed dietary supplements of royal jelly for 16 weeks found that they had an increase in lifespan, possibly from a reduction in oxidative damage to their cells and tissues. Royal jelly is often found as an ingre-dient in other bee products, such as melbrosia, which is a mixture of royal jelly, flower pollen, and fermented bee pollen. Studies indicate that melbrosia may have promise for easing menopausal symptoms including headache, urinary incontinence, vaginal dryness, anxiety, irritability, and hot flashes.

Last but not least are numerous studies indicating that bees' most popular product—honey—has antibacterial effects and that when applied topically it may be useful in treating burns and preventing infection. A particular type of honey from New Zealand, called Manuka honey, may have especially effective antibacterial properties. Studies suggest that Manuka honey may fight the *Helicobacter pylori* bacteria that cause gastrointestinal ulcers.

Do remember, though, that while all of the bee products described here are generally considered safe, any type of bee product may trigger an allergic reaction. Therefore, be careful about using these products if you have allergies, especially to bee stings, honey, or the particular flower that is the source of a bee pollen product.

A later trial, which seemed to show that the heart rate, breathing, and perspiration of subjects taking bee pollen returned more rapidly to normal than those of subjects taking a placebo, got some proponents excited. However, since this trial was not done in a "double-blind" manner—in which neither the investigators nor the subjects would know whether they were getting pollen or placebo—many felt that it could not yield accurate results.

Studies indicate that Cernilton, a proprietary blend of bee pollen extract, may be useful for treating chronic prostatitis by reducing swelling, relaxing muscles in the urethra, and preventing prostate cells from growing. Other studies suggest that bee pollen may reduce symptoms of benign prostatic hyperplasia, but more research is needed on this.

Bee pollen has also been touted as preventing hay fever, but there is no evidence to support this claim. Worse yet, if you're allergic to pollen—as are many people with hay fever— you might have a dangerous and even life-threatening allergic reaction if you use it.

For additional information on specific health conditions and how you can treat them with supplements, see Part 3 of this book, beginning on page 309.

HOW IT WORKS
The body digests, absorbs, and metabolizes the various vitamins, minerals, carbohydrates, and other nutrients found in bee pollen, but apart from providing these nutrients, the way in which bee pollen works is unknown.

HOW TO TAKE IT
Bee pollen is available in many different forms including capsules, chewable tablets, regular tablets, granules, powder, and liquid. Optimal dosages of bee pollen are unknown.

LOOK OUT FOR THIS!
Bee pollen supplements may cause allergic reactions—including the potentially life-threatening allergic reactions known as *anaphylactic reactions*—in people with allergies or sensitivities to pollen, and such people should strictly avoid bee pollen supplements.

Pregnant or breastfeeding women and children should avoid taking bee pollen.

WHAT TO AVOID

There are no known interactions of bee pollen with other supplements, drugs, or herbs.

BETA-SITOSTEROL

BETA-SITOSTEROL BELONGS TO A FAMILY of plant-based compounds called phytosterols, which are closely related to cholesterol (which comes almost exclusively from animal products). Beta-sitosterol is the most abundant phytosterol in the human diet and is found in a wide variety of fruits, vegetables, nuts, and seeds. Everything with peanuts in it—peanut oil, peanut butter, and peanuts themselves—packs more beta-sitosterol than almost any other food we regularly consume.

WHAT IT DOES

Beta-sitosterol has joined a fairly well substantiated list of herbs that alleviate the symptoms of benign prostatic hyperplasia (BPH), known more commonly as enlargement of the prostate. It has been shown to be effective in relieving such symptoms of BPH as inflammation and urine retention.

Although it may seem paradoxical because beta-sitosterol is so closely related to cholesterol, studies have shown that phytosterols can reduce blood levels of LDL ("bad") cholesterol, as well as total cholesterol levels. Studies have also shown it to be effective in lowering cholesterol in familial hypercholesterolemia.

Other potential uses of beta-sitosterol include the prevention of colon, breast, and prostate cancers. Some studies also suggest that beta-sitosterol may prevent weakening of the immune system caused by endurance exercise (such as long-distance running) by reestablishing a balance between the hormone cortisol, which breaks down muscle tissue, and dihydroepiandrosterone (DHEA), which helps rebuild it. More research is needed to support these uses.

For additional information on specific health conditions and how you can treat them with supplements, see Part 3 of this book, beginning on page 309.

HOW IT WORKS

It's not exactly clear how beta-sitosterol helps with the symptoms of BPH. However, beta-sitosterol has been shown to bind to prostate tissues and to counteract the metabolism of substances called prostaglandins, which are involved in the body's pain and inflammation responses.

As for reducing blood levels of LDL cholesterol, it is precisely because beta-sitosterol is related to cholesterol in chemical structure that it seems to work in this way. It blocks the normal absorption of dietary cholesterol in the gastrointestinal tract, reducing the amount of cholesterol that is transported to the bloodstream, and increases the amount of cholesterol eliminated from the gastrointestinal tract.

HOW TO TAKE IT

Beta-sitosterol is available as a supplement in capsules and tablets. Generally, practitioners recommend between 60 and 135 milligrams a day, divided into three doses, for treating BPH. Be patient: Positive effects of beta-sitosterol can take up to 4 weeks to emerge. In clinical research, anywhere from 500 milligrams to 10 grams a day of beta-sitosterol has been found to reduce high levels of cholesterol. Food sources of beta-sitosterol include peanuts, pumpkin seeds, avocados, rice bran oil, and wheat germ and wheat germ oil.

Be sure to take beta-sitosterol on an empty stomach, 1 hour before meals.

LOOK OUT FOR THIS!

Side effects of beta-sitosterol may include indigestion, gas, and diarrhea or constipation.

Pregnant or nursing women should not take beta-sitosterol supplements.

WHAT TO AVOID

Herbs and Dietary Supplements: Some evidence suggests that beta-sitosterol can interfere with the absorption of beta-carotene, lycopene, and vitamin E. Therefore, consider avoiding beta-sitosterol supplementation if you're trying to boost your intake of these important nutrients.

Food: Animal fats such as milk may inhibit the absorption of beta-sitosterol.

BETAINE

BETAINE IS A COMPOUND FOUND IN FISH, beets, broccoli, spinach, and some kinds of beans, and the body metabolizes it from choline, yet betaine itself isn't defined as essential for human health. However, that's really only a matter of technical definition, because research is making clear that through a variety of complex effects on the body's chemistry, betaine and related compounds are indeed very important for keeping cells and tissues in good shape and protecting them from disease.

WHAT IT DOES

One form of betaine, called betaine hydrochloride (HCl), can aid digestion in people who are deficient in hydrochloric acid, known more commonly as stomach acid, and essential for digestion. Studies indicate that people with such chronic problems as asthma, allergies, and gallstones may not produce enough stomach acid, which is vital to the breakdown of proteins and the delivery of nutrients through the small intestine. Some practitioners suggest that betaine HCl may also help relieve heartburn, heal ulcers, and reduce excessive gas, although more research is needed to confirm these findings.

Another form of betaine, called betaine trimethlyglycine, plays a vital supporting role in combating homocysteine, a potentially harmful amino acid, and identified in recent years as a major culprit in increasing the risk of a variety of cardiovascular problems, including heart disease, stroke, and peripheral vascular disease (which decreases blood flow to the legs). Betaine and other closely related nutrients also keep the liver healthy and protect the kidneys; betaine can help protect against liver damage and perhaps even reverse it.

Betaine has also been found to relieve dryness of the mouth, and is now being added as an ingredient in some toothpastes.

For additional information on specific health conditions and how you can treat them with supplements, see Part 3 of this book, beginning on page 309.

HOW IT WORKS

For people with low levels of stomach acid, betaine HCl functions as a replacement source of hydrochloric acid, helping to stimulate the digestive system.

Betaine also plays a fascinating role in maintaining proper liver function and helping cells to replicate. It works together with choline (an essential nutrient), as well as with folic acid (vitamin B_9), vitamin B_{12}, and other nutrients, to contribute the chemical entity known as a methyl group, which subsequently facilitates a variety of important chemical processes.

In addition to supporting normal liver function, betaine protects the liver from damage in two ways: by preventing fat from being deposited in the liver and by speeding up the removal of fatty material from the liver.

HOW TO TAKE IT

In addition to its food sources (fish, legumes, beets, broccoli, and spinach), betaine is also available as a dietary supplement in powder, capsule, and tablet form. Betaine HCl is often measured in grains or milligrams and recommended in dosages of 5 to 10 grains or 325 to 650 milligrams daily with meals, although higher dosages may be taken under a doctor's supervision. Betaine HCl may work best when taken along with a protein.

Although the optimal intake of betaine trimethylglycine is unknown, dosages may range from 375 to 3,000 milligrams daily. For the best results take betaine together with folic acid and vitamins B_6 and B_{12}.

LOOK OUT FOR THIS!

Most people do not experience side effects from betaine supplements, but rare side effects may include nausea, vomiting, and diarrhea. Stop using betaine or reduce your dosage and consult a doctor if you have any of these reactions.

Betaine trimethylglycine and betaine HCl, although related, are different compounds and shouldn't be confused. Only those with a deficiency of hydrochloric acid should take betaine HCl, and it is essential that people with heartburn or ulcers consult a doctor before taking betaine HCl, since it may help treat them but may also worsen them.

Children and pregnant or nursing women shouldn't take betaine or betaine HCl.

WHAT TO AVOID

Medication: Since some practitioners feel betaine HCl can worsen ulcers and heartburn, you should avoid this supplement if you are taking nonsteroidal anti-inflammatory drugs (NSAIDs) or other medications associated with an increased risk of peptic ulcers.

BILBERRY (*VACCINIUM MYRTILLUS*)

This small, blue/black or purple berry—a relative of the American blueberry, cranberry, and huckleberry—is harvested in Europe from wild stands and also grows wild in scattered regions of the United States. While alleged reports by British bomber pilots during World War II claimed a marked improvement in night vision after eating bilberry jam and prompted the further investigation of bilberry's effect on vision, this story may be no more than a myth. While most of bilberry's acclaim comes from its antioxidative effects on eye-related disorders, this herb has also shown beneficial results in treating vascular disorders.

WHAT IT DOES

Bilberry extracts are credited with improving a variety of visual and vascular disturbances, including diabetic and hypertensive retinopathy, cataracts, glaucoma, nearsightedness, and macular degeneration, but these uses have not been definitively documented in scientific studies. Bilberry does appear to have anticancer properties in preliminary studies and may also have some astringent, "anti-bruising," antiseptic, antiedema, and anti-inflammatory properties. It is used in the treatment of vascular disorders such as bruising, varicose veins, and hemorrhoids. It may be useful in treating and preventing hemorrhoids associated with pregnancy. The dried fruit of bilberry has been used in traditional European medicine to treat diarrhea, constipation, and vomiting. It is also a popular remedy for the topical relief of minor mucous membrane inflammations, such as sore throats, and for sinusitis. The German Commission E (see page 16) permits the use of bilberry fruits for the treatment of acute diarrhea, particularly in children, and for treatment of mild inflammation of the mucous membranes of the mouth and throat. While bilberry leaves have been used to control blood sugar levels in people with diabetes, the efficacy and safety of bilberry leaves is questionable and therefore is best avoided at present.

For additional information on specific health conditions and how you can treat them with supplements, see Part 3 of this book, beginning on page 309.

HOW IT WORKS

Ripe bilberry fruit and its extracts contain a potent class of the flavonoid pigments called anthocyanosides (or anthocyanidins). These compounds help build strong capillaries (the small vessels that transport blood from arteries to veins), and bilberry, with its anthocyanosides, may help in a number of eye diseases in which capillary damage is a main factor. Anthocyanosides also help boost the production of pigments that help the eyes adjust to light changes. They also help reduce the risk of blood clots. Bilberry is also rich in tannins, which act as both an anti-inflammatory agents and astringents. Bilberry is credited with helping to ease diarrhea by reducing intestinal inflammation.

HOW TO TAKE IT

Bilberry may be taken in a variety of forms. The berries may be eaten fresh or dried, and in Europe they are used in liquers, flavorings for sorbet, and crepes, pies, tarts, and jams. The dried ripe fruits may be eaten daily but may be difficult to find in the United States. Bilberry tablets or capsules may be taken by mouth, and pressed juice from the berries can be prepared at home or purchased commercially. Bilberry can be used externally by boiling the fruit in water to make a decoction. A typical dose of bilberry tablets or capsules ranges from 240 to 600 milligrams of an extract standardized to contain 25% anthrocyanosides daily, 1 to 2 milliliters twice a day in tincture form, or 20 to 60 grams of the dried fruit per day.

Note: Only dried bilberries themselves or dried bilberry preparations are recommended for the treatment of diarrhea, since fresh bilberries may act as a laxative.

LOOK OUT FOR THIS!

There are no known health concerns when taking bilberry supplements. However, the long-term safety and side effects of bilberry have not been extensively studied. Also avoid ingesting the leaf itself, since it may be toxic.

People with diabetes or bleeding disorders should consult their doctor before taking bilberry supplements, and high doses of bilberry leaf extract can cause digestive upset, skin rash, and drowsiness.

WHAT TO AVOID

Medication: The German Commission E (see page 16) monograph on bilberry fruits lists no known contraindication, interactions with

BIOTIN

Most healthy people receive adequate amounts of biotin from their diet. If you like filberts, you're in luck. A half-cup of filberts is packed with 51 micrograms of biotin. Read on for other sources of biotin.

▶ Almonds, bananas, brewer's yeast, cauliflower, cooked eggs, filberts, grapefruit, liver, milk, mushrooms, salmon, sardines, soy, strawberries, sweet potatoes, and watermelon.

other drugs, or side effects. Because of a theoretical increased risk of bleeding, take bilberry cautiously if you are using any anticoagulant or antiplatelet medications such as warfarin. Also use caution if you are taking medication for hypoglycemia, since bilberry may theoretically reduce blood sugar levels.

BIOTIN

FOR MANY PEOPLE, BIOTIN IS SYNONYMOUS with healthy hair and nails, and it can be found in many beauty products such as shampoos, hair conditioners, and nail polishes. Although deficiencies of biotin are rare, raw eggs contain a protein called avidin, which binds to biotin and prevents the body's absorption of this nutrient. However, although this can be a problem for people who consume raw eggs, don't eliminate scrambled or boiled eggs from your breakfast routine, since cooking renders the protein-binding qualities of avidin powerless.

Biotin supplementation is not necessary for most people. Not only do most people get enough biotin through their diet, but bacteria in the far end of the small intestine synthesize biotin as well. However, biotin is depleted by many antibiotics and headache medications containing butalbital (Fioricet, Fiorinal).

WHAT IT DOES

Note that the therapeutic uses of biotin are highly preliminary and require additional research.

While most of biotin's acclaim comes from its ability to strengthen hair and nails, there is limited scientific support to back these claims. Several studies indicate that biotin may help treat dry, brittle nails and hair. And while biotin is commonly recommended for treating cradle cap in infants, there are no studies confirming its efficacy for this.

Early research shows that biotin may have some promise for treating diabetes, in that it may reduce blood sugar levels in people with type 1 and type 2 diabetes, as well as decrease the symptoms associated with diabetic neuropathy, a complication of diabetes in which nerve damage causes pain, burning, itching, tingling, and numbness of the legs, feet, arms, or hands.

Biotin, in combination with chromium picolinate (see page 77), may also lower heart disease risk in people with diabetes.

For additional information on specific health conditions and how you can treat them with supplements, see Part 3 of this book, beginning on page 309.

HOW IT WORKS

Biotin aids a number of enzymes that convert food into usable energy. It is also necessary for various other functions, including the conversion of fats and carbohydrates into fatty acids and glucose and the breakdown of protein into amino acids.

Biotin may also be involved in the synthesis of insulin, which is why it may help in controlling blood-sugar levels in people with diabetes.

In theory, biotin may work to strengthen hair and nails by helping to form "cross links" between the molecules of the protein found in hair known as keratin, which constitutes most of the structure of hair and nails.

HOW TO TAKE IT

The need for biotin is highest in pregnant and nursing women. See the table on the next page for the recommended daily intakes (RDIs) of biotin.

Biotin is a member of the B-complex vitamin group (a term given to a group of 8 important B vitamins). Most general-purpose multivitamin and mineral supplements contain the full range of B vitamins (be sure to check the label to see which B vitamins a supplement contains). A supplement that contains biotin (alone) is usually not necessary.

People who may require additional, supplemental biotin include those with genetic biotin deficiency disorders and pregnant women.

Biotin supplements are available in capsule and tablet form. For people with diabetes, recommended dosages of biotin range from 7,000 to 15,000 micrograms daily. A dosage of 3,000 micrograms daily is often recommended for improving the condition of hair and nails. Consult your doctor to determine an appropriate dosage of biotin.

LOOK OUT FOR THIS!

Biotin is generally a safe supplement, even when taken at high dosages. Maximum safe dosages, however, have not been established for children, pregnant or nursing women, and people with liver or kidney disease. Consult your doctor before taking dosages of biotin above the recommended daily intake (see page 47).

Since biotin is water-soluble, excess levels are excreted in the urine, reducing the chance of toxicity from this vitamin.

AGE/CONDITION	RECOMMENDED DAILY INTAKE (RDI)*
Infants	
0–5 months	5 mcg
6–11 months	6 mcg
Children	
1–3 years	8 mcg
4–8 years	12 mcg
9–13 years	20 mcg
Males and Females	
14–18 years	25 mcg
19 years and older	30 mcg
Pregnant Women	30 mcg
Nursing Women	35 mcg

For more information on RDIs, see Want to Know More About Intake? on page 8.

WHAT TO AVOID

Medication: People taking antiseizure medications may require higher dosages of biotin. Biotin should be taken 2 to 3 hours after taking antiseizure medications. If you take such medications, consult your doctor to determine an appropriate dosage of biotin.

BLACK COHOSH

NATIVE AMERICANS AND CHINESE herbalists used the root of the black cohosh plant *(Cimicifuga racemosa)* to alleviate menstrual cramps, labor pain, and menopause—and even used it as an insect repellent. Chinese herbalists also used this plant to treat headaches, sore teeth and gums, sore throat, mouth sores, measles, and shortness of breath. Black cohosh's most notable uses are in a wide range of gynecologic conditions, including the symptoms of menstruation and menopause. One popular remedy for menstrual cramps, which your grandmother probably knew was Lydia Pinkham's Elixir, sold from the 1870s to the 1950s, and which contained black cohosh and alcohol.

WHAT IT DOES

In recent years, black cohosh has been widely used to ease menstrual discomfort, specifically in women with endometriosis (growths or lesions on the uterine wall), painful menstrual periods, mood swings, and headaches. Its popularity is greater in Europe than in the United States, and it has been approved by the German Commission E (see page 16) for these uses. Black cohosh's effectiveness and safety have been confirmed by long-term clinical experience and controlled clinical trials. Black cohosh has also become popular as a natural alternative to estrogen replacement therapy in the alleviation of menopausal symptoms such as hot flashes, mood swings, night sweats, palpitations, and vaginal dryness. A recent study found it effective for menopausal complaints, when combined with St. John's wort. Another study found almost identical effects when comparing black cohosh to transdermal estrogen. A third study found black cohosh to be particularly effective in the early stages of menopause.

For additional information on specific health conditions and how to treat them with supplements, see Part 3 of this book, beginning on page 309.

HOW IT WORKS

The precise chemical constitution of black cohosh remains unclear, and its effects on estrogen receptors and hormone levels have not been fully explained. However, it appears that black cohosh may act in a manner similar to estrogen in certain parts of the body such as the brain (where mood swings and hot flashes are experienced) and the vagina, consequently soothing menstrual and menopausal symptoms.

HOW TO TAKE IT

Black cohosh is available in capsules, tablets, a liquid tincture that can be mixed with water, and a dried root that can be simmered in water to make a decoction. The typical recommended dosage of black cohosh is 40 milligrams of a standardized extract three times a

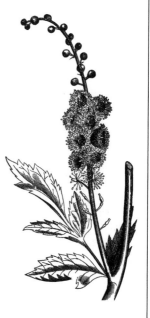

day. When taken in dried root form, the dosage of black cohosh is 1.5 to 9 grams daily, boiled as a decoction.

Note: Do not confuse black cohosh with blue cohosh, an herb that may produce similar effects, but which contains potentially toxic chemicals and whose full effects have not been thoroughly tested.

LOOK OUT FOR THIS!

Black cohosh is generally considered safe for adults. The use of black cohosh is not suitable for children and women who are pregnant or nursing, because of its hormone-like effect. Individuals with a history of blood clots, stroke, or seizure disorders should consult their doctors before using black cohosh.

Side effects of black cohosh are rare but occasionally may include headaches, gastrointestinal discomfort, nausea, vomiting, dizziness, a slow heart rate, visual disturbances, and excess perspiration.

WHAT TO AVOID

Medication: There are no known drug interactions with black cohosh. However, women using estrogen replacement therapy should consult their doctor before taking black cohosh, because side effects have been noted with this combination. Also people who are allergic to aspirin or other salicylates should not take black cohosh, since it contains small amounts of salicylic acid.

BORON

BORON IS A TRACE MINERAL FOUND in many tissues in the human body, but primarily concentrated in the bones, the spleen, and the thyroid gland. Recently, boron has been marketed for a number of therapeutic purposes. Some experts say it is essential to the functioning of the brain and that it enhances memory, cognitive functions, and hand-eye coordination. Boron is also promoted for bone and joint health, particularly in women. Some researchers say it reduces the incidence and symptoms of arthritis. Boron has even become a popular supplement in the bodybuilding world, where its proponents claim that it helps build strength and muscle mass and boosts levels of the hormone testosterone, which also contributes to muscle growth. Yet despite the apparent excitement surrounding boron, scientific evidence for its use as a supplement is lacking, and doctors do not generally recommend it as a supplement.

WHAT IT DOES

Studies indicate that boric acid—a chemical compound derived from boron—has antiseptic and antiviral properties. Several studies indicate that boric acid, when used in suppository form, may help in treating chronic vaginal yeast infection, especially when such infection has persisted despite the use of conventional antifungal medications. Other studies indicate that boric acid may prevent relapses of vaginal yeast infection in women who are prone to chronic yeast infections.

Boron's potential uses are mainly in bone and joint health. Whether boron has a biomechanical role in strengthening bone is not yet known, but it does help to increase the absorption of calcium—a mineral essential to bone health.

Recent experimental evidence shows that boron may also help the body to better absorb and utilize magnesium, vitamin D, and copper, possibly contributing to bone density. Consequently, boron is sometimes recommended for people with osteoporosis and osteoarthritis. However, more research is needed to support these preliminary findings.

Some researchers suspect that boron supplements may prevent or alleviate arthritis, since people with arthritis often appear to have low levels of boron. More evidence is needed to support this hypothesis.

Boron has also been promoted for its possible role in hormone production. For example, people who live in parts of the world with boron-rich diets seem to have consistently higher testosterone levels. But in this case too, studies have not shown boron supplements to be effective in boosting testosterone levels.

For additional information on specific health conditions and how you can treat them with supplements, see Part 3 of this book, beginning on page 309.

HOW IT WORKS

Boric acid may fight yeast infections by restoring the acid-base balance in the vagina, thus creating an environment in which yeast cannot grow and thrive.

A number of studies have shown no effect of boron supplements in either men or women. However, scientists are examining the possibility that boron can improve bone density and strength by increasing the levels of hormones such as estrogen or testosterone after menopause and in other circumstances.

FOOD SOURCES

BORON

If your diet consists mostly of meat and poultry, there is a good chance that you are not getting much boron, since it is found mainly in foods of plant origin. To boost your boron levels, increase your intake of non-meat foods, including green vegetables and fresh fruits. Read on for other boron-containing foods.

▶ Cooked dried beans and peas, dark green, leafy vegetables, grape juice, legumes, non-citrus fruits such as blueberries, peaches, or plums, and nuts.

HOW TO TAKE IT

Boron is found in relatively high levels in foods that come from plants (see Food Sources, page 51). Adding these foods to your diet should increase the levels of boron in your body. Often, boron is found in drinking water (although the amounts vary considerably, depending on location).

Boron as a supplement is available in capsule and tablet forms. The most common commercially available form of boron is boric acid, which has been used as a mild antiseptic and eyewash, but there is no well-researched evidence that these uses are safe or effective.

Boric-acid suppositories are available over-the-counter for treating vaginal yeast infection.

No recommended dietary allowance has been established for boron.

LOOK OUT FOR THIS!

In small doses, boron is considered safe for adults. Dosages above 50 milligrams per day, however, are potentially toxic. Symptoms of boron toxicity may include appetite loss, nausea, vomiting, skin rashes, lethargy, and diarrhea.

Because of a lack of research on their safety, boron supplements are not recommended for children or for women who are pregnant or nursing.

WHAT TO AVOID

Medication: In theory, boron may interfere with the effects of estrogen-active medications. Therefore, women taking birth-control pills or hormone replacement therapy should consult their doctor before taking boron supplements.

Herbs and Dietary Supplements: Magnesium may interfere with the effects of boron.

BOSWELLIA

THE BOSWELLIA TREE *(Boswellia serrata),* native to India, North Africa, and the Middle East, produces a gummy sap under its bark that has traditionally been used to treat a variety of conditions, including skin disorders, wounds, and varicose veins. According to Christian belief, Jesus was presented with three gifts from three wise men to celebrate his birth; one of the gifts—frankincense—is made of resin from the boswellia tree. The aromatic resin was used as incense and was considered very valuable. In traditional Chinese medicine, boswellia is often used together with myrhh, another gift of the three wise men, for pain resulting from trauma, swelling, and muscle spasms.

WHAT IT DOES

Today, evidence suggests that boswellia may have anti-inflammatory properties. Based on this evidence, it is believed that boswellia may be useful for bursitis, carpal tunnel syndrome, osteoarthritis, rheumatoid arthritis, tendonitis, asthma, and other inflammatory conditions. Some studies have shown that boswellia is equivalent to ibuprofen or aspirin in its ability to reduce swelling. In traditional Chinese medicine, boswellia is used to treat pain and inflammation of the gums, mouth, and throat, and it can be found as an ingredient in natural mouthwashes.

Recent studies suggest that boswellia may also be an effective treatment for inflammatory bowel disease, Crohn's disease, and ulcerative colitis. One study found boswellia to be as effective as a standard medication used for the treatment of ulcerative colitis. A similar study examined boswellia in chronic colitis and found it effective for this condition as well. Yet another study determined that boswellia is effective and safer than medication traditionally used to treat Crohn's disease.

Boswellia has traditionally been used to treat acne, bacterial and fungal infections, boils, wounds, scars, and varicose veins and cosmetically to tone the skin and smooth wrinkles. One study suggested that boswellia has broad antibiotic properties as well. More studies are needed to test boswellia's efficacy in these conditions.

For additional information on specific health conditions and how you can treat them with supplements, see Part 3 of this book, beginning on page 309.

HOW IT WORKS

The active ingredients in boswellia are called boswellic acids. In theory, they inhibit the body's synthesis of certain enzymes called leukotrienes that contribute to inflammation and pain.

HOW TO TAKE IT

Boswellia is available in tablet and capsule form. To help control pain or stiffness attributed to inflammation, it should be taken as needed. The typical dose of boswellia is 150 to 400 milligrams of a standardized extract taken three times a day, but some studies have used dosages as high as 1,200 milligrams three times a day. Consult your doctor to determine an appropriate dosage of boswellia for you. It may be important to take boswellia with a fatty meal, so the body can better absorb and utilize the herb.

LOOK OUT FOR THIS!

Side effects of boswellia may include stomach complaints such as nausea, acid reflux, and other gastrointestinal conditions, as well as dermatitis.

Boswellia is generally considered safe. Individuals with kidney or liver diseases should consult their doctor before takingboswellia. Do not use boswellia to treat asthma, unless under the supervision of a doctor.

Boswellia is not suitable for children or for women who are pregnant or nursing, because there is little study-based information about its safety in these populations.

WHAT TO AVOID

Medication: Consult you doctor if you are taking leukotriene inhibitors, antineoplastic agents, lipid-lowering agents, fat-soluble medications, nonsteroidal anti-inflammatory drugs (NSAIDs), or antifungal agents, since boswellia may interfere with these medications.

Herbs and Dietary Supplements: If you are taking glycosaminoglycans, antiproliferative agents, antifungal agents, or lipid-lowering agents, theoretically they might interact with boswellia, but this is generally no cause for concern.

BROMELAIN

PINEAPPLES ARE GOOD FOR YOU. This might seem like an obvious statement, but there is more to it than you might know. The stems of pineapples are the main source of bromelain, an enzyme that provides many benefits, from aiding digestion to speeding recovery time after surgery. Bromelain was first produced in Japan and Hawaii and is now widely used everywhere.

WHAT IT DOES

Bromelain is a proteolytic (or protein-digesting) enzyme that may work as a digestive aid in some people. While other proteolytic enzymes are often recommended as digestive aids, evidence suggests that bromelain is better absorbed by the body and may have the best effect.

Bromelain also works as an anti-inflammatory agent and may be used to help speed tissue repair and recovery after surgery and healing of athletic injuries including sprains, strains, back pain, arthritis, bursitis, tendonitis, and carpal tunnel syndrome. Bromelain may also ease a variety of respiratory infections because of its ability to decrease inflammation in the respiratory system and reduce the thickness of mucus.

When applied topically, bromelain may clean burns as well as speed the recovery time from burns and bruises.

Other suggested uses of bromelain include treatment of chronic obstructive pulmonary disease (COPD), phlebitis (swelling of a vein, often accompanied by blood-clot formation), chronic venous insufficiency (abnormal circulation characterized by reduced return of blood from the legs to the trunk), conjunctivitis, hemorrhoids, urinary tract infections, and ulcerative colitis.

For additional information on specific health conditions and how you can treat them with supplements, see Part 3 of this book, beginning on page 309.

HOW IT WORKS

As a digestive enzyme, bromelain works along with the body's own digestive enzymes, therefore reducing many of the side effects of poor digestion (such as gas, cramps, and diarrhea). Unlike other digestive enzymes, bromelain works directly in the stomach and the small intestine, significantly increasing its effectiveness as a digestive aid.

Bromelain also appears to have benefits throughout the body, including reducing inflammation, working to counteract abnormal blood clotting, and enhancing the immune system. Bromelain also thins blood and mucus, which is why this enzyme may help people with respiratory infections. A recent German study found bromelain effective for children with acute sinusitis.

HOW TO TAKE IT

Unless you enjoy eating pineapple stems, you may have to stick to supplements when it comes to taking bromelain. Bromelain supplements are available as oral tablets and topical oil-based creams. The recommend dosages differ according to the form of supplement used, so be sure to read and carefully follow the label directions.

Bromelain is often measured in milk-clotting units (MCU) or gelatin-dissolving units (GDU). One GDU is the equivalent of 1.5 MCU. Some doctors recommend taking a starting dose of 3,000 MCU of bromelain three times a day for several days, followed by a maintenance dose of 2,000 MCU three times daily.

Be sure to choose an oral brand of bromelain that is "enteric-coated" in order to prevent premature digestion of this enzyme in the stomach. Some experts advise taking oral bromelain on an empty stomach, since some foods (such as soybean and potato protein) may reduce its effects.

LOOK OUT FOR THIS!

Bromelain appears to be a safe supplement, with few side effects. Occasionally, it may cause gastrointestinal problems (mild heartburn, stomach upset, and diarrhea), an increased heart rate (at higher doses), irritation of mucous membranes, menstrual problems, and drowsiness or sedation.

Allergic and asthmatic reactions to bromelain have been reported, mainly in people allergic to pineapples, honeybee venom, latex, birch pollen, carrot, celery, fennel, cypress pollen, grass pollen, rye flour, or wheat flour.

The safety of bromelain has not been established for young children, pregnant or nursing women, or people with severe liver or kidney disease.

Bromelain should be used cautiously by people with heart disease and those with bleeding disorders and by people at risk for developing ulcers.

WHAT TO AVOID

Medication: Unless advised by a doctor, bromelain may not be suitable for people taking anticoagulant agents (such as warfarin). Bromelain may increase the absorption of some antibiotics (especially amoxicillin and tetracycline) and increase the action of some anticancer drugs, cholesterol-lowering drugs, and drugs that cause drowsiness, such as lorazepam, diazepam, phenobarbital, codeine, and certain antidepressants.

CALCIUM

IN 2001, THE NATIONAL INSTITUTES of Health (NIH) announced a "calcium crisis" in the United States, revealing that only 13.5 percent of girls and 36.3 percent of boys between the ages of 12 and 19 are getting the recommended daily amount (RDA) of calcium. Since about 90 percent of bone mass is established between these two ages, an inadequate intake of calcium increases these children's risk for osteoporosis and other bone diseases later in life.

And children aren't the only ones with low intakes of calcium; most experts agree that adults are also not receiving adequate intakes of this important nutrient.

WHAT IT DOES

Aside from its well-known role in maintaining healthy teeth and bones (a well-controlled study showed that calcium did prevent fractures in elderly woman, as long as they were compliant with taking it on a regular basis), recent research indicates calcium may promote

FRIENDS AND FOES

We need **calcium** for healthy bones, but **vitamin D** is equally important, since it helps the body absorb the calcium. There's no need to take the two together in one pill for the combination to be effective, although doing so may be more convenient than taking two separate pills.

I have heard a lot about coral calcium supplements and the various health benefits they are purported to provide. Is there any truth to these claims?

Q & A

Coral calcium supplements are widely promoted in health-food stores, infomercials, and on the Internet. Claims for coral calcium supplements have run the gamut of their supposed benefits, from curing and treating Alzheimer's disease, cancer, and lupus, to being the best source of calcium for your bones. Endless as they are, the claims are untrue.

Coral calcium is a relatively expensive supplement, and there is no evidence to support the claims made by manufacturers of this supplement. One company made

such outlandish claims that a trade group of supplement manufacturers asked the government to step in and stop them. As a result, the Federal Trade Commission (FTC) pressed charges against the company and some others; yet even though evidence about coral calcium supplements is lacking, manufacturers continue to make unsubstantiated claims.

There is no reason to believe the hype about coral calcium: It is not a magical supplement. You can get the same benefits from a generic calcium supplement and spend the money you save on something more worthwhile.

weight loss. Studies have found that higher calcium intakes are related to lower body fat and body weight in both adults and children, as well as to reduced weight gain in midlife.

Other recent studies have shown that men who eat more calcium-rich foods reduce their risk of colon cancer. Women who take daily supplements of calcium carbonate can alleviate unpleasant premenstrual symptoms such as pain and tenderness, bloating, mood swings, and food cravings.

Calcium also has a beneficial impact on blood pressure. Not only may a deficiency in calcium lead to high blood pressure, but people with high blood pressure may experience a reduction in blood pressure with calcium supplementation. Pregnant woman should be sure to get enough calcium, since a recent study demonstrated that sufficient calcium intake decreases infant mortality and other pregnancy-related illnesses.

Among the other conditions in which calcium may be beneficial are attention deficit hyperactivity disorder (ADHD), canker sores, headaches, heartburn, high cholesterol, and gum disease, although more research is needed to substantiate these claims.

For additional information on specific health conditions and how you can treat them with supplements, see Part 3 of this book, beginning on page 309.

HOW IT WORKS

The calcium that our bodies store in our teeth and bones—which accounts for over 99 percent of the calcium in our bodies—takes part in an ongoing exchange of minerals with our bloodstream. Our bones are constantly releasing calcium and other minerals into the bloodstream, where these minerals play various important roles.

When calcium levels in the blood run low, the body pulls the calcium it requires from our bones, which can leave the bones weakened and fragile over time. One result of this may be osteoporosis.

HOW TO TAKE IT

The need for calcium increases with age. See the table on next page for the recommended daily intakes (RDIs) for calcium.

AGE/GENDER/ CONDITION	RECOMMENDED DAILY INTAKE (RDI)*
Infants	
0–6 months	210 mg
7–12 months	270 mg
Children	
1–3 years	500 mg
4–8 years	800 mg
9–18 years	1,300 mg
Males and Females	
19–50 years	1,000 mg
51 years and over	1,200 mg
Pregnant Women	1,000 mg
Nursing Women	1,000 mg

For more information on RDIs, see Want to Know More About Intake? on page 8.

Note: The body can't absorb more than 500 milligrams of calcium at a time. People taking calcium supplements should divide their dosages for maximum effectiveness.

As a supplement, calcium is relatively inexpensive, readily available, and well tolerated. Chewable tablets, and calcium powders and solutions are more easily absorbed than hard, compressed tablets. Calcium comes in many forms, but they differ in terms of the amount of calcium they contain, how well they are absorbed by the body, and how much they cost.

■ *Calcium citrate*—Probably the form of calcium that is most easily absorbed and digested by the body. It's considered particularly effective in preventing osteoporosis.

■ *Calcium carbonate*—Less expensive than calcium citrate but perhaps not as effective in preventing osteoporosis. Also somewhat more difficult to absorb for people without sufficient stomach acid. Best taken with meals.

■ *Calcium formate*—Recent studies suggest that this may be more absorbable than even calcium citrate, but this form is not yet widely available.

CALCIUM

The best way to get the amount of calcium you need is through the foods you eat. Some herbs, spices, and seaweeds are rich in calcium as well. Read on to discover some high-calcium foods and herbs.

▶**Herbs:** Basil, cinnamon, dill weed, fennel, fenugreek, ginseng, kelp, marjoram, oregano, parsley, poppy seed, sage, and savory.

▶**Foods:** Blackstrap molasses, bok choy, brazil nuts, broccoli, calcium-fortified juices, collard greens, dried figs, green, leafy vegetables such as kale, milk and milk products, nuts, oysters, sardines with bones, soybean flour, Swiss chard, tahini, wheat-soy flour, and whole grains.

■ *Calcium gluconate*—Not recommended. This form of calcium contains low concentrations of calcium, so you have to take more of the supplement to get the recommended amounts.

■ *Calcium lactate*—Not recommended. This form of calcium contains low concentrations of calcium, so you have to take more of the supplement to get recommended amounts.

■ *Calcium chloride*—Not recommended because it may irritate the gastrointestinal tract.

■ *Calcium phosphate*—Not recommended because it's difficult to absorb.

■ *Calcium-rich mineral water*—May be a useful way for some people to get their daily dose of supplemental calcium.

Note: Calcium supplements that are products of oyster shell, dolomite, and bone meal should be avoided as they may contain traces of lead, mercury, or arsenic.

Calcium deficiency is usually detected through bone-density tests. People who have chronically low calcium intakes; children, adolescents, and seniors; postmenopausal women; people who have recently experienced prolonged bedrest or who diet frequently; and those who have low intakes of vitamin D are good candidates for calcium supplementation.

LOOK OUT FOR THIS!

People with sarcoidosis or high levels of calcium in their blood should not take calcium as a supplement. If you have kidney disease, chronic constipation, colitis, diarrhea, stomach or intestinal bleeding, irregular heartbeat, or heart problems, consult a doctor before taking calcium.

For most people, calcium loss from the body is largely undetectable. In rare cases of severe calcium deprivation, symptoms include muscle spasms or cramping (typically in the hands or feet), hair loss, dry skin and nails, numbness, tingling or burning sensations around the mouth and fingers, constipation, nausea and vomiting, headaches, confusion, yeast infections, anxiety, convulsions and seizures, muscle and bone pain, and poor tooth and bone development. Many postmenopausal women have no idea they're not getting enough calcium until a bone-density scan or X ray reveals bone loss, or worse, a bone break.

Until recently, people with a history of kidney stones had been advised to stick to a low-calcium diet. A new study has changed this recommendation: experts now suggest that normal amounts of calcium and a reduced intake of animal protein and salt may provide even more protection from kidney stones. If you have a history of kidney stones, consult your doctor before taking calcium supplements.

WHAT TO AVOID

Medication: Certain medications can deplete levels of calcium in the body including antibiotics, aluminum-containing antacids, butalbital-containing analgesics, corticosteroids, digoxin, colchicines, antifungal drugs, and diuretics. Consult your doctor to determine if you require an adjustment to your calcium dosage.

Herbs and Dietary Supplements: Do not take iron supplements at the same time as you take calcium, since calcium interferes with the absorption of iron. Regular large doses of calcium may also interfere with the absorption of zinc and magnesium.

CALENDULA

CALENDULA OFFICINALIS, OR CALENDULA, as it is more commonly called, is the botanical name for pot marigold, a daisy-like herb that blooms for many months, usually from early spring to the first frost of fall. In fact, this flower's lengthy flowering season could well be the reason for the name "calendula," since in Latin, *calend* means month. Both the flowers and the leaves and stem of calendula have been used for centuries to treat a variety of ailments.

Grow This!

Even if you don't have a green thumb, calendula (pot marigolds) are a cinch to grow. You can buy them from your local garden center, order them from an herb nursery, or easily grow them from seed. Place calendula seeds in a sunny spot and they'll grow into plants 12 to 18 inches high, blooming month after month until the frost sets in.

- **Light:** Full sun to light shade.
- **Temperature:** Cool weather (70° F).
- **Water:** Calendulas require only moderate watering. Once they're established, you only need to water calendulas if the soil dries between rains. Keep the soil moist. You may have to water calendulas more frequently if they are in direct sunlight for extended periods of time.
- **Repotting:** You can grow calendula directly in the garden or plant them in pots or in window boxes filled with potting soil or well-drained garden loam that is enriched with thoroughly decayed organic matter and fertilizer with a high phosphorus content. If you plan to use the flowers medicinally, make sure to snap off mature flowers before they start to wilt. Pull off the petals and soak them in water for a few minutes to allow dust and small insects to float off.

WHAT IT DOES

Evidence suggests that calendula, when applied topically, is an effective treatment for various skin disorders, including eczema and other skin irritations and burns. Preliminary evidence also suggests that when taken in the form of eardrops, calendula may reduce the pain of ear infections. A recent study indicated that calendula may also be useful in the treatment of venous leg ulcers. Calendula was recently shown to be effective in preventing acute dermatitis during the treatment of breast cancer with radiation.

Popular and historical uses of calendula include the successful treatment of acne, anemia, bruises, bee and wasp stings, cramps, headache, hemorrhoids, mouth sores, nausea, rashes, sore throat, tinnitus, warts, and yeast infections, although many of these uses are scientifically unsubstantiated and require further study.

For additional information on specific health conditions and how you can treat them with supplements, see Part 3 of this book, beginning on page 309.

HOW IT WORKS

Calendula is believed to possess anti-inflammatory, antibacterial, antiviral, antitumor, and wound-healing properties (by repairing damaged tissue, in part by stimulating the production of new blood vessels). Additional research is needed to understand more about calendula's therapeutic effects.

HOW TO TAKE IT

Calendula flowers are available in the form of powder, gel, ointment, eye solution, tea, tincture (calendula dissolved in alcohol), shampoo, soap, and hand cream. The herb is also available as an ointment. The recommend dosages differ according to the form of supplement used, so be sure to read and carefully follow the label directions.

LOOK OUT FOR THIS!

When taken properly, calendula causes very few side effects. In a few cases, allergic reactions of the skin have occurred when a tincture of 10 percent calendula has been used. If you are allergic to plants such as ragweed, chrysanthemums, marigolds, or daisies, you may experience an allergic reaction to calendula. When taken in high doses, calendula can cause drowsiness and reduce blood pressure.

Calendula is not recommended for children or for women who are pregnant or nursing.

WHAT TO AVOID

There are no known interactions of calendula with other drugs, herbs, or supplements.

CAT'S CLAW

DEEP IN THE AMAZON RAINFORESTS, indigenous people have been using cat's claw vine *(Uncaria tomentosa)* to treat a variety of health problems for centuries. Known in Spanish as "uña de gato," the plant takes it name from the sharp, curved thorns that grow on the vine. But it's the bark and root of the cat's claw plant that contain the curative compounds. In recent years, some herbalists have praised cat's claw for its supposedly unlimited healing powers, calling it "the miracle herb from the rainforest of Peru." But be careful—most of the claims are not yet scientifically verified and are in need of additional research.

WHAT IT DOES

Studies suggest that cat's claw is as effective as anti-inflammatory agent for various conditions including rheumatoid arthritis, osteoarthritis, and carpal tunnel syndrome. Other studies have shown that cat's claw may be effective in boosting the immune system and speeding the healing of wounds, including the lesions associated with oral and genital herpes outbreaks.

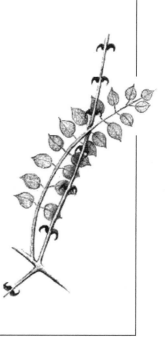

Cat's claw has also been used to treat disorders such as human immunodeficiency virus (HIV) and acquired immune deficiency syndrome (AIDS), rheumatism, gastric ulcers, gastrointestinal disorders including diverticular disease, and tumors and even as a contraceptive.

For additional information on specific health conditions and how you can treat them with supplements, see Part 3 of this book, beginning on page 309.

HOW IT WORKS

The bark of the cat's claw root contains a group of chemicals called oxindole alkaloids, which have inflammation-fighting properties.

Cat's claw also contains sterols, which many researchers believe is the reason for the herb's anti-inflammatory effects. More research is needed to understand exactly how cat's claw works.

HOW TO TAKE IT

In addition to *Uncaria tomentosa* is *Uncaria guianensis*, a second main species of cat's claw. While both species are used medicinally, the former is recommended for rheumatoid arthritis while the latter is often used for osteoarthritis.

Extracts of cat's claw root bark are available as capsules, tablets, powders, tinctures, and creams. Also, the bark of the vine can be crushed to make a tea. In fact, the Ashanika Indians of Peru have long regarded this tea as a sacred beverage—but beware, it's bitter. Dosages of this herb vary, but often range from 20 to 1,000 milligrams daily, depending on the condition and form of the supplement you are taking.

Note: The effectiveness of cat's claw root bark can vary significantly, depending on what time of year that section of the plant was harvested. Also, some supplements use parts of the plant other than the root, which is where the most active compounds are concentrated. Look for standardized supplements made from the root.

LOOK OUT FOR THIS!

Cat's claw tea may cause mild nausea because of its bitter taste.

Cat's claw is not recommended for women who are pregnant or nursing, children, or people with liver or kidney disease.

WHAT TO AVOID

There are no known interactions of cat's claw with other drugs, herbs, or supplements.

CAYENNE

IF YOU ADD CAYENNE PEPPER TO YOUR FOOD because you like it spicy, you're getting some unexpected health benefits along with that tingling sensation. Cayenne seasoning—which comes from the cayenne shrub *(Capsicum frutescens, Capsicum annuum)*—has been used for centuries for its therapeutic effects. Cayenne is just one name for this spice, which is also known as chili pepper, paprika, red pepper, Tabasco pepper, habanero pepper, and more. Although the sensation it produces is hot, cayenne actually works by stimulating part of the brain that lowers the body's temperature. In hot climates, many people eat fiery foods because these help them to handle the heat by inducing perspiration, which cools the body. Cayenne has been an important ingredient in traditional Indian Ayurvedic, Chinese, Japanese, and Korean medicines as a treatment for digestive problems, muscle pain, and frostbite, as well as for appetite stimulation.

WHAT IT DOES

Studies show that when taken orally, cayenne's active ingredient—capsaicin—relieves excess gas, helps curb appetite, and may increase the metabolism of dietary fats, thus promoting weight loss.

When applied to the skin topically as a cream or ointment, cayenne acts as a powerful pain reliever. It is used externally for various kinds of pain, including the pain of arthritis, shingles, headaches, and the nerve damage associated with diabetes. Some people apply cayenne topically to children's fingers to deter them from sucking their thumbs or biting their nails, as the taste can be perceived as unpleasant.

Other studies have suggested that cayenne may be helpful in treating duodenal ulcers, but this is controversial because study results are conflicting. Other preliminary uses of cayenne include the treatment of aspirin-induced stomach upset and the management of overactive bladder, but more study is needed to confirm these findings. One fascinating study found that a capsaicin plaster applied to a Korean hand-acupuncture point decreased post-operative sore throat.

For additional information on specific health conditions and how you can treat them with supplements, see Part 3 of this book, beginning on page 309.

HOW IT WORKS

The active ingredient in cayenne is capsaicin, but other important ingredients include carotenoids, vitamins A and C, and flavonoids. Research has shown that capsaicin relieves pain topically by interfering with a pain transmitter known as "substance P" that carries sensory messages through the nervous system to the brain.

At the same time, capsaicin also produces what's known as a counterirritant effect, in which a mild irritation on the surface of the skin distracts the brain from feeling pain in other areas.

Cayenne may aid in digestion by promoting the secretion of gastric acid in the stomach. In terms of weight loss, cayenne may speed the body's metabolism of fats and carbohydrates, as well as increase activity in the sympathetic nervous system, thus curbing appetite.

HOW TO TAKE IT

Cayenne may be consumed raw or cooked. Dried cayenne pepper comes in a powdered form and is added to food and stirred into juice, tea, and even milk. A cayenne infusion can be made by pouring 1 cup of boiling water over one-half to 1 teaspoon of cayenne powder and letting this mixture sit for 10 minutes. You can then mix 1 teaspoon of the resulting infusion with a cup of water and drink it up to four times a day. As an oral dietary supplement, cayenne is sold in the form of tablets and capsules. General dosage recommendations for cayenne range from 500 to 1,000 milligrams, taken up to three times daily.

For topical use, cayenne may be found in gels, ointments, creams, roll-ons, and occasionally as a tincture. The cream usually comes in two strengths, 0.025 percent and 0.075 percent, and is applied two or three times daily. When purchasing a cream, it should contain at least .02 percent capsaicin. Follow individual product labels for application instruction.

Be careful: Capsaicin cream can cause a burning sensation during its first few applications. Never apply topical capsaicin to cracks or open sores or to mucous membranes—as anyone knows who has ever chopped a chili pepper and then touched their eyes. Inhalation of capsaicin can also cause severe irritation. Always wash your hands immediately after applying cayenne-containing creams, unless your hands are the area being treated.

A Patch to Relieve Arthritis Pain

Did You Know?

The cayenne ingredient responsible for relieving arthritis and neuralgia-associated pains—capsaicin—is available in the form of a patch. This patch, which is applied topically, heats upon contact with the skin, providing temporary relief from pain (see How It Works, page 65). While capsaicin is already a well-known treatment for pain relief in arthritis and neuralgia, some people have found topical capsaicin-containing ointments or creams to be too messy or troublesome to apply repeatedly. The patch is an attractive alternative because it can be applied in the morning and forgotten about until bedtime.

Cayenne is generally considered safe, with no side effects. Occasional rashes have been reported.

WHAT TO AVOID

Medication: Consult your doctor before taking cayenne for a long period of time with angiotensin converting enzyme (ACE) inhibitors, aspirin, blood-thinning medications such as warfarin and low-molecular-weight heparin, theophylline, monoamine oxidase (MAO) inhibitors, and blood-pressure-lowering medications.

CHAMOMILE

THE MEDICINAL USE OF THE chamomile plant (German *[Matricaria recutita];* Roman *[Chamaemelum nobile]*) goes back thousands of years to the ancient Egyptians, Romans, and Greeks. Today chamomile is one of the most widely used ingredients in herbal remedies. In Europe it's often used as a digestive aid, to treat mild skin conditions, menstrual cramps, and insomnia and to relieve tension. In the United States, 90 percent of the chamomile imported is used in teas, although it's also a popular ingredient in beauty products.

The small, daisy-like flower of the chamomile plant is crushed and steamed to extract a blue oil, which contains ingredients that may reduce swelling and limit the growth of bacteria, viruses, and fungi. Despite its popularity, however, surprisingly little scientific research has been done on chamomile in human beings to support many of its medicinal uses.

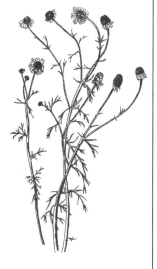

Both the more popular German (or Hungarian) chamomile and the rare and more expensive Roman or English chamomile are members of the *Asteraceae* family, with includes ragweed, echinacea, and feverfew, and the two kinds of chamomile have many of the same medicinal properties. However, German chamomile has been studied far more intensively than Roman chamomile, even though both are used in teas, ointments, and other medicinal preparations.

WHAT IT DOES

Studies have shown that German chamomile may reduce inflammation, speed the healing of wounds, reduce muscle spasms, and act as a mild sedative. Other, more preliminary studies have shown that chamomile may have antimicrobial properties, and as a result, may help combat bacterial infections. Several studies comparing the topical use of chamomile to cortisone cream for treating eczema found that chamomile was more effective.

The German Commission E (see page 16) has approved the use of chamomile for a variety of ailments—topically for bacterial skin infections; orally for gastrointestinal spasms and inflammatory diseases of the gastrointestinal tract; and as an inhalant, for respiratory infection and inflammation.

For additional information on specific health conditions and how you can treat them with supplements, see Part 3 of this book, beginning on page 309.

HOW IT WORKS

Chamomile contains flavonoids that may have anti-inflammatory and antispasmodic effects. More research is needed to determine exactly how chamomile works.

HOW TO TAKE IT

Chamomile is available as dried flower heads, and in liquid extract, tincture, capsule, tablet, and topical cream preparations, and as a tea. You can make chamomile tea by steeping 2 to 3 teaspoons of chamomile flower in 1 cup of boiling water for 10 minutes.

Dosages of chamomile vary with the condition being treated and how the herb is being taken. Chamomile is usually taken three to four times a day between meals. You may take up to two capsules, each containing 300 to 400 milligrams of standardized chamomile extract, three times daily.

Chamomile-containing creams may be applied topically three or four times a day. To make an inhalant, pour 1 cup of boiling water over 3 to 10 grams of dried herb and let it steep for 5 to 10 minutes (if you are using a chamomile tincture, add 15 milliliters of chamomile tincture to 2 cups of boiling water) and deeply inhale the steam vapor.

Chamomile is also popular as a mouth gargle to treat inflammation of the mucous membranes in the mouth and throat and as a soothing bath additive. It can also be found in face creams, drinks, hair dyes, shampoos, and perfumes.

LOOK OUT FOR THIS!

Chamomile is generally considered safe by the U.S. Food and Drug Administration (FDA); however, there have been reports of allergic reactions in individuals who have eaten or come into contact with chamomile preparations, including at least one case of a life-threatening allergic reaction. Some experts have doubted these reports, and believe that the affected individuals were exposed to ragweed or to products contaminated with "dog chamomile"—a highly allergenic and foul-tasting plant that resembles chamomile. People with allergies to birch pollen, mugwort, or plants belonging to the aster family may also be allergic to chamomile.

Because chamomile can cause drowsiness or sedation, use caution when taking it if you are driving or operating heavy machinery. In very high doses, chamomile may cause vomiting.

WHAT TO AVOID

Medication: Chamomile may increase the effect of warfarin, heparin, clopidogrel, ticlopidine, and pentoxifylline.

CHASTEBERRY

CHASTEBERRY, ALSO KNOWN AS VITEX *(Vitex agnus-castus)*, received its common name from the ancient Greeks and Romans, who believed that this plant promoted chastity and who used it to suppress sexual desire. The medicinal parts of the chasteberry plant are the reddish black, ripe dried fruit and the dried leaves. Chasteberry has been a popular supplement in Germany for years, but only recently has it become known in the United States.

WHAT IT DOES

The German Commission E (see page 16) has approved the use of chasteberry for tempering symptoms of premenstrual syndrome (PMS), including irritability, depression, headache, and breast tenderness, and symptoms of menopause, including hot flashes and mood changes. A recent study that compared fluoxetine (Prozac) with chasteberry extract for PMS found that while fluoxetine was more successful in relieving psychological symptoms, chasteberry was more effective in relieving the physical symptoms of PMS.

Chasteberry may also aid in infertility, as well as help the body regain its natural hormonal balance and restore ovulation after women discontinue using birth control pills.

Preliminary research suggests that chasteberry may help reduce hormone-related acne, suppress appetite, increase milk production during nursing, and alleviate insomnia; however, more research is needed to confirm these possibilities. There is no scientific evidence to back claims for chasteberry as effective in enhancing breast shape or size. A recent study found that a CO_2 extract of chasteberry was as effective as a mosquito, biting fly, flea, and tick repellent!

For additional information on specific health conditions and how you can treat them with supplements, see Part 3 of this book, beginning on page 309.

HOW IT WORKS

Research indicates that chasteberry may aid in gynecological discomfort by reducing the secretion of prolactin, a hormone made and released by the pituitary gland in the brain. High prolactin levels are believed to be responsible for premenstrual symptoms as well as infertility.

The active ingredients in chasteberry are thought to be iridoid glycosides, flavonoids, and volatile oils, but it's not clear exactly how they function. It appears, though, that chasteberry inhibits the release of the hormone called follicle stimulating hormone (FSH), which acts to promote the growth and release of egg cells from the ovary, while promoting the release of another hormone, called luteinizing hormone (LH), that is also needed for ovulation. This action, called the "corpus luteum hormone effect," increases progesterone levels and helps to regulate estrogen levels. Regulated progesterone and estrogen levels promote regular menstrual cycles and may prevent acne.

HOW TO TAKE IT

Chasteberry is available in a variety of forms, including capsules, tablets, tinctures, and extract.

There is no established daily recommended dosage for chasteberry, but the typical dose for liquid extract is 40 drops each morning, and for capsule form, 175 to 225 milligrams of an extract standardized to contain 0.5 percent agnuside per day. Studies indicate that chasteberry may be more effective if taken with black cohosh or omega-3 fatty acids.

Note: Chasteberry does not take effect immediately. A duration of 3 months is recommended for its use in easing PMS, and 5 to 7 months may be needed before effects are noticed in treating infertility. For most other conditions, symptoms may begin to subside after only 2 months of using chasteberry.

LOOK OUT FOR THIS!

Chasteberry is generally considered safe for adults. The use of chasteberry is not suitable for children or pregnant women. Women who are nursing should consult their doctor before taking chasteberry because it may disrupt the cessation of menstruation that normally accompanies breastfeeding. Also, nursing mothers may experience an early return to fertility when taking chasteberry.

Occasional, mild side effects of chasteberry include gastrointestinal disturbances, headaches, skin rash, hair loss, fatigue, agitation, dry mouth, rapid heartbeat, nausea, and increased menstrual flow.

WHAT TO AVOID

Medication: It is not advisable to take chasteberry with bromocriptine or other medications that affect prolactin levels, hormones such as estrogen or progesterone, or medications that affect endocrine activity. If you are taking any of these medications, consult your doctor before taking chasteberry. Chasteberry may also interfere with the hormonal activity of oral contraceptives and hormone-replacement therapy.

CHOLINE

THE B VITAMIN KNOWN AS CHOLINE had long been "waiting in the wings" for recognition of the many ways in which it can enhance human health. In 1998, that recognition came when the Food and Nutrition Board of the U.S. National Academy of Sciences named choline an essential nutrient and outlined the recommended amount that people should take each day (see the recommended daily intake, page 73). Choline plays a role in just about every system in the body, from the brain and liver to the heart. It can be made naturally in the body, although the amount the body makes is not sufficient to meet daily requirements. Experts once believed that the body could use other nutrients, such as folate and vitamins B_6 and B_{12}, as substitutes for choline. But they now

CHOLINE

You don't have to go far to find foods containing choline. In fact, an average daily diet contains 500 to 1,000 milligrams of this important B vitamin. Read on for healthy ways to increase your dietary intake of choline.

▶ Brewer's yeast, cabbage, cauliflower, egg yolks, legumes, oatmeal, oranges, organ meats, potatoes, wheat germ, and whole milk.

know that this is not the case, and recommend that people get choline independently from either food or supplements.

WHAT IT DOES

Research has suggested several promising uses for supplemental choline. Several well-designed studies found that one form of choline, called choline alfoscerate, produced improvement in people with mild to moderate Alzheimer's disease. Another substance closely related to choline, called citcholine or CDP-choline, if taken immediately after a stroke and continued, may slightly improve the chances for full recovery.

Animal studies have indicated that the presence of adequate amounts of choline during pregnancy and nursing can help ensure healthy brain development in infants and can even have positive long-term effects on brain functions such as memory.

Supplementation with phosphatidylcholine (PC) or pure choline, both constituents of lecithin, have been found to enhance the effect of interferon and to have liver-protecting effects in people with hepatitis B and hepatitis C. Other studies have indicated that PC may be helpful for people with liver inflammation from alcohol consumption or the use of certain prescription medications.

Preliminary studies suggest that choline may also help to prevent cancer. However, although animal studies have shown that cancer rates rise with diets that have a very low content of choline, there is no evidence that choline supplements will reduce these rates. Lethicin or pure choline may also help people with bipolar disorder.

For additional information on specific health conditions and how you can treat them with supplements, see Part 3 of this book, beginning on page 309.

HOW IT WORKS

Choline, as phosphatidylcholine (PC), is a vital part of cell membranes (the outer coating of cells that selectively controls the contents exiting and entering the cell) and so helps keep cells intact and functioning properly. PC also aids in the metabolism of fats and the way in which fat is moved from the liver. Choline also plays a critical role in making acetylcholine, one of several chemical substances known as neurotransmitters because they are essential for sending nerve signals in the brain and nervous system, and in brain function.

Thus, choline plays an important role in functions such as movement, coordination, and muscle stimulation and contraction. It is also important for other brain functions including thought, memory, and intellect.

In terms of cancer prevention, choline is a source of methyl in the body, a substance that is vital for copying the deoxyribonucleic acid (DNA) and ribonucleic acid (RNA) that make up the genetic material in every cell. It has been suggested that a diet with a low choline content may cause an error in the copying of DNA and RNA, leading to damaged genes and perhaps the growth of cancer.

HOW TO TAKE IT

Choline may be obtained from food or through supplementation. For pregnant women, dietary sources of choline (see below) are preferred over nutritional supplements.

Choline is available in capsule or tablet form. Choline is also an ingredient is some infant formulas. Studies of choline have used dosages ranging from 1 to 30 grams daily. This range in dosage simply reflects the various forms in which choline is available and the different amount of active ingredient in each product.

How much choline you need every day will depend on your age, gender, and condition. See the table below for the recommended daily intakes (RDIs) of choline.

AGE/GENDER/CONDITION	RECOMMENDED DAILY INTAKE (RDI)*
Infants	
0–6 months	125 mg
7–12 months	150 mg
Children	
1–3 years	200 mg
4–8 years	250 mg
9–13 years	375 mg
Males	
14 years and older	550 mg
Females	
14–18 years	400 mg
19 years and older	425 mg
	(continued)

AGE/GENDER/ CONDITION	RECOMMENDED DAILY INTAKE (RDI)* (continued)
Pregnant Women	450 mg
Nursing Women	550 mg

For more information on RDIs, see Want to Know More About Intake? on page 8.

The safe upper limit for choline is 3.5 grams per day for adults. There have been no maximum safe dosages set for young children, pregnant or nursing women, or people with severe liver or kidney disease.

LOOK OUT FOR THIS!

Choline supplementation is generally considered safe. Few side effects occur when choline supplements are taken in daily doses of up to 3 grams, although occasionally nausea or diarrhea may occur. At higher doses (around 5 grams), some people have reported a "fishy body odor" as well as excessive sweating, hypotension (low blood pressure and lightheadedness), and depression. To avoid the fishy odor, switch to phosphytidylcholine.

WHAT TO AVOID

There are no known interactions of choline with other drugs, herbs, or supplements.

CHONDROITIN

IMPLY PUT, THE SUBSTANCE that makes the cartilage in your joints resilient is chondroitin, more properly known as chondroitin sulfate. It's one of the basic building blocks of most connective tissue, and it plays an important role in keeping joints supple and healthy. Thus, it would seem only logical that one way to treat diseases such as osteoarthritis, which damages cartilage or makes it less resilient, would be to take a chondroitin supplement. Until recently, however, many researchers contended that when taken orally, chondroitin was too large a substance to be absorbed through the digestive tract, and that supplements of it were therefore basically worthless. However, the latest studies indicate that the body can indeed absorb chondroitin taken as supplements and that it really does work to help treat the pain and inflammation of worn and damaged joints—and may even keep osteoarthritis from getting worse.

WHAT IT DOES

Chondroitin supplements help relieve the pain and joint stiffness associated with osteoarthritis. In one study, test subjects taking chondroitin were able to increase their walking speed by as much as 50 percent over the course of the study. Other studies have indicated that chondroitin may help prevent further damage to the knee joint in patients with osteoarthritis. The evidence is mounting that chondroitin may actually slow or even stop the progression of osteoarthritis, in addition to reducing the pain and inflammation that accompany it. A recent study in the *New England Journal of Medicine* (the GAIT trial) found that people with moderate to severe knee arthritis benefited most from chondroitin.

Chondroitin is often also recommended for other ailments, such as tendonitis, sprains and strains, and carpal tunnel syndrome, because of its ability to heal tissue and reduce pain and swelling.

There is some evidence that chondroitin may also help patients with atherosclerosis, lower blood levels of cholesterol, and protect against blood clotting, but studies of these effects are so far are inconclusive.

For additional information on specific health conditions and how you can treat them with supplements, see Part 3 of this book, beginning on page 309.

Not All Chondroitin Is Created Equal

Did You Know?

There's a bewildering array of chondroitin supplements on the market and choosing the wrong supplement may mean decreased absorption and less effectiveness of chondroitin. You may want a supplement in which chondroitin is combined with glucosamine, although studies are inconclusive as to whether this will increase the benefit. But you should know that a study has shown that many supplements don't pack the amount of chondroitin they advertise on the box, and some may have virtually no chondroitin at all!

Look for a brand of chondroitin that has undergone independently performed quality control tests, called "assays." Also, because varieties of chondroitin with a lower molecular weight are likely to be more fully absorbed, choose products with smaller molecules (less than 16,900 daltons).

HOW IT WORKS

There are several theories about how chondroitin works. It may work by resupplying connective tissue with the "building-block" material of this tissue, thus enabling cartilage to repair itself. Other evidence suggests that chondroitin blocks the action of enzymes that damage cartilage, thereby reducing cartilage damage and slowing the progression of osteoarthritis. And chemical analysis indicates that chondroitin may stimulate the production of hyaluronic acid, a substance that lubricates joints and helps maintain their mobility.

HOW TO TAKE IT

Since the only dietary source of chondroitin is animal cartilage—otherwise known as gristle—you're unlikely to get much from the foods you eat. Many oral chondroitin supplements come in combination with glucosamine, which is thought to have similar beneficial effects in osteoarthritis, and the two agents may enhance each other's effects. Methylsulfonylmethane (MSM) is also often added to this supplement. Very few studies have been performed on MSM, but at least one recent study suggested that it might be effective for osteoarthritis pain in the knee.

The typically recommended dosage is 1,200 milligrams a day with meals, and although some suppliers suggest taking this divided into either two or three separate doses, there is no evidence that taking it all at once is any less effective. Don't expect results right away: You probably won't feel the benefits of chondroitin until you've been taking it daily for 2 to 4 months.

LOOK OUT FOR THIS!

Chondroitin appears to have no serious side effects. Minor side effects include such gastrointestinal complaints as heartburn and mild nausea.

Unless your doctor advises you, don't take chondroitin if you have hemophilia or other bleeding problems, or if you're about to go into labor or have surgery, because of its possible anticoagulant effects.

Because the long-term safety of chondroitin has not been studied, children and pregnant or nursing women should not take this supplement unless advised to do so by a doctor.

Medication: Although studies are inconclusive about whether chondroitin has an anticoagulant effect, it's best to avoid combining it with blood-thinning medications such as aspirin or warfarin, unless specifically instructed by your doctor.

Herbs and Dietary Supplements: The weight-loss supplement chitosan may interact with chondroitin in a manner that decreases chondroitin's absorption.

CHROMIUM

CHROMIUM IS A HEAVY METAL, one of the basic elements found in nature, and it is used to make steel alloys and in the plating of other metals, which is what gives them a "chrome" finish. In trace amounts, however, chromium is also essential to human health, contributing to proper growth and helping the body metabolize food. Some estimates indicate that as many as 90 percent of Americans get less than the recommended amount of chromium from dietary sources, and chromium deficiency is known to affect the elderly, people with poor diets or a high intake of sugar in their diets, people who exercise a great deal, and those who are chronically under stress.

WHAT IT DOES

Chromium's role in helping the body to metabolize food is responsible for its potential benefit in the treatment of diabetes. Because chromium helps insulin to increase the uptake of glucose into cells, it can lower blood sugar levels and help to treat or prevent the condition known as insulin resistance (see Diabetes, page 410); chromium also appears to reduce the amount of insulin needed by people with diabetes.

Chromium has also been shown to improve cholesterol levels, particularly in people with high cholesterol. One study found that in men taking beta-blocker drugs, chromium supplements helped raise HDL ("good") cholesterol levels, and in people with obesity or diabetes, chromium has been shown to lower triglyceride levels by as much as 20 percent.

Although some claims that chromium is a "fat burning" substance are unjustified, it does appear to alter the breakdown of fats

FOOD SOURCES

CHROMIUM

There's a lengthy list of food sources for chromium, but the best sources are foods that most people don't eat, namely brewer's yeast and calf's liver. Read on for other high-chromium foods.

▶ Beer, black pepper, bran cereal, cheese, coffee, lean meat, molasses, thyme, and whole-grain bread and cereal.

and may thus help reduce weight, particularly in obese people. A recent study suggests that chromium may help reduce carbohydrate cravings in people who are depressed.

Because insulin resistance and elevated blood sugar levels have been associated with heart disease, the ability of chromium to regulate insulin and blood sugar may help prevent heart disease. One study found that taking chromium supplements reduced the risk of heart attack. Preliminary observations have also shown that chromium may improve mood in people who are taking the antidepressant medication setraline (Zoloft) for dysthymic disorder, a type of depression. More research is needed to explore chromium's effects in these areas.

For additional information on specific health conditions and how you can treat them with supplements, see Part 3 of this book, beginning on page 309.

HOW IT WORKS

Researchers are still investigating precisely how chromium helps regulate blood sugar and insulin levels. Scientists refer to chromium as a "cofactor" of insulin, which means that it serves as a kind of key to the cell membrane, unlocking it so that insulin can carry glucose from the bloodstream into the cell. Researchers theorize that chromium may increase the number of insulin receptors in cells, in essence making cells more sensitive to insulin—the opposite of what insulin resistance does. Chromium may also keep the liver from extracting too much insulin from the bloodstream.

People with a high sugar intake may have a deficiency in chromium, because sugar increases the amount of chromium in the bloodstream and subsequently, increases its excretion in the urine.

HOW TO TAKE IT

See the table below for the adequate daily intakes (AIs) of chromium.

AGE/GENDER/ CONDITION	ADEQUATE DAILY INTAKE (AI)*
Infants	
0–6 months	0.2 mcg
7–12 months	5.5 mcg

AGE/GENDER/ CONDITION	RECOMMENDED DAILY INTAKE (RDI)*
Children	
1–3 years	11 mcg
4–8 years	15 mcg
Males	
9–13 years	25 mcg
14–18 years	35 mcg
19–50 years	35 mcg
51 years and older	30 mcg
Females	
9–13 years	21 mcg
14–18 years	24 mcg
19–50 years	25 mcg
51 years and older	20 mcg
Pregnant Women	
14–18 years	29 mcg
19 and older	30 mcg
Nursing Women	
14–18 years	44 mcg
19 and older	30 mcg

For more information on AIs, see Want to Know More About Intake? on page 8.

Therapeutic doses of chromium range from 200 to 1,000 micrograms (mcg) a day, with the higher amount recommended for patients with type 2 diabetes (but be sure to consult your doctor). Chromium is available in tablet and capsule form and can be taken from one to three times a day. Note that the long-term safety of high doses of chromium is unknown. See Look Out for This! on page 80.

Chromium obtained from brewer's yeast is believed to be one of the forms of chromium best absorbed by the body. Look for high-chromium brewer's yeast, often available in powder, tablet, or capsule form. High-quality brewer's yeast powder contains up to 60 micrograms of chromium in every tablespoon. Chromium picolinate is also thought to be well absorbed.

LOOK OUT FOR THIS!

Because industrial chromium is a heavy metal, some researchers have expressed concern that in general, chromium might build up to toxic levels in the body if taken in too large an amount or for an extended period of time. However, the form found in food and supplements do not have any clearly demonstrated toxic effects. Several anecdotal reports indicate that excessive amounts of chromium may cause kidney or liver damage or anemia, but animal studies have not confirmed these findings.

Recommended doses appear safe, but high doses of chromium may interfere with the effectiveness of insulin and have caused stomach irritation, itching, and flushing.

WHAT TO AVOID

Medication: Because chromium may enhance the effectiveness of a wide variety of diabetes medications, you may be able to reduce your diabetes medication if you're also taking chromium, but be sure to consult your doctor before you begin taking it. Aspirin and nonsteroidal anti-inflammatory drugs (NSAIDs) may increase the absorption of chromium; antacids (such as Tums and Maalox) may decrease the absorption of chromium.

COENZYME Q10

UBIQUINONE, ANOTHER NAME for coenzyme Q10 (CoQ10), comes from the word "ubiquitous," meaning "everywhere"—a fitting moniker since CoQ10 is found in every single cell of the body. However, the amount of CoQ10 produced in the body decreases with age and with the development of certain diseases such as heart disease, Parkinson's disease, and asthma. Scientists have been studying CoQ10 for many years—the Japanese first discovered its benefits for treating heart conditions in the 1960s. Since then, it has been widely used in Europe, Israel, and Japan. In fact, CoQ10 has become one of the most popular dietary supplements available today.

WHAT IT DOES

Many studies have been conducted on the health effects of CoQ10 supplementation, often reaching conflicting results. The best evidence for a benefit of supplemental CoQ10 is its ability to significantly reduce symptoms of congestive heart failure. CoQ10 is also useful in managing high blood pressure, easing angina, and warding off coronary artery disease, and it may speed recovery time after coronary artery bypass surgery. Trials have also shown that taking CoQ10 after having a stroke helps alleviate symptoms and may prevent the recurrence of strokes. Other studies suggest that CoQ10 taken prior to elective heart surgery may be useful. One important recent study suggests that C0Q10, taken in combination with acetyl-n-carnitine, and omega-3 fatty acids may be useful in the treatment of macular degeneration. Another recent study found that CoQ10 could help prevent migraines.

CoQ10 is sometimes recommended to treat male infertility because it may increase sperm count and sperm movement. Many naturopathic doctors recommend taking CoQ10 for treating breast cancer, and preliminary studies show that this enzyme may also have a beneficial effect against prostate tumors.

Other studies show that CoQ10 may be effective in tempering symptoms of fibromyalgia and gum disease. Research suggests that CoQ10 may also be useful in Parkinson's disease, diabetes, bronchitis, and emphysema.

Preliminary research suggests that CoQ10 may help strengthen the immune system and improve exercise endurance, although more studies are needed to substantiate these potential benefits.

CoQ10 may also help protect against the side effects of certain prescription medications including certain psychiatric drugs, blood-pressure-lowering medicatations, and statin-cholesterol lowering drugs. These medications deplete the body's store of CoQ10.

For additional information on specific health conditions and how you can treat them with supplements, see Part 3 of this book, beginning on page 309.

HOW IT WORKS

Experts believe that CoQ10 works by improving the production of energy in cells, especially cells that require significant amounts of energy, such as those located in the heart. CoQ10 is also a powerful antioxidant, meaning that it can reduce the effect of the free radical molecules that damage cells in the body.

FRIENDS AND FOES

Taking **vitamin E** along with **CoQ10** may be a smart move. Studies have shown that these two substances can work together to achieve greater benefits.

HOW TO TAKE IT

It is important to know that CoQ10 should never be taken in place of any regular medication, but rather in addition to it, when appropriate. In fact, many studies have shown that CoQ10, when taken in conjunction with standard prescription medications such as drugs for high blood pressure, may allow in time a reduction in the dosage of prescription medications and even their elimination under a doctor's supervision.

In most studies, the usual dose of CoQ10 ranges from 30 to 300 milligrams each day, often divided into two or three doses. However, some studies have used even higher doses, suggesting that dosages as high as 1,200 milligrams a day may have positive effects.

CoQ10 is available in softgel capsules, wafers, tablets, and powder-filled capsules. Since CoQ10 is fat-soluble (requiring fat to be absorbed by the body), an oil-based softgel form may improve its absorption over a dry form such as tablets. Absorption of CoQ10 supplements also improves when they are taken with food.

LOOK OUT FOR THIS!

No serious side effects have been reported with CoQ10 supplementation, although some people taking high doses of this enzyme (more than 200 milligrams per day) have experienced nausea, heartburn, diarrhea, abdominal pain, headache, and dizziness.

CoQ10 appears to be a safe supplement. However, pregnant and nursing women should avoid taking CoQ10 supplements since no long-term studies have assessed its safety for them. Additionally, people with severe illnesses such as cancer and kidney failure should not use CoQ10 unless advised to do so by their doctor.

WHAT TO AVOID

Medication: CoQ10 may reduce the effectiveness of the blood-thinning drug warfarin. If you are taking warfarin, be sure to speak to your doctor before taking CoQ10. Statin drugs such as lovastatin, prescribed to reduce cholesterol levels, lower the levels of CoQ10 in the body.

CONJUGATED LINOLEIC ACID

LINOLEIC ACID IS ONE OF THE ESSENTIAL fatty acids that the body does not produce but does require in order to help regulate blood clotting, blood pressure, heart rate, and immune response. By slightly changing its molecular structure, linoleic acid becomes "conjugated linoleic acid" or CLA. CLA is an unsaturated, omega-6 fatty acid, found primarily in beef, lamb, dairy products, poultry, and eggs. CLA is also found in vegetable oils. Most CLA supplements are made from safflower or sunflower oils.

WHAT IT DOES

Athletes have long used CLA to improve strength and body composition by increasing the ratio of lean mass to fat in the body. But while CLA may help burn fat, build muscle, and boost calorie consumption, most of the studies in which it has shown such effects have been conducted on animals. The results of human studies of CLA have been mixed. In one study of already lean weightlifters (with 14 percent body fat), CLA supplements had no significant effect on overall weight or fat mass. However, in small studies, CLA did help obese men to lose an inch of abdominal fat and some overall weight. Nevertheless, the amount of weight lost (2 to 4 pounds over a 12-week period) was not enough to reduce the health risks associated with obesity.

Some exciting new animal and laboratory research with CLA shows that it may have use against cancer, cardiovascular disease, atherosclerosis, food allergies, high cholesterol, and high triglycerides (another type of fat in the blood), but more human studies are needed to confirm these benefits. CLA may also be useful in reducing the risk of breast, prostate, colorectal, lung, skin, and stomach cancer. Studies that have examined the role of CLA supplements on the immune system have documented minimal effect.

For people with obesity, CLA may be a relatively safe, nonstimulant supplement that improves body composition slightly and boosts thermogenesis—the rate at which the body burns calories—although both animal and human studies report conflicting results.

For additional information on specific health conditions and how you can treat them with supplements, see Part 3 of this book, beginning on page 309.

HOW IT WORKS

In theory, CLA increases the body's production of prostaglandins and growth hormone, which in turn builds muscle, boosts blood circulation to both muscle and fat tissue, and mobilizes body fat to be burned. In animal studies, CLA has reduced LDL ("bad") cholesterol and triglyceride levels, reduced glucose intolerance, and slowed the growth of various cancers.

HOW TO TAKE IT

CLA is available in capsule and liquid form. The daily requirement of CLA is unknown, but in the few human studies conducted on CLA, doses typically ranged from 2 to 5 grams of CLA daily. This makes choosing a reputable brand critical, since these relatively high doses of CLA carry the risk of ingesting high levels of potentially toxic contaminants along with it. Most researchers chose the brand of CLA called TonalinTM for their studies.

LOOK OUT FOR THIS!

CLA is generally safe, although some people experience heartburn or nausea at doses of 2 grams a day or more. The safety of CLA supplements is still unknown, and they are not recommended for children or for women who are pregnant or nursing. It may be necessary to take CLA for up to 2 years to see results with decreasing body fat.

Anyone with cardiovascular disease or obesity should consult their doctor before taking CLA supplements. People with liver disease, type 2 diabetes, or insulin resistence should not take CLA.

WHAT TO AVOID

There are no known interactions of CLA with other supplements, herbs, or prescription drugs.

COPPER

or some people, copper is more often associated with electrical wiring, pipes, pennies, and the Statue of Liberty than it is with the human body. However, this essential trace mineral serves some very important purposes in the body. The importance of copper was first discovered in Peru, where a group of malnourished children with anemia did not respond to iron supplementation but did respond to copper supplementation. Not only can a deficiency in copper cause anemia, but this mineral plays an integral role in bone strength, brain development, immune function, iron transport, and the health of developing infants.

WHAT IT DOES

Copper is often recommended for people taking high doses of zinc, iron, or vitamin C, since these minerals and this vitamin may reduce copper levels in the body. Injections of copper are used to treat a condition known as Menke's disease, in which the body cannot properly regulate the metabolism of copper, causing it to accumulate in low levels in the liver and brain and in high levels in the kidney and intestines.

Most of the evidence for the therapeutic benefit of copper supplements is experimental but compelling. Some studies suggest that copper deficiency may contribute to the development and progression of osteoporosis. Thus, supplemental copper may be beneficial for the treatment of osteoporosis.

Since a deficiency in copper has been shown to lead to cardiovascular disease, some experts believe that copper may also be useful in preventing and treating heart disease in people who have even slight deficiencies of this mineral. Preliminary studies show that copper may reduce hardening of the arteries caused by high cholesterol. More research is needed to examine copper's role in cardiovascular health.

Copper has been suggested as a treatment for both osteoarthritis and rheumatoid arthritis, since these conditions involve a copper deficiency. Copper may increase the growth of cells that make cartilage in the joints.

For additional information on specific health conditions and how you can treat them with supplements, see Part 3 of this book, beginning on page 309.

HOW IT WORKS

While only small amounts are needed in the body, copper supports many important biological functions. Copper aids in the production of red blood cells, nerve fibers, collagen (a main component of bones, skin, joints, and ligaments), and melanin (a pigment in the

FOOD FACTORS

COPPER

A little bit of copper goes a long way. Since the body requires only small amounts of copper, eating a diet with foods containing copper is the healthiest way to maintain needed levels of this mineral. Cooking foods in copper cookware will also increase your copper intake. Read on for more copper-containing foods.

▶Beef, black pepper, blackstrap molasses, cashews, clams, crab, green leafy vegetables, kidneys, lentils, liver, lobster, mussels, nuts, oysters, pistachios, shellfish, soybeans, squid, unsweetened baker's chocolate, and whole grains.

hair and skin), and it promotes bone growth, as well as the body's ability to use sugar.

Interestingly, copper works both as an antioxidant, in that it neutralizes the cell- and tissue-damaging molecules known as free radicals, and as a pro-oxidant, in that it promotes damage by free radicals and may contribute to conditions such as Alzheimer's disease.

HOW TO TAKE IT

Although copper is an important element in many biochemical processes, it can be very toxic when taken at high levels. See the table below for the recommended daily intakes (RDIs) of copper.

AGE/CONDITION	RECOMMENDED DAILY INTAKE (RDI)*
Infants	
0–6 months	200 mcg
7–12 months	220 mcg
Children	
1–3 years	340 mcg
4–8 years	440 mcg
14–18 years	890 mcg
9–13 years	700 mcg
Males and Females	
19 years and older	900 mcg
Pregnant Women	1,000 mcg
Nursing Women	1,300 mcg

For more information on RDIs, see Want to Know More About Intake? on page 8.

A slight deficiency in copper is very common among Americans, since most only get 50 percent of their copper from their diet. Symptoms of copper deficiency include a loss in hair and skin color, kinky-textured hair, anemia, fatigue, low body temperature, cardiovascular problems, and a reduced resistance to infection.

Copper supplements are available in tablet form. Most general-purpose multivitamin and mineral supplements contain copper (be sure to check the label). However, studies suggest that cupric oxide—a type of copper commonly found in multivitamin/mineral supplements—may be poorly absorbed by the body. As a result, other forms of copper, including copper sulfate, cupric acetate, and alkaline copper carbonate, may be preferable to cupric oxide.

Copper supplements should be taken 2 to 3 hours apart from iron and vitamin C so that they don't interfere with the absorption of these latter two nutrients. High doses of zinc can cause a copper deficiency. If you are taking high doses of zinc for a prolonged period of time, consult your doctor about whether you may need additional copper supplementation.

Human immunodeficiency virus (HIV) medications may deplete levels of copper in the body. Ask your doctor about copper supplementation if you are taking HIV medication.

LOOK OUT FOR THIS!

Copper can be toxic when taken in high doses. See the table below for the maximum safe dosages of copper.

AGE/CONDITION	MAXIMUM SAFE DOSAGE
Children	
1–3 years	1,000 mcg
4–8 years	3,000 mcg
9–13 years	5,000 mcg
14–18 years	8,000 mcg
Males and Females	
19 years and older	10,000 mcg
Pregnant or Nursing Women	10,000 mcg

Maximum safe dosages of copper have not been established for people with liver or kidney disease. Side effects of copper include nausea and vomiting, diarrhea, and stomach pain.

Copper supplements should not be taken by people with Wilson's disease, a condition in which the body accumulates high levels of copper.

People who are taking high doses of iron, zinc, or vitamin C should wait 2 hours before taking copper supplements.

SUPPLEMENTAL TRIVIA

In the 1990s, athletes from China—never known before for its prowess in either aquatic or track and field events—set several world records in running and swimming. Chinese women runners won gold medals in the 1,500, 3,000, and 10,000 meter races at one world championship and, in a later race, shaved a remarkable 42 seconds off the previous world record for 10,000 meters. *Their secret?* According to their coach, the entire team was on a supplement regimen that included cordyceps as one of its ingredients. Drug tests proved negative for any banned performance-enhancing substances, and the Chinese athletes' records were ratified as valid by an international athletic federation.

WHAT TO AVOID

Medication: People taking penicillamine and trientine should consult their doctor before taking copper supplements, since copper may interfere with the absorption of these medications, and they may interfere with the absorption of copper.

CORDYCEPS

IT GROWS IN THE MOST BIZARRE OF PLACES, and some of the claims about its beneficial effects seem at first to be equally extraordinary. But scientific research indicates that the Chinese mushroom cordyceps *(Cordyceps sinesis)*—which sprouts from the head of a rare Tibetan caterpillar—does indeed have several verifiable therapeutic benefits. Extracts of cordyceps are now grown on soybeans and other nutrient sources. Research has demonstrated that cordyceps may relieve such lung conditions as asthma, boost libido, and perhaps even improve athletic performance. Test results also suggest that it may have positive effects on liver and kidney function, may benefit the cardiovascular and immune systems, and may even help to fight cancer.

WHAT IT DOES

Cordyceps appears to have a wide variety of biological and pharmacological effects. Studies show that it improves the ability of the lungs to use oxygen, and clinical trials indicate that, particularly in the elderly, it reduces fatigue while improving memory and cognitive ability and increasing the sex drive. Its ability to reduce fatigue and boost energy levels suggests that it may indeed improve athletic performance.

Cordyceps also seems to improve liver and kidney function. It has been shown to stimulate metabolism in the liver, have therapeutic effects in patients with chronic hepatitis B, help patients with cirrhosis of the liver, and have several beneficial effects on the functioning of the kidneys.

The immune system also appears to benefit from supplements containing cordyceps. In particular, cordyceps seems to boost the numbers of helper T cells, which are essential to several immune functions, while animal studies indicate that it can help suppress the autoimmune disease lupus.

With regard to the cardiovascular system, studies of cordyceps suggest that it may lower blood pressure and reduce the risk of dangerous blood clotting. It has also been shown to help counteract irregular heartbeat and reduce heart rate. Perhaps most exciting of all is evidence that cordyceps can inhibit the growth of several types of cancer cells; one study showed that it inhibited the spreading of lung cancer to the liver, and another study demonstrated that it helped to stop the growth of melanoma, a type of cancer of the skin. More studies are needed to test the efficacy of cordyceps on these conditions.

For additional information on specific health conditions and how to treat them with supplements, see Part 3 of this book, beginning on page 309.

HOW IT WORKS

Scientists have identified two chemical compounds in cordyceps—deoxyadenosine and mannitol—that may account for its effects on lung function, energy levels, and sex drive. In addition, animal studies indicate that cordyceps increases the ratio of adenosine triphosphate to inorganic phosphate in the liver, an action that may improve the body's ability to produce energy.

Other studies have found that cordyceps may increase the body's uptake of oxygen, as well as raising the body's anaerobic threshold—the level at which muscles need more oxygen to keep functioning. Both of these effects could account for improved athletic performance and resistance to fatigue.

Animal studies suggest that cordyceps stimulates the production of hormones by the adrenal glands, releasing natural steroids into the

Odd Ingredients Used in Traditional Chinese Medicine

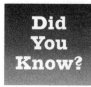

Did You Know?

In traditional Chinese medicine, the name for cordyceps means "winter bug, summer herb." The fungus and the carcass of the insect larva it was grown on are often used together as an herb.

Chinese medicine is based upon the principles of the yin and the yang in which the yin is often associated with cold, dark, passive, and wet, and the yang is often associated with hot, bright, active, and dry. In traditional Chinese medicine, yin and yang tonics are often used to provide adequate balance between a person's yin and yang. Cordyceps is considered a "yang tonic," used for drying, warming, and invigorating the yang.

Other unusual yang tonics used in traditional Chinese medicine include such seemingly odd ingredients as gecko (a male and female pair are used), the velvet of the young deer antler, and the infamous "yin yang hou," also known as "licentious goat wort" or "horney goat weed." Other ingredients used are the sexual organs of a male seal, stalactite tips, seahorses, and sea slugs (sea cucumbers). Keep in mind, you will not find these ingredients in your local health food store!

body. This may account for the effect of cordyceps on libido, although a direct connection has yet to be proven.

The cardiovascular effects of cordyceps may be attributed to a protein constituent of this mushroom that helps relax blood vessels, and which may also have an antioxidant effect, scavenging the free radical molecules that damage cells in the body.

HOW TO TAKE IT

Cordyceps is available as a dietary supplement in capsule form. The typical dosage recommendation is from 4 to 15 grams daily.

Practitioners of traditional Chinese medicine typically prescribe cordyceps in conjunction with other herbs that also target specific conditions and work synergistically.

LOOK OUT FOR THIS!

The safety of cordyceps in pregnant or breastfeeding women and children is not known.

WHAT TO AVOID

More study is needed to determine whether and how cordyceps interacts with other drugs, herbs, and supplements, although studies suggest that cordyceps may have blood-thinning effects. Consult your doctor before taking cordyceps if you are taking any blood-thinning medications or herbs.

CRANBERRY

Did you know that the delicious cranberry sauce you eat on Thanksgiving is chock full of health benefits? The Pilgrims had the right idea—they learned about the usefulness of cranberries *(Vaccinium macrocarpon)* from local Indian tribes and adopted the berries as their own, using them to make poultices and dyes. Today, many women can attest that drinking cranberry juice is their first line of defense in preventing urinary tract infections.

WHAT IT DOES

Cranberries are best known for their effectiveness in preventing urinary tract infections. However, they may also be useful for men with prostatitis (an inflammation of the prostate) caused by recurrent urinary tract infection.

Because of its ability to block bacteria from clinging to the bladder wall in urinary tract infections, researchers have speculated that cranberry may prevent *Helicobacter pylori*—the bacteria that cause ulcers—from adhering to the stomach wall, and a recent controlled study confirmed this.

Because of their tart flavor, cranberries may be effective in stimulating taste buds in people with a loss of appetite.

Preliminary research suggests that cranberries may also prevent plaque from developing on the teeth and gum disease. Cranberries are also loaded with antioxidants and may thus help prevent cancer (see Did You Know? below), heart disease, and stroke. Cranberry may also inhibit the growth of urinary tract bacteria that have been implicated in the cause of rheumatoid arthritis.

Cranberry will also increase vitamin B_{12} in people who take proton-pump inhibitors such as omeprazole.

For additional information on specific health conditions and how to treat them with supplements, see Part 3 of this book, beginning on page 309.

HOW IT WORKS

Most of cranberry's medicinal powers come from anti-adhesive properties that can prevent harmful bacteria from adhering to various part of the body. While early studies credited the acidic content of cranberries with preventing urinary tract infections, modern studies show that it is these anti-adhesive properties of cranberries that prevent infectious bacteria from collecting on the bladder wall. A compound in cranberries called proanthocyanidin has been found to prevent bacterial infection.

Cranberry May Have Tumor-Fighting Properties

Did You Know?

In a preliminary study at the University of Massachusetts, reported in the *Journal of Agricultural and Food Chemistry,* researchers observed that an extract of whole cranberry may be able to stunt the growth of tumor cells. Two compounds were identified as successful agents in inhibiting such tumor-cell growth, which specifically involved breast, prostate, lung, cervical, and leukemia cells grown in the laboratory. Researchers observed that cranberry was strongest in its effect against breast tumor cells, whose growth it inhibited by 50 percent. The evidence suggests that the tumor-fighting activity of cranberry stems from its anti-inflammatory properties, and further research on this is planned. Look for further studies on the anti-inflammatory and tumor-fighting properties of cranberries.

A study reported in the *Journal of the American Dental Association* found that cranberries also contain a unique substance—known as a high-molecular-weight nondialysable material (NDM)—that may be able to reverse and inhibit the growth of plaque and gum-disease-causing oral bacteria on the teeth and gums.

HOW TO TAKE IT

Cranberries may be purchased fresh and then cooked at home. Sweeten them to your taste with the natural sweetener Stevia; the unsweetened berries may be a bit too tart for most taste buds. Cranberry juice is a more convenient option than fresh berries, although most cranberry juice cocktails sold in grocery stores contain high quantities of sugar, which may reduce some of the positive health effects of the cranberry. Look for 100 percent juice blends, such as cranberry-grape (also rich in antioxidants) or apple-cranberry, or choose unsweetened cranberry juice.

Canned cranberry sauce is another option, although it too contains large amounts of sugar; you may benefit by making a homemade cranberry sauce, since this will let you have more control over the sugar content of the sauce.

Cranberry is also available in capsule and tea form. Usual doses of cranberry in capsule form range from 300 to 500 milligrams of a cranberry juice concentrate, taken two to three times daily.

LOOK OUT FOR THIS!

Cranberry in is an extremely safe supplement, with no known side effects. However, if taken in extremely large quantities (3 to 4 liters

Grow This!

You may be surprised to discover that you can grow cranberries in your own backyard. New varieties of cranberry don't require the bog conditions most people associate with the growing of cranberries. Moreover, since cranberries can be stored in the refrigerator for up to 2 months, you can store the fruit you grow as it ripens in the summer.

■ **Light:** Full sun

■ **Temperature:** Cranberry plants cannot stand temperatures of 30° F or less.

■ **Water:** Water cranberries as you would any other garden plant. Contrary to popular belief, they do not like to be saturated. The soil should be moist to the touch, but not saturated.

Cranberries thrive in acidic soil. If your soil is acidic enough to grow blueberries, azaleas, and rhododendrons, it's perfect for the new cranberry varieties. Otherwise, you can make your soil more acidic by incorporating peat in your soil, watering with a vinegar-water mixture (2 tablespoons of vinegar to 1 gallon of water), or adding elemental sulfur according to package directions. Keep cranberry plants evenly moist in mulch with peat compost or shredded leaf mulch. Look for these varieties in nursery catalogs that specialize in fruit.

per day), cranberry juice may cause diarrhea or other gastrointestinal problems.

People with kidney stones should be cautious when taking cranberry supplements, since the berry contains the compounds known as oxalates which can produce kidney stones; if taken in moderation, however, cranberries may help reduce the risk of kidney stones.

People with diabetes or glucose intolerance should make sure they purchase sugar-free forms of cranberry juice.

WHAT TO AVOID

There are no known interactions of cranberry when taken with other drugs, herbs, or supplements.

CREATINE

CREATINE IS AN AMINO ACID made in the body and which plays a key role in generating energy at the cellular level. The body converts creatine into a substance called phosphocreatine, which stores energy for use by the muscles. Most people's bodies make adequate amounts of creatine naturally. The popularity of creatine as a supplement is due to its potentially beneficial effects in bodybuilding. This does not hold true, however, for lower intensity, repetitive endurance activities like cycling and running. Of all the myriad sports supplements on the market, creatine is the one with the most scientific credibility.

Creatine is especially helpful for high-intensity physical activities that require short bursts of energy such as weightlifting, football, soccer, basketball, jumping, and sprinting. Taking creatine may also help with other athletic activities; it can improve training with weights, which itself enhances overall athletic performance.

WHAT IT DOES

The best evidence for creatine in exercise shows that this nonessential amino acid may enhance performance in athletic activities that require repeated, short bursts of high-intensity activity such as basketball.

Studies indicate that creatine may also help maintain muscle mass and prevent the wasting of muscle strength that occurs with old age, conditions such as acquired immune deficiency syndrome (AIDS),

---

RESTORATIVE RECIPES

HOMEMADE CRANBERRY SAUCE

Next Thanksgiving, give your family a healthy and delicious alternative to store-bought cranberry sauce. This homemade sauce is sugar-free, packed with the healing properties of cranberries, and very easy to make.

Ingredients
4 cups fresh cranberries
3/4 cup apple juice
2 ripe pears, cored and sliced
1 cup raisins
1 teaspoon liquid stevia (an all natural sweetener)

Directions: Combine all the ingredients in a medium-size, heavy saucepan and bring the mixture to a boil over medium heat. Reduce the heat to low, cover, and simmer for 10 minutes, stirring occasionally. Chill the sauce completely before serving.

the degeneration of muscle that takes place when a limb is injured, congestive heart failure, illnesses that affect the energy-producing mitrochondria in cells, and muscular dystrophy; some studies have found that creatine improves strength and the ability to perform daily activities in people with muscular dystrophy.

Although evidence once suggested that creatine had the potential to slow the progression of amyotrophic lateral sclerosis (ALS)—also known as Lou Gehrig's disease—as well as promote strength in people with ALS, a study done in 2003 found that supplementation with creatine had no positive effects on people with this condition.

Preliminary evidence suggested that creatine may reduce weight by lowering the proportion of body-fat to muscle; however, there is little subsequent evidence to support this. Preliminary evidence also suggests that creatine may reduce triglyceride levels in the blood, but more research into this possibility is needed. Studies suggest that creatine may be useful in the treatment of congestive heart failure. Researchers are presently examining the role of creatine in the treatment of Parkinson's disease.

For additional information on specific health conditions and how you can treat them with supplements, see Part 3 of this book, beginning on page 309.

HOW IT WORKS

Creatine provides energy for muscles by bonding with the substance known as phosphate in muscle tissue to produce a substance called phosophocreatine. This then transfers its phosphate to another substance, known as adenosine diphophate, to create adenosine triphosphate, which fuels muscle activity and helps boost performance.

Creatine also seems to transfer water from other body tissues to muscle tissue, making muscles larger. It is still unclear whether the muscles simply become bigger from swelling with water, or actually add new muscle tissue, which would be preferable.

HOW TO TAKE IT

Creatine comes in powder, liquid, effervescent tablet, and wafer form. Creatine in the form of creatine monohydrate may be best absorbed in the body and better tolerated in the stomach than other forms of this amino acid. You can also increase your dietary intake of creatine by eating wild game, lean red meat, and fish (including salmon and tuna).

For exercise enhancement, a typical dose of creatine is a starting dose of 15 to 30 grams daily for 3 to 4 days followed by a maintenance dose of 2 to 5 grams daily.

Be sure to drink 8 to 12 glasses of water daily while taking creatine. Because creatine causes the muscles to store water, the body needs extra water to prevent dehydration and cramping. Creatine seems to be absorbed better when taken with glucose, fructose, or a high-carbohydrate drink such as fruit juice.

Creatine may enhance the effects of other bodybuilding supplements, including whey and glutamine.

LOOK OUT FOR THIS!

Several athletic organizations, including the National Collegiate Athletic Association (NCAA), forbid their members from using creatine supplements. Many other organizations frown upon the use of creatine and other performance-enhancing drugs.

Some studies suggest that people taking pure creatine supplements may be at risk for kidney damage, in addition to an impaired ability to form creatine naturally. As a result, some doctors believe that the only safe way to take creatine is as part of a performance-enhancing regimen that includes other supplements, although more research is needed to test this theory.

There is also increasing disapproval of the commercial marketing of creatine supplements to teenagers, who may be vulnerable to misleading claims for this supplement. A study found that teenagers who take creatine often exceed the dosage indications for this supplement. Furthermore, the safety of creatine has not been tested in people under the age of 19 years.

When taken at recommended dosages, creatine is generally considered safe for adults, with few side effects. Occasional side effects may include muscle cramps, muscle tears, dehydration upset stomach, and diarrhea.

Individuals with kidney disorders, especially those who must undergo dialysis, and people at risk for dehydration should consult a doctor before taking creatine. People who are trying to lose weight should check with their healthcare provider before taking creatine, since it encourages water retention.

The long-term safety effects of creatine have not been studied. Children, teenagers, and pregnant or nursing women should not take creatine.

WHAT TO AVOID

Medication: Creatine, when taken in conjunction with cimetidine, diuretics, probenecid, or nonsteroidal anti-inflammatory drugs (NSAIDs) such as ibuprofen, may increase the risk of kidney damage.

Food: Caffeine may inhibit the effects of creatine.

DANDELION

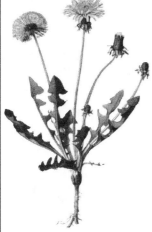

AS A CHILD, YOU MAY HAVE THOUGHT that dandelions *(Taraxacum officinale)* were magic—you probably remember blowing the tops off dandelions that had gone to seed and making a wish as the seeds dispersed into the air. As an adult, you may think of dandelion as an annoying weed that ruins the look of your front lawn, but dandelion is also considered an herb with many valuable medicinal uses. This yellow flower grows all over the Northern hemisphere, and the leaves can be harvested for their health potential throughout the flowering season. The dandelion was first mentioned for its medicinal properties by Arabian physicians in the tenth and eleventh centuries. Traditionally, the roots and leaves have been used to aid digestive and liver problems.

WHAT IT DOES

The leaves of the dandelion plant are loaded with nutrients, including vitamins A, C, D, and B-complex vitamins, as well as iron, magnesium, zinc, potassium, manganese, copper, choline, calcium, boron, and silicon. As a result, dandelion is often recommended for people who require additional nutrients. Lab studies indicate that dandelion root–infusion increases the growth of beneficial intestinal bacteria.

The roots of the dandelion plant are commonly used as an appetite stimulant, as an aid to digestion, and for the relief of mild constipation, while the leaves are used as a diuretic and may be helpful for reducing water retention. The German Commission E recommends dandelion for the treatment of gallstones.

Early laboratory studies suggest that dandelion may also have anti-inflammatory and antioxidant properties. In traditional herbal medicine, dandelion is used to treat eczema. Dried, roasted dandelion roots have even been used as a substitute for coffee, and parts of the root are used to make wines. Other preliminary studies suggest that dandelion may help regulate blood sugar. More research is needed to test these uses of dandelion.

For additional information on specific health conditions and how you can treat them with supplements, see Part 3 of this book, beginning on page 309.

HOW IT WORKS

As a diuretic, dandelion works to increase urine production by promoting the excretion of salts and water from the kidneys. It has an advantage over other diuretic substances because it's also a good source of potassium.

The active components in dandelion include eudesmanolide and germacranolide. Research has indicated that the dandelion ingredients taraxol, taraxerol, taraxasterol, stigmasterol, beta-sitosterol, caffeic acid, and p-hydroxyphenylacetic acid may also contribute to dandelion's therapeutic effects. More research is needed to determine exactly how these active components work therapeutically.

HOW TO TAKE IT

Dandelion herb and roots are available fresh or dried in a variety of forms, including tinctures, prepared teas, and capsules. Dandelion can be brewed into a tea, distilled into a wine, and even fermented and made into a beer. The roots are used to make a substitute for coffee. Young dandelion leaves add flavor to salads or can be sautéed with garlic.

A typical dosage of dandelion root infusion ranges from 2 to 8 grams taken three times daily; and a typical dosage of dandelion leaf infusion ranges from 4 to 10 grams taken three times daily. Dosages vary according to the form of dandelion taken, so be sure to read individual labels for specific dosage information.

A word of caution: Be careful with wild dandelion leaves and don't eat dandelion leaves found on the lawn, since they have probably been treated with pesticides and herbicides.

SUPPLEMENTAL TRIVIA

Dandelion takes its name from the leaves of certain varieties of this plant. If you stretch your imagination, the leaves look somewhat like the teeth of a lion, which in French would be *dent de lion*. The other name for dandelion is *pis-en-lit*, which is translated as "wet the bed." Dandelion leaves have diuretic properties, hence the name.

LOOK OUT FOR THIS!

Dandelion is generally considered safe, with few side effects. Some individuals may develop an allergic reaction from touching the plant, while others may develop mouth sores.

People with allergies to chamomile and yarrow should use dandelion carefully, since they may be at increased risk for an allergic reaction.

Individuals with gallbladder problems and gallstones should consult their doctor before taking dandelion.

Pregnant and breastfeeding women should consult their doctor before taking dandelion supplements.

WHAT TO AVOID

Medication: Consult your doctor before taking dandelion with lithium and quinolone-type antibiotics such as ciprofloxacin, since it may worsen the side effects of these drugs.

DEVIL'S CLAW

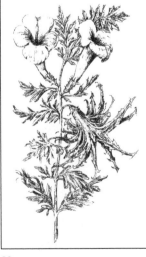

WHEN YOU SEE THE SMALL, anchor-like hooks that cover its fruit, you'll know why devil's claw *(Harpagophytum procumbens)* is sometimes referred to as the "grappling hook plant." The Khoisan people of the Kalahari Desert in southern Africa used this leafy perennial for thousands of years as a pain and fever remedy, digestive stimulant, and topically as a treatment for skin problems. When devil's claw was introduced to European colonists in the 1900s, it became a popular treatment for easing arthritis-related pain and inflammation.

WHAT IT DOES

While evidence supporting the therapeutic powers of devil's claw requires further investigation, it is most often used for arthritis-related pain. Various studies have found that devil's claw may help reduce pain and improve mobility in osteoarthritis. Some studies have found that devil's claw may even be as effective as certain prescription medications for treating osteoarthritis, and low-back pain. Preliminary studies also indicate that devil's claw may be useful for rheumatoid arthritis.

The German Commission E (see page 16) has approved devil's claw for arthritis, tendonitis, and back pain, as well as for appetite loss and heartburn.

A recent laboratory study found that devil's claw may fight the organism that causes malaria. To treat skin injuries and disorders, the dried tubers and roots of the devil's claw plant are traditionally ground up and made into an ointment. More studies are needed to confirm the effects of devil's claw on these conditions.

For additional information on specific health conditions and how to treat them with supplements, see Part 3 of this book, beginning on page 309.

HOW IT WORKS

Devil's claw contains iridoid glycosides, like harpagoside, which are thought to work in the body as anti-inflammatory agents. They also are believed to stimulate the secretion of gastric juices and the production of bile.

HOW TO TAKE IT

Devil's claw is available in capsules, tablets, liquid extracts, tinctures, and topical ointments. You can also make a tea from the dried roots, but beware, devil's claw is extremely bitter.

Dosages of devil's claw vary depending on the condition you are treating; consult your doctor about what is appropriate for you. A typical dosage of devil's claw is 600 to 1,200 milligrams three times a day of a preparation standardized to contain 3 percent iridoid glycosides or 50 to 100 milligrams of harpagoside.

LOOK OUT FOR THIS!

Devil's claw is generally considered safe when taken in recommended doses, with few side effects. High doses may cause gastrointestinal problems. If taken for prolonged periods, devil's claw may become toxic.

People with stomach ulcers, duodenal ulcers, or gallstones should consult their doctor before taking devil's claw, since it may promote the excretion of acid in the stomach.

Devil's claw has not been studied in children or in pregnant or breastfeeding women, and should be avoided in these groups.

WHAT TO AVOID

Medication: Consult your doctor before taking devil's claw with blood-thinning medications such as warfarin or any anticoagulant or antiplatelet medication.

DHEA

DHEA (DEHYDROEPIANDROSTERONE) is a common hormone produced in the adrenal glands, the gonads, and the brain. Because the level of DHEA in the body naturally peaks around the age of 25 and then starts to decline, researchers have recently studied the potential role of this hormone in the aging process. Some overenthusiastic supplement manufacturers have even called DHEA a "fountain of youth" supplement. Scientific studies haven't supported these claims, and mainstream scientists warn people to be cautious when taking DHEA. Because of the false claims for DHEA's benefits, the FDA banned its sale as a supplement in the mid-1980s, but it has since come back on the market and is extremely popular, particularly for boosting athletic performance.

DHEA is completely banned in the United Kingdom and Canada. Also, the International Olympic Committee and the National Football League have banned the use of DHEA by athletes because in high amounts its effects are similar to those of anabolic steroids.

WHAT IT DOES

Because the amount of DHEA in the body declines with age, some researchers have speculated that boosting this amount with supplemental DHEA will slow the effects of aging, such as the deterioration of muscles, bone loss, the loss of endurance and strength, and the loss of libido. One study showed that people who took DHEA supplements for a 6-month period experienced increased muscle mass and an overall feeling of well-being. While some studies suggest that low levels of DHEA may increase the risk of heart disease and cancer, other studies indicate that higher levels of DHEA are associated with an increased risk of breast and prostate cancer.

Studies conducted on seniors suggested that long-term supplementation with DHEA may improve female sexual function. Men with erectile dysfunction who have low levels of DHEA also seem to benefit from supplementation with this hormone.

Many of the benefits of DHEA have been seen in women. A substantial amount of research suggests that DHEA may reduce the symptoms of lupus in women, including fatigue, pain, and inflammation. Studies also indicate that supplementation with DHEA may prevent osteoporosis in postmenopausal women and women with anorexia nervosa. Some recent studies indicate that DHEA may benefit men with osteoporosis. Still other studies suggest that DHEA may reduce symptoms of menopause.

A double-blind, placebo-controlled study showed that DHEA helped improve the effect of certain medications used to treat schizophrenia.

Other possible uses of DHEA include treating depression and burns, improving symptoms of adrenal failure (such as hormone levels, sex drive, increased capacity for exercise, and overall improvements in well-being and quality of life), boosting the immunizing effects of vaccines, easing symptoms of chronic fatigue syndrome and various autoimmune diseases (including rheumatoid arthritis), preventing obesity, and improving overall well-being in people with multiple sclerosis. More research is needed to establish the value of DHEA in these settings.

For additional information on specific health conditions and how you can treat them with supplements, see Part 3 of this book, beginning on page 309.

HOW IT WORKS

DHEA is an androgen or male steroid hormone that the body converts into other hormones such as testosterone, estrogen, progesterone, or cortisol. The precise way in which DHEA works is still largely unknown.

HOW TO TAKE IT

Caution: DHEA should be used only under a doctor's supervision. Ask your doctor to check your DHEA-S level. This test will help determine if you need to take this supplement.

As a supplement, DHEA is available in capsules, powders, tablets, chewing gum, drops for use under the tongue, and topical creams. Dosages of DHEA vary depending on the form administered and the condition being treated; be sure to check individual product labels for dosage information.

Be forewarned, however, that the amount of DHEA in commercial supplements can vary widely. One study found that the amount ranged from 0 to 150 percent of the content stated on the label.

Most DHEA supplements are synthetically manufactured from soybeans. DHEA cannot be found in food, despite a common misconception that DHEA comes from wild yam. Although DHEA may be produced by using wild yam extract, the body cannot convert wild yam into DHEA. Many supplement manufacturers have tried to sell wild yam supplements as "natural DHEA," which is inaccurate, and these products are ineffective in raising blood levels of DHEA.

LOOK OUT FOR THIS!

As noted earlier, DHEA should be used only with a doctor's supervision. Long-term use of DHEA has not been studied. Occasional side effects of DHEA include fatigue, nasal congestion, acne, and headaches. Also, some forms of masculinization may occur in women who use DHEA, including growth of facial hair, hair loss, increased sweating, weight gain around the waist, and a deepening of the voice. For men, side effects may include breast development and breast tenderness. Men may also experience higher blood pressure, testicular wasting, and heightened aggression. Some studies indicate that DHEA may contribute to artherosclerosis.

People under the age of 40 should not take DHEA supplements unless their DHEA levels are known to be low. People taking DHEA should have their blood levels monitored every 6 months.

People with prostate, breast, uterine, and ovarian cancer, or a family history of any of these cancers, should not take DHEA. Children and pregnant or nursing women should not take DHEA.

WHAT TO AVOID

Medication: Consult your doctor before taking DHEA together with zidovudine, barbiturates, cisplatin, metformin, heart medications, steroids, or estrogen.

DIGESTIVE ENZYMES

ENZYMES ARE ESSENTIAL to every step of digestion. There are three kinds of digestive enzymes: Those that digest protein, those for fats, and those for carbohydrates. All are made in the body by the pancreas. Enzymes that digest the proteins in food are called "proteolytic enzymes," or "proteases," and are the most studied of these enzymes.

WHAT IT DOES

Many people's bodies seem to produce all the digestive enzymes they need for breaking down and absorbing nutrients. But supplements are invaluable for people with pancreatic disease, cystic fibrosis, Crohn's disease, celiac disease, and other conditions that cause specific enzyme deficiencies.

Studies of the use of digestive enzymes to treat general indigestion and its symptoms of bloating and gas, as well as irritable bowel syndrome and heartburn, have also shown mostly positive results for supplemental enzymes, although with some mixed results. Some practitioners of alternative medicine believe that the leakage of undigested protein into the bloodstream ("leaky gut") is the culprit in food allergies and autoimmune diseases like lupus and rheumatoid arthritis. Although these practitioners may advise proteolytic enzymes for these reasons, research has not yet been done on these conditions.

Curiously, one of the most well studied and documented uses for proteolytic enzymes is in treating low back pain, neck pain, and athletic sprains and strains. There is also evidence that proteolytic enzymes move into the bloodstream and provide anti-inflammatory benefits and pain relief for peeople with osteoarthritis and shingles (herpes zoster), and those who have just had surgery. In one study, proteolytic enzymes taken with cancer treatment extended the lifespan of pancreatic cancer patients. Recent studies have compared digestive enzymes with nonsteroidal anti-inflammatory drugs (NSAIDs) and found the two to be equally effective for the treatment of arthritis of the hip and knee.

For additional information on specific health conditions and how to treat them with supplements, see Part 3 of this book, beginning on page 309.

HOW IT WORKS

A healthy pancreas makes two primary enzymes that digest proteins: trypsin and chymotrypsin. These two proteolytic enzymes can also be extracted from the pancreatic tissue of animals such as pigs and oxen. Pineapple and papaya (also used as meat tenderizers) are the two major plant sources of proteolytic enzymes as nutritional supplements. Pineapple stems are the source of the enzyme bromelain (see also page 54), while unripe papaya provides a second enzyme, papain. Whatever their source, all of these proteolytic enzymes act as catalysts that act in the intestine to break down proteins into their smaller and more absorbable constitutents, known as amino acids and peptides. Besides the sources named here, digestive enzymes can also be made from fungi or bacteria.

Enzymes that digest fats are called lipases, and enzymes that digest carbohydrates are called amylases. Pancreatin, a substance taken from animals, provides all three kinds of digestive enzymes—proteolytic enzymes, lipases, and amylases. Another enzyme, lactase, breaks down lactose (milk sugar) for people with lactose intolerance.

HOW TO TAKE IT

Makers of supplemental enzymes label their potency in various ways, as well as in milligrams, but you'll want to look for "activity units," which is a better indicator of an enzyme's digestive potency than is the weight of enzyme in the product. The U.S. Pharmacopeia (USP) standard for pancreatin potency is 25 USP units of protease, 2 USP units of lipase, and 25 USP units of amylase. A brand labeled "2x" has twice the enzyme potency of this USP standard.

For pancreatic insufficiency, 3 to 4 grams of 4x pancreatin taken with each meal may improve digestion, although people with serious pancreatic disease may need medically supervised higher doses of this enzyme.

Because stomach acid may break down digestive enzymes, some doctors advise taking them throughout each meal rather than simply before the meal, and buying enzyme supplements with an enteric coating so that the enzymes themselves won't break down until they reach the intestine.

LOOK OUT FOR THIS!

Digestive enzymes are generally safe, although they can cause heartburn, stomach irritation, constipation, or diarrhea. People with ulcers may not be able to tolerate supplemental enzymes at all. Because many brands of digestive enzyme brands derive their pancreatin from pork, and accordingly label it as "porcine," people wanting to avoid pork should read labels carefully. In such cases, brands of vegetarian enzymes are also available.

Consult your doctor if you have a disease that causes malabsorption of foods. In this case you may need a brand of enzyme with a maximum lipase and minimum protease content, since protease can digest the lipase in a supplement.

Some studies have shown that in children with cystic fibrosis, supplemental enzyme preparations can lead to a serious bowel condition called fibrosing colonopathy. For this reason, enzyme therapy for children with cystic fibrosis requires medical supervision.

WHAT TO AVOID

Medication: If you're taking a sedative or antibiotic medicine, you should avoid bromelain, since it can affect these medications. Both bromelain and papain can boost the effects of blood-thinning drugs.

Herbs and Dietary Supplements: Pancreatin can interfere with the absorption of folate (one of the B vitamins), so talk with your doctor if this is a concern.

DONG QUAI

THE DONG QUAI PLANT *(Angelica sinensis)* grows at high altitudes in the cold, damp mountainous regions of China, Korea, and Japan. The thick roots have many traditional medicinal uses. A relative to celery and parsley, dong quai is sometimes called "female ginseng" because of its use in gynecological health. It is one of the most popular herbs used in traditional Chinese medicine for both premenstrual and menopausal problems.

WHAT IT DOES

In traditional Chinese medicine, dong quai is used to treat pain, purify the blood, regulate the menstrual cycle, and treat cough and constipation. Western countries have embraced dong quai because of its apparent ability to ease menstrual and menopausal problems, but it may be that it works best in combination with other herbs, as the Chinese use it. An Israeli study found a preparation containing dong quai and chamomile to be effective for symptoms of menopause.

Preliminary studies suggest that dong quai may also be beneficial for abnormal heart rhythms, angina, accumulation of platelets in blood vessels, liver ailments, urination problems, and constipation. Other studies suggest that dong quai may inhibit tumor growth, but more research is needed to confirm these claims. A recent study preformed in China found that dong quai could be useful in the treatment of ulcerative colitis.

For additional information on specific health conditions and how to treat them with supplements, see Part 3 of this book, beginning on page 309.

HOW IT WORKS

The active ingredients in dong quai appear to be the compounds called coumarins, ferulic acid, and ligustilide, all of which affect blood flow and prompt muscle relaxation.

The success of dong quai for treating gynecological symptoms has suggested that it may have phytoestrogen properties, which researchers are studying.

HOW TO TAKE IT

Dong quai is available in a variety of forms, including tablets, powders, dried root extracts, topical oil, dried leaf, leaf tincture, and leaf extract.

There are no standard or well-studied recommended doses of dong quai. In Chinese traditional medicine, from 3 to 15 grams of raw dong quai herb are used to make a tea, although even for this dong quai is often mixed with other herbs.

LOOK OUT FOR THIS!

Dong quai is generally considered safe for adults. Dong quai is not suitable for children since it has not been sufficiently studied in this age group. Women who are pregnant or nursing should avoid using dong quai because of its possible hormonal effects.

Given the potential ability of dong quai to increase bleeding, women taking it for premenstrual symptoms should stop taking it as soon as menstruation begins. At high doses, dong quai may cause headaches and gastrointestinal distress.

WHAT TO AVOID

Medication: Consult your doctor before taking dong quai with blood-thinning medications such as warfarin, antiplatelet drugs such as clopidogrel, nonsteroidal anti-inflammatory drugs (NSAIDs) such as ibuprofen, hormonal medications, oral contraceptives, hormone replacement therapy, and selective estrogen receptor modulators (SERMs). Dong quai contains furanocoumarins, the compounds also found in grapefruit juice and which inhibit an enzyme called cytochrome P450 that helps the body to metabolize drugs.

Food: People with allergies to caraway, carrot, celery, dill, or parsley should not use dong quai.

ECHINACEA

A NATIVE AMERICAN MEDICINAL PLANT, echinacea *(Echinacea purpurea, Echinacea angustifolia, Echinacea pallida)* is one of the most popular herbal remedies on the market. It gets its name from the prickly scales in the seed head at the center of the flower, which look like the spines of an angry hedgehog—*echinos* is Greek for hedgehog. Commercial preparations of echinacea are made from the flowers, stems, leaves, and roots of the plant. Native Americans used echinacea to treat all types of infections and wounds, and it gained esteem in the United States in the 18th and 19th centuries. However, after the introduction of antibiotics in the 1930s, echinacea lost its popularity. Today, however, echinacea is one of the most popular herbal supplements in the United States, and many people consider it as the herbal equivalent of vitamin C.

WHAT IT DOES

Today echinacea is used mainly to fight the symptoms of upper respiratory tract infections such as the common cold and flu, sore throat, cough, and fever, as well as to boost the immune system. A number of studies have confirmed that when taken for 8 to 10 days beginning at the first sign of a cold, echinacea can effectively reduce cold symptoms or shorten their duration. One popular way to take echinacea is continuously, as a supplement, throughout the cold and flu season or after exposure to infection, although this approach to taking echinacea is slightly controversial; some experts believe that echinacea cannot stimulate the immune system on a continuous basis. This theory may be more myth than fact, however, with decades of research supporting echinacea's long-term use, and neither modern nor traditional reference sources support any long-term-use limitations of the herb.

Aside from its use for treating cold, flu, and respiratory infection, preliminary studies suggest that when applied topically, echinacea may be useful for treating herpes virus sores. Echinacea is also an excellent topical anesthetic for sore throats and is found in a number of herbal products for use in the treatment of that condition.

The endless list of additional conditions that echinacea may be useful for treating includes breast pain, burns, meningitis, urinary tract infection, Lyme disease, mouth inflammation, human immunodeficiency virus (HIV), allergies, arthritis, and eczema.

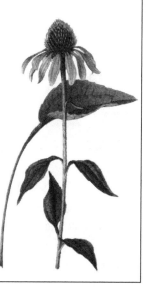

For additional information on specific health conditions and how to treat them with supplements, see Part 3 of this book, beginning on page 309.

HOW IT WORKS

Several studies suggest that echinacea stimulates the growth and activity of cells of the immune system and boosts the body's defenses against bacteria and viruses. However, the exact way in which echinacea works to strengthen the immune system is unknown.

Other studies have found that echinacea might possibly have anti-inflammatory and wound-healing properties. The exact chemical compounds that make echinacea effective have not been identified.

HOW TO TAKE IT

Commercial echinacea preparations vary widely in their echinacea content. Since researchers are still unsure about what active component makes echinacea beneficial, standardization may not be relevant in terms of the effectiveness of a particular echinacea preparation. The best evidence shows that products made with *E. purpurea*, which come from the flowers, leaves, and stems of this plant, are most effective. However, be aware that products made from the root of *E. purpurea* don't seem to have any benefits. The varying effectiveness of different types of echinacea may explain the wide variation in anecdotal reports about the effectiveness of echinacea.

Echinacea is available as capsules, tablets, tinctures, dried root, extracts, ointments, and teas. You can even buy echinacea juice. Some herbalists believe that echinacea is more effective when taken in liquid form, although there is no scientific basis for this claim.

Supplements Don't Always Contain What Their Labels Claim

Did You Know?

Echinacea is an extremely popular supplement in the United States, accounting for 10 percent of dietary supplement sales. However, many echinacea products found in your local drugstore may not contain exactly what they claim.

A study done to determine what echinacea supplements contained in order to assess their quality found that 10 percent of the 59 products analyzed contained no echinacea at all! Only 52 percent of the products assayed had contents consistent with the information on the label. And of 21 standardized products, only nine met the quality standard stated on the label. You know that you have a potent product if the tincture makes your tongue go slightly numb.

Bottom line? Don't believe everything you read about supplements. Make sure to shop wisely and distinguish reputable supplement manufacturers from less reputable ones so that you get the most for your money.

Dosages vary depending on the form of echinacea you are taking, so be sure to read product labels for individual dosage information.

Recent studies indicate that unrefined echinacea (made from whole, unrefined roots of the plant) is not effective in treating colds.

LOOK OUT FOR THIS!

Echinacea is generally considered safe, with few side effects. Occasionally it can produce an allergic reaction (especially in people allergic to this and other members of the *compositae* family, which includes the asters), and people with asthma or allergies may be at a particular risk for such reactions.

Women who are pregnant or nursing, people with liver and kidney disease, and children should not take echinacea unless instructed to do so by a doctor, since its safety in these populations has not been firmly established.

WHAT TO AVOID

Medication: Consult your doctor before taking echinacea at the same time as immunosuppressant medications including corticosteroids (such as prednisone), cyclosporine, amiodarone, methotrexate, and ketoconazole. Echinacea may interact adversely with drugs that are metabolized in the liver. Echinacea should be used with caution by highly allergic individuals.

ELDERBERRY

IF YOU'VE GOT ROOTS IN RURAL AMERICA, you or someone you know probably used to—and maybe still does—make elderberry wine, bake elderberry pies, or concoct elderberry preserves. Although tasting these homespun favorites may have delighted your taste buds, you may not have realized that you might also have been doing something good for your health. The flowers and black or blue berries of elderberry bushes have long been a part of traditional herbal treatments for colds, infections, and pain relief (red elderberries have no medicinal benefit). Current research is examining whether extracts of elderberry may have even more important therapeutic effects.

Nevertheless, elderberry needs to be treated with care. If it's not prepared properly—if the berries aren't cooked, for example, or if the leaves, stems, or roots are included in preparations to be taken internally—it can cause nausea and sometimes more severe reactions.

WHAT IT DOES

Traditionally, elderberry extracts have been used to treat colds and the flu, sinus infection, bronchitis, sore throat, and cough, and a few studies support these practices. In a placebo-controlled, double-blind study conducted in Israel during an influenza outbreak, people treated with elderberry had more resistance to the flu strain that caused the outbreak than those who took a placebo. Furthermore, the group treated with elderberry had symptoms for 4 days less than those who took a placebo.

Studies have found that herbal preparations containing elderberry may relieve symptoms of sinusitis by reducing the inflammation of mucous membranes and decreasing nasal congestion better than medications often prescribed for these conditions.

Preliminary laboratory research has also shown that an extract made from elderberry leaves, when combined with St. John's wort and soapwort, not only inhibited influenza virus but also herpes simplex virus. (However, ingesting elderberry leaves is not recommended.) As one result of these findings, researchers are investigating whether elderberry may be a viable treatment for cold sores and other forms of herpes, as well as for infection by human immunodeficiency virus (HIV).

For additional information on specific health conditions and how to treat them with supplements, see Part 3 of this book, beginning on page 309.

HOW IT WORKS

The flowers and berries of elderberry contain flavonoids, most notably quercetin, that have antioxidant effects and may also boost the immune system (see also Quercetin, page 236). Studies with animals indicate that elderberry flowers have anti-inflammatory properties as well.

Some research has shown that elderberry both stimulates the immune system and inhibits the growth of viruses. Some studies indicate that elderberry extract works by binding to the influenza virus and preventing it from entering cells in the body.

HOW TO TAKE IT

Elderberry is available as dried flowers for making a tea, as a syrup made from extracts of black or blue elderberries, and as capsules. Practitioners recommend making the tea by steeping 3 to 5 grams of dried flowers in a cup of boiling water for 10 to 15 minutes and drinking up to three cups a day. Typical doses of elderberry extract syrup are 1 to 2 tablespoons taken twice a day for 3 days. *Note:* Some practitioners recommend against giving elderberry syrup to children because of the high sugar content. Standardized extracts of elderberry in capsule form should contain 28 percent anthocyamins and be taken in dosages of 4 grams a day divided into three doses.

LOOK OUT FOR THIS!

Elderberry flowers are generally considered safe. Rare side effects may include stomach upset or nausea.

Do not use unripe or raw parts of the elderberry plant; if consumed in large amounts it may cause diarrhea or vomiting.

Do not use elderberry if you know you're allergic to honeysuckle or to plants in the honeysuckle family.

WHAT TO AVOID

Medication: If you're taking a diuretic, you may want to consult a doctor before taking elderberry, because its long-term use has been shown to increase urine production, which a diuretic also does. There is also evidence that elderberry can lower blood sugar levels and should not be taken in combination with diabetes medications without first consulting your doctor. Also, animal studies indicate that elderberry may exacerbate adverse reactions to some forms of chemotherapy.

Herbs and Nutritional Supplements: Because elderberry has potential diuretic effects, use it with caution if you're taking other diuretic herbs, including artichoke, celery, corn silk, couchgrass, dandelion, horsetail, juniper berry, kava, shepherd's purse, uva ursi, or yarrow. Since elderberry may also work as a laxative, use it wisely with herbs that also have this effect.

EUCALYPTUS

THE CHANCES ARE THAT EUCALYPTUS *(Eucalyptus globules)* is in the mouthwash you use, the cough drops you take when you've got a cold, and the over-the-counter cream you rub on aching joints. The dried leaves and extracted oil of this plant are also herbal remedies in their own right, with a good track record for treating several different conditions.

For certain people—most notably children—eucalyptus, especially in high amounts, can be poisonous and has even been known to be fatal. See the cautions and warnings about its use under Look Out for This! page 113, especially if you plan to use preparations that involve ingesting eucalyptus oil.

WHAT IT DOES

Besides being an ingredient in a variety of products for oral hygiene, relieving coughs and colds, and soothing minor aches and pains, eucalyptus is used on its own to treat both respiratory problems and joint and muscle soreness. The German Commission E (see page 16) has approved eucalyptus oil taken internally or inhaled for the treatment of inflammation of the mucous membrane of the respiratory tract, as well as for relieving nasal congestion and cough.

Eucalyptus may be applied topically for a variety of uses, one of which is for relieving respiratory congestion. Studies also suggest that when eucalyptus is applied to the temples and forehead, it may help relieve tension headaches. Eucalyptus oil is present in over-the-counter decongestant products such as Vicks VapoRub Ointment.

Eucalyptol, which is derived from eucalyptus and is contained in eucalyptus oil, is used in many over-the-counter cough drops and mouthwashes. Studies suggest that eucalyptus may protect teeth against plaque-causing bacteria, and because of this, essential oil of eucalyptus is an ingredient of certain toothpastes.

In addition to these uses of eucalyptus and its oil, Germany has licensed eucalyptus tea for the relief of bronchitis. The German Commission E (see page 16) has approved topical preparations of eucalyptus for "rheumatic complaints." Besides this, eucalyptus may be helpful for treating headaches and ear infections.

Eucalyptus Repels Insects

Did You Know?

The eucalyptus plant is the main food of the furry marsupials known as koalas, of Australia, who eat so much of it that some of the oil is excreted onto their skin surface. Scientists suspect that the eucalyptus oil may help protect koalas from various parasites. In this regard, laboratory studies have shown that eucalyptus oil repels certain types of biting insects and live mites. Some studies have found that eucalyptus may even be as effective as diethyltoluamide, an ingredient commonly found in insect repellents.

To make a eucalyptus-based insect repellent, mix 1 fluid ounce (30 milliliters) of eucalyptus oil with 2 to 3 cups of lukewarm water, and apply the mixture topically to keep bugs away.

Try making a eucalyptus-containing insect repellent next summer, or better yet, if you live in a warm climate, try planting some eucalyptus on the patio to keep the bugs away!

For additional information on specific health conditions and how you can treat them with supplements, see Part 3 of this book, beginning on page 309.

HOW IT WORKS

Although scientists don't know for sure how eucalyptus works, studies have given them some indications. The active ingredient in the oil, eucalyptol, appears to have antibacterial and fungicidal effects, as well as being anti-inflammatory. It also acts as an expectorant. Some researchers theorize that the anti-inflammatory properties of eucalyptol may result from its action as an antioxidant, destroying the cell- and tissue-damaging molecules known as free radicals. The oil may serve to counteract irritation of respiratory passages. It also appears to increase blood flow and increase skin and muscle temperature—which may explain the effectiveness of eucalyptus in relieving minor joint and muscle aches—and to inhibit production of the hormone-like compounds known as prostaglandins that, among other effects, cause inflammation.

HOW TO TAKE IT

Diluted eucalyptus oil can be taken internally, inhaled in steam, or applied topically in an ointment. The dried leaves of eucalyptus can be made into a tea. The maximum daily dose of the oil if taken internally is 0.3 to 0.6 grams. Be sure to read the cautions about overdosing with eucalyptus in the Look Out for This! section, which is below.

For inhalation, 2 to 3 drops of eucalyptus oil may be infused into boiling water and the steam inhaled. Topical preparations consist of 5 to 20 percent of the essential oil in oil-based formulations or 5 to 10 percent of the essential oil in alcohol-based formulations. A few drops of the essential oil can also be rubbed into the skin, but first see the cautions in the Look Out for This! section, below.

LOOK OUT FOR THIS!

Undiluted eucalyptus oil is toxic. Less than one teaspoonful can be fatal when ingested. Signs of poisoning include seizures, delirium, dizziness, burning in the intestines, nausea, diarrhea, and a feeling of suffocation.

Eucalyptus should not be used by children, pregnant or nursing women, or people with liver disorders or kidney problems.

SUPPLEMENTAL TRIVIA

The eucalyptus tree, which is native to Australia, was first used medicinally by Australian Aborigines. The eucalyptus tree is one of the tallest trees in the world, and can grow up to heights of 300 feet. One eucalyptus tree, found near Melbourne, Australia, was more than 318 feet tall!

Because studies have shown that eucalyptus can affect blood sugar levels, people with type 2 diabetes should not use eucalyptus oil without a doctor's supervision.

In addition to the side effects mentioned above, eucalyptus oil used topically may cause allergic skin reactions and when ingested in excess may cause nausea, vomiting, and diarrhea.

WHAT TO AVOID

Medication: Eucalyptus oil causes liver enzymes to work more actively, which may weaken or shorten the effects of other medications. Since eucalyptus oil can depress the central nervous system, it may add to the effects of any sedatives. It may also add to the effects of hypoglycemic medications used for treating diabetes.

EVENING PRIMROSE OIL

IT IS VERY MISLEADING that the evening primrose *(Oenothera biennis)* is actually not a member of the primrose family, but a willow herb. True to part of its name at least, the flowers of the evening primrose plant do open at dusk and close when exposed to direct sunlight. Native Americans boiled the root of the plant and used the leaves to make a poultice for bruises and hemorrhoids. Modern remedies that use this plant are based on the oil extracted from the seeds.

WHAT IT DOES

Today, evening primrose oil is particularly known for its use in women's health—for relieving premenstrual symptoms, discomfort from fibrocystic or swollen breasts, and menopausal symptoms such as hot flashes. However, most scientific studies of the effects of evening primrose have not been large enough to be conclusive.

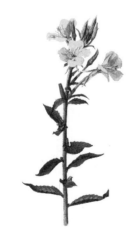

The oil of evening primrose is also widely used topically, especially in Europe, to soothe the itchiness associated with some skin conditions, such as eczema. It also seems to have potential benefits for soothing allergic skin rashes or hives. Preliminary studies support these claims.

Preliminary research suggests that evening primrose oil may ease symptoms of arthritis and bursitis because of its potential ability to reduce inflammation. Other potential uses of evening primrose oil include treatment for diabetic neuropathy, dry eyes, high cholesterol, and alcoholism and to promote weight loss. However, studies have given inconclusive results about its benefits in these conditions, and more research is needed to confirm these findings.

For additional information on specific health conditions and how to treat them with supplements, see Part 3 of this book, beginning on page 309.

HOW IT WORKS

The active ingredient in evening primrose oil is an omega-6 fatty acid known as gamma-linolenic acid (GLA). The body itself normally makes this fatty acid, fueled by the linolenic acid it gets from food. But in some cases, such as diabetes, eczema, or premenstrual syndrome, the body does not properly convert fatty acids into GLA and requires an additional source of this acid.

GLA acts as an anti-inflammatory agent, promoting relief from inflammation or swelling in various places in the body.

HOW TO TAKE IT

Evening primrose oil is a clear, golden yellow oil extracted from the seeds of the plant. It is available as capsules or as an oil, and is standardized to contain 8 percent GLA. General dosage recommendations for evening primrose oil range from 3 to 6 grams daily. When ingested, evening primrose oil should always be taken with food to prevent stomach upset.

Keep evening primrose oil in the refrigerator and out of direct sunlight so that the oil does not become rancid. The recommended dosages differ according to the form of supplement used, so be sure to read and carefully follow the label directions for a particular supplement. Some suggest taking an omega-3 supplement along with evening primrose oil in a 1:4 ratio.

Other ways to get a good dose of GLA are by taking borage oil, which is derived from the seeds of the borage plant *(Borago officinalis)*, and black currant *(Ribes nigrum)* seed oil.

LOOK OUT FOR THIS!

Side effects of evening primrose oil are rare, but may occasionally include headache, mild nausea, and abdominal pain.

Evening primrose oil is generally considered safe for adults. However, safe dosages for children, women who are pregnant or nursing, and people with liver or kidney disease have not yet been determined. Consequently, you should consult your doctor before using evening primrose oil.

WHAT TO AVOID

Medication: Evening primrose oil may increase the effects of certain medications. Consult your doctor before taking evening primrose oil with antibiotics, chemotherapy, cyclosporine, nonsteroidal anti-inflammatory drugs (NSAIDs), phenothizine drugs for schizophrenia, anesthetics, and anticonvulsant medications.

Herb and Dietary Supplements: Consult your doctor before taking evening primrose oil with blood pressure–lowering herbs.

FENUGREEK

IF YOU'VE EVER EATEN INDIAN CURRY, then you've probably consumed fenugreek *(Trigonella foenumgraecum)*—a practically indispensable ingredient in cooking on the Indian subcontinent. Fenugreek is also a favorite in North African and Middle Eastern dishes. In fact, it has been used as both a culinary and medicinal herb for thousands of years.

Fenugreek seeds taste slightly like celery, burnt sugar, or maple and are used to make imitation vanilla, butterscotch, and rum flavorings. Fenugreek seeds are also the main ingredients in imitation maple flavoring.

WHAT IT DOES

The leaves and seeds of the fenugreek plant have traditionally been used to make extracts and powders believed to serve a variety of medicinal purposes, including the treatment of indigestion, baldness, menstrual pain, and postmenopausal vaginal dryness, as well as for the stimulation of lactation in pregnant women. There are, however, few studies in medical literature examining these uses.

Today, the German Commission E (see page 16) approves the use of fenugreek as an appetite stimulant and for reducing skin inflammation. Fenugreek may also be useful in treating constipation, since it provides fiber in the diet.

Several studies show that fenugreek may also be effective in reducing blood sugar and lowering cholesterol levels. It also has a positive effect in reducing excess lipids in the blood, a condition known as hyperlipidemia. Several studies have indicated that fenugreek improves glucose control and reduces blood cholesterol levels in people with diabetes.

Some herbalists believe that fenugreek can aid upper respiratory inflammation and congestion, but these claims are anecdotal and have not been scientifically studied. Preliminary animal studies suggest that fenugreek seeds may prevent colon cancer. More research is needed to explore this potential use of fenugreek.

For additional information on specific health conditions and how to treat them with supplements, see Part 3 of this book, beginning on page 309.

HOW IT WORKS

Fenugreek seeds contain a soluble fiber called mucilage, which may help slow digestion and the absorption of food from the intestine. This in turn can slow the increase in blood sugar levels that follows a meal.

Fenugreek's effects in lowering lipid levels may be due to ingredients called saponins, which increase cholesterol secretion in the gastrointestinal tract, thereby reducing cholesterol levels in the serum.

HOW TO TAKE IT

Fenugreek is available as a supplement in capsule, tablet, and powder forms. Because of the bitter taste of fenugreek, the capsule form may be the easiest to take. There is no standardized recommended dosage of fenugreek. The German Commission E (see page 16) recommends a dosage of 6 grams of fenugreek daily.

Fenugreek can be easily sprouted and added to salads when taken fresh, although it may be too bitter for some taste buds. Fenugreek seeds are packed with vitamins A, B, C, and E, and the minerals calcium, iron, magnesium, and zinc, to name just a few.

LOOK OUT FOR THIS!

Fenugreek should be used with caution in children, and only under a doctor's supervision. Pregnant or nursing women should not take fenugreek unless advised by a doctor.

Fenugreek is generally considered safe for adults. Individuals allergic to chickpeas should avoid fenugreek.

Side effects of fenugreek may include mild gastrointestinal upset and sweating.

WHAT TO AVOID

Medication: If you are taking any oral medications, speak with your doctor before using fenugreek, because its mucilaginous fiber content and high viscosity may interfere with the normal absorption of

---

RESTORATIVE RECIPES

FENUGREEK RICE

To reap the health benefits of fenugreek and please your palate at the same time, try this Indian dish. It's packed with delicious spicy flavors and healing properties.

Ingredients

3 tablespoons vegetable broth

1 teaspoon cumin

1/3 cup chopped onion

2 potatoes, diced

1 bunch fresh fenugreek leaves, chopped

2 cups long grain brown rice, presoaked

3 3/4 cups water

1 green chili, chopped

1 teaspoon garam masala (This is a spice blend that can be found in the international section of your grocery store.)

Directions: In a large skillet, heat the vegetable broth and sauté the cumin and onion until the onion becomes soft. Add potatoes and fenugreek to the skillet; cover and cook over medium heat for 5 minutes, stirring occasionally. Add the rice, water, salt, and chili. Do not cover the pan. Bring the water to a boil. Once the water is boiling, reduce the heat to low, cover the pan, and simmer for 20 to 30 minutes or until the rice is tender. Sprinkle with garam masala.

many medications. Fenugreek may also interfere with the effects of diabetes medications and blood-thinning medications such as warfarin and cardiac glycosides such as digoxin.

FEVERFEW

FEVERFEW *(Tanacetum parthenium)* is a plant with fragrant, featherlike flowers. A member of the daisy family with a vibrant yellow flower, feverfew was used in European folk medicine to alleviate symptoms of everything from fever and arthritis to labor difficulties, stomachaches, and asthma. The name itself comes from the Latin word *febrifugia* or "fever reducer."

In the 1980s, feverfew gained popularity among herbalists in Britain as an alternative treatment for migraine headaches when the widely respected British journal *Lancet* published a study of its apparent benefits. This prompted additional studies of feverfew to determine its effectiveness. Recent studies, using various proprietary extracts, appear to confirm these results. In spite of some conflicting reports, feverfew remains a widely sold herbal supplement in the United States in mainstream retail outlets.

WHAT IT DOES

Feverfew is primarily used to treat migraine headaches, as well as the nausea and vomiting often associated with these headaches. However, if stopped too abruptly, feverfew may actually cause rebound headaches and joint stiffness; slowly reducing the dosage of this herb may prevent such problems.

Laboratory studies suggest that feverfew may have some anti-inflammatory properties, and as a result, some herbalists recommend taking feverfew to reduce arthritis-related pain. Feverfew may also be an effective insect and bee repellent.

For additional information on specific health conditions and how you can treat them with supplements, see Part 3 of this book, beginning on page 309.

HOW IT WORKS

Researchers believe that the dried leaves of feverfew contain sesquiterpene lactones, which are the active ingredients of this herb. Parthenolide, a major component member of these compounds, may inhibit smooth-muscle contraction, preventing the constriction of blood vessels in the brain that some experts believe to be the cause of migraines.

Although more research is needed to understand the role of feverfew as an anti-inflammatory agent, some researchers believe that it reduces inflammation by inhibiting the body's production of histamine.

HOW TO TAKE IT

Feverfew is available as fresh and dried leaves and as capsules, tablets, and liquid extracts.

In the form of fresh, powdered leaves, feverfew may be taken as often as three times a day in doses of 380 milligrams. When taken in the form of freeze-dried leaves, dosages of 25 milligrams daily are often recommended. In capsule form, a feverfew supplement standardized to contain 250 micrograms of parthenolide is often recommended for once-daily use. You may also make a tea from feverfew leaves. But beware: boiling feverfew leaves will increase this herb's bitterness. Instead, put 2 to 8 leaves in a cup of boiled water and drink it once daily.

As much as 2 weeks may be needed before the therapeutic effects of feverfew are noticed.

Note: There is a wide variability in commercial feverfew products, partly because the parthenolide content of this herb can vary according to the geographical origin of the plant, the stage of the plant's life at the time of its harvest, the parts of the plant used to make a product, and how the plant material was stored.

LOOK OUT FOR THIS!

Feverfew can alter the menstrual cycle and increase bleeding. Pregnant and nursing women should not take feverfew.

Occasional side effects associated with feverfew can include abdominal pain, dry mouth, indigestion, flatulence, diarrhea, nausea, vomiting, and nervousness. Individuals who chew feverfew leaves may experience mouth ulcers, temporary loss of taste, and swelling of the lips, tongue, and mouth.

Individuals who are allergic to chamomile, ragweed, yarrow, chrysanthemum, marigold, and daisy will also probably be allergic to feverfew and shouldn't take it. Handling the leaves of the feverfew plant may cause an allergic reaction on the skin in some sensitive people.

WHAT TO AVOID

Medication: Be sure to consult your doctor before taking feverfew with blood-thinning medications such as warfarin; nonsteroidal anti-inflammatory drugs (NSAIDs) such as ibuprofen and aspirin; and antiplatelet drugs such as clopidogrel.

FIBER

FIBER IS PROBABLY SOMETHING that you know is good for you, but you may not know exactly what it is and how it can benefit your health. Found in the stems, leaves, and seeds of plants, fiber (also called roughage) consists of long chains of sugar molecules linked to one another. Because the body can't digest or absorb fiber, it can work its way through the digestive system. There are two types of fiber—soluble fiber, which partially dissolves in water, and insoluble fiber, which doesn't dissolve in water and moves through the digestive system more quickly than soluble fiber.

Fiber from food sources is usually a mixture of both soluble and insoluble fiber, while supplements often contain either one kind of fiber or the other. Eating more fiber-rich foods is the best way to ensure you get enough fiber. But if you don't make the right dietary choices or if you have certain medical conditions, such as irritable bowel syndrome, supplements may be used to provide your body with the extra fiber it requires.

WHAT IT DOES

Fiber provides a wide range of health benefits. You may be well aware of its role in preventing and relieving constipation. Both insoluble and soluble fiber help keep your bowels moving.

Many studies have shown that by lowering your total cholesterol and LDL ("bad") cholesterol, soluble fiber reduces the chances of developing heart disease. Soluble fiber can also help lower blood sugar levels and reduce the risk of developing type 2 diabetes.

Other benefits of a high-fiber diet may include a lower risk for getting such conditions as hemorrhoids, irritable bowel syndrome, diverticular disease, and gallstones.

For many years, experts believed that insoluble fiber helped to prevent colon cancer. But three large, recent studies have shown that this may not be entirely true. But don't give up on fiber just yet! Even if studies have shown that it's not the whole picture in preventing colon cancer, it may still be part of this picture.

Fiber may also be a healthy addition to a weight-loss plan, with studies indicating that people whose diets have a high-fiber content in their diets may weigh less than those with low fiber intakes.

For additional information on specific health conditions and how you can treat them with supplements, see Part 3 of this book, beginning on page 309.

HOW IT WORKS

Fiber's ability to prevent and treat constipation is due in large part to its water-attracting ability. Fiber soaks up water, which keeps stools moist, helping them to move through and out of your bowels. Insoluble fiber helps to promote soft, bulky stools that move more quickly out of your bowels.

Scientists don't know exactly why soluble fiber reduces cholesterol levels in the blood, but they think that it has to do with bile—a substance that is released by the liver and permits fat to be digested. After digestion, most bile is reabsorbed by the body. Soluble fiber decreases the amount of bile that is reabsorbed, forcing the liver to produce more bile. Because bile contains cholesterol, this increased

Calculating Food and Fiber Content

Need help choosing the best sources of fiber in your diet? Reading the food label can tell you the amount of dietary fiber in a particular product. Below are the fiber contents of some foods.

Food	Fiber Content (grams)
Split peas (cooked, 1 cup)	16.3
Kidney beans (red, boiled, 1 cup)	13.1
Chickpeas (canned, 1 cup)	10.6
Buckwheat or kasha (cooked, 1 cup)	9.6
Raspberries (raw, 1 cup)	8.4
Broccoli (boiled, 1 cup)	4.5
Oatmeal (instant, cooked, 1 cup)	4.0

Food	Fiber Content (grams)
Apple (medium, with skin)	3.7
Brown rice (cooked, 1 cup)	3.5
Banana (raw, medium)	3.1
Almonds (sliced, 1/4 cup)	2.4
Carrot (raw, medium)	2.2
Whole wheat bread (1 slice)	1.9
Popcorn (air-popped, 1 cup)	1.2

Other high-fiber foods include all whole grains, vegetables such as acorn squash (winter squash), beans, cruciferous vegetables (such as broccoli, cabbage, and kale), berries (such as blackberries and blueberries), pears, and apples.

production of bile takes more cholesterol out of the blood. In addition, soluble fiber can be partly broken down by bacteria in the intestine. This process generates substances called fatty acids that reduce the livers production of cholesterol.

HOW TO TAKE IT

The best sources of dietary fiber are fruits and vegetables, nuts and legumes, and whole-grain foods. The recommended intake of fiber for adults is 20 to 40 grams per day. You can calculate the dosage of fiber for children over age 2 by taking the childs age and adding 5 grams (for example, if a child is 7 years old, their recommended dosage would be 12 grams).

Fiber supplements include psyllium, which is made from the husks of the psyllium plant, as well as methylcellulose and polycarbophil, which are forms of cellulose (the substance that makes up the cell walls of plants).

Recommended dosages of fiber are as follows:

■ Psyllium supplements: Take 7 grams in 8 ounces of liquid, as often as up to three times per day.

■ Methylcellulose: Take 10.2 grams in 8 ounces of liquid, as often as three times per day.

■ Polycarbophil: Take 1 gram (or 2 caplets) per day. Do not exceed 4 grams per day.

Increase your fiber intake gradually over a period of a few weeks so that your digestive system can adjust to it; this can help reduce any side effects (see below). Be sure to drink plenty of water too, since fiber works best when it absorbs water. Without plenty of water along with fiber, you might become constipated.

LOOK OUT FOR THIS!

Taking fiber in the recommended doses is considered safe, although you may experience some mild side effects such as bloating or excessive gas.

Some people have an allergy to certain fiber sources such as wheat or psyllium and must obtain their fiber from other sources, such as fruits and vegetables or nuts and legumes.

WHAT TO AVOID

Fiber has no known interactions with other drugs, supplements, or herbs.

5-HTP

ITS FULL NAME IS A CLASSIC chemical tongue twister: 5-hydroxytryptophan. But it's pretty easy to say how important 5-HTP is for human health. The body creates 5-HTP from the amino acid tryptophan, a component of the protein in many foods, and uses it in turn to produce serotonin, an important chemical produced in the brain and spinal cord, which acts as a neurotransmitter substance that carries messages between nerve cells. People who don't have enough serotonin, or whose serotonin isn't doing its job properly, can suffer a wide variety of ailments, from depression and other mood disorders to insomnia, headaches, and chronic pain.

Given serotonin's wide-ranging effects, it's not surprising that antidepressant medications, which treat mood disorders by acting on serotonin, can also treat pain, headache, and insomnia, and for some time, doctors have prescribed these medications accordingly. Unfortunately, though, many prescription antidepressants come with bothersome side effects. The good news about 5-HTP in supplemental form is that it duplicates almost all of the positive effects of prescription antidepressants without some of the negatives. Thus, for many people, 5-HTP is a welcome alternative to prescription drugs.

WHAT IT DOES

Clinical research suggests that 5-HTP supplements can help treat many of the same conditions alleviated by prescription antidepressants, including depression, migraines and other headaches, obesity, insomnia, and fibromyalgia. In several small studies, 5-HTP was compared to the prescription antidepressant fluvoxamine (Luvox), a member of the class of drugs known as "serotonin-specific reuptake inhibitors" (SSRIs) because they delay the resorption of serotonin by the nerve cells that secrete it, thus allowing it to exert its effect over a longer period of time. Over the course of 6 weeks, 5-HTP proved to be just as effective as fluvoxamine, while causing fewer and less intense side effects.

Moreover, in a 6-month trial, migraine headaches were relieved by 5-HTP just as well as by a standard migraine medication, although 5-HTP didn't seem to help children with migraines as much. And while there's some evidence that it can reduce the pain from other types of headaches, 5-HTP was not found to work well against tension-type headaches in women.

5-HTP may have promise as a treatment for obesity and to encourage weight loss in adults. Several studies have shown that 5-HTP helped overweight women to lose weight. One group of women lost 2 percent of their body weight during an initial period when they took no other steps to lose weight; after that, when they also followed a weight-loss diet, they lost 3 percent of the body weight they'd started at.

Interestingly, 5-HTP caused participants in one study to eat less even though they weren't deliberately trying to. Those taking a placebo consumed an average of 2,300 calories a day; those taking 5-HTP consumed only 1,800 calories. That's effortless dieting!

People with depression can sometimes have problems sleeping, and studies have shown that, as with prescription antidepressants, 5-HTP can help alleviate insomnia stemming from depression.

For additional information on specific health conditions and how you can treat them with supplements, see Part 3 of this book, beginning on page 309.

HOW IT WORKS

In almost all cases in which 5-HTP has been effective, this has come from the ability of this supplemental amino acid to raise levels of serotonin in the brain and throughout the body. Like antidepressants, 5-HTP does this either by binding to the receptors for serotonin on the surfaces of nerve cells and causing the body to synthesize more serotonin, or by inhibiting the reuptake of serotonin by nerve cells; when this reuptake of serotonin is blocked, the serotonin remains active, continuing to transmit signals from one nerve cell to another, as noted above.

In addition to these effects, 5-HTP also appears to have pain-relieving properties. This is partly because of its effects on serotonin production, which helps to control pain, but it may also be because 5-HTP reinforces other pain-relieving agents in the body, such as endorphins. 5-HTP also helps serotonin to function normally in blood vessels, which may account for its positive effect on migraine headaches.

Research has indicated that some forms of insomnia may be related to a deficiency of tryptophan, the amino acid that the body uses to make 5-HTP. Therefore, 5-HTP supplements may help relieve sleeplessness by enabling the body to make more tryptophan.

As for weight loss with 5-HTP, researchers think that it may partly result from 5-HTP creating a feeling of satiety after eating.

HOW TO TAKE IT

Eating foods that contain tryptophan won't raise your levels of 5-HTP enough to be of therapeutic value, for which supplements of 5-HTP are probably your best bet.

The amount of 5-HTP you need varies with the condition for which you want to use it. In almost all cases, though, once it begins to work you may be able to reduce the dosage.

Dosages of 5-HTP depend on the condition for which it is being used, but often range from 100 to 900 milligrams daily, divided into two or more doses. 5-HTP should be taken on an empty stomach.

LOOK OUT FOR THIS!

Do not use 5-HTP without consulting your doctor if you're pregnant or nursing or if you have diabetes, high blood pressure, cardiovascular disease, or an autoimmune disorder such as scleroderma.

The Tryptophan Ban and the Safety of 5-HTP

Did you ever wonder why you can no longer purchase supplements containing tryptophan—the amino acid from which 5-HTP is made? In 1989, the U.S. Food and Drug Administration (FDA) banned the sale of tryptophan as an amino acid supplement and in 1990, banned its sale as a dietary supplement, claiming that it caused a rare and deadly flu-like condition called eosinophilia myalgia syndrome (EMS). What may actually have been responsible for this EMS was a genetically engineered binder used in the manufacture of tryptophan, which studies have suggested may cause EMS.

Nevertheless, in 1998, researchers at the Mayo Clinic found that many store-bought 5-HTP supplements contained impurities, a finding that was later confirmed by the FDA, raising concerns about the safety of 5-HTP, and among these impurities was Peak X. Because of this discovery of Peak X in 5-HTP products and because of its possible link to EMS, the FDA advised supplement manufacturers to implement rigorous manufacturing controls and tests to prevent the selling of products containing impurities.

Interestingly, after the Mayo clinic reported its findings, the National Nutritional Foods Association (NNFA)—which used independent contractors to test 5-HTP supplements—was unable to replicate the Mayo Clinic's results. Moreover, despite the Mayo Clinic's findings of 5-HTP contamination, 5-HTP supplements have been widely used around the world for the past 20 years, and with the exception of only 1 unresolved case in Canada, extensive other studies have not found Peak X contaminants in 5-HTP supplements.

Although 5-HTP typically causes fewer side effects than prescription antidepressant medications, some people who take it report mild gastrointestinal complaints such as heartburn, flatulence, a feeling of fullness or rumbling sensations in the stomach, and mild nausea.

Taking too much 5-HTP may theoretically cause the condition known as serotonin syndrome, which occurs when there is too much serotonin in the body—although this condition has never been reported with 5-HTP supplementation in humans. Symptoms of this syndrome include rapid heartbeat, confusion, anxiety, muscle jerks, and loss of coordination. If any of these side effects occur, stop taking 5-HTP and consult your doctor.

WHAT TO AVOID

Medications: 5-HTP may interact adversely with carbidopa, a drug used to treat Parksinson's disease, and cause a skin condition similar to scelorderma. Zolpidem, a drug used to treat insomnia, may cause hallucinations in combination with 5-HTP.

The following medications shouldn't be taken with 5-HTP because the combined effects could produce too much serotonin in the body or increase the risk of other adverse effects: antidepressant medications of the selective serotonin reuptake inhibitor (SSRI) type; monoamine oxidase inhibitors (MAOIs); methysergide and cyproheptadine, which act to block the effects of the amino acid known as 5-hydroxytryptamine (5-HT)—a relative of 5-HTP; the 5-HT receptor agonists naratriptan, sumatriptan, and zolmitriptan; and tramadol, whose effects are similar to those of 5-HTP.

Both methyldopa and phenoxybenzamine may interfere with the conversion of 5-HTP to serotonin.

FLAXSEED

FLAX *(LINUM USITATISSIMUM)* is an incredible plant: It has been used for 10,000 years to make clothing and paper, as well as traditional medicines. About the size of sesame seeds, flaxseeds are either tan or dark brown, and can be cold-pressed to make flaxseed oil. Although many of its medical claims aren't yet fully proven, flaxseed is one of those natural products that's popular because it's still a safe, inexpensive way to boost your intake of essential fatty acids.

WHAT IT DOES

Most research with flaxseed has focused on its effects on heart disease, high cholesterol, and cancer, but from a scientific standpoint, chronic constipation remains the most solid, proven use for flaxseed. Along with its use for colon health, flaxseed shows promise in several other areas: It may enhance the function of the immune system, provide antioxidant protection against free radicals, and confer anti-inflammatory benefits. An expert panel recently advised the use of flax for people who have colons damaged by laxative use, and those who have irritable bowel syndrome, diverticulitis, and enteritis, as well as chronic constipation.

As for heart health, only a mild reduction of LDL ("bad") cholesterol is a consistent research finding with the use of flaxseed. Although animal research shows that flaxseed may reduce high blood pressure and the build-up of atheroschlerotic plaque that leads to heart attack or stroke, human studies have reached contradictory conclusions about its effects on HDL ("good") cholesterol, high cholesterol levels (hyperlipidemia), triglycerides levels, and blood pressure.

Other conditions for which flaxseed is being studied include lupus and associated kidney disease, mastalgia (breast pain), menopause, diabetes and hyperglycemia, human immunodeficiency virus (HIV) infection, prostate cancer, and bipolar disorder.

For additional information on specific health conditions and how you can treat them with supplements, see Part 3 of this book, beginning on page 309.

HOW IT WORKS

The seeds and the oil of the flax plant have different benefits. Both are rich sources of alpha-linoleic acid, an essential fatty acid not found in most vegetable oils. Alpha-linoleic acid is a precursor of omega-3 fatty acids, which have long been associated with heart health. But while alpha-linoleic acid can sometimes be converted in the body to the essential fatty acids found in fish oil (eicosapentaenoic acid [EPA] and docosahexaenoic acid [DHA]), this conversion appears to be limited. Curiously, flaxseed contains linoleic acid, an omega-6 fatty acid, that seems to inhibit alpha-linoleic acid's conversion to omega-3 fatty acids. Therefore, substituting flaxseed for fish oil is not a good way of getting omega-3 fatty acids.

Only the seeds of the flax plant contain the fiber that provides colon health and laxative properties. The seeds work by swelling, becoming gelatinous, and triggering peristalsis—the muscular contractions in the gastrointestinal tract that move food and waste through the tract—thus speeding the transit time of foods. One study showed that ground flaxseed worked better than psyllium for relieving constipation.

Besides this, only the seeds (not the oil) of flax contain lignan, a substance currently being studied for possible anticancer benefits. Studies have shown that lignan has both estrogen receptor agonist properties, acting like an estrogen on the receptors for this hormone on the surfaces of cells, and estrogen-receptor antagonist properties, acting in an opposite manner to block the action of these receptors. Therefore, it's not clear whether flaxseed boosts or blocks estrogen reception in the human body. Some animal studies show increased breast tumor size after consumption of flaxseed; others show a decrease. Human prostate cancer studies are just as contradictory: One such study associated taking alpha-linoleic acid with an increased risk of prostate cancer; another showed no effect. It's clear that as a phytoestrogen, flaxseed does affect hormone levels, but exactly how it works is still unknown.

HOW TO TAKE IT

Flaxseed can be eaten whole or can be ground into a flour or powder. Flaxseed oil is also available, in liquid or capsule form. The oil can be used in salad dressing or drizzled over vegetables, although it's more expensive than fresh flaxseeds and lacks their fiber content and possible anticancer benefits. Raw flaxseeds are more potent than flaxseed oil; cooking with flaxseed oil or baking with flaxseed flour degrades its strength. Defatted flaxseed provides only the fibrous hulls of the seeds without the essential oils.

As a general supplement for providing essential fatty acids, 1 tablespoon (15 grams) of whole or crushed flaxseeds can be taken two or three times a day. Be sure to drink 8 to 10 ounces of water per tablespoon, since flaxseed can swell and block the digestive system if you do not have enough water in your system. Alternatively, take 1 to 2 tablespoons (15 to 30 milliliters) of flaxseed oil.

One tablespoon of flaxseed oil provides about 7 grams of alpha-linoleic acid and 130 calories (mostly in unsaturated fats). If you're buying capsules of flaxseed oil, read the label carefully, since the alpha-linoleic acid dose per capsule can be confusing: A "1,000 milligram flaxseed oil" capsule might contain only 500 milligrams of alpha-linoleic acid.

If you're preparing your own flaxseed oil, it's best to grind whole flaxseed daily in a coffee or spice grinder, because once the oil oxidizes it becomes rancid very quickly unless refrigerated. Store flaxseed oil and capsules in a dark, airtight container in the refrigerator or freezer, since light, heat, and oxygen quickly make the oil rancid. If flaxseed oil smells at all bad, it has probably lost its potency. Whole flaxseed is usually safe in a cool, dry place for up to 12 months, and ground flaxseed and flaxseed oil are usually safe in the refrigerator for up to 3 months or in the freezer for 6 months.

Keep in mind that flaxseed oil is sometimes called "linseed oil," which is used to make paints and other nonedible materials, so check the label to be sure you're buying a food product.

LOOK OUT FOR THIS!

High doses of flaxseed taken for longer than 4 months may cause potassium deficiency, which can lead to muscle weakness and heart-rhythm irregularity. Immature flax pods are poisonous, so buy flaxseed at a reputable store. No data exist on the long-term use of flaxseed, although in one study flaxseed at normal doses appeared safe to take for 5 years. Megadoses of over 100 grams (7 tablespoons) per day of flaxseed may cause digestive distress.

Consult your doctor before taking flaxseed if you have a history of digestive problems (such as diverticulitis), irritable bowel syndrome, bleeding disorders, diabetes, or hypertension.

WHAT TO AVOID

Medication: In general, take any prescription medication at least 1 or 2 hours before or 2 hours after consuming flaxseed, since its laxative effect can lessen the absorption of medication. Because flaxseed oil appears to delay blood clotting, avoid taking it with antiplatelet medications such as clopidogrel or ticlodipine, or with anticoagulants like heparin and warfarin. As a phytoestrogen, flaxseed may theoretically disrupt oral contraceptive effects and hormone replacement therapies. It can also boost the effects of stool softeners and blood-pressure-lowering medications.

Herbs and Dietary Supplements: Flaxseed may interfere with the absorption of vitamins, minerals, and other supplements, so take these 1 or 2 hours before or 2 hours after taking flaxseed. Flaxseed may increase the effects of St. John's wort, valerian, niacin, garlic, guggul, and fish oil.

FOLIC ACID

FOLIC ACID (VITAMIN B$_9$) IS A B VITAMIN that deserves a whole lot of attention. Bountiful in green vegetables, some fruit, beans, and wheat germ, folate can prevent birth defects, promote heart health, and even protect against some cancers. When folate is used in supplements or fortified foods, it's called folic acid. Because dietary folates can be easily destroyed by cooking and processing and since many people do not eat enough folate-rich foods, folate deficiency is considered to be one of the most common nutritional deficiencies. Consequently, these supplemental sources are often necessary to obtain the many important health benefits that folate can provide.

WHAT IT DOES

Convincing evidence supports the role of folate in ensuring the health of mothers and their babies. Adequate folate levels have been found to reduce the risk of neural tube defects such as spina bifida and anencephaly (in which the spine and brain fail to develop normally). Folic acid supplements may also prevent other birth defects, including heart defects, cleft lip or cleft palate, and urinary tract defects. Sufficient folate intake may also reduce the risk of early miscarriage. Pregnant women who take folic acid supplements are also less likely to have high blood pressure.

Folic acid may play a role in preventing cardiovascular disease. A large study published in 2002 found that people who took the most folic acid had a lower risk of stroke and heart disease than those taking little folic acid. Some experts say that increased folate intake has reduced deaths caused by heart disease in as many as 50,000 people per year. However, recent studies found that taking B vitamins after a heart attack and for the treatment of vascular disease might do more harm than good. Be sure to consult with your doctor if you have recently had a heart attack and are thinking about taking this supplement.

Folic acid achieves this success by keeping the levels of homo-cysteine (an amino acids byproduct that may lead to heart disease) from rising, especially when it is taken together with vitamins B_6 and B_{12}.

Since preliminary research suggests that high homocysteine lev-els in the body may increase the risk for developing Alzheimer's dis-ease, folic acid supplementation may also help to prevent this condition.

In cases of anemia caused by folic acid deficiency, supplementa-tion with this nutrient is important for restoring healthy folic acid levels.

Recent studies have shown that a high folate intake may play a role in reducing the risk of colon cancer, particularly when taken for many years. There is also some evidence that it protects against cer-vical cancer and breast cancer in certain women (such as those who are heavy consumers of alcoholic beverages).

Folic acid has been found to interact in beneficial ways with certain medications. For example, a recent study found that folate supplements may enhance the effectiveness of antidepressant medications. Folic acid supplements may also reduce nausea, and vomiting, liver problems, and other side effects of methotrexate (Trexall), a drug used to treat cancer, rheumatoid arthritis, and psoriasis.

Preliminary evidence indicates that folic acid may help prevent cataracts, as well as combat gout, infertility in men, and restless legs syndrome.

Other, although weaker, evidence suggests a role for high-dose folic acid in treating bipolar disorder, osteoarthritis (when taken with vitamin B_{12}), rheumatoid arthritis, osteoporosis, seborrheic dermatitis, vitiligo (uneven loss of skin pigmentation), migraine headache, and periodontal disease and points to the need for further study of this important vitamin.

For additional information on specific health conditions and how you can treat them with supplements, see Part 3 of this book, beginning on page 309.

HOW IT WORKS

Folate is involved in many vital processes in the body. Its vital role in DNA production, nervous system maintenance, and healthy cell

SUPPLEMENTAL TRIVIA

In just over a decade, folate has had an enormous impact on the health of babies in the United States. Efforts to increase the intake of folate finally began in 1992, when the U.S. Public Health Service urged all women of childbearing age to take at least 400 micrograms of folate every day. In 1998, food manufacturers were required to begin fortifying refined grain products to help women meet the recommended levels of folate. Since then, there has been a 25 percent reduction in the number of neural tube defects in the United States, and the lives of about 4,000 children have been saved.

division may be responsible for its prevention of certain birth defects. In terms of preventing cancer, folate may have the ability to prevent unhealthy cell division. And in matters of cardiovascular health, folate may have the ability (when taken together with vitamins B_6 and B_{12}) to reduce levels of homocysteine in the blood, thereby reducing the risk of heart disease and stroke, as noted earlier.

HOW TO TAKE IT

Your need for folic acid rises with age and is greatest for pregnant and nursing women. See the table below for the recommended daily intakes (RDIs) of this important nutrient.

AGE/GENDER/ CONDITION	RECOMMENDED DAILY INTAKE (RDI)*
Infants	
0–6 months	65 mcg
7–12 months	80 mcg
Children	
1–3 years	150 mcg
4–8 years	200 mcg
Males	
9–13 years	300 mcg
14 years and older	400 mcg
Females	
9–13 years	300 mcg
14 years and older	400 mcg
Pregnant Women	600 mcg
Nursing Women	500 mcg

For more information on RDIs, see Want to Know More About Intake? on page 8.

Folate is a part of the B-complex vitamin group (a term given to a group of eight important B vitamins), and most general purpose multivitamin and mineral supplements contain the full range of B vitamins (be sure to check the label).

The upper safe limit for folic acid from supplements or fortified foods is 1,000 micrograms per day. Higher doses can mask the symptoms of a vitamin B_{12} deficiency (a type of anemia), allowing nerve damage to develop. This is of particular concern for older people. If you plan to take more than 400 micrograms of folate per day, be sure to have your vitamin B_{12} levels checked first.

People who may need to take a folic acid supplement include women of childbearing age, pregnant women, people with alcoholism, people taking certain medications (such as anticonvulsants or other medications that interfere with the action of folate), people with a diagnosed folate deficiency, and those with liver disease or who require dialysis for kidney problems.

LOOK OUT FOR THIS!

When taken at recommended levels, folic acid is very safe, although some people have developed fever, shortness of breath, skin rash, or in rare cases, diarrhea, with this supplement. When taken in very high doses (over 5,000 micrograms), folic acid can cause loss of appetite, nausea, flatulence, and abdominal bloating. If you have cardiovascular disease or a history of stroke, be sure to consult with your doctor before taking a folate supplement.

WHAT TO AVOID

Medication: Certain medications can interfere with your body's absorption of folic acid. These include aspirin and other anti-inflammatory medications, antacids, histamine blockers, sulfa antibiotics, oral contraceptives, bile-acid sequestrants such as cholestyramine and colestipol, nitrous oxide, high-dose triamterene, oral hypoglycemic medications, steroids, and decongestants containing pseudoephedrine. People taking the medication known as pancreatin as well as folic acid should separate their doses of one from the other by at least 2 hours to avoid absorption problems.

Folic acid may interfere with antiseizure medications such as valproic acid, carbamazepine, primidone, and phenytoin and thus cause seizures. If you are taking any of these medications, be sure to consult your doctor before taking folic acid supplements.

As mentioned above, adding folic acid to methotrexate treatment for certain conditions may be beneficial. However, be sure to consult your doctor before taking folic acid supplements, since they may also decrease the effectiveness of methotrexate.

Herbs or Dietary Supplements: People taking digestive-enzyme supplements should separate their doses of these from folic acid by at least 2 hours to avoid absorption problems.

FOOD SOURCES

FOLATE

Although folate is abundant in many foods, it is easily destroyed by cooking and processing. A diet rich in fruits, vegetables, and grains should supply an ample amount of folate. Some of the foods listed below are good choices. When it comes to vegetables, eat them raw or lightly steamed, since the cooking process destroys folate.

▶Asparagus, beans, beef liver, brewer's yeast, dark, green, leafy vegetables (for example, broccoli, brussels sprouts), kelp, oranges and other fruits, rice, soybeans, and soy flour.

Be aware that supplemental forms of folic acid (supplements and fortified foods) may be better absorbed than folate from food. Avoid relying on "fortified foods" such as breakfast cereal to obtain your daily folate, since many of these foods contain large amounts of refined sugars.

GARLIC

GARLIC *(ALLIUM SATIVUM)* MAY be bad for your breath (and toxic to vampires!) but it's good for your health. Americans spent $61 billion on garlic in the year 2000, making this pungent bulb one of the most popular herbs in the United States, both as a conventional food and as a dietary supplement. Garlic has been regarded as a medicinal remedy for centuries—an Egyptian papyrus from 1550 BC mentions its benefits. Yet garlic wasn't really studied in Western medicine until the 1930s. Today, this "stinking rose" is believed to promote heart health as well as provide a variety of other potential health benefits.

WHAT IT DOES

Garlic has shown medicinal potential in several areas, and may have antibacterial, antiviral, antifungal, anticancer, and antiparasitic properties. Garlic may even be useful in the treatment of sickle-cell anemia.

Studies have shown that garlic may prevent heart attacks. In a controlled study, 423 people who had a previous heart attack were either given garlic oil extract or no treatment over the course of 3 years. Those who were given the garlic oil had a significantly lower risk of having a second heart attack.

Garlic may also have medicinal potential in preventing colds. Although people have been touting the cold-fighting potential of garlic for years, it wasn't until 2001 that scientific evidence supported this claim. In a 12-week, double-blind, placebo-controlled study conducted between November and February, 146 people were given either garlic extract or a placebo. Those who took the extract were about two-thirds less likely to catch a cold than those who took the placebo. Furthermore, those who took garlic recovered from their colds an average of one day sooner than those who did not.

Numerous trials have suggested that garlic is an effective treatment for hyperlipidemia (excess lipids in the blood) and for age-related vascular disorders—taking garlic may lower the levels of both total cholesterol and LDL ("bad") cholesterol in the blood. Garlic is also commonly used to prevent the buildup of atherosclerotic plaque in the arteries and to reduce high blood pressure.

Because of its power as an antibacterial and antifungal agent, garlic is often recommended for killing the intestinal bacteria that may cause diarrhea and urinary tract infections, and the fungi that cause yeast infection and athlete's foot.

Because of its antibacterial properties, preliminary research suggests that garlic may kill the *Helicobacter pylori* bacteria that cause ulcers. Garlic may also reduce the risk of developing colon and stomach cancers. Preliminary studies are beginning to examine the role of garlic treatment and prevention of gastric cancer.

Research also suggests that garlic may help to maintain proper blood-sugar levels in people with diabetes.

For additional information on specific health conditions and how you can treat them with supplements, see Part 3 of this book, beginning on page 309.

HOW IT WORKS

Garlic contains various sulfur compounds, including the substances known as alliin and alliinase, which are converted into another substance known as allicin. Allicin is the chemical that gives garlic its unmistakable odor, but it may also provide the health-fortifying properties of this herb. Sulfur compounds—isolated from the raw cloves of garlic—appear to have infection-fighting properties and may protect the heart, but the precise mechanism by which garlic helps lower cholesterol is unknown.

Aside from allicin, garlic contains compounds called clutamylcysteines and fructans. These compounds are credited with garlic's blood-pressure-lowering effects.

Studies show that garlic may contain enzymes that can reduce levels of lipids in the blood and inhibit platelet adhesion—the process in which blood platelets form blood clots—resulting in improved heart health.

Garlic, may also have antifungal and antibacterial abilities when applied topically. Preliminary evidence suggests that a compound derived from garlic, called ajoene, may help soothe athlete's foot.

HOW TO TAKE IT

Garlic is available in tablet, capsule, powder, tincture, and oil forms. In preparing food, raw garlic is generally more potent than cooked garlic, and fresh garlic is more potent than old garlic.

The German Commission E (see page 16) recommends taking 4 grams (or 1 clove) of fresh garlic daily for lipid-lowering effects.

The amounts of allicin and other important ingredients in both fresh and commercial garlic products vary widely. If you choose to

SUPPLEMENTAL TRIVIA

During World War I, garlic was widely used as an antiseptic dressing for battle wounds. Since cotton was in short supply, peat moss (sphagnum moss) was used as a substitute for covering wounds! During World War II, garlic was often referred to as "Russian penicillin" because of its use to replace antibiotics, which were in short supply.

take garlic in capsule form, try to choose a product standardized to contain 1.3 percent allicin or 5,000 to 6,000 milligrams of "allicin potential."

Allicin potential is a term given to a process that manufacturers use to make the allicin in garlic more potent in the body. Allicin potential is measured by adding water to garlic products that contain alliin and alliinase in order to determine how much allicin they will yield in the body.

Some studies suggest that aged garlic extract may be more useful than other types of garlic for preventing cancer.

LOOK OUT FOR THIS!

Side effects of garlic may include mild gastrointestinal problems such as heartburn and nausea, upset stomach, bloating, bad breath, body odor, and a stinging sensation on the skin from handling too much garlic.

Other side effects may include headache, fatigue, appetite loss, muscle aches, dizziness, and allergies.

The use of garlic is considered safe for adults and children. Garlic is presumed to be safe for pregnant women and breastfeeding women, but pregnant or breastfeeding women should consult their doctor before taking garlic supplements.

Avoid taking garlic before surgery, since it poses a risk of causing excess bleeding.

WHAT TO AVOID

Medication: Be sure to consult your doctor before taking garlic with aspirin, anticoagulants and antiplatelet drugs, nonsteroidal anti-inflammatory drugs (NSAIDs), antihypertensive drugs, certain diabetes medications, hypoglycemic drugs, saquinavir—a protease inhibitor—thyroid drugs and iodine, and lipid-lowering drugs because garlic may intensify the effects of these medications.

GINGER

WHILE YOUR EXPERIENCE WITH GINGER *(Zingiber officinale)* may be limited to the tasty accompaniment of your favorite sushi dish, herbalists in Asian, Indian, and Arabic cultures have been using ginger since ancient times for a vast array of ailments, including gastrointestinal disturbances, inflamed joints, and heart conditions. Not only is ginger a valuable resource when cooking—especially when preparing a marinade for beef or chicken—this potent spice can be a saving grace for anyone feeling nauseous or suffering from diarrhea.

When used sparingly, this wonderful herb can hit the spot, whether it's a spice you crave or a desperately needed antidote to motion sickness.

WHAT IT DOES

Given the safety of ginger, it is often a welcome alternative to over-the-counter medications for combating nausea. In many studies, ginger has outperformed prescription medications in its ability to stop nausea, without causing sedation and the other side effects commonly associated with anti-emetic drugs. And for people who have motion sickness, taking ginger 30 minutes before traveling just might nip queasiness in the bud. Ginger has also been shown to be an effective and safe supplement for reducing nausea during early pregnancy. And a study testing the efficacy of ginger on postoperative nausea and vomiting found that it was as effective as the drug metoclopramide (Reglan) for treating nausea.

Ginger may also be useful in treating other gastrointestinal problems, such as irritable bowel syndrome, digestive problems, and excessive gas.

Although evidence for such an effect is limited, ginger, because of its power as an anti-inflammatory agent, may have promise for decreasing the pain and swelling that accompanies various forms of arthritis and joint inflammation. Some laboratory studies suggest that ginger may be more potent than aspirin for reducing inflammation.

Although no human studies exist for documenting ginger's effectiveness as a heart-protecting agent, preliminary animal studies have shown that ginger may have a positive effect against unwanted blood clotting, as well as reducing cholesterol levels.

A staple of traditional Chinese medicine, ginger is often recommended for treating colds and flu. Because of its potential ability to kill certain bacteria and viruses, ginger may indeed be useful for treating colds, flu, and sinusitis.

For additional information on specific health conditions and how you can treat them with supplements, see Part 3 of this book, beginning on page 309.

GROW THIS!

Ginger is very easy to grow at home from a piece of the root, which you can purchase at a health food store. Use regular potting soil and put the root down horizontally. Barely cover it, and make sure to keep the soil moist and warm, but not wet. It's that simple!

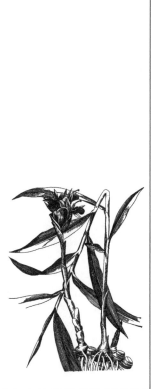

HOW IT WORKS

Rather than acting on the brain, as do many over-the-counter medications, ginger reduces nausea by slowing the pathway from the stomach to the brain that stimulates nausea.

Ginger may aid digestion by increasing the action of peristalsis, the muscle contraction in the digestive tract that pushes food through the digestive system.

HOW TO TAKE IT

Ginger products are made from fresh or dried ginger root. Common forms of ginger include capsules, liquid extract, tincture, oil, tea, powder, and fresh or dried root. A simple way to take ginger at home: Take a piece of fresh root and squeeze it with a garlic press to extract the juice.

For most purposes, the standard dosage of ginger is 1 to 4 grams daily, divided into two to four doses.

LOOK OUT FOR THIS!

Few side effects have been reported in people taking high doses of ginger (more than 6 grams); they include heartburn, bloating, and gas. Ginger may occasionally cause heartburn when taken in lower dosages.

Pregnant women and people with gallstones should consult a doctor before taking ginger, although ginger is generally thought to be an extremely safe herb. Ginger should not be given to children under 2 years of age.

WHAT TO AVOID

Medication: Excessive doses of ginger may interfere with cardiac, antidiabetic, or anticoagulant medications and herbs. Some evidence exists that ginger may interfere with heartburn, ulcer, and antireflux medications.

GINKGO BILOBA

GINKGO BILOBA (ALSO CALLED GINKGO) is called a "living fossil" because it's believed to be the oldest surviving tree species on earth—about 200 million years old. Ginkgo was first mentioned in 1436, during the Chinese Ming dynasty, for treating respiratory ailments, for improving circulation and digestion, and for boosting memory. Most preparations of ginkgo come from the dried, green leaf of *ginkgo biloba,* easily recognized by its split lobes. Unlike most herbs, an extract from the ginkgo leaf and not the leaf itself is used for medicinal purposes. This extract—*Ginkgo biloba* extract (GBE)—is one of the most popular herbs in Europe and the United States.

WHAT IT DOES

The German Commission E (see page 16) has approved the use of ginkgo for treating memory loss, tinnitus, vertigo, and disorders of blood circulation. Studies show that ginkgo has beneficial effects on dementia, poor memory, and poor concentration, as well as on certain cardiovascular and circulatory problems, such as the leg pain known as intermittent claudication.

Ginkgo may also be helpful in overcoming sexual dysfunction associated with taking the selective serotonin reuptake inhibitor (SSRI) class of drugs for depression, but not all studies have found it to have beneficial effects for this purpose.

Although further research is needed, ginkgo has also shown potential for alleviating symptoms of vascular reactivity to cold exposure as well as for battling hypoxia, or oxygen shortage, and deafness related to the part of the ear known as the cochlea. While ginkgo has also shown potential for alleviating symptoms of altitude sickness, several recent studies were unable to confirm this application. Although study results are conflicting, preliminary research suggests that ginkgo may reduce symptoms of tinnitus, and may be as effective as the prescription medication pentoxifylline (Trental) for treating sudden deafness.

The potential benefits of ginkgo may also extend to the eyes, with studies indicating that the antioxidant effects of this herb may improve vision in people with glaucoma, cataracts, and macular degeneration.

Among its other purported benefits, ginkgo may ease fibrocystic breast pain, fibromyalgia (when taken together with coenzyme Q10), cyclic edema, asthma, Raynaud's disease, and premenstrual syndrome and may enhance the effectiveness of antipsychotic medications while reducing their side effects. It may also help in treating equilibrium disorders and reduce blood pressure during times of stress.

For additional information on specific health conditions and how to treat them with supplements, see Part 3 of this book, beginning on page 309.

HOW IT WORKS

Ginkgo's widespread effectiveness in treating a variety of seemingly unrelated conditions may come from its ability to improve blood flow to the brain and other parts of the body, as well as to improve the metabolism in cells.

The flavonoids and terpenoids in ginkgo may explain some of its therapeutic functions. Flavonoids have antioxidant effects and aid in cleansing the body by eliminating cell- and tissue-damaging free radicals and in maintaining healthy cells. Terpenoids improve blood flow and reduce the possibility of blood clots by dilating blood vessels and increasing blood flow to the brain and extremities.

HOW TO TAKE IT

As a supplement, ginkgo is commercially available in capsules, tablets, and tinctures. It is most frequently used in the form of concentrated *Ginkgo biloba* extract (GBE) standardized to contain 24 percent flavonoids and 6 percent terpenoids. Standard doses of ginkgo are usually 120 to 160 milligrams daily.

LOOK OUT FOR THIS!

Side effects of ginkgo may include occasional gastrointestinal problems, headaches, dizziness, palpitations, and skin reactions.

Ginkgo, when taken in small doses, is considered safe for adults. The use of ginkgo is not suitable for children or for women who are pregnant or nursing. People with severe liver or kidney disease, bleeding disorders, and who have a history of seizures should also avoid taking this herb. Discontinue using ginkgo 2 weeks before scheduled surgery, since it has blood-thinning effects and may increase the risk of bleeding.

WHAT TO AVOID

Medication: Ginkgo may not be safe to take with blood-thinning drugs such as aspirin and warfarin or with anticonvulsants, cyclosporine, the monoamine oxidase inhibitor (MAOI) class of antidepressants, papaverine, thiazide diuretics, or trazodone. Consult your doctor if you are taking any of these medications, since ginkgo may intensify their blood-thinning effects.

GINSENG

THE CHANCES ARE GOOD that if you have heard of only one herb, it's ginseng. Ginseng is one of the most commonly and widely used medicinal herbs. In the year 2000, Americans spent about $62.5 million on ginseng. In fact, though, ginseng is not really one herb—the term "ginseng" refers to several species of the plant genus *Panax*. The two most commonly used supplements in this genus are American and Asian each of which contains a different profile of chemical substances. Siberian ginseng is a distant cousin to the panax species.

Both American and Asian ginseng *(Panax ginseng and Panax quinquefolium)* belong to the genus Panax, and have tan-colored, gnarly roots with stringy shoots that can sometimes look like human arms and legs. Ancient herbalists thought that this shape meant that the root could cure human ailments, and it has been used in many cultures as a "cure-all." In fact, *Panax* is the Latin word for "all illness." The Chinese regard ginseng as the king of herbs: something that brings not just good health to those who take it, but also wisdom.

Siberian ginseng *(Eleutherococcus senticosus)*, also know as *Acanthopanax senticous,* is entirely different from American and Asian ginseng. It is a different plant with a different chemical makeup. However, Siberian ginseng has been promoted in Russia as a less expensive alternative to Asian ginseng—which is nearly extinct in the wild as a result of overharvesting—because it was believed to have the same health benefits. While the active ingredients in Siberian ginseng, eleutherosides (similar to ginsenosides in the panax species) are thought to increase stamina, not all studies have demonstated this. Preliminary studies indicate that Siberian ginseng appears to stimulate the immune system, and in vitro studies of cell cultures indicate antiviral activity against influenza A. However, more research is needed to confirm this.

WHAT IT DOES

Ginseng is widely advertised as the "cure-all" that the Chinese believed it to be—and that, coupled with the three different species of this herb that are sold as supplements, can make it puzzling to decipher just what ginseng *can* do. Largely, ginseng is used to help curb fatigue and to improve concentration and focus.

Some researchers consider ginseng an adaptogentic herb. Adaptogentic herbs are essentially herbs that combat stress through

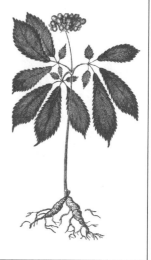

SUPPLEMENTAL
TRIVIA

Written records of the use of ginseng in China date back to 100 AD. In ancient times, ginseng was considered a royal plant, and Asian rulers reserved its use for themselves. During the Chin dynasty in China, people who were caught stealing ginseng from the emperor's stash were beheaded, and both their family and belongings were confiscated.

nonspecific actions and create balance in the entire body. That means that whether you are healthy or sick, an adaptogentic herb should help protect your body from stress.

Ginseng appears to help balance blood glucose levels for people with type 2 diabetes. A double-blind, placebo-controlled study of 36 individuals who had all recently been diagnosed as having type 2 diabetes found that 200 milligrams of ginseng once a day improved blood glucose levels, concentration, and physical performance after 8 weeks of therapy. Ginseng may also be beneficial for maintaining blood sugar levels in nondiabetic people. Further research is being conducted to test ginseng's effect on blood glucose levels.

Human trials suggest that ginseng may also be beneficial in boosting the immune system. In one double-blind, placebo-controlled study of 227 participants, people who were given 100 milligrams of ginseng a day showed a significantly lower frequency of colds and flu than the placebo group. A subsequent study obtained similar results; regular ingestion of ginseng reduced the number and severity of colds. And yet another study found ginseng effective in preventing upper respiratory tract infections in institutionalized elderly persons. Ginseng may also increase the ability of people with chronic obstructive pulmonary disease (COPD) to exercise.

Perhaps one of ginseng's most famous uses is for enhancing mental function. In several studies, ginseng has displayed an ability to modestly improve cognition. These benefits have been seen in people of all ages and in sick as well as in healthy individuals. One study found that American and Asian ginseng improved thought processes. Specifically, the two ginsengs seemed to improve people's ability to detect errors and proofread. Some studies suggest that ginkgo may increase the memory-enhancing effect of ginseng when these herbs are taken together. While this evidence is promising, many researchers are not convinced of the cognitive-enhancing potential of ginseng, and more research is needed to confirm this property of the herb.

The variety of ginseng known as Asian red ginseng may help treat erectile dysfunction. Besides improving the immune system of people with human immunodeficiency virus (HIV) and acquired immune deficiency syndrome (AIDS), when taken on a long-term basis, Asian red ginseng may delay resistance to the medication zidovudine (zidovudine; AZT) in people with HIV infection.

Other studies indicate that ginseng may be helpful for treating gout and fibromyalgia. On the other hand, research on the effects of Asian and American ginseng on attention deficit hyperactivity disorder (ADHD), alcohol intoxication, cancer, cardiovascular disorders, depression, fertility and sexual performance, menopause, mood enhancement, and respiratory function has been inconclusive.

Preliminary research suggests that ginseng may help improve sperm count and sperm motility in men with infertility. Ginseng may also increase appetite, especially when the loss of appetite is due to fatigue or illness.

For additional information on specific health conditions and how you can treat them with supplements, see Part 3 of this book, beginning on page 309.

HOW IT WORKS

The active ingredients in American and Asian ginseng are called ginsenosides. Siberian ginseng does not contain ginsenoides, which is why it is considered to be the milder, less potent form of ginseng. Ginsenoides seem to target several tissues in the body, producing several different effects, such as altering blood flow to the brain, modifying the levels of certain neurotransmitters, and possibly exerting mild hormonal effects.

HOW TO TAKE IT

Ginseng comes in several forms, including powder, capsules, and either fresh or dried root in water or alcohol mixtures. Dried, unprocessed ginseng root is called white ginseng and is often considered more calming than with the processed root; ginseng that has been cured by steaming in aconite juice is called red ginseng and is considered more warming.

Be aware that some commercial ginseng products contain very little ginseng. The plant must be grown for 5 years before it can be harvested, which means that it can be very expensive. Top-quality ginseng products are standardized on the basis of their ginsenoside content and should contain 4 to 5 percent ginsenosides (for American and Asian ginseng) or 0.5 to 1.0 percent eleutherosides (for Siberian ginseng).

Dosages of ginseng vary, so be sure to check individual product labels for dosage information.

Note: Make sure to distinguish between Asian (white and red) and American ginseng varieties (called *panax*) and Siberian ginseng. Although there's some overlap, they have different actions and side effects.

Ginseng should not be taken for more than a 3-month period without a resting period before taking it again.

LOOK OUT FOR THIS!

Ginseng is generally considered to be safe. No reports have suggested that ginseng is harmful for pregnant or nursing women. People with low blood sugar levels should be cautious about taking ginseng because it may reduce blood sugar levels. Anyone with acute illness or diabetes should also use caution when taking ginseng and should consult their doctor before doing so.

Use of ginseng should be stopped at least a week before surgery, since it may have blood-thinning properties and may also lower blood sugar levels, which can be problematic for people who are fasting before surgery.

WHAT TO AVOID

Medication: Consult your doctor before taking American or Asian ginseng with blood-thinning agents, haloperidol, morphine, or phenelzine and other monoamine oxidase inhibitors (MAOIs) for depression. Use with caution if you are taking insulin or oral hypoglycemic medication.

GLUCOSAMINE

WHAT HAPPENS WHEN YOU JOIN an amino acid with a sugar? In the case of glucosamine—which is made from the amino acid glutamine and glucose (the main sugar found in blood)—you get an amino-sugar, also called an aminopolysaccharide. Glucosamine is produced naturally by the body, and its main role is to help build cartilage, so it's no surprise that some researchers believe that glucosamine supplements may reduce the pain and inflammation associated with the joint disease osteoarthritis.

WHAT IT DOES

Glucosamine's best-known use is for treating joint pain and increasing mobility in people with mild to moderate osteoarthritis. Studies show that while it may not work as quickly as over-the-counter pain relievers such as ibuprofen and aspirin, glucosamine may have similar pain-relieving effects to these drugs. Additionally, many people experience fewer side effects with glucosamine than with conventional arthritis medications. And unlike many other treatments for arthritis, glucosamine may have the ability to prevent further joint damage by this disease, slowing the progression of the disease. While several recent studies were unable to find benefit for glucosamine in the treatment of osteoarthritis of the knee, another group of studies found that glucosamine helped decrease osteoarthritis progression in postmenopausal women with knee arthritis.

Preliminary studies show that glucosamine may also be effective in treating osteochondritis of the knee, a condition that affects the cartilage in the knee and is related to osteoarthritis.

Many studies of glucosamine's effects on osteoarthritis give it in combination with chondroitin sulfate. It is not yet clear which compound is more effective in treating arthritis, or if these two supplements have synergistic effects when they are combined. An ongoing study (called the Glucosamine/Chondroitin Arthritis Intervention Trial) sponsored by the U.S. National Institutes of Health is designed to learn more about these supplements when taken individually and in conjunction with one another. (For more information on chondroitin, see page 74.)

Some athletes use glucosamine to prevent muscle and tendon injuries; however, there are no scientific studies to support these uses.

For additional information on specific health conditions and how to treat them with supplements, see Part 3 of this book, beginning on page 309.

HOW IT WORKS

In theory, glucosamine works by maintaining the cartilage in joints and repairing damage to joints. Glucosamine may also stimulate cartilage cells (or chondrocytes) to create healthy, new cartilage.

HOW TO TAKE IT

Glucosamine is available in three forms—glucosamine sulfate, glucosamine hydrochloride, and N-acetyl glucosamine—all of which are available in capsules and tablets. There is no evidence that one form is better than another. Glucosamine is also sold as a combination supplement with chondroitin sulfate.

A typical dose of glucosamine for the treatment of osteoarthritis is 1,500 milligrams daily, divided into three doses. Keep in mind that several weeks may be needed for glucosamine to begin working.

LOOK OUT FOR THIS!

Glucosamine is generally a safe supplement. Mild side effects include gastrointestinal complaints such as heartburn, diarrhea, and stomach pain.

However, glucosamine is often made from the shells of shrimp, lobster, and crab, which can cause sometimes serious allergic reactions. If you are allergic to shellfish or eat a kosher diet, look for a supplement whose label states that it is shellfish free.

While some research shows that glucosamine may increase insulin resistance and affect glucose tolerance, recent studies indicate that it does not have this effect. Just to be sure, however, people with diabetes should speak with their doctor before using glucosamine.

WHAT TO AVOID

There are no known interactions between glucosamine and other supplements, herbs, or prescription medications.

GLUTAMINE

GLUTAMINE—ALSO KNOWN AS L-GLUTAMINE—is the most common amino acid in the human body and is involved in more metabolic processes than any other amino acid. It plays a major role in the health of the immune system, digestive tract, and muscle cells. The body manufactures glutamine from glutamic acid (another amino acid) in the liver.

Certain people are susceptible to glutamine deficiencies, which are often caused by health conditions or temporary infections. People who suffer from liver cirrhosis or cancer, or who experience weight loss because of human immunodeficiency virus (HIV) or acquired immunodeficiency syndrome (AIDS), often have glutamine deficiencies.

Other factors—such as intense exercise, infections, and surgery—may trigger glutamine depletion. For example, some scientific studies suggest that glutamine supplements may prevent endurance athletes from catching colds or getting infections after periods of major athletic exertion—a common occurrence. On the basis of this theory, glutamine supplements are extremely popular with athletes eager to boost their performance, maintain muscle mass, and prevent illness.

Ironically, not much solid research has been done on the use of glutamine for athletes—even though they are the biggest consumers of glutamine supplements. Glutamine may be useful in the treatment of children with sickle-cell anemia because of its ability to decrease resting energy expenditure, thereby increasing body weight and nutritional status.

WHAT IT DOES

When the body is under stress, the immune system becomes more susceptible to infection, perhaps because the body has not manufactured enough glutamine to replace what's been lost. Scientific studies support the use of glutamine to maintain muscle mass and boost the immune system of critically ill patients, as well as for people recovering from extensive burns, major surgery, trauma, or anyone with intestinal problems, such as gastritis, ulcers, and colitis. Individuals with problems in the intestinal lining may also benefit from glutamine.

Glutamine is also being studied as a therapy for angina, various digestive conditions, food allergies, and alcoholism. Studies are revealing that glutamine may help reduce side effects of chemotherapy, such a peripheral neuropathy. One study found that glutamine could reduce the oral inflammation occurring in pediatric stem cell patients.

For additional information on specific health conditions and how to treat them with supplements, see Part 3 of this book, beginning on page 309.

HOW IT WORKS

Glutamine is stored in muscle tissues throughout the body, and is constantly being converted to glucose and used for energy. It is particularly important as a fuel for the cells lining the intestines.

When converted to a related substance called glutamate and combined with a substance called N-Acetylcysteine (see page 213), glutamine helps the body to synthesize glutathione, an antioxidant.

HOW TO TAKE IT

Glutamine supplements are commercially available in powder form and as capsules. The powder is tasteless and can be mixed with water,

---

FOOD SOURCES

GLUTAMINE

Looking to boost your intake of glutamine through your diet? Make sure to eat plenty of high-protein foods packed with this important amino acid, including the foods listed below.

▶ Beans, beef, cheese, chicken, cod, crab, eggs, ham, lobster, macadamia nuts, oyster, salmon, shrimp, trout, turkey, and walnuts.

but don't add it to hot or acidic liquids such as orange juice, since it may change their chemical composition. Dosages of glutamine range from 1 to 10 grams daily.

LOOK OUT FOR THIS!

Few side effects are associated with glutamine supplementation. Occasionally, constipation may occur. To counter this side effect, drink at least 10 glasses of water a day when taking glutamine supplements. People who have chronic constipation might also want to take some type of soluble fiber while taking glutamine.

Glutamine is generally considered a safe supplement, although pregnant and nursing women should consult their doctor before taking it. Additionally, people with kidney or liver problems, or those undergoing chemotherapy, should avoid glutamine.

WHAT TO AVOID

Medication: Consult your doctor before taking glutamine with antibiotics for stomach ulcers, or with antiseizure medications such as carbamazepine, phenobarbital, phenytoin, primidone, and valproic acid, since glutamine may interfere with the effects of these drugs.

GLUTATHIONE

YOU MIGHT FIND GLUTATHIONE just a bit frustrating. It's a small protein molecule that's found in virtually every one of your cells. Your body manufactures it from three amino acids, the most significant of which is cysteine. Glutathione plays such a significant role in human health—performing many vital functions and helping to prevent and protect against disease—that it has been aptly dubbed a "naturally occurring universal drug."

Unfortunately, we tend to become deficient in glutathione as we age. Glutathione supplements are available, but even more unfortunately, studies show that glutathione taken orally is almost entirely destroyed by the digestive process.

There is hope, however. At least one patented product based on whey protein appears to supply the body with the building blocks it needs to make enough glutathione. And you can also boost your levels of glutathione with N-Acetylcysteine (NAC; see page 213), whey protein, or alpha lipoic acid (see page 29).

WHAT IT DOES

Glutathione may be the body's most important antioxidant, routinely fighting off the onslaught of cell-damaging oxygen free radicals. Antioxidants have been found to keep cells and tissues healthy and may help prevent heart disease and cancer. In particular, some research has indicated that glutathione may help fight colon cancer.

Our bodies take in many harmful substances from the environment, including heavy metals such as mercury and lead, pesticides, air pollutants, and harmful breakdown products, or metabolites, of medications. Glutathione has been called the body's main detoxifying agent. It is found in particularly high concentrations in the kidneys, liver and lungs, sites where toxins can accumulate, and it is in these locations that glutathione is most likely to deal with these harmful substances.

Glutathione also helps keep the immune system functioning properly. The greater tendency of older people to get sick may come from their bodies' having less glutathione. Some studies suggest that people with diseases such as acquired immune deficiency syndrome (AIDS) and others that damage the immune system may benefit from getting extra glutathione into their systems.

Other conditions that may be treated with glutathione are male infertility caused by a lack of mobility of sperm, noise-induced hearing loss, high blood pressure in people with diabetes, Parkinson's disease, chronic rhinitis, and cystic fibrosis. It is also possible that glutathione may reduce the undesirable side effects of the chemotherapy medication cisplatin (Platinol-AQ).

Some health conditions are associated with a deficiency of glutathione. These include human immunodeficiency virus (HIV), cirrhosis of the liver, alcoholic pancreatitis, Crohn's disease and gastrointestinal inflammation, pulmonary diseases, acute heart attack, diabetes, Parkinson's disease, and Alzheimer's disease.

For additional information on specific health conditions and how you can treat them with supplements, see Part 3 of this book, beginning on page 309.

HOW IT WORKS

Most of glutathione's beneficial effects are due to its role as a potent antioxidant. Cells produce energy in structures called mitochondria, where they "burn" glucose as fuel by using oxygen. By-products of this process are oxygen free radicals, which can damage parts of cells and may even cause mutations in deoxyribonucleic acid (DNA), the giant molecular substance that carries the genetic code. Glutathione works chemically to neutralize free radicals.

Besides this, the immune system benefits from glutathione in a couple of ways. Glutathione protects the immune system through its antioxidant action, and it helps carry nutrients to two important types of immune cells, lymphocytes and phagocytes.

Researchers think that noise-induced hearing loss may in part result from so-called oxidative stress, in which cells and tissues are damaged by free radicals. Through its antioxidant action, glutathione may help treat this condition.

HOW TO TAKE IT

Although glutathione is available in oral form as a supplement, studies indicate that when taken in this way it is broken down by the digestive system and therefore is not absorbed in its whole, useful form for use by cells. However, some studies have found that an aerosol version of glutathione can help with the treatment of cystic fibrosis and may help address glutathione deficiency in AIDS patients. In some cases, intravenous administration of glutathione may be helpful. All of these uses of glutathione require medical supervision.

You may be able to raise your glutathione levels by taking NAC (see page 213). The antioxidant alpha lipoic acid (ALA; see page 29) may also raise levels of glutathione in the body, especially in patients with HIV infection. According to some studies, whey protein may raise levels of glutathione in the body.

You may also be able to increase your supply of glutathione by taking 500 milligrams of vitamin C a day. One study showed that this amount of vitamin C raised blood levels of glutathione by as much as 50 percent in 2 weeks, whereas diets with a low content of vitamin C were found to decrease glutathione levels.

Dietary glutathione may be found in fresh and frozen fruits and vegetables, fish, meat, asparagus, avocado, and walnuts.

LOOK OUT FOR THIS!

Pregnant or nursing women should consult their doctor before taking glutathione supplements.

If you're taking an immunosuppressant medication, consult your doctor before trying any kind of glutathione-raising supplement.

If you have an allergy to milk proteins, do not take whey protein supplements, since they may raise glutathione levels.

WHAT TO AVOID

There are no known interactions of glutathione when taken orally with other drugs, herbs, or supplements.

GOLDENSEAL

IT WAS THE NATIVE AMERICAN TRIBES, specifically the Cherokee and Iroquois, who discovered the healing properties of the goldenseal plant *(Hydrastis canadensis)* and shared them with early American settlers. They used goldenseal to treat skin diseases, stomach ailments, and tired, irritated eyes. The name "goldenseal" comes from the gold-colored scars on the roots of the plant, which resemble the wax seals used on envelopes in the nineteenth century.

In the mid-1990s, word spread that drinking goldenseal tea would mask illegal drugs in the blood and urine. Although it wasn't true, the rumor gave a huge boost to sales of goldenseal. Unfortunately, goldenseal crops were drastically over-harvested, and the plant became nearly endangered. Today, the international trade in goldenseal is closely monitored for this reason.

WHAT IT DOES

Goldenseal is one of the top-selling herbal products in the United States and is found in dozens of dietary supplements and remedies for just about everything under the sun, from bad breath and the common flu to cancer. However, more scientific studies are needed to evaluate its effects on humans.

Often sold together with echinacea (see page 107), goldenseal is commonly found in remedies for hay fever, colds, the flu, and upper respiratory infections, and it can boost the immune system. Goldenseal is also used as an antiseptic for minor cuts and scrapes. Another use of goldenseal is as a mouthwash for sore throats and canker sores and to soothe upset stomach and aid digestion. It may also be helpful for urinary tract infections and diarrhea. Scientific evidence

FRIENDS AND FOES

Beware of faulty advertising for goldenseal! Many products that are labeled "goldenseal" may contain "goldenseal herb," which is produced from the leaves of the goldenseal plant rather than from the root. The leaves contain significantly less of the alkaloids usually found in the root, making such products virtually useless.

is beginning to document the antibiotic properties of goldenseal, although more clinical studies are needed. And keep an eye on this one: In experiments with mice, goldenseal was found to increase bone mineral density and therefore may be useful in the treatment of osteoporosis. Additionally, goldenseal and other berberine compounds are being studied for benefits in the treatment of heart arrhythmias and heart failure.

For additional information on specific health conditions and how you can treat them with supplements, see Part 3 of this book, beginning on page 309.

HOW IT WORKS

Goldenseal contains a number of alkaloid compounds in its roots, stems, and leaves. It is suspected that these alkaloid compounds may be the active ingredients in goldenseal. The main compounds in goldenseal, berberine and hydrastine, have been shown to dilate blood vessels and may act as antibacterial agents, with the potential to kill germs and bacteria that come in direct contact with the herb, as in the gastric mucosa (including the oral cavity), the skin and the urinary tract. It does not appear to be a systemic antibiotic. Goldenseal has demostrated in vitro antibiotic properties against *H. pylori,* the bacteria that cause ulcers; several important pathogenic oral bacteria; and skin bacteria such as staph, strep, and pseudomonas.

HOW TO TAKE IT

Goldenseal is commercially available in the form of tablets, capsules (that contain powdered root), alcoholic tinctures, liquid extracts, and topical creams, gels, ointments, and powders.

Dosages of goldenseal vary depending on the form of supplement taken; be sure to check the product label for dosage information. Goldenseal is not meant to be used long-term.

LOOK OUT FOR THIS!

Side effects of goldenseal, especially when it is taken in high doses, may include nausea, nervousness, vomiting, depression, sun sensitivity, and diarrhea.

Goldenseal is generally considered safe for use in adults. The use of goldenseal is not considered suitable for children and women who are pregnant or nursing. Also, people with severe kidney or liver disease, high blood pressure, cardiovascular disease, or inflammation of the stomach should consult their doctor before taking goldenseal.

WHAT TO AVOID

Medication: Goldenseal may increase the anticoagulant effects of certain anticoagulants including heparin. If you are taking an anticoagulant drug, consult your doctor before using goldenseal.

GOTU KOLA

THE LEAVES AND STEMS of the gotu kola plant *(Centella asiatica)* have been a popular medicinal herb for thousands of years in India, China, and Indonesia, where they are mainly used to heal wounds and treat skin diseases such as leprosy and psoriasis.

In Thailand, gotu kola is used to make a soft drink. In the Singhalese language of Sri Lanka, "gotu" means cup-shaped and "kola" means leaf. People in Sri Lanka noted that elephants often ate the gotu kola plant, and since elephants were known for their longevity, it was thought that the plant might also be healthy for humans. This led to a Singhalese proverb, "Two leaves a day keep old age away."

Note that gotu kola should not be confused with the kola nut, which is an active ingredient in Coca Cola and contains caffeine. Gotu kola has no caffeine and is not a stimulant.

WHAT IT DOES

The most well-studied use of gotu kola is in treating the symptoms of varicose veins and swelling caused by weak veins or veinous insufficiency. Many experts believe that gotu kola is useful in treating varicose veins because it strengthens connective tissues, which suggests that it may be helpful in treating various skin conditions. Gotu kola has been recommended as a treatment for hemorrhoids (a form of varicose veins), bruises, stretch marks caused by pregnancy, and scars, but further research is needed to confirm the effectiveness of gotu-kola in these cases.

Other studies indicate that gotu kola may ease diabetic circulatory problems and may also prevent leg swelling caused by air travel.

Studies with rats indicate that gotu kola may enhance memory and learning and suggest that it may be effective in treating Alzheimer's disease. Traditionally, gotu kola has been used as a mild sedative, memory-improving agent, and brain tonic. However, more human research is needed to test gotu kola's effect on memory in humans.

For additional information on specific health conditions and how you can treat them with supplements, see Part 3 of this book, beginning on page 309.

HOW IT WORKS

Gotu kola contains a blend of compounds—asiaticoside, asiatic acid, and medecassic acid—that seem to have antioxidant effects. Specifically, they seem to have a beneficial effect on connective tissues, where they may stimulate the synthesis of collagen to regenerate tissues and strengthen the veins.

HOW TO TAKE IT

Gotu kola is commercially sold as capsules, tablets, tinctures, ointments, dried herbs, and teas. A typical dosage of gotu kola ranges from 20 to 60 milligrams taken three times daily of an extract containing 40 percent asiaticoside, 29 to 30 percent asiatic acid, 29 to 30 percent madecassic acid, and 1 to 2 percent madecassoside.

Note: It may take 4 weeks of using gotu kola to note any significant benefits.

Gotu Kola May Help Ease Anxiety

Did You Know?

In traditional Ayuvedic medicine—an ancient healing system of India—gotu kola has been used to temper anxiety. It is believed to develop the "crown chakra," which, in Ayurvedic medicine, is the energy center at the top of the head, and to create balance between the hemispheres of the brain.

Western medicine tested the traditional theory about gotu kola and anxiety in a double-blind controlled study. At the beginning of the study, half of the 40 participants were given a placebo and half were given gotu kola. Using the concept that easy startling is related to anxiety, researchers subjected the participants to sudden loud noises and measured their startle response. Those participants who were given gotu kola exhibited a significantly reduced startle response compared to those who received placebo. While these results are promising, more research is needed to support gotu kola's role in anxiety.

LOOK OUT FOR THIS!

Gotu kola is generally considered safe, with few side effects. These can include skin allergies, sun sensitivity, burning sensations, headaches, stomach upsets, nausea, dizziness, and drowsiness.

Gotu kola is not recommended for children, pregnant or breastfeeding women, or people with severe liver or kidney disease.

Individuals with a history of precancerous or cancerous skin lesions should not take gotu kola because one of its major components, asiaticoside, has been associated with the growth of tumors in mice.

WHAT TO AVOID

Medication: Consult your doctor before taking gotu kola with sedative drugs, central nervous system (CNS) depressants, oral hypoglycemic drugs and insulin, lipid-lowering agents, corticosteroids, and phenylbutazone.

GRAPE SEED EXTRACT

FOR MANY PEOPLE, THE SEEDS found in grapes are a mere inconvenience. However, Mother Nature may have had the right idea about putting seeds in grapes, as researchers have discovered. Grapes have a long history of medicinal use by the ancient Egyptians, ancient Greek philosophers—who used grape leaves as astringents to heal conditions such as diarrhea and varicose veins—and European folk healers. Now researchers are discovering that most of the grape's untapped healing powers have been locked in its seeds. While eating grape seeds may not be the answer, grape seed extract (GSE) can effectively deliver a dose of the healthy benefits that grape seeds have to offer.

WHAT IT DOES

As an antioxidant, GSE reduces cell- and tissue-damaging free radical molecules and oxidative stress. As a result, GSE may help reduce the risk of cancer and cardiovascular disease and the effects of aging. While most studies of GSE have been conducted in a laboratory, preliminary results about its health benefits are very promising. One fascinating recent study performed in Japan found that GSE was useful in the treatment of melasma, a.k.a. chloasma (an acquired hyperpigmentation of sun-exposed areas of skin, which most commonly appears in women in their reproductive years).

Early studies show that a group of compounds in GSE, called oligomeric proanthocyanidins (OPCs), may be effective in treating chronic venous insufficiency, a condition in which there is reduced return of blood from the feet and legs to the heart, as well as varicose veins. Some studies show that OPCs may reduce the swelling and leg pain associated with these conditions. OPCs have also been recommended as a treatment for hemorrhoids, which are a form of varicose veins; however, more research on this is necessary.

A recent study of 40 people with high cholesterol showed that those who were given a combination of GSE and chromium for 2 months had a reduction in their total and LDL ("bad") cholesterol levels. More studies are needed to determine GSE's effectiveness in lowering cholesterol levels.

Early studies with mice show that GSE may have the potential to reduce systolic blood pressure. More research is being conducted to see if GSE has this same effect on humans.

Other potential uses of the OPCs contained in GSE include the ability to reduce inflammation after surgery and to strengthen connective tissues in the skin and reduce the effects of aging. Additionally, OPCs may improve vision for people with macular degeneration, and are also being studied to determine their potential benefits in treating impaired night vision, lupus, bruising, periodontal disease, and cirrhosis of the liver.

For additional information on specific health conditions and how to treat them with supplements, see Part 3 of this book, beginning on page 309.

HOW IT WORKS

OPCs are a group of compounds chemically known as flavonoids or polyphenols. Most supplements containing OPCs come either from GSE or from pine bark extract, both of which have a high concentration of these compounds. However, some consider GSE a better source of OPCs than pine bark.

GSE increases levels of antioxidants in the blood. It also neutralizes free radicals and may reduce or prevent some of the damage they cause.

Early research shows that GSE may have anti-inflammatory, anticarcinogenic or cancer-fighting properties, and antiatherogenic effects, with the ability to prevent fat deposits from building up in the arteries. Researchers believe that these properties can be attributed to the antioxidant activity of GSE.

HOW TO TAKE IT

GSE is available in tablet, capsule, and fluid extract form. When purchasing GSE, be sure that the product is standardized to contain 80 to 95 percent OPCs. A typical dose of GSE is 50 to 100 milligrams daily, while dosages of 150 to 300 milligrams daily may be recommended for treating illnesses.

LOOK OUT FOR THIS!

GSE has been thoroughly tested and deemed an extremely safe, essentially nontoxic supplement. Rare side effects include gastrointestinal distress and allergic reaction.

Maximum safe dosages of GSE for children, pregnant or nursing women, and people with liver or kidney disease have not been established. Make sure to consult a doctor to determine an appropriate dosage for you.

WHAT TO AVOID

Medication: Individuals taking blood-thinning medications such as warfarin, heparin, clopidogrel, ticlopidine, pentoxifylline, or aspirin should consult a doctor before taking GSE, since it may increase the risk of bleeding.

GREEN TEA

THE *CAMELLIA SINENSIS* PLANT is the source of the three main types of tea: black, oolong, and green. The difference lies in the ways these plants are processed: black tea leaves are fully fermented, which destroys some of their active ingredients; oolong tea leaves are partly fermented; and green tea leaves are not fermented at all.

Studies show that green tea contains the highest concentration of polyphenols, which may have a variety of health benefits. No wonder green tea is second only to water in the category of most consumed beverages in the world!

WHAT IT DOES

While more research is needed, it appears that green tea may help to prevent certain types of cancer (including breast, cervical, and prostate cancer, cancers of the liver and digestive system, and certain types of leukemia). While one recent study found that green tea

SUPPLEMENTAL TRIVIA

Tea drinkers, rejoice! Researchers have long suspected that drinking at least 1 cup of tea a day may lead to weight loss, and recent evidence supports this theory, suggesting that drinking tea habitually—especially for ten years or more—may actually reduce the percentage of total body fat and waist-to-hip ratios. Studies also suggest that habitual tea drinkers have higher bone mineral density, particularly in the lower back, spine, and hip regions. Your daily cup of tea may not only be promoting a slimmer waist, it may be contributing to healthy bones.

prevented the progression of prostate intraepithelial neoplasia (a premalignant condition of the prostate), another study found that green tea had only minimal impact on prostate cancer refractory to hormone treatment. It has been recommended for cancer patients undergoing chemotherapy or radiation, on the basis of research suggesting that white blood cell counts are better maintained in cancer patients who drink green tea.

Both animal and human studies suggest that green tea extract may promote weight loss, although some recent studies have not demostrated this effect.

Scientists believe that green tea's antioxidant effects may provide some protection for the body's immune system. Green tea may help treat atherosclerosis, high cholesterol, inflammatory bowel disease, diabetes, and liver disease. However, more research is needed to support these claims.

Studies indicate that when applied topically, green tea may act in a unique way to protect the skin from the harmful effects of the sun. Unlike most sunscreens, green tea may protect skin cells from damage by reactivating dying skin cells. This healthful botanical may have a promising future when it comes to preventing skin cancer.

Preliminary studies suggest that green tea, when used as an adjunctive treatment with UV-A radiation for treating psoriasis, may protect the skin from damage caused by UV radiation exposure.

For additional information on specific health conditions and how you can treat them with supplements, see Part 3 of this book, beginning on page 309.

HOW IT WORKS

The health benefits of green tea are thought to come from a family of polyphenols (catechins) and flavonols, chemicals that neutralize cell- and tissue-damaging free radical molecules and which may have antioxidant, anticancer, and tumor-preventing properties as well as antibiotic effects.

Some research suggests that polyphenols may have a greater antioxidant effect than vitamin C. If they have a downside, it is that they give green tea its somewhat bitter flavor.

Research suggests that green tea may contribute to weight loss by causing prolonged thermogenesis (heat production) in the body.

Green tea extract may also reduce fat digestion by inhibiting certain digestive enzymes.

HOW TO TAKE IT

Green tea is commonly sold as dried tea leaves or tea bags. It is also available in capsule form and as an extract derived from the leaves and leaf buds of the tea plant. Green tea or its components may be found in a variety of health products, including toothpaste, mouthwash, and skin creams.

Dosages of green tea supplements vary widely depending on the product; be sure to read product labels for dosage information. A typical dosage is 100 milligrams of an extract standardized to contain a minimum of 90 percent total tea catechins and providing a minimum of 70 percent epigallocatechin gallate (EGCG). It is unclear whether taking the extract is as effective as drinking the tea.

LOOK OUT FOR THIS!

Green tea is generally considered safe, with few side effects. Even as much as 20 cups per day has not been linked to significant side effects.

However, be aware that even though it contains significantly less caffeine than black tea, green tea does have some caffeine, which makes it a mild stimulant. As with any food or drink containing caffeine, excess amounts can cause side effects, including irritability, restlessness, insomnia, heart palpitations, and dizziness. Caffeine overdose can cause nausea, vomiting, diarrhea, headaches, and loss of appetite.

It is possible to buy decaffeinated green tea and decaffeinated green tea extract, but the extraction methods may alter the amount of active ingredients, and if a chemical extraction is used, it may leave chemical residues. If the tea is not organically grown and treated, its products may contain pesticide and herbicide residues. Be sure to choose an organic extract that is standardized for total polyphenol content and catechin concentration.

Individuals with heart problems, kidney disorders, stomach ulcers, and psychological disorders, such as anxiety, should consult their doctor provider before taking green tea.

Infants, young children, and pregnant or nursing women should not take green tea.

WHAT TO AVOID

Medication: Consult your doctor before taking large amounts of green tea with adenosine, beta-lactam antibiotics (such as penicillins and cephalosporins), benzodiazepines, beta-adrenergic blocking drugs, blood-thinning medications, clozapine, ephedrine, lithium, monoamine oxidase inhibitors (MAOIs), oral contraceptives, and phenylpropanolamine. If you are undergoing chemotherapy, consult your doctor before taking green tea supplements.

GUARANA

WHILE IT MAY SOUND MYSTERIOUS and exotic, guarana is mostly thought of as a source of caffeine. The seeds of this South American shrub are ground to make an extract that locals have used in the Amazon rainforest to stay alert, reduce fatigue, and treat arthritis, diarrhea, menstrual headaches, and hangovers, and it has been used as an aphrodisiac. Also called "Brazilian cocoa," guarana seeds by weight contain twice the amount of caffeine as coffee beans. For the sake of comparison: While tea has more caffeine than coffee (by weight), the average cup of tea contains only one-half to one-third the amount of caffeine as a cup of coffee.

WHAT IT DOES

While the active ingredient in guarana was thought to be mostly caffeine (some manufacturers call it guaranine to give consumers the impression that it's rare and exotic), there may be more to it than that. In fact, one recent study found that guarana (by itself or combined with ginseng) improved task performance, in spite of the low caffeine level (9 milligrams; the average cup of coffee has 75 milligrams of caffeine). Previous studies had not demonstrated this effect.

Preliminary animal studies suggest a protective effect against liver cancer. Other studies have begun to demonstrate significant antibiotic and antioxidant properties of guarana. Animal studies suggest that guarana may help protect against gastric injury caused by nonsteroidal anti-inflammatory drugs (NSAIDs) and alcohol.

Guarana has had a reputation for being an herbal speed and diet pill. Rather than taking guarana alone for weight loss, dieters have found a more effective tool in the "ECA stack," a combination of ephedra (which has been banned by the U.S. Food and Drug Administration [FDA]), caffeine, and aspirin. Taken together, the ECA stack can increase the body's metabolic rate and calorie consumption to twice what ephedrine alone could do. But ephedra, for this purpose, has been banned by the FDA because it can be very dangerous. Therefore, do not use these products in conjunction under any circumstances, since their use may have fatal effects.

Guarana does in fact have more caffeine content by weight than does coffee (but again, so does tea). Since the FDA banned ephedra for weight loss, other products have come on the market that combine bitter orange and guarana. These products are no safer than the ones banned by the FDA and ought to be avoided. Guarana may be toxic when used at high concentrations or in large doses.

For additional information on specific health conditions and how you can treat them with supplements, see Part 3 of this book, beginning on page 309.

HOW IT WORKS

The activity of guarana often occurs more gradually than that of coffee or tea, and it often lasts for 1 to 3 hours. Besides caffeine, other active ingredients in guarana include the alkaloids theobromine and theophylline, which may also be found in coffee and tea. The tannins in guarana act as astringents (substances that remove water from tissues and cause them to contract), which may be why guarana was traditionally used to treat diarrhea.

HOW TO TAKE IT

Guarana is available in capsule, liquid, and tablet form, and may also be bought fresh in the form of its seeds. A typical guarana supplement provides 50 to 200 milligrams of caffeine per day. To make a cup of guarana tea containing about 50 milligrams of caffeine, boil a cup of water with one-fourth to one-half teaspoon of crushed guarana seed or resin for 10 minutes. The safe dosage range of 180 to 450 milligrams of caffeine a day is equivalent to 500 to 1,000 milligrams of guarana extract.

Guarana and caffeine are generally safe for most healthy people when taken at normal doses. No major health problems are associated with taking up to 400 milligrams of caffeine divided into several doses throughout the day, which is the equivalent of 3 or 4 cups of brewed coffee. However, some people have side effects with even one cup.

LOOK OUT FOR THIS!

Too much caffeine can cause irritability, insomnia, anxiety, heart palpitations, headaches, high blood pressure, and dehydration from frequent urination. Because of the effects of caffeine, anyone with heart palpitations, circulatory or kidney problems, muscle spasms, hyperthyroidism, or anxiety should consult their doctor before taking guarana or caffeine.

Pregnant women should avoid guarana—and all other sources of caffeine. Nursing women may also want to avoid caffeine since it can cause sleeping problems in their infants.

WHAT TO AVOID

Medication: Because it's a diuretic, guarana, if overused, can cause hypokalemia (potassium deficiency), which in turn can increase the toxicity and side effects of certain medications, especially heart medications like digoxin.

Discuss taking caffeine or guarana with your doctor if you're taking medication for your heart or kidneys or if you're being treated for anxiety or panic disorder.

GUGGUL

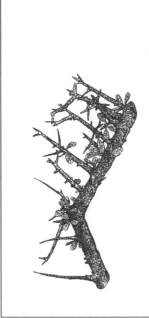

GUGGUL (IT RHYMES WITH "FRUGAL") has been used in India since as early as 600 BC. It's a staple in Ayurvedic medicine, approved in India for the treatment of high cholesterol and triglyceride levels, two factors associated with heart disease. But research is still underway when it comes to how effectively guggul lowers these blood fats for Westerners.

Also known as gum guggul, guggulu, or African myrrh, guggul is made from the thorny *Commiphora mukul* shrub found in India. Most older studies of guggul, especially those done in India, show it to have positive cholesterol-lowering effects. But an American study of guggul in August 2003 showed that it increased levels of LDL ("bad") cholesterol and caused no real change in total cholesterol, triglycerides, or HDL ("good") cholesterol. These conflicting results may have been due to genetic or dietary differences between Indian and Western cultures.

WHAT IT DOES

In one of the most promising studies of guggul, a daily dose of 100 milligrams of guggulsterones taken with diet therapy produced decreases of almost 13 percent, 12 percent, and 11 percent, respectively, in the ratios of LDL cholesterol, triglycerides, and total cholesterol to HDL cholesterol.

Because it has anti-inflammatory qualities, guggul has also been used to treat osteoarthritis, rheumatoid arthritis, and a severe kind of acne called nodulocystic acne vulgaris. Of these, guggul has shown solid evidence of benefit only in treating acne. Although recently marketed for obesity, guggul remains unproven as a weight-loss aid. Guggul is also being studied for possible anticoagulant and antioxidant effects. In Egypt, guggul is being studied for its ability to eradicate intestinal parasites.

For additional information on specific health conditions and how you can treat them with supplements, see Part 3 of this book, beginning on page 309.

HOW IT WORKS

The active ingredients in guggul are guggulsterones (specifically, guggulsterone E and Z), derived from the fatty substances known as guggulipids in the gum resin of the plant. How guggulsterones lower the blood levels of fats like cholesterol and triglycerides is still unknown. Initial laboratory studies suggest that they may work by changing cholesterol metabolism or excretion, or by affecting liver enzymes, thyroid function, or bile-acid regulation in the body.

HOW TO TAKE IT

Standardized guggul extracts contain from 2.5 to 5 percent guggulsterones. Typical dosages for reducing high cholesterol and triglyceride levels are 25 milligrams of 2.5 percent guggulsterone extract taken three times a day or 50 milligrams taken twice a day, for 12 to 24 weeks. The most promising study of guggul for nodulocystic acne used 25 milligrams of guggulsterone twice a day for 6 weeks.

Guggulsterone also comes in tablet form as a gum resin and as a preparation called fraction A, although some researchers believe that guggul is safer and more effective when taken as a standardized extract rather than in gum resin form. Keep in mind that commercial brands vary widely in their content of active guggul components; independent testers found from 4 to 74 percent of the supposed active ingredients in different guggul products.

LOOK OUT FOR THIS!

A reputable brand of standardized guggul is generally considered safe for taking by healthy adults in normal doses for up to 6 months. In rare cases, guggul may cause allergic skin reactions, diarrhea, nausea, or headache, but these side effects disappear after stopping guggul. One published case report documented severe muscle damage (rhabdomyolysis) while taking guggul. Some people may find guggul hard to digest.

Guggul may reduce the platelet aggregation responsible for blood clotting, so consult your doctor before taking guggul if you're at risk of having a bleeding disorder. Stop taking guggul two days prior to surgery. Because guggul also appears to have thyroid-stimulating properties in animals, anyone with a thyroid condition may want to avoid guggul.

No data exist on the safety of guggul for pregnant or nursing women, children, or people with serious kidney or liver disease.

WHAT TO AVOID

Medication: Guggul appears to lessen the efficacy of the beta-blocker drug propranolol, although no studies have been done of guggul taken with other beta-blockers. Since guggul also interferes with the calcium-channel blocker diltiazem, anyone taking guggul with this medication should watch for even slight changes in blood pressure or heart rate.

GYMNEMA

SWEET THINGS DON'T TASTE SWEET for a while after you've chewed the leaves of the gymnema plant *(Gymnema sylvestre)*, and apparently gymnema has the same effect on "sweetness" in the blood: An herbal remedy made from the leaves of this plant is apparently very good at lowering blood sugar levels. Gymnema has been used for at least 2,000 years in India, where this woody plant grows, to treat diabetes. Its name in Hindi, *gurmar,* couldn't be more appropriate: It means "destroyer of sugar."

WHAT IT DOES

Both long practice in traditional Indian medicine and modern clinical investigations in India and the West support the notion that gymnema lowers levels of blood sugar, thereby helping to control type 2, or non-insulin-dependent, diabetes. The effect is more gradual than with prescription hypoglycemic (blood-sugar-lowering) medications; in one study, gymnema showed no effect on fasting blood glucose levels for up to 45 minutes. That could be an advantage, because some medications that work quickly can cause a precipitous drop in blood sugar levels and create serious adverse reactions, including faintness, dizziness, weakness, and even loss of consciousness. In the long term, though, gymnema has been found to keep blood sugar levels under control to such an extent that some type-2 diabetic participants in one study were able to stop taking their prescription hypoglycemic drugs. (Most practitioners don't recommend this and suggest that gymnema serve as a complement to conventional treatments for type 2 diabetes until blood sugar levels are consistently normal.)

Gymnema has also been found to raise insulin levels in the blood, meaning that it is also beneficial for controlling type 1 diabetes, or insulin-dependent diabetes. Participants in a study of gymnema for type 1 diabetes were able to reduce their requirement for externally supplied insulin by 50 percent. Practitioners don't suggest that gymnema can replace the insulin used to treat type 1 diabetes, but that it instead serve as an effective adjunct to insulin.

Although the first research efforts with gymnema focused on its effects on diabetes, investigators noticed that it also lowered total cholesterol, LDL ("bad") cholesterol, and triglycerides. In one study that lasted more than a year and a half, participants receiving gymnema had an 18 percent decrease in their total cholesterol levels and a 16 percent decline in their triglyceride levels.

Because gymnema keeps sweet things from tasting sweet, some investigators have suggested that it might be a good way to encourage weight loss. A craving for sweets is the downfall of many overweight and obese people.

In traditional Indian medicine, gymnema has been credited with a wide variety of therapeutic benefits. It has been used to treat stomach problems, constipation, liver disease, gout, and malaria. It is also used as an aphrodisiac and an antidote for snake bites. There is no scientific evidence to support these uses.

For additional information on specific health conditions and how you can treat them with supplements, see Part 3 of this book, beginning on page 309.

HOW IT WORKS

Animal research suggests that gymnema may lower blood sugar levels by facilitating glucose uptake by the body's cells. It may also keep adrenaline from stimulating the liver to produce excess glucose.

Several theories exist about how gymnema raises insulin levels. Insulin is secreted into the blood by beta cells in the pancreas. These cells don't function properly, or may actually be damaged or destroyed, in people with type 1 diabetes. Research with animals suggests that gymnema may regenerate these cells, increasing their number. Other investigators, however, contend that gymnema doesn't cause the body to produce more insulin, but rather increases the effectiveness of insulin that's already present. Still others think gymnema stimulates existing beta cells in the pancreas to release more insulin into the blood.

Gymnema is thought to lower cholesterol either by decreasing its synthesis or increasing the rate at which it is metabolized; gymnema may also interfere with the absorption of fats in the intestinal tract.

HOW TO TAKE IT

Gymnema is available as a water-soluble extract made from the leaves of the plant or as a leaf powder. You can also use patented products containing gymnema extract. The recommended dosage for treating both type 1 and type 2 diabetes is 500 milligrams taken twice a day, for a total of 1,000 milligrams daily, or 2 to 3 grams of leaf powder, in divided doses.

Gymnema should be taken with meals. Because gymnema's effects are gradual, you should expect to keep taking it for several days before you see results.

Note: If you have either type 1 or type 2 diabetes, you should take gymnema only under the supervision of your doctor. You may need to reduce the amount of insulin you're taking or adjust your prescription hypoglycemic medication.

LOOK OUT FOR THIS!

Even though gymnema may be less likely to cause a sudden and dangerous hypoglycemic reaction than prescription medications that work more quickly, gymnema may, with time, be so effective at lowering your blood sugar that it lowers it too much. Watch for the symptoms of an adverse hypoglycemic reaction, which include headache, faintness, weakness, and dizziness, and consult your doctor if any of these symptoms develop.

Safe dosages of gymnema have not been determined for children, pregnant or nursing women, or people with liver or kidney disease.

WHAT TO AVOID

Medication: If you are taking insulin or prescription medication to control blood sugar, you may need to reduce the dosage of your medication, since gymnema may increase its effects, possibly causing hypoglycemia. Gymnema may increase the effects of cholesterol-lowering drugs.

HAWTHORN

HAWTHORN *(CRATAEGUS MONOGYNA, Crataegus laevigata, Crataegus oxyacantha,* and *Crataegus pentagyna),* a relative to the rose, is a thorny shrub that can grow 5 to 15 feet tall, dons white and pink flowers, and has prickly branches. This plant grows in the temperate climates of Europe, Asia, and North America. The hawthorn leaf and fruit have been used medicinally for centuries all over the world, including China and Europe. Today, hawthorn preparations are among the most popular botanical medicines for cardiovascular ailments in Europe. Hawthorn was originally used in Europe to treat kidney and bladder problems. In traditional Chinese medicine, the fruit of the hawthorn shrub is used to help digest meals containing greasy meats.

WHAT IT DOES

Hawthorn has an impressive ability to expand blood vessels and increase the amount of oxygen-rich blood flowing through the body. Consequently, hawthorn is best known for its use in cardiovascular health. Laboratory and animal studies have shown that it may help cut down plaque formation in the arteries and improve blood flow to the heart. This may not only reduce the risk of heart disease but may also prevent stroke. In many, but not all, human studies, patients with congestive heart failure who took hawthorn supplements showed better overall heart function and exhibited greater stamina than those who did not. Hawthorn is an effective and low-risk herb for people with coronary heart disease, atherosclerosis, hypertension, or hypercholesterolemia.

Hawthorn may be useful for more than matters of the heart. Preliminary studies suggest that its antioxidant properties may help reduce swelling and heal tissue damaged by sprains and strains. As a circulatory stimulant, hawthorn may also improve symptoms of sexual dysfunction and reduce hypertension.

For additional information on specific health conditions and how to treat them with supplements, see Part 3 of this book, beginning on page 309.

HOW IT WORKS

Studies have shown that hawthorn contains flavonoids and other compounds that help dilate the blood vessels leading to the heart, thus increasing the flow of oxygen to this important muscle and strengthening the heart's pumping action. When blood vessels are dilated, their resistance to blood flow is decreased, and blood can flow more freely through the entire body. As an antioxidant, hawthorn may help maintain arterial walls so they remain elastic and able to expand so as to accommodate the flow of blood.

HOW TO TAKE IT

Hawthorn is available in a variety of forms, including capsule, tincture, liquid, and solid extract. The usual dosage of hawthorn, in solid extract form, is 300 to 600 milligrams a day; capsules are available in 100-milligram doses, and it is recommended that 1 capsule be taken two or three times a day. In liquid form, the suggested dosage is 0.5 to 1 milliliters three times a day, and with a tincture, the recommended dosage is at 1.0 to 2.0 milliliters of a 1:5 hawthorn extract in 45 percent alcohol, taken three times a day.

A tea can be made from the dried leaves, flowers, and berries of hawthorn but watch out—hawthorn has a very bitter taste.

Hawthorn is often sold in combination with ginkgo, but the effectiveness of this combination in various ailments is unknown.

Note: Up to 6 months may be needed to reap the full benefits of hawthorn.

LOOK OUT FOR THIS!

Hawthorn is considered a safe supplement, but is not suitable for women who are pregnant or nursing. Additionally, individuals with cardiovascular problems should not use hawthorn without first consulting their doctor.

Side effects of hawthorn are rare and consist primarily of mild stomach upset and occasional skin rash.

WHAT TO AVOID

Medication: Hawthorn may interfere with some heart medications, such as digoxin, and with antihypertensive medications, coronary vasodilators, alpha-receptor agonists, or cholesterol-lowering agents. People taking any of these medications should consult their doctor before taking hawthorn.

HORSE CHESTNUT

YOU'RE PROBABLY FAMILIAR WITH THE horse chestnut *(Aesculus hippocastanum)*, a tall, erect tree with spreading branches that produce beautiful blooms in the spring and small nuts with a dark, polished skin in the autumn.

Native Americans have been using the seeds of the nuts for centuries, roasting, peeling, and mashing them, then leaching them in lime to make them less toxic. In Europe, the nuts are a common feed for horses and cattle, hence the name of this tree.

WHAT IT DOES

There is strong evidence that an extract from the seeds of the horse chestnut tree, called horse chestnut seed extract (HCSE), helps in treating chronic venous insufficiency, a condition marked by water retention in the legs, varicose veins, leg pain, itching, and skin ulcers.

Other studies suggest that horse chestnut may be helpful for reducing hemorrhoids, which are actually a type of varicose vein, as well as treating edema (water retention) by reducing inflammation and swelling.

Horse chestnut also appears to have laboratory antiviral properties against influenza.

For additional information on specific health conditions and how to treat them with supplements, see Part 3 of this book, beginning on page 309.

HOW IT WORKS

The active ingredient in horse chestnut, which is called aescin, works as an anti-inflammatory agent and also safeguards veins by protecting the body's stores of collagen and elastin, two proteins integral to vein health.

While more research is needed to fully understand the role of aescin, some researchers believe that besides having anti-inflammatory activity it may prevent the release of certain enzymes in the body (particularly glycosaminoglycan hydrolases), thus preventing them from causing vein damage.

HOW TO TAKE IT

Horse chestnut is available as capsules, tablets, and tinctures. It is also available in a topical gel that is sometimes recommended for treating bruises, but no scientific studies support this use.

The raw or unprocessed seeds, leaves, bark, or flowers of the horse chestnut tree should not be eaten or made into a tea, since they contain esculin, which may be toxic. When properly prepared, horse chestnut seed extract does not contain esculin.

A typical dosage recommendation for horse chestnut is 300 milligrams, taken 2 or 3 times daily, of a preparation standardized to contain 50 milligrams of aescin per dose.

LOOK OUT FOR THIS!

When taken properly, horse chestnut is generally considered safe, with few side effects. Occasionally, it may produce severe itching, nausea, and stomach complaints.

Topical forms of horse chestnut (such as the gel described above) should not be applied to open wounds. Most experts say that oral forms of horse chestnut other than HCSE should be avoided.

People with kidney problems should not take horse chestnut without first consulting their doctor. Because horse chestnut increases the risk of low blood sugar levels, people with diabetes and on antidiabetic medications should consult their doctor before taking horse chestnut.

Children and women who are pregnant or nursing should not take horse chestnut.

WHAT TO AVOID

Medication: Consult your doctor before taking horse chestnut with blood-thinning drugs such as warfarin or heparin, antiplatelet drugs such as clopidogrel, or nonsteroidal anti-inflammatory drugs (NSAIDs) such as ibuprofen, since it may increase the effects of these medications.

HUPERZINE A

WHAT DO CAFFEINE AND CODEINE have in common with huperzine A (HupA)? All three are medicinally active chemicals called alkaloids, derived from plants. HupA is an extract of a Chinese moss (*Huperzia serrata*) used in traditional Chinese medicine to treat fever, inflammation, pain, and tendonitis. First isolated from this moss by Chinese scientists in 1948, HupA is now sold over the counter as a dietary supplement. However, HupA is much more akin to a drug than to an herb, in being a potent chemical compound that is highly purified in a laboratory.

WHAT IT DOES

HupA has shown promise as a memory booster, especially in people with Alzheimer's disease. It can also improve mental function in healthy people. More research is needed to test HupA's traditional uses as a fever-reducing and anti-inflammatory agent.

For additional information on specific health conditions and how you can treat them with supplements, see Part 3 of this book, beginning on page 309.

HOW IT WORKS

HupA may improve memory and mental function bcause of its effect on a neurotransmitter called acetylcholine. Acetylcholine transfers nerve impulses (messages) from one nerve cell to the next. Normally, acetylcholine is broken down and replenished in the nerve cells that use it. In memory disorders such as Alzheimer's disease, acetylcholine may be broken down too quickly so that it becomes deficient and the "message" is too weak or can't be sent properly. HupA appears to play a part in slowing the breakdown of acetylcholine so that nerve impulses can be properly transferred.

HOW TO TAKE IT

HupA should only be used under a doctor's supervision.

HupA comes in the following forms: "A" and "B," and (-) and (+). The most effective form of huperazine is (-) huperzine A—look for it on the label.

Since HupA is a powerful substance, the recommended dosage is only 50 micrograms taken twice a day. However, in studies of people with Alzheimer's disease, dementia, and age-related memory loss, doses of 100 to 200 micrograms 2 or 3 times a day have been used safely and effectively.

LOOK OUT FOR THIS!

Side effects of HupA include headaches and dizziness. Raw preparations of the huperzine moss have been known to cause liver and kidney toxicity in a few isolated cases. Be sure to use a purified extract of HupA in order to avoid these potential side effects.

HupA should not be taken by children or women who are pregnant or nursing.

HupA should not be used by people with high blood pressure, serious liver or kidney disease, seizure disorders, irregular heartbeat, asthma, irritable bowel syndrome, or malabsorption syndromes.

WHAT TO AVOID

Medication: HupA may increase the effects of acetylcholinesterase inhibitors (such as donepezil, tacrine, physostigmine, and pyridostigmine) and of anticholinergic drugs, such as bethanechol.

IPRIFLAVONE

THERE'S JUST NO BONES ABOUT IT: Ipriflavone may help prevent, slow, and possibly even reverse osteoporosis. After menopause, many women's bones become significantly less dense and more brittle, which can cause a notable hunching of the back and a good deal of bone pain, and can also lead to crippling fractures, especially of the spine. Because of its crippling effects, doctors have long sought effective treatments for osteoporosis, and while the data for ipriflavone in treating this condition are somewhat contradictory, it may have promise. In Japan, ipriflavone is widely used to treat osteoporosis.

Ipriflavone is a synthetic substance that belongs to the family of substances known as flavonoids, which are present in many plants, and belongs to the subgroup of this family called isoflavones. For supplemental use, it is derived from a soy compound called daidzein.

Ipriflavone is found in some foods, such as soy sauce, but in amounts that are far too small to have any therapeutic value. Supplements, however, are available over the counter.

WHAT IT DOES

Ipriflavone may stop the loss of bone caused by osteoporosis, and may help to grow new bone. Studies have indicated that ipriflavone may be effective for stopping such bone loss, particularly when it's taken in conjunction with calcium. Other studies indicate that in women with osteoporosis, ipriflavone may also increase bone density, reduce the likelihood of vertebral fractures, and ease bone pain.

In one study, postmenopausal women whose bones were less dense than normal but who had not yet developed osteoporosis were divided into two groups, one receiving ipriflavone and the other a placebo; both groups also received 1,000 milligrams of calcium a day. After 2 years, bone density in the spine had decreased by 4.9 percent in the placebo group but hadn't decreased at all in the ipriflavone group. In another study of similar groups of women, those receiving ipriflavone actually had a gain in bone density of 1 percent—a small amount but one that could be significant over time. One study found that ipriflavone was more effective than vitamin D in preventing osteoporosis in people who had experienced a stroke.

Ipriflavone has also been shown to prevent osteoporosis in women taking corticosteroid medications, which can cause bone loss, and has been found to curtail the sometimes rapid loss of bone density that occurs in women who have had their ovaries removed.

Although estrogen-replacement therapy has also been used to try to prevent osteoporosis in menopausal women, it carries an increased risk of causing uterine and breast cancer. However, when ipriflavone and estrogen are taken together, they prevent osteoporosis somewhat more effectively than when either is used alone.

However, not all studies with ipriflavone have shown positive results with its use against osteoporosis: A double-blind study published in the *Journal of the American Medical Association* found that ipriflavone was not successful in treating osteoporosis, and in Canada, ipriflavone is not recommended for the treatment of this bone-threatening disease.

Preliminary research suggests that ipriflavone may be helpful as a treatment for other bone conditions, including Paget's disease— a metabolic bone disease that causes bone destruction and bone deformity, hyperparathyroidism—a condition in which the parathyroid gland produces an excess of parathyroid hormone, causing calcium to be leached from the bones, and otosclerosis—a condition in which abnormal bone growth in the ear may lead to hearing loss.

For additional information on specific health conditions and how you can treat them with supplements, see Part 3 of this book, beginning on page 309.

HOW IT WORKS

Bones need calcium, and ipriflavone appears to facilitate the incorporation of calcium into bone. That's why it may be best to take calcium and ipriflavone together. Ipriflavone also appears to restore a balance between two types of cells found in bone—a balance that osteoporosis disturbs. One of these two types of bone cells, known as *osteoclasts,* break down bone and cause it to be resorbed, while the second type of cells, known as *osteoblasts,* form new bone. Ipriflavone inhibits the action of osteoclasts and encourages the action of osteoblasts, thus helping to preserve and even add new bone to what exists.

Ipriflavone holds a special advantage over other types of soy-based isoflavones. Most soy isoflavones have effects similar to estrogen in the body and potentially carry the same risks, increasing the chances of uterine and breast cancer. But ipriflavone is specifically synthesized in a way that enables it to have bone-stimulating effects without causing any of the adverse results that may be associated with soy isoflavones.

HOW TO TAKE IT

Ipriflavone is available as an over-the-counter supplement in capsules of 100, 200, and 300 milligrams each. The recommended dose is 600 milligrams a day, taken either twice or three times a day, along with a daily total of 1,000 milligrams of calcium. Ipriflavone is absorbed better when taken with food.

LOOK OUT FOR THIS!

A small but significant number of women (29 out of 132 in one study) who took ipriflavone experienced a reduction in the number of the white blood cells called lymphocytes that circulate in the blood and which play a crucial role in the immune system. Many practitioners recommend that anyone taking ipriflavone routinely have a count done of their white blood cells to be sure it doesn't fall below normal.

Because of its potential effects on the immune system, ipriflavone should not be taken by people whose immune system is compromised in any way—such as by a person who is infected with human immunodeficiency virus (HIV) or who has any another immunodeficiency disease.

Ipriflavone is metabolized in the kidneys, so consult your doctor about an appropriate dosage of this supplement for you if you have kidney disease.

WHAT TO AVOID

Medications: Because ipriflavone can reduce the white blood cell count, corticosteroids and other immune-suppressing medications should not be taken while it is being used—and vice versa. Ipriflavone may raise blood levels of the asthma medication theophylline. Other drugs that are metabolized in the liver—including tolbutamide, phenytoin, and warfarin—may also be affected when taken together with ipriflavone.

IRON

IRON IS AN ESSENTIAL MINERAL that your body needs every day to function at its best. Without enough iron, people can suffer from the deficiency of red blood cells known as anemia, and from learning problems, fatigue, and depression. In fact, iron deficiency is one of the most common nutritional deficiencies in the world (see When Micronutrients Are Missing, page 6), with children, teenage girls, menstruating or pregnant women, and the elderly at the greatest risk for developing it. Fortunately, there are many ways to ensure you and your family are getting enough iron, either through food or, when necessary, with iron supplements.

WHAT IT DOES

Iron supplementation is a widely accepted and effective treatment for people with confirmed iron deficiency, including women who have heavy menstruation or endometriosis. Keeping iron levels in the blood within a proper range is also extremely important for pregnant women, since their bodies produce an increased number of

SUPPLEMENTAL TRIVIA

Long before Popeye, the benefits of iron were well known. In 4000 BC the Persian physician Melampus gave iron supplements to sailors to replenish the iron they lost from bleeding wounds suffered during sea battles.

red blood cells during pregnancy. Two small studies have shown that the use of iron supplements in people with slightly low iron stores can significantly improve their performance during exercise.

Preliminary studies suggest that iron may also be helpful in treating attention deficit disorder, as well as dry coughs caused by the angiotensin-converting enzyme (ACE)–inhibiting drugs used to treat high blood pressure, although more research in these areas is needed.

For additional information on specific health conditions and how to treat them with supplements, see Part 3 of this book, beginning on page 309.

HOW IT WORKS

Iron is needed for the formation of hemoglobin, the protein in red blood cells that carries oxygen to every part of the body, and for myglobin, a form of hemoglobin in muscles that helps muscle cells to store oxygen. Iron also plays a vital role in producing energy, making the neurotransmitting substances known as serotonin and dopamine which transfer nerve impulses from one nerve cell to the next. Iron is also important for keeping the immune system healthy, and forming collagen—an essential component of the connective tissue in tendons, ligaments, bones, and cartilage.

HOW TO TAKE IT

See the table below for the official recommended daily intakes (RDIs) of iron.

AGE/GENDER/ CONDITION	RECOMMENDED DAILY INTAKE (RDI)*
Infants	
0–6 months	0.27 mg
7–12 months	11 mg
Children	
1–3 years	7 mg
4–8 years	10 mg
Males	
9–13 years	8 mg
14–18 years	11 mg
19 years and older	8 mg

AGE/GENDER CONDITION	RECOMMENDED DAILY INTAKE (RDI)*
Females	
9–13 years	8 mg
14–18 years	15 mg
19–50 years	18 mg
50 years and older	8 mg
Pregnant Women	27 mg
Nursing women	
18 years or younger	10 mg
19 years and older	9 mg

For more information on RDIs, see What to Know More About Intake? on page 8.

Healthy people can usually get enough daily iron by eating a well-balanced diet containing iron-rich foods (see Food Sources, alongside). Most general purpose multivitamin and mineral supplements also contain iron (be sure to check the label).

Specific iron supplements are usually needed only by people with diagnosed iron deficiency. If you suspect that you may have iron deficiency (for example, if you constantly feel tired or weak), see your doctor, who may recommend that you take iron supplements. On the other hand, taking too much iron can pose serious health risks (see below).

Iron supplements are available in capsule, tablet (including extended release), chewable tablet, and solution forms. Researchers recently warned against using inorganic iron (often added to enrich foods with iron, as with white flour and breakfast cereals), because the body cannot effectively use it and it may build up to toxic levels in the blood.

LOOK OUT FOR THIS!

When taken at recommended doses, iron supplements are quite safe; their side effects are generally mild, but may extend to nausea, vomiting, diarrhea, constipation, dark-colored stools, and abdominal pain. You can reduce the chance or severity of these side effects by taking the supplement in divided doses with food. Although it may be easier to swallow, iron taken in liquid form may stain your teeth.

FOOD SOURCES

Food sources provide two different types of iron: *heme iron,* which is obtained from meat, poultry, and fish, and which is easily absorbed by the body, and *non-heme iron,* which is obtained from vegetables, fruits, and grains, and is more difficult for the body to absorb than heme iron. Acidic foods, such as tomatoes, are a good source of iron when cooked in iron or stainless steel cookware (from which some iron leaches into these foods).

Heme Iron Sources
▶Beef, clams, egg yolks, fish, red meat, lamb, liver (beef, pork, and chicken), kidneys, mussels, pork, poultry, sardines, shrimp, and turkey.

Non-Heme Iron Sources*
▶Beans, dried fruits, enriched pastas and breads, leafy green vegetables (especially spinach), nuts, and peas.

Note: Be sure to eat foods rich in vitamin C—including oranges, pineapple, citrus juices, kiwi, brussels sprouts, broccoli, peppers, and tomatoes—when consuming non-heme-iron-containing foods so as to help your body to better absorb the non-heme iron.

Contrary to popular belief, certain sources of iron may not be well-absorbed by the body. Spinach is a notable example: while spinach contains iron, it also contains a compound called oxalate, which renders the iron nonabsorbable by the body. Therefore, if you're looking to boost your intake of iron, spinach may not be the key.

Studies suggest that iron taken in doses above the recommended doses may play a role in stroke-related brain injury, increase complications of pregnancy, and increase the risk of cancer and heart disease (although this claim is highly controversial). However, children can be poisoned by an overdose of iron supplement, so be sure to safely store such supplements well out of their reach.

People with hemachromatosis or hemosiderosis (conditions that result in too much iron in the body), hemolytic anemia (in which red blood cells are destroyed prematurely), or who have had several blood transfusions should not take iron.

People who consume alcohol in large amounts, are planning to conceive, are currently pregnant or nursing, or are over age 50 with a family history of heart disease, and those with gastrointestinal diseases such as peptic ulcer disease, enteritis, colitis, pancreatitis, hepatitis, and kidney disorders, should consult their doctor before taking any supplements, including iron.

WHAT TO AVOID

Medication: Antibiotics in the quinolone or tetracycline families, angiotensin-converting enzyme (ACE) inhibitors such as captopril, histamine blockers, proton pump inhibitors, levodopa, thyroid hormones, and methyldopa may reduce the body's ability to absorb iron. If you take any of these medications, wait at least 2 hours before taking iron.

Herbs and Dietary Supplements: Avoid taking high doses of vitamin C while taking iron supplements, since it can cause the body to absorb too much iron. Conversely, zinc, calcium, soy, copper, and manganese can reduce the body's absorption of iron. If you take any of these supplements, be sure to wait at least 2 hours before taking iron.

Food: A number of foods may interfere with iron absorption, including tea, coffee, red wine, phytates (substances found in food products that are unleavened, including pita bread, matzoh, wheat germ, vanilla extract, cacao powder, oats, and nuts), and soy protein.

KAVA

ALTHOUGH IT MAY NOT TASTE like a fine cabernet or chardonnay, kava *(Piper methysticum)* is used in the South Sea Islands as the social equivalent of wine—a drink that helps you unwind. Today kava is popular in the United States and Europe for the same reason—it creates a feeling of relaxation, and without the mental fogginess or nasty hangover associated with alcoholic drinks.

WHAT IT DOES

In the United States, kava is used for its tranquilizing effect. Several studies show that kava has strong properties as a relaxant and antianxiety agent, and that it may have an effect equal to that of certain antianxiety medications with fewer side effects and without the effect known as tolerance, which can make a drug ineffective. Kava helps elevate mood and contributes to a sense of well being and contentment. It is also used to combat insomnia, stress, and restlessness.

Because kava even seems to ease certain aches and pains, it has been useful in easing symptoms of fibromyalgia as well as prostate problems.

For additional information on specific health conditions and how to treat them with supplements, see Part 3 of this book, beginning on page 309.

HOW IT WORKS

The active ingredients in the kava root are substances known as kavalactones, which depress the central nervous system and can have a soothing effect on emotions, resembling that of alcohol, but without the disorienting effects.

Note: The actual content of kavalactone can vary significantly from one kava plant to another, depending on the growing, harvesting, and processing conditions. When purchasing kava, be sure to buy a standardized form that lists the total kavalactone content per pill.

I heard that kava was banned by the U.S. Food and Drug Administration (FDA) because it can cause liver damage. Is this true, and is it safe to take kava supplements?

In recent years, reports have linked kava with severe liver damage, prompting regulatory agencies in Europe and the United States to warn consumers about the potential risks associated with this supplement. Still, kava remains one of the most popular herbs sold in the United States, with sales totaling over $40 million dollars annually. In 2002, the FDA issued an advisory about the potential risk of liver failure associated with kava products, but it did not officially ban kava from being sold as a supplement. Although some specific kava-containing products have been removed from the market because they were deemed unsafe, kava is a legal supplement in the United States, although it is banned in Canada. It is worth remembering that many people have been using kava for the past 30 years without apparent safety problems.

HOW TO TAKE IT

Caution: Kava should only be used under a doctor's supervision.

In the modern manufacture of kava supplements, the roots of the plant are dried and ground into a powder, then packed into capsules or tablets, blended into drinks, or dissolved in a tincture or extracts. The German Commission E (see page 16) recommends a maximum dose of 300 milligrams daily of kava.

Be sure to look for kava products that contain at least 70 percent kavalactones for maximum effectiveness.

LOOK OUT FOR THIS!

The most common side effect linked to kava is stomach ache. Other side effects include drowsiness and dizziness; in rare cases, and if taken for prolonged periods, kava may cause itching, scaling, and yellowing of the skin.

Kava taken under a doctor's supervision is considered safe for adults. The use of kava is not suitable for children or women who are pregnant or nursing. Kava should not be taken before driving or operating heavy equipment. People with liver or kidney disease should consult their doctor before taking kava supplements.

WHAT TO AVOID

Medication: Kava may enhance the effects of medications used to treat seizures, sleep disturbances, or anxiety. People taking barbiturates, psychopharmacological drugs, or other substances that act on the central nervous system should consult their doctor before taking kava. Also, kava may increase the risk of unpleasant side effects of certain medications for schizophrenia or Parkinson's disease.

Food: If taken with alcohol, kava may hasten or intensify the feeling of being inebriated.

LACTOBACILLUS ACIDOPHILUS

MILLIONS OF BACTERIA MAKE their home in the human digestive system, steadily doing the necessary work of breaking down and digesting the various foods we eat. While most people think of all bacteria as "bad," some bacteria are useful for maintaining good health. *Lactobacillus acidophilus* (also called acidophilus) is a key species of good bacteria that populate our digestive tract, specifically the small or lower intestine. Because it is associated with health, acidophilus is sometimes called a "probiotic" (meaning "pro-life"). Not only do these "friendly bacteria" aid us in digesting vitamins and minerals, they help make conditions unfavorable for bad bacteria and stop them from growing.

WHAT IT DOES

Besides aiding in digestive health, acidophilus can be used as a remedy for various ailments of the digestive tract, such as stomach upsets and ulcers, and to treat vaginal yeast infections and urinary tract infections. Acidophilus has been shown to help suppress the level of *H. pylori*, the bacteria that can cause stomach and intestinal ulcers. People with irritable bowel syndrome may also benefit from acidophilus. Acidophilus may also play a role in preventing food allergies. Studies suggest that because of it ability to promote healthy digestion, acidophilus may help the intestines to properly absorb various foods as well as affecting the body's response to various foods.

Since acidophilus has the ability to replenish the body with good bacteria, it is often recommended for people with diarrhea, who lose both good and bad bacteria from their digestive tract in their stool. Acidophilus is also used in managing a variety of conditions in which levels of good bacteria in the body may become low, including eczema and chronic fatigue syndrome.

By replenishing the body with good bacteria, and keeping a healthy balance of bacteria in it, acidophilus may keep the immune system

Do all types of yogurt have equal amounts of acidophilus?

Q & A

When it comes to acidophilus, it is important to choose your yogurt wisely. All yogurt contains curdled milk and two kinds of "good" bacteria—*Lactobacillus thermophilus* and *Lactobacillus bulgaricus,* but not all yogurts contain acidophilus. Be sure to check the label when choosing yogurt, to make sure that acidophilus is clearly marked as one of the ingredients. Also, if the yogurt has been heat treated or pasteurized after being cultured, it won't have any remaining beneficial bacteria. Be sure to look for a statement such as "contains live cultures" on the label. Organic yogurt without preservatives or artificial sweeteners is the healthiest choice.

Note: When yogurt ages, the acidophilus count, or population of these bacteria, is depleted. Always purchase yogurt well before its expiration date, and don't let it sit in your refrigerator for too long if you want to reap the probiotic benefits.

healthy, allowing it to successfully fight various disease-causing bacteria. Studies are demonstrating enhanced effects for vaccinations against viruses when used along with acidophilus and other probiotics. Teeth and gums will benefit as well, since people with poor oral health have been found to have low levels of *Lactobacilli*. Even perennial allergic rhinitis symptoms have been diminished with the use of acidophilus. And recent studies have confirmed that taking probiotics containing acidophilus along with antibiotics helps to maintain the level of these important intestinal bacteria in the gut. *Lactobacillus acidophilus* has been demonstrated to help prevent canker sores.

For additional information on specific health conditions and how to treat them with supplements, see Part 3 of this book, beginning on page 309.

HOW IT WORKS

Because it is capable of resisting destruction by acid and bile—both of which are critical for the digestion and absorption of nutrients—acidophilus can survive the long, arduous journey through the intestinal tract.

Acidophilus works to keep a healthy balance of bacteria in the body by producing certain compounds, including lactic acid, hydrogen peroxide, and acetic acid, that make the intestine more acidic, and thus prevent certain harmful bacteria from reproducing. Acidophilus also

Important Tips for Purchasing Acidophilus

Did You Know?

One of the challenges for people taking acidophilus supplements has been identifying those products that contain live bacteria and are free from contamination. As with many supplements, standardization of lactobacillus products has been an ongoing challenge. Various factors that can affect the quality of acidophilus include storage conditions and the length of time the product has been on the shelf. Read on for some tips to help you shop for acidophilus wisely.

■ Many acidophilus products require refrigeration to maintain their potency. Always check the label for storage directions.

■ Most acidophilus products have the number of "living cells" listed on the side panel of the bottle. The number of living cells decreases with time, so be sure to purchase a product that is as far away from its expiration date as possible. Do not buy acidophilus if there is no expiration date on the label.

■ Acidophilus in coated-capsule form may be a good choice for people with more severe stomach symptoms, since the coating allows the supplement to pass through the digestive tract without breaking down before it reaches the intestines.

■ Milk-free acidophilus, which is often cultured from soy, may be a favorable choice to people with lactose intolerance.

produces substances called bacteriocins, which work as natural antibiotics in the body and fight invading organisms that could cause illness.

HOW TO TAKE IT

Acidophilus may be taken in capsule, tablet, powder, or liquid form, or ingested in yogurt. Since acidophilus are a live bacteria, they may need to be refrigerated. Check the label for important storage information. For yeast infections, acidophilus may be used in suppository form.

Dosages of acidophilus are measured in organisms or colony forming units (CFUs) rather than grams or milligrams. General dosage recommendations for acidophilus often range from 1 to 2 billion live organisms or CFUs daily. Sometimes, dosages of 10 billion live organisms or CFUs are recommended for a short period of time, to restore the balance of bacteria in the digestive system, such as, after taking an antibiotic medication.

Note: When taking acidophilus to replace intestinal bacteria destroyed by antibiotics, wait 3 hours after taking any antibiotic, since the antibiotic may kill acidophilus if the two are taken together.

LOOK OUT FOR THIS!

Acidophilus is generally safe to take on a regular basis. However, if you have a gastrointestinal ailment such as Crohn's disease or ulcerative colitis, you should consult your doctor before taking acidophilus. Caution is also advised about using acidophilus for people with damaged intestines, a weakened immune system, or an overgrowth of intestinal bacteria.

Some people taking acidophilus may experience abdominal discomfort, or gas.

Pregnant and nursing women should consult with their doctor before taking acidophilus.

WHAT TO AVOID

Medication: It is advisable to take acidophilus 3 hours after taking an antibiotic. People using antacids should wait 30 to 60 minutes before taking acidophilus, since it may not be able to survive the acidic conditions in the stomach. Acidophilus may reduce the effect of sulfasalazine, often prescribed for irritable bowel syndrome, though further study of this is needed.

FRIENDS AND FOES

Making sure that all the various bacteria in the gastrointestinal tract coexist in harmony is the key to optimum digestive and gynecological health. For a variety of reasons, including the use of antibiotics, the level of acidophilus in the intestinal tract and in the vagina can sometimes drop steeply, which upsets this delicate balance. For example, although an antibiotic may be necessary for treating a bacterial infection, the antibiotic kills bacteria indiscriminately, often depleting the system of good bacteria. Maintaining the right level of acidophilus helps keep the numbers of disease-promoting bacteria and yeast in the body within their proper limits. You can boost the level of acidophilus bacteria in your digestive tract (and also in the vagina) by taking acidophilus supplements or by consuming cultured yogurt or fermented milk.

Some experts believe that taking acidophilus in conjunction with fructo-oligosaccharides—long-chain sugars found in onions, bananas, Jerusalem artichokes, asparagus, and garlic—may help boost the healthful effects of acidophilus by speeding the rate of its growth.

LAVENDER

BEST KNOWN AS A RELAXATION- and sleep-promoting ingredient in massage oils and aromatherapy products, lavender has been used worldwide for centuries. Ancient Egyptian mummies were bathed in it (for the ultimate sleep), and it is currently used in herbal medicines, soaps, cosmetics, and tea. Of the many species of lavender, English lavender *(Lavandula angustifolia)* is the most prevalent.

WHAT IT DOES

Although it has many anecdotal uses, lavender is most commonly used to relieve anxiety and depression, promote sleep, and ease perineal discomfort after childbirth. Lavender may also have antibiotic, anti-inflammatory, antifungal, antispasmotic, and anticancer properties, and recent studies are beginning to confirm these claims. In one study conducted at Wesleyan University using healthy young sleepers, lavender appeared to increase sleep quality and give a more restful night's sleep. A British study came to similar conclusions.

Want to get more done at work? A Japanese study found that lavender oil aroma, but not jasmine, when used during "recess" periods, prevented deterioration of concentration. Anxious in the dentist's office? One study found that an ambient odor of lavender and orange oil diminished anxiety more than quiet music. And yet another study found that lozenges flavored with oils of lavender and lemon balm created a relaxed state in healthy volunteers.

In traditional herbal medicine, lavender was considered effective for "nervous stomach"—what doctors today might call gastritis or irritable bowel syndrome (IBS). The German Commission E (see page 16) has recently approved lavender for treating IBS as well as for insomnia and general intestinal discomfort.

Herbalists also use lavender essential oil topically as an antiseptic treatment for acne. Use it sparingly on a cotton swab, or look for cleansing lotions that contain lavender essential oils. Preliminary studies suggest that lavender oil may increase the sense of well-being when used in a bath or promote relaxation and enhance concentration when used as a topical gel. Another study found that lavender tincture, when combined with prescription antidepressant medication, may be more effective in relieving symptoms of depression than prescription medication alone. And although the findings are varied, lavender may ease agitation in people with severe dementia when administered as an aromatherapy. Early studies also suggest that when used in a footbath, lavender may improve blood flow and calm the nervous system. A more recent study found that lavender oil applied during acupressure massage gave added benefit in the short-term relief of neck pain.

Many essential oils have potent antibiotic and antiparasitic properities, and recent studies are determining that lavender is no different. Studies are now finding that in vitro, lavender has the ability to eliminate the human protozoal pathogens *Giardia duodenalis* and *Trichomonas vaginalis,* and the yeast *Candida albicans* (both the oral and vaginal varieties). A bit of lavender oil added to your dandruff shampoo may help treat the condition by utilizing the antifungal properties of lavender. And if all that doesn't excite you about lavender, consider that early studies indicate that lavender has properties that help prevent stroke and bloot clots.

For additional information on specific health conditions and how you can treat them with supplements, see Part 3 of this book, beginning on page 309.

HOW IT WORKS

A flower rich in volatile oils (oils that evaporate easily), lavender contains over 100 chemical components, including linalool, perillyl alcohol, limonene, cineole, camphor, tannins, coumarins, and flavonoids.

So far, most studies of lavender as an oral formulation have been on animals or with cell cultures. In animals, linalool has reduced levels of glutamate, a neurotransmitter that excites the brain, while boosting the calming neurotransmitter gamma-aminobutyric acid (GABA). Animal researchers are also studying perillyl alcohol and limonene for their possible anticancer uses, as well as cineole to lower cholesterol.

In preliminary human trials with cancer patients, oral perillyl alcohol (POH) has seemed promising for stabilizing the progression of advanced tumors that didn't respond to other treatment.

HOW TO TAKE IT

Lavender is available as dried flowers or a liquid extract for oral use, and as concentrated lavender oil for external use. In general, lavender oil should not be taken orally. However, highly diluted oil may be found in candies and chewing gum.

Typical doses of lavender for aromatherapy are 2 to 4 drops of extract in 2 to 3 cups of boiling water; it's safe to inhale these vapors a few times a day. Some people find that sprinkling their pillows with water-diluted lavender can help them sleep; others tuck lavender sachets beside their pillows. Or, use a commercially available aromatherapy device to help volatize (distribute) the oil's scent while you sleep or work.

For massage, use 1 to 4 drops of lavender extract per tablespoon of massage oil. For perineal discomfort after childbirth, add 6 drops of lavender oil, or up to one-half cup of dried leaves and flowers, to each bath.

To make lavender tea, steep 2 teaspoons of dried flowers in 1 cup of boiling water for 15 minutes; drink this as many as three times a day. Or use one-half to three-fourths of a teaspoon of tincture, up to three times a day.

Because lavender isn't standardized, and each species of the flower has different active ingredients, some lavender products may seem stronger or weaker than others. If the recommended doses do not seem effective, you may have a weaker version and may increase the dose.

LOOK OUT FOR THIS!

Lavender is generally safe and well tolerated when taken in the usual amounts. A few people have an allergic skin reaction to lavender products.

Although externally applied lavender is generally assumed to be safe, women should be cautious about taking lavender orally during pregnancy or breastfeeding, since no safety data are available.

WHAT TO AVOID

There are no known interactions of lavender when taken with other drugs, herbs, or supplements.

L-CARNITINE

FORGET WHAT YOU'VE HEARD about L-carnitine—also known simply as carnitine—at the gym or in your weight-loss group. The really good news about this amino acid derivative is something you're more likely to hear at your doctor's office. Although studies haven't supported claims that carnitine can improve your staying power during workouts, or help you lose weight, they do show that it can have therapeutic benefits for a surprisingly wide range of medical conditions, from diabetes and heart disease to chronic fatigue syndrome, human immunodeficiency virus (HIV) and acquired immune deficiency syndrome (AIDS), infertility and cancer. Carnitine may be useful for the fatigue associated with interferon treatment for hepatitis C and for the fatigue associated with multiple sclerosis. In fact, several studies have indicated that it may be useful for alleviating the fatigue associated with multiple sclerosis. One study found that L-carnitine worked better than amantadine, a medication typically used for this purpose.

Carnitine is a natural compound manufactured in the liver and kidneys from the amino acids lysine and methionine. Most healthy people produce enough carnitine—or get enough from dietary sources such as meat and dairy products—to supply the body's needs. The body requires lysine, methionine, vitamin C, niacin (vitamin B_3), and vitamin B_6 (pyroxide) to produce carnitine. But certain conditions, such as liver and kidney problems, as well as certain medications, can cause a carnitine deficiency or can interfere with the action of carnitine, making supplementation necessary.

Carnitine comes in three forms: L-carnitine, which affects muscles; L-acetylcarnitine, which affects brain function and memory; and L-propionylcarnitine, which affects the heart and brain. L-carnitine is the recommended form for supplementation.

WHAT IT DOES

Carnitine plays a vital role in helping the body turn fat into energy. Stored in the skeletal muscles, heart, brain, and sperm, it helps supply energy to a wide variety of tissues and organs.

Supplementation with carnitine is primarily used for several different heart and circulatory conditions. Patients with exercise-induced angina who take carnitine can exercise longer and more intensely without pain. Studies also indicate that people with atherosclerosis who get painful leg cramps when walking (sometimes called intermittent claudication) may benefit from taking carnitine as a supplement. Carnitine may also help prevent some of the complications that can occur after a heart attack, and may actually reduce the amount of damage done to the heart muscle by a heart attack. It may also make a subsequent heart attack less likely, and help prevent congestive heart failure after an attack.

For people with type 2 diabetes, carnitine may help the body control blood sugar levels and prevent injury to the nerves of the heart. It may also help prevent complications when people with diabetes undergo heart surgery. Carnitine may help prevent nerve damage in children with diabetes. Some, but not all, studies also indicate that carnitine supplements may improve sperm count and mobility, and thus may help correct male infertility.

A few studies have shown that the form of carnitine called acetyl-L-carnitine may have beneficial effects in the initial stages of Alzheimer's disease; it may also help prevent mild depression in the elderly. However, because other studies have shown that carnitine may actually make symptoms worse in the later stages of Alzheimer's disease, it should be taken only under the supervision of a doctor.

Preliminary studies indicate that carnitine may help reduce cholesterol and triglyceride levels; one study found this to be the case in people undergoing dialysis. Other studies show that carnitine may be useful for treating chronic obstructive pulmonary disease (COPD), which includes bronchitis and emphysema, as well as for chronic fatigue syndrome, muscle pains, and hyperthyroidism (overactive thyroid gland). Carnitine may also be useful for reducing the side effects of some commonly prescribed anti-HIV medications, since many of these medications deplete carnitine.

Carnitine appears to be useful in the treatment of nerve damage. Recent studies confirm that carnitine is useful in the treatment of antiretroviral-induced peripheral neuropathy. People undergoing chemotherapy for cancer may also benefit from carnitine's ability to treat peripheral neuropathy. Carnitine also diminishes the symptoms associated with diabetic neuropathy.

Carnitine appears to offer a protective effect from brain damage seen in people with cirrhosis of the liver. It may also help prevent lung and heart problems in children with sickle-cell anemia.

For additional information on specific health conditions and how to treat them with supplements, see Part 3 of this book, beginning on page 309.

HOW IT WORKS

Carnitine transports long-chain fatty acids to the energy-producing components of cells, known as mitochondria, and helps the mitochondria metabolize those fatty acids to produce energy. This may account for the positive effects of carnitine on patients with atherosclerosis and COPD, in whom it seems to make the muscles around the lungs and in the legs work more efficiently, without actually improving blood flow. Carnitine also appears to block the action of excess thyroid hormone in cells, accounting for its potentially beneficial effects in patients with hyperthyroidism.

HOW TO TAKE IT

Carnitine may be prescribed by your doctor, especially in cases in which a specific disease or inherited condition has caused a deficiency of it (see Did You Know? below). Dosages of carnitine for supplementation vary with the condition being treated. Typically, adults take anywhere from 500 to 1,000 milligrams three times a day. When taken in the form of acetyl-L-carnitine, dosages often range from a total of 1 to 3 grams daily in tablet or capsule form, divided into several doses. In liquid form, L-carnitine should be drunk slowly with or after meals to help avoid stomach upset.

Note: A form of carnitine known as D-carnitine is sometimes found in over-the-counter supplements. This form of carnitine is physiologically inactive in humans and may actually displace the active form, L-carnitine, in tissues. This can lead to muscle weakness and other undesirable side effects and is particularly a problem if you have a diagnosed carnitine deficiency. Avoid supplements containing D-carnitine.

LOOK OUT FOR THIS!

Carnitine supplements rarely cause side effects, but some people experience nausea and diarrhea when taking more than 5 grams a day.

Making Up for Lost Carnitine

Did You Know?

A number of health conditions and some medications can cause deficiencies of carnitine and may lead your doctor to prescribe a carnitine supplement. Alcohol-induced liver disease, for example, can prevent existing levels of carnitine from functioning properly, causing a buildup of fat in the liver; supplemental carnitine may help reduce this buildup. Kidney dialysis patients may also have lower-than-normal levels of carnitine, and eating disorders such as anorexia may deplete the body of carnitine.

There are also a number of medications that may reduce levels of carnitine in the body. These include allopurinol, anticonvulsant medications (such as carbamazepine), phenytoin, topirimate, and valproic acid, HIV medications (such as zidovudine), and barbiturate medications (such as phenobarbitol and secobarbital).

If you are taking any of these medications or have any of the health conditions listed above, consult your doctor about taking supplemental carnitine.

Because carnitine blocks the action of thyroid hormone, individuals with borderline or low levels of thyroid hormone should take carnitine supplements only under the supervision of a doctor.

The greatest source of carnitine may be dairy products and red meat. People who have low intakes of meat and dairy products (such as vegans) may also have low carnitine intakes.

Pregnant women should take carnitine supplements only if advised to do so by their doctor.

WHAT TO AVOID

Medication: See Did You Know? on previous page.

LEMON BALM

THE LEAVES OF THE LEMON BALM *(Melissa officinalis)* plant are so fragrant and refreshing that the medieval king Charlemagne ordered it to be planted in the gardens of every monastery in his realm. But lemon balm has an even more ancient history as a medicinal plant. Both the Greeks and Romans used it as a treatment for wounds, and herbalists throughout the ages have prescribed it for everything from sleeping problems to anxiety and "nervous stomach." It is often used as a digestive aid to alleviate gas (carminative), to induce sweating when one is sick (diaphoretic), and to lower a fever (febrifuge). Modern practitioners have found solid evidence for at least some of these uses.

WHAT IT DOES

Lemon balm may be applied topically or taken orally. Topical applications containing lemon balm have been found to reduce flare-ups of both genital and oral herpes, and one study indicated that lemon balm salves could help cold sores heal more rapidly. When applied to the face and arms, the essential oil of lemon balm has been noted to calm patients with severe cases of dementia, and applications to the temples are a traditional treatment for insomnia.

Taken internally, lemon balm has been found to help with insomnia and ease anxiety. In a clinical trial, a combination of lemon balm and valerian extracts had effects similar to the prescription sleep medication triazolam (Halcion), helping patients to fall asleep more easily and improving the quality of their sleep. Two additional clinical trials found that either a similar combination or lemon balm

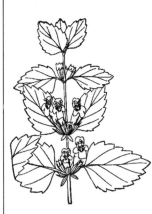

alone decreased experimentally-induced stress in healthy volunteers. Lemon balm also appears to have gas-relieving properties in the gastrointestinal system. Lemon balm is so gentle that it's used in infants; a recent study found that a combination of lemon balm, fennel, and chamomile, when used for 1 week, reduced colic in breastfed infants.

Laboratory studies have suggested that lemon balm may be an effective treatment for hyperthyroidism (overactivity of the thyroid gland) and may also have activity against human immunodeficiency virus (HIV), and also herpes simplex virus type 2 (genital herpes), but no clinical trials have yet supported these possibilities.

For additional information on specific health conditions and how to treat them with supplements, see Part 3 of this book, beginning on page 309.

HOW IT WORKS

The active components of lemon balm have several attributes that explain its observed therapeutic effects. Laboratory tests show that lemon balm has antiviral properties; the presumed action is that its components—including flavonoids and phenolic acids—prevent viruses from attaching to cells. Lemon balm also appears to have some in vitro antibiotic and antifungal properties. Other studies indicate that by blocking hormonal signals from the brain, lemon balm reduces the excessive stimulation of the thyroid gland that occurs in hyperthyroidism.

The terpenes, or volatile oils, that help produce lemon balm's pleasant aroma are thought to be responsible for its calming effects and its ability to relieve intestinal distress. The use of lemon balm in aromatherapy for patients with dementia is often combined with massage, which may cause calming effects as much as lemon balm itself.

Grow This!

The lemon balm plant is a favorite of bees, as is attested in its botanical name—*Melissa*—which translates to "honey bee" in Greek. Lemon balm, an herbaceous perennial belonging to the mint family, is very easy to grow, and often grows wild in sunny fields along roadsides. The lemon-scented leaves of the plant can be added to soups, salads, sauces, fish, and meat, providing a delicious lemon flavor.

Light: Full sun or partial shade.

Water: Lemon balm will be most fragrant if it is grown in a rich, moist soil; however, it also tolerates poor, sandy soils, and full sun.

You may propagate lemon balm by dividing the root mass or from cuttings. The species can also be propagated from seed.

HOW TO TAKE IT

Lemon balm is available as an essential oil and in cream preparations for topical application. For treating flare-ups of herpes, one suggested method is to apply the cream thickly to lesions up to four times a day. Inhalations of the essential oil are thought to have sedative effects.

Lemon balm is also available in tea and capsule form. To treat insomnia and calm the stomach, practitioners recommend using 1.5 to 4.5 grams of the herb per cup of tea and to drink several cups a day, as needed. Recommended dosages for the capsule form of lemon balm vary widely. Some authorities suggest taking 200 milligrams a day to treat insomnia, but at least one study found beneficial effects at dosages ranging from 300 to 900 milligrams taken once a day.

LOOK OUT FOR THIS!

If you have glaucoma, do not use the essential oil of lemon balm, and avoid any preparations containing the volatile oils of this herb. Animals studies indicate that lemon balm may increase pressure in the eye.

WHAT TO AVOID

There are no known interactions between lemon balm and other herbs, drugs, or dietary supplements.

LICORICE

THE ROOTS AND UNDERGROUND stems of the licorice plant *(Glycyrrhiza glabra)* have been used to treat a variety of illnesses in both Eastern and Western medicine, from the common head cold and respiratory ailments to stomach problems, inflammatory disorders, skin diseases, and liver problems. In Greek, licorice is known as "sweet root," and in Chinese, "sweet grass." In fact, it contains a compound that is about 50 times sweeter than table sugar, but which some researchers say is more than 150 times sweeter. The sweetness comes from an ingredient called glycyrrhizic acid, which also has important health benefits. In spite of the sweet taste, licorice has been found to inhibit the growth of *Streptococcus mutans*, the bacteria that cause dental caries. And that's not all: Two recent studies found that licorice has properties that may be useful in the treatment of breast and prostate cancer.

WHAT IT DOES

Licorice is often used to prevent and treat stomach ulcers, heartburn, acid reflux, and excessive gastrointestinal gas. In Europe and Japan, medical doctors prescribe a synthetic form of licorice for stomach ulcers, and some animal studies and early trials in humans support this use. A combination containing licorice and an antacid called Caved-S, is commonly sold in Europe. Animal studies suggest that licorice may reduce the stomach irritation and risk of stomach ulcers commonly associated with use of aspirin. One study found that chewable licorice tablets, in the form of deglycyrrhizinated licorice (DGL), were as effective as the medication cimetidine (Tagamet) in healing ulcers.

Topically, licorice-containing gels and ointments may be used for treating herpes simplex, herpes zoster (shingles), and eczema. Gargling with licorice mouthwash may help to heal canker sores, although licorice supplements may also be recommended for this condition.

Herbalists sometimes recommend licorice for people with respiratory infections and cough. The German Commission E (see page 16) has approved licorice for the treatment of cough, bronchitis, and gastritis.

Nevertheless, the health benefits of licorice are still in debate. People who regularly consume large amounts of licorice—more than 20 grams per day—may risk raising the level of the hormone aldosterone in their blood, which can lead to headaches, high blood pressure, and heart problems. DGL is often preferred to whole licorice because it has fewer such side effects.

Some research suggests that licorice may play a role in treating heart disease. In one study, licorice root extract taken for only 1 month lowered blood levels of total cholesterol, LDL ("bad") cholesterol, and triglycerides. Licorice may also play a role in treating individuals infected with the human immunodeficiency virus (HIV) and encephalitis. In Japan, licorice is used to treat hepatitis.

For additional information on specific health conditions and how to treat them with supplements, see Part 3 of this book, beginning on page 309.

HOW IT WORKS

Licorice has a number of active ingredients, but the one most studied is glycyrrhizin, which has been shown in laboratory studies to reduce inflammation, promote the secretion of mucus, soothe throat, lung, and bronchial membranes, and stimulate the adrenal glands. However, when taken at high doses, glycyrrhizin may cause water retention, high blood pressure, and a loss of potassium. As a result, many manufacturers have begun to produce the variety of licorice called deglycyrrhizinated licorice (or DGL), which does not contain glycyrrhizin.

HOW TO TAKE IT

Licorice is available in capsules, chewable tablets, as a liquid for oral use in drop form, and as a tea. It comes in two varieties: as whole licorice and in the chemically modified form of DGL. Many healthcare providers prefer the DGL form, since it's gentler on the stomach and does not trigger undesirable side effects (see How It Works, above). DGL does not have compounds in whole licorice that stimulate the adrenal glands.

For adults and older children with sore throats, a piece of licorice root may be chewed. The beneficial effects of chewing on the root are far greater than chewing on licorice candy, since the candy often contains artificial flavoring, without any real licorice. Certain types of licorice candy may contain actual licorice, but the amount is not standardized.

Licorice tea is also a remedy for sore throat, and licorice is also available in cough syrups, gum, and beverages, and is even a common additive in tobacco products including cigarettes, cigars, and chewing tobacco.

Short-term dosages of licorice usually range from 5 to 15 grams daily. Licorice should not be used for more than 4 to 6 weeks without medical supervision.

LOOK OUT FOR THIS!

Some side effects may occur when taking even the recommended doses of licorice, such as muscle pain and numbness in the arms and legs. High doses may be linked to serious side effects, including a condition called pseudoaldosteronism, which causes headaches, fatigue, high blood pressure, and can lead to heart attacks. Too much licorice may also cause water retention, which leads to leg swelling and other problems.

People with high blood pressure, obesity, diabetes, or kidney, heart, or liver conditions, and men with decreased libido or other sexual dysfunctions, should not take this supplement.

Young children and pregnant or nursing women should not take licorice, but DGL doesn't carry the same risks as licorice.

WHAT TO AVOID

Medication: Taking licorice with thiazide or loop diuretics may lead to potassium loss. Licorice may also interfere with the effectiveness of corticosteroid medications. Licorice is not recommended for people taking cardiac glycosides (such as digoxin) without a doctor's advice. Consult your doctor before taking licorice if you are taking angiotensin-converting enzyme (ACE) inhibitors, insulin, laxatives, or oral contraceptives.

LUTEIN

LUTEIN IS A NATURAL YELLOW PIGMENT found in such foods as egg yolks and some yellow fruits and vegetables, but most abundantly in green vegetables. And like its more famous cousin, beta-carotene, it has important health properties, safeguarding the body against the harmful effects of cell- and tissue-damaging free radicals molecules. But lutein also has a unique benefit that should make it an important part of everyone's preventive health regimen: It protects our eyes and may actually prevent the development of cataracts and an even more serious condition called macular degeneration, which affects a very important part of the eye.

WHAT IT DOES

Lutein, like beta-carotene, is a carotenoid—a naturally occurring pigment that's essential to human health. Aside from protecting against free radicals, recent studies indicate that lutein's special role is to protect the eyes, reducing the risk of cataracts and macular degeneration, one of the leading causes of blindness in aging adults.

In fact, research shows that people with the highest consumption of spinach, which has an especially high content of lutein, had a whopping 90 percent lower risk of developing age-related macular degeneration. Popeye's greatest strength may have been his eyesight!

There's also evidence that lutein consumption may protect against and combat certain forms of cancer, particularly breast, colon, lung, and ovarian cancers. And animal studies indicate that it

FOOD SOURCES

The best way to reap the benefits of lutein is to get it naturally from the foods you eat. It shouldn't be too hard to introduce more lutein into your diet because it is abundant in so many vegetables. You can easily increase your lutein intake by simply eating more greens. Read on for some foods that are rich in lutein.

▶ Broccoli, collard greens, egg yolks, kale, leek, peas, romaine lettuce, spinach, and yellow corn.

may protect the skin from the damaging rays of ultraviolet light. Preliminary research also suggests that lutein's antioxidant properties make it effective against atherosclerosis, but the results of various human studies of this are inconclusive.

For additional information on specific health conditions and how to treat them with supplements, see Part 3 of this book, beginning on page 309.

HOW IT WORKS

Lutein is the main pigment in the macular region of the eye, located near the center of the retina. Over time, the ultraviolet rays of sunlight damage this pigment, setting the stage for further cell damage, which causes macular degeneration. But lutein, when absorbed into the bloodstream, becomes concentrated in the eye, replacing lost pigment and protecting the macular region of the eye. Scientists also think lutein's antioxidant effects provide an additional measure of protection to the eye.

Lutein may fight cancer in two ways: By increasing the death rate of cancer cells and by reducing the growth of blood vessels supplying tumors.

HOW TO TAKE IT

If you're not keen on eating your greens, you might want to opt for a lutein supplement. Capsules are available in 6- and 20-milligram doses, and studies indicate that anywhere from 5 to 30 milligrams a day is a good idea. As with many other supplements, lutein is best taken with food to decrease the chance of stomach upset and increase its rate of absorption. Lutein-enriched eggs and yellow carrots may turn out to be the most absorbable sources of this nutrient.

LOOK OUT FOR THIS!

The U.S. Food and Drug Administration (FDA) has not established maximum safe dosage levels of supplemental lutein for young children, pregnant or nursing women, or people with severe kidney or liver disease. People in these groups should limit their intake of lutein to 5 milligrams a day.

Unlike other carotenoids, lutein is not converted into vitamin A, so do not take this supplement to treat a vitamin A deficiency. Also, taking lutein supplements may decrease absorption of beta-carotene.

Some popular multivitamin supplements now contain lutein, but in very small amounts. One brand includes only 250 micrograms, about 20 times less than the minimum amount thought to be adequate.

WHAT TO AVOID

Medication: Cholestyramine and colestipol may decrease the absorption of lutein.

Food: Mineral oil, orlistat, pectin, and the fat substitute Olestra may decrease the absorption of lutein.

LYCOPENE

THE RED IN TOMATOES COMES from lycopene, and a growing body of evidence suggests that this member of the carotenoid family is good for a lot more than one of nature's prettiest food colors. A high intake of lycopene has been linked to preventing some of the worst scourges of human health, from cancer to cardiovascular disease.

Since the first indications that lycopene might be a potent disease-preventive agent, it has been extensively studied, but most of these investigations aren't as conclusive as researchers would like because they're based on observations of people's diets rather than on rigorous double-blind studies. Nevertheless, there's enough of a connection between lycopene and preventive success to warrant your attention—and perhaps an extra helping of tomato sauce on your next dish of pasta.

WHAT IT DOES

With the provision that the studies of it aren't definitive or all in agreement, the evidence for lycopene's potential benefits makes a long and impressive list. First and perhaps most significantly, like other carotenoids such as beta-carotene, lycopene has been linked to reducing the risk of various forms of cancer. One study found that elderly Americans with a diet high in tomatoes—and therefore presumably rich in lycopene—were 50 percent less likely than average to get cancer.

Lycopene appears to have a unique ability among carotenoids to improve the odds against getting prostate cancer. In one study, men

TOMATO-CARROT SOUP

Try this rich soup that is sure to delight your taste buds and add some extra lycopene to you your diet. This flavorful soup is especially enjoyable in the winter.

Ingredients

1 tablespoon olive oil

1 cup sliced scallions

1 clove garlic, minced

3 cups unstrained canned
  tomatoes, chopped

1 cup carrot juice

$1/2$ teaspoon ground cumin

$1/4$ teaspoon ginger

$1/4$ teaspoon black pepper

$1/2$ cup evaporated milk

1 teaspoon fresh basil

Directions: In a medium saucepan, sauté scallions and garlic in oil over low heat. Stir occasionally for 3 minutes or until scallions are soft. Stir in tomatoes and their juice; let them cook for 5 minutes, stirring occasionally. As the mixture becomes thick, add carrot juice, cumin, ginger, and black pepper. Do not cover the pan; let the ingredients simmer for 5 minutes. Add evaporated milk and cook for 1 minute, but do not let the milk boil. Sprinkle basil on top of the soup just before serving.

who had the highest intake of lycopene in their diet had a 21 percent less chance of developing prostate cancer than those with the lowest intake. Men who consumed more than 10 servings of tomatoes a week did even better, having a 35 percent lower risk than men eating only 1.5 servings. And among patients with prostate cancer, levels of lycopene in the blood are often lower than average. While some recent studies have not been able to find that greater lycopene-tomato product consumption provides protection from prostate cancer, another recent study indicated that lycopene therapy appears to be effective and safe in the treatment of hormone refractery prostate cancer.

High levels of lycopene also seem to reduce the risk of cancers other than prostate cancer. The chance of developing cancers of the gastrointestinal tract was 30 to 60 percent lower in the top quarter of people in one study who ate the most tomato-based products; colorectal cancer risk was 50 percent lower in the top third. Conversely, in one studied group of women, the 75 percent who ate the least amount of tomatoes had as much as a 4.7 times greater risk of developing cancer of the cervix. A study in India recently found that lycopene supplements could be an effective treatment for oral leukoplakia (a potentially precancerous condition of the mucus membranes of the mouth).

Both lung cancer and breast cancer appear to be less frequent in high tomato consumers, but the evidence is somewhat less compelling than for the other forms of cancer mentioned previously.

Several other conditions seem to respond to lycopene. Researchers in Europe have noted a 48 percent lower risk of cardiovascular disease among people with the highest levels of lycopene in the blood. An Israeli study indicated that the natural antoxidants from tomato extract were able to reduce blood pressure in patients with mild to high blood pressure who had never taken any medication. Because it's a powerful antioxidant, some observers have suggested that lycopene may help prevent age-related macular degeneration. While lycopene may also help reduce exercise-induced asthma through antioxidant action, a recent study found no effect on lung function after exercise and clinical difficulty in breathing in young athletes. Observational studies indicate that diets high in carotenoids are inversely associated with type 2 diabetes and impaired glucose metabolism. Lycopene appears to act as a photoprotectant and may be able to diminish sun damage caused by UV light. It may also be able to prevent DNA damage in certain white blood cells. Increased levels of lycopene and other beta-carotenoids may help decrease respiratory disease in elderly people. Overall, more research is needed to determine lycopene's effectiveness in these cases.

HOW IT WORKS

Most research suggests that lycopene's antioxidant properties—its ability to counteract the cell-damaging effects of free radicals—account for its presumed effects in reducing the risk of cancer, heart disease, and macular degeneration. In patients who have already developed prostate cancer, increasing their levels of lycopene has been noted to slow tumor growth. Lycopene's special status among carotenoids in reducing the risk of certain cancers is supported by its presence in higher levels than other carotenoids in the lungs, prostate, and colon, as well as in the blood, skin, liver, and adrenal glands.

Interestingly, research indicates that raw tomatoes don't raise lycopene levels as much as products containing cooked tomatoes, such as tomato sauce and ketchup. Scientists think this may be because the cooking process breaks down plant tissues, releasing carotenoids and thus allowing them to be more easily absorbed.

HOW TO TAKE IT

Although you might be tempted to get your daily dose of lycopene from a supplement, so as to know precisely how much you're getting, keep this in mind: Lycopene supplements are notoriously expensive, and several studies indicate they don't work as well as lycopene obtained from the diet. Although lycopene supplements are readily available on the market, most experts agree that the best source of this carotenoid is tomato-based foods. But keep in mind that cooked tomato products give your body lycopene in the most readily absorbable form. In fact, some studies show that raw tomatoes and tomato juice don't do much to raise blood levels of lycopene. In more delicious news, one study found that the addition of olive oil to diced tomatoes during cooking greatly increases the absorption of lycopene. Additionally, lycopene absorption appears to be much greater if your salad contains oil in the dressing. Tomatoes aren't the only source of lycopene: You can also get lycopene from pink grapefruit, guava, and watermelon.

Although lycopene does appear to have positive effects, don't forget that it has not been subjected to any well-controlled studies. It's possible that people who eat a lot of foods rich in lycopene may have a

---

SUPPLEMENTAL TRIVIA

Just what you needed—another reason not to eat doughnuts and other baked goods! The caramelization process that helps brown cookies, processed cereals, pastries, and doughnuts links sugar and lysine molecules together. The result? Your body absorbs less lysine. So if your diet has a high content of these foods, you may develop a lysine deficiency.

generally healthier lifestyle that might account for their lower incidence of cancers and heart disease. So don't assume that you can just pig out on pizza and slather your hot dogs or hamburgers with extra ketchup to get the benefits of lycopene that studies seem to suggest.

The U.S. Food and Drug Administration (FDA) hasn't established a minimum daily requirement, but observational studies suggest that 6.5 milligrams a day may have disease-preventive effects. Some practitioners recommend levels as high as 20 to 40 milligrams a day.

Lycopene-rich foods include tomatoes, pink grapefruit, fresh papaya, watermelon, and apricots. Tomato paste is the most concentrated source of lycopene.

Laboratory studies suggest beneficial interactions between lycopene and both lutein and vitamin E. Taking lutein and lycopene together may offer improved antioxidant action, and vitamin E works with lycopene to more effectively inhibit the growth of prostate cancer cells.

LOOK OUT FOR THIS!

Lycopene is considered a generally safe supplement. If you're allergic to tomatoes, consult your doctor before taking lycopene supplements.

People who smoke 25 or more cigarettes a day have significantly lower than average levels of lycopene.

WHAT TO AVOID

Medication: Studies indicate that lycopene is actually transported through the bloodstream by LDL ("bad") cholesterol—the cholesterol associated with increased risk of heart disease. If you are taking a cholesterol-lowering medication such as fluvastatin, you may have lower levels of lycopene in your system. But it's not clear whether this is a problem.

Food: Olestra, a fat substitute available in some commercially prepared low-fat foods, may reduce lycopene levels in the blood by as much as 30 percent.

LYSINE

YOU PROBABLY GET ALL THE LYSINE you need from your diet without even knowing it. But if you have herpes, you might want to think about getting extra lysine through a supplement.

Lysine is one of a few amino acids—the basic building blocks of protein—that are deemed "essential," meaning the body can't produce them on its own but must get them from dietary sources such as food or supplements. Lysine plays an important role in keeping the body's tissues healthy, is needed for normal growth, and helps regulate a proper balance of nitrogen in the body.

WHAT IT DOES

As a crucial component of many different proteins, lysine is important for building and repairing tissues, and it also helps the body synthesize hormones, enzymes, and antibodies. In particular, it's one of the main ingredients in collagen, the material from which cartilage and other connective tissues are made.

Supplementation with lysine is reported to help prevent recurrences of herpes attacks, caused by the herpes simplex virus, and is prescribed by doctors for people who experience frequent cold sores. It may also help treat genital herpes, although the evidence for its benefit in this condition is less compelling. Although some practitioners recommend taking lysine at the first sign of a herpes flare-up, others contend that it's only useful when taken preventively.

Some researchers have suggested that lysine also keeps blood vessels healthy and builds muscles, but no studies have confirmed this. There is also some preliminary evidence that lysine may help prevent osteoporosis or even be useful in treating it, but most researchers feel that more studies are needed to confirm this benefit.

For additional information on specific health conditions and how you can treat them with supplements, see Part 3 of this book, beginning on page 309.

HOW IT WORKS

There's good scientific evidence for how lysine helps in combating herpes flare-ups. It apparently keeps the herpes simplex virus from replicating, and laboratory studies suggest it does so by blocking another amino acid, arginine, that the virus uses to reproduce. The fact that lysine keeps the virus from proliferating may explain why it's good for preventing recurrences of herpes but not effective for treating attacks once they've begun. (Some studies use L-lysine in combination with zinc for the treatment of herpes.)

Although researchers are still studying whether lysine might be a good treatment or preventive measure for osteoporosis, they do know that it helps the digestive tract absorb calcium and that it reduces the amount of calcium excreted in urine. By increasing and conserving the body's store of calcium, lysine may help prevent the bone loss associated with osteoporosis. L-lysine, when taken in combination with L-arginine, may be useful in the treatment of anxiety.

HOW TO TAKE IT

Most of us get enough lysine from the food we eat. It's found in a wide variety of foods, including meat, dairy products, fish, eggs, and legumes (primarily beans, peas, and lentils). Therefore, lysine deficiency is rare in healthy people. However, if you're a vegetarian and don't eat a lot of legumes, or if you're an athlete who exercises vigorously, you may require a lysine supplement. Doctors have also found that burn patients have high requirements for essential amino acids to help their bodies rebuild tissue.

Lysine is a part of many daily multivitamin supplements. The recommended daily amount for general health is 5.5 milligrams per pound of body weight. Lysine is also available (alone) in capsule or tablet form, in doses of 500 milligrams. If you have herpes, the recommended dosage for reducing flare-ups is from 1 to 3 grams a day.

LOOK OUT FOR THIS!

Safe levels of supplemental lysine have not been established for children or for pregnant or nursing women. In fact, animal studies indicate that high levels of lysine may actually stunt growth. You don't need to worry about getting too much lysine from your diet, but don't give lysine supplements to children.

Avoid lysine supplementation if you have kidney or liver problems, because taking individual amino acids can put an extra strain on those organs. You should also stay away from lysine supplements if you have diabetes or an allergy to the proteins found in wheat, milk, or eggs.

Other animal studies have shown that high doses of lysine can increase the risk of developing gallstones, and may raise cholesterol levels. People taking extremely high doses of lysine—as much as 15 to 40 grams a day—have reported having abdominal cramps and diarrhea.

WHAT TO AVOID

Food: Because of the evidence that lysine works against herpes by blocking arginine, stay away from foods containing arginine, such as chocolate, peanuts, and other nuts and seeds, if you are taking lysine for herpes.

MAGNESIUM

THE HEALING PROPERTIES of the mineral magnesium have been recognized for centuries. In 1695, an article described the healing properties of salts found in the mineral-rich waters of Epsom, England. They were called "Epsom salts" in English, and on the European continent, *"salt anglicum."* The active ingredient was magnesium.

Whether you consume it in your daily food, take dietary supplements, or soak in it at night, magnesium is vital for maintaining good health. Internally, magnesium helps every organ in the body do its job—particularly the heart, muscles, kidneys, and lungs. Unfortunately, most adults in the United States fail to consume adequate amounts of magnesium in their diets.

WHAT IT DOES

Magnesium assists metabolic processes throughout the body. It plays an important role in regulating blood pressure; is involved in the metabolism of energy, and enhances the synthesis of proteins; and it also helps regulate calcium levels as well as those of copper, zinc, potassium, vitamin D, and other important nutrients. It keeps your muscles and nerves in good shape, your heart beating steadily, and your teeth and bones strong. In fact, magnesium is needed for the actions of more than 350 enzymes in the body.

When taken in conjunction with calcium supplements, magnesium improves calcium absorption, which helps increase bone density and prevent conditions such as osteoporosis.

That old medical standby—milk of magnesia—is an effective treatment for constipation. The active ingredient is magnesium hydroxide, which is also an effective antacid and remedy for an upset stomach.

Studies show that magnesium is helpful in preventing migraine headaches, hearing loss, and kidney stones, and (along with potassium) for treating high blood pressure, angina, dysmenorrheal (painful periods), leg cramps during pregnancy, and premenstrual syndrome.

FOOD FACTORS

MAGNESIUM

Magnesium is contained in many foods, but usually in extremely small amounts. Additionally, the soil in which food is grown may be depleted of magnesium, so that its levels in such foods are lower than they should be. Eating the following foods can help you to incorporate magnesium into your diet.

▶ Almonds, apricots, bananas, bran, cocoa and bitter chocolate, coconut, dates, dried figs, dried seaweed, Florida avocado, green leafy vegetables, lentils, legumes, pumpkin seeds, shellfish, spinach (cooked), wheat germ, and whole grains.

Magnesium supplementation may also act as a mood stabilizer and be useful in the treatment of sleep disorders associated with aging. Magnesium helps regulate the "biological clock" and the regulation of sleep in general.

Supplemental magnesium may help regulate blood sugar levels in people with diabetes. Several studies have found that blood levels of magnesium are low in people with type 2 diabetes, and that supplementation with magnesium may help improve insulin sensitivity in cases when magnesium levels are low.

Magnesium may play an important role in controlling a normal rhythm of the heart; studies indicate that intravenous magnesium-sulfate may be an effective adjunct treatment for persons with atrial fibrillation. And, if given during cardiac bypass surgery, magnesium may help prevent damage to the heart.

Prior studies document that intravenous magnesium is useful in the treatment of an acute asthma attack. Now some preliminary studies indicate that magnesium sulfate, when used in a nebulizer, may also aid in the treatment of asthma. Research also suggests that high levels of dietary magnesium may be associated with lower levels of certain types of cancer, including prostate and stomach cancers. Other studies indicate that diets with a high intake of magnesium may contribute to greater bone density and a lower risk of osteoporosis, while diets low in magnesium may increase the risk of heart disease.

Supplementation with magnesium reduces pregnancy-induced hypertension, high blood pressure, seizures, and water retention; increases tolerance to stress; and helps prevent sleep disorders, including those associated with aging. Night terrors, sleepwalking, sleep-talking, and teeth grinding are all sleep disturbances associated with magnesium deficiency.

Moreover, magnesium has also been suggested as a treatment for an array of ailments, including Alzheimer's disease, attention deficit hyperactivity disorder (ADHD), fatigue, fibromyalgia, high cholesterol, periodontal disease, rheumatoid arthritis, and stroke.

For additional information on specific health conditions and how to treat them with supplements, see Part 3 of this book, beginning on page 309.

HOW IT WORKS

Magnesium assists several vital enzymes in helping convert carbohydrates, proteins, and fats into energy. It also plays a role in conducting nerve impulses, enabling proper function of the heart and other muscular structures. Magnesium contributes to bone heath because of its ability to increase the body's absorption of calcium.

HOW TO TAKE IT

See the table below for the recommended daily intakes (RDIs) of magnesium. Note that most magnesium researchers recommend twice the RDA amount.

AGE/GENDER/ CONDITION	RECOMMENDED DAILY INTAKE (RDI)*
Infants	
0–6 months	30 mg
7–12 months	75 mg
Children	
1–3 years	80 mg
4–8 years	130 mg
9–13 years	240 mg
Males	
14–18 years	410 mg
19–30 years	400 mg
31 years and older	320 mg
Females	
14–18 years	360 mg
19–30 years	310 mg
31 years and older	320 mg
Pregnant Women	
19–30 years	350 mg
31–50 years	360 mg
Nursing Women	
19–30 years	310 mg

*For more information on RDIs, see Want to Know More About Intake? on page 8.

Unfortunately, most people are not getting enough magnesium even when eating a balanced diet. Supplemental magnesium is even more important for people with conditions that cause excessive urinary loss of magnesium, chronic malabsorption, severe diarrhea, and chronic or severe vomiting.

People with diabetes who do not control this condition properly may also require magnesium supplements, because an increased amount of magnesium is lost in the urine. People with alcoholism are usually magnesium deficient as well, as are people with low levels of calcium and potassium; often, increasing the intake of magnesium will help improve the absorption of calcium and potassium.

As a commercial supplement, magnesium is available in many forms. Magnesium citrate, magnesium gluconate, magnesium glycinate, and magnesium lactate are all more soluble and more easily absorbed into the body than magnesium oxide (which is a good source for people with constipation). It's best to take magnesium supplements with food.

LOOK OUT FOR THIS!

People with kidney disease should not take magnesium unless supervised by their doctor.

Ingesting too much magnesium in your food is extremely rare, but overdosing can happen to people who take large amounts of milk of magnesia—excess magnesium can have a laxative effect.

People who have kidney failure or heart block, or who have had an ileostomy, should not take magnesium supplements.

WHAT TO AVOID

Medication: Do not take magnesium supplements with amiloride or with oral diabetes medications without a doctor's supervision. If you are taking tetracycline antibiotics or nitrofurantoin, separate your dosage of these medications from magnesium by 2 hours to avoid absorption problems. If you are taking any type of heart medication, consult your doctor before taking magnesium, since it may lower your need for the drugs.

MASTIC

MASTIC—A SAP THAT COMES from the stem and leaves of the mastic tree *(Pistacia lentiscus)*—has had many commercial uses over the years, from a breath freshener and liquor-flavoring agent to a paint stabilizer. Its medicinal properties have been long recognized as well. The ancient Greeks used mastic in the form of chewing gum after meals to help prevent heartburn, nausea, and ulcers. In fact, they valued mastic so highly that anyone caught stealing it would be punished with ear, nose, or limb amputation.

WHAT IT DOES

Studies have shown that mastic is effective in both preventing and treating ulcers of the stomach and intestines, easing their symptoms and promoting tissue healing. It can also ease the symptoms of indigestion and heartburn, and may reduce bad breath. In vitro studies indicate that *Pistacia lentiscus* may have a role in the treatment of colon cancer. A recent study found that chewing mastic gum was an effective treatment against the bacteria that cause dental caries.

The resin of the mastic tree works to repel mosquitos. Among its other uses, mastic has been applied externally to treat boils, ringworm, and muscle stiffness; however, more study is needed to confirm the value of these uses.

For additional information on specific health conditions and how to treat them with supplements, see Part 3 of this book, beginning on page 309.

HOW IT WORKS

Mastic works to restore normal acid levels in the stomach by reducing stomach secretions. It has been shown not only to stop the growth of *Helicobacter pylori*—a bacterial infection that is responsible for most stomach ulcers, as well as other disorders of the gastrointestinal system—but also to kill this organism, possibly by making it more vulnerable to the body's immune system.

HOW TO TAKE IT

Mastic is available in capsule, oil, toothpaste, and mouthwash form.

The mastic sold as a dietary supplement is made up of oils obtained by distilling the sap, leaves, and twigs of the mastic tree. Typical doses range from 1 to 3 grams per day.

LOOK OUT FOR THIS!

When taken as directed (1 to 3 grams per day), mastic does not appear to produce serious side effects, although its use in small children may cause diarrhea.

WHAT TO AVOID
Mastic has no known interactions with other drugs, herbs, or supplements.

MELATONIN

LOOKING FOR A GOOD NIGHT'S SLEEP? Melatonin supplements may be just what the sandman had in mind. Melatonin is a natural hormone produced by the pineal gland in the brain. During the day, this gland produces serotonin, a chemical that relays messages between nerve cells in the brain; at night, it produces melatonin, which triggers sleep. The darker the room, the more melatonin your pineal gland produces. When you're having sleeping problems, melatonin supplements can provide a nonaddictive and inexpensive alternative to chemical sleeping aids and can help you to get your internal clock back on track.

WHAT IT DOES
Although the evidence is somewhat contradictory, many studies show that melatonin supplements are highly effective in helping people with sleep disturbances (caused by jet lag, for instance) adjust to a new schedule. Melatonin may also be helpful for other types of insomnia, including insomnia related to shift work. It may also be a way to increase daytime activity in institutionalized elderly people. Some studies have used melatonin with children. In fact, one study found that melatonin administered to children can be effective in reducing anxiety associated with surgical anesthesia. Another study found melatonin to be effective in children with seizures and sleep disturbance. However, be sure to speak with your pediatrician before administering this to your child.

A study of people who regularly used prescription benzodiazepine-type sleeping pills found that melatonin helped them to stop using these drugs, which can have more side effects than does melatonin.

Additional studies have explored the benefits of melatonin beyond sleep. Two studies found that melatonin reduced anxiety in people undergoing surgery. A recent, small study suggests that melatonin may reduce tardive dyskinesia, a syndrome marked by involuntary movements of the face, limb, and trunk muscles and often caused by medications used to treat Parkinson's disease and psychosis. Tinnitus (ringing in the ears) is a difficult condition to treat. A recent study reported some success using melatonin to treat people experiencing tinnitus, particularly those who suffer from disturbed sleep. Melatonin may also be useful in the treatment of chronic fatigue syndrome. People with irritable bowel syndrome, even if they sleep normally, may have improvement in symptoms by taking melatonin. Melatonin may also be useful in the prevention of migraine and the treatment of traumatic brain injury. Melatonin may also be helpful for preventing anxiety before surgery, with fewer side effects than sedating medication that's typically given.

Other preliminary evidence (mostly involving animal studies) suggests that melatonin may be useful for preventing and treating some types of cancer (when combined with conventional cancer treatments), as well as for preventing heart disease and the overall effects of aging.

Additionally, early findings suggest that melatonin may reduce the pain associated with fibromyalgia and may help prevent stroke. Although these findings are promising, they must be subjected to more research.

For additional information on specific health conditions and how to treat them with supplements, see Part 3 of this book, beginning on page 309.

HOW IT WORKS

Melatonin lowers the body's core temperature, producing an immediate hypnotic (sleep-like) state, which in turn causes sleep. When taken in very high doses, melatonin works as an antioxidant, reducing the harmful effects of cell- and tissue-damaging free radical molecules. It may also increase levels of some cancer-fighting cytokines—substances made by the body's own immune system.

HOW TO TAKE IT

Caution: Melatonin should be used only under a doctor's supervision.

Melatonin is available as capsules, liquid, lozenges, sublingual tablets (tablets that are placed under the tongue until dissolved), timed-release tablets, and tea.

In studies of melatonin and sleep disturbances, doses of 1 to 10 milligrams have been effective. The dose you take depends on the severity of your sleep problem. Keep in mind that safety studies have only assessed melatonin taken over a short period of time (for example,

28 days). It is not known whether melatonin is safe if taken over a longer period.

The optimal dosage of melatonin for conditions other than those described here is unknown.

LOOK OUT FOR THIS!

Side effects of melatonin include drowsiness, decreased attention, and balance problems for about 6 hours after taking it. Be sure that you don't operate a car or other machinery for several hours after taking a melatonin supplement. Other side effects associated with melatonin include stomach discomfort, headache, and morning grogginess.

Melatonin supplements, particularly when taken at high doses, may also impair fertility, reduce sex drive in males, damage the retina of the eye, and cause hypothermia—an abnormally low body temperature.

Melatonin can also produce depression and psychotic episodes when used with certain antidepressant medicines. Experts recommend that people with depression or at risk for developing it should avoid melatonin.

Since the long-term safety of melatonin has not been studied, children, pregnant or nursing women, and people with serious liver or kidney disease should not take this supplement unless advised by a doctor that it is safe to do so. People at risk for cardiovascular disease or with a history of seizures should also steer clear of melatonin supplements, unless advised by a physician.

WHAT TO AVOID

Medication: Melatonin may interact with the antidepressant fluoxetine (see above). It may increase the effects and side effects of sedating medications (such as benzodiazepines and antihistamines) and interfere with the effectiveness of corticosteroids.

Food: When taken with alcohol, melatonin may produce increased sedative and side effects.

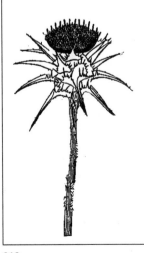

MILK THISTLE

A NATIVE MEDITERRANEAN PLANT with prickly leaves and red-purple flowers, the milk thistle plant *(Silybum marianum)* has been used since ancient times to treat a range of aliments, particularly those associated with the liver and gallbladder. It has also been used as a remedy for snakebites, jaundice, and other diseases.

Traditionally, milk thistle was thought to improve lactation in nursing mothers, perhaps because of the milky streaks on the plant's leaves, which were said to carry the milk of the Virgin Mary. Milk thistle is also edible and was once cultivated as a vegetable. The young leaves make an excellent salad—just make sure to first remove the prickly parts!

WHAT IT DOES

Milk thistle has been shown to protect liver tissue, aid in the regeneration of damaged liver tissue from cirrhosis and infectious hepatitis, and decrease levels of cholesterol in the liver and in bile. Milk thistle may also be useful as an adjunctive treatment for people with alcoholic liver disease, which is marked by severe inflammation of the liver.

Milk thistle is also the most powerful antidote to poisoning by deathcap mushrooms *(Amanita phalloides)*, which are among the most deadly mushrooms on the planet. Studies have shown that milk thistle completely counteracts the toxic effects of this mushroom when given within 10 minutes of the mushroom's ingestion. Even when taken within 24 hours, milk thistle can significantly reduce the risk of liver damage and death from the deathcap mushroom.

Milk thistle may also be helpful for treating psoriasis, because of its ability to improve liver function and by slowing the body's production of the substances known as leukotrienes—which are often present in excess in people with psoriasis.

Preliminary studies are being done of milk thistle's effectiveness when taken in conjunction with chemotherapy for people with prostate and other types of cancer. Some studies suggest that milk thistle may slow the growth of prostate cancer cells, although more research is needed to back these preliminary findings. Other studies suggest that milk thistle may be effective against certain types of bacteria and against viral hepatitis. Good news: Recent studies indicate that milk thistle does not appear to adversely affect the metobolism of important medications such as indinavir (an HIV treatment), certain anticancer drugs, and digoxin (a cardiac medication).

For additional information on specific health conditions and how to treat them with supplements, see Part 3 of this book, beginning on page 309.

HOW IT WORKS

The active ingredients in milk thistle are a group of flavonoid compounds that are collectively called silymarin, and which have antioxidant properties that protect the liver. A substance called silybin (the strongest of the flavonoid compounds in silymarin), can prevent or counteract damage caused by alcohol, acetaminophen, and other toxins. Milk thistle also promotes the regeneration of liver tissue by increasing protein synthesis in the liver.

Milk thistle enhances the process by which the liver detoxifies alcohol and many other toxins, achieving this by inhibiting Phase I detoxification (see Detoxification, page 406) and protecting against the depletion of glutathione, an important element in the detoxification process. Milk thistle may also have anti-inflammatory effects, and it may inhibit certain inflammation-causing agents in the body.

The other ways in which milk thistle works are not completely understood.

HOW TO TAKE IT

The crushed or powdered seeds of the milk thistle plant are sold commercially in the form of capsules, tablets, liquid extracts, and tinctures. Most milk thistle products are standardized to contain 70 to 80 percent silymarin. Dosages of milk thistle vary, depending on the form of administration. Typical dosages of milk thistle range from 140 to 280 milligrams of silymarin, taken three times daily.

Keep in mind that milk thistle is not water soluble and that taking this herb in the form of a tea is therefore not effective.

LOOK OUT FOR THIS!

Milk thistle is generally a very safe supplement with few side effects. Some people may experience a mild laxative effect after taking milk thistle for long periods of time. People with allergies to plants in the aster family may have allergic reactions to milk thistle.

Since no formal guidelines have been established for the use of milk thistle by children, women who are pregnant or nursing, and people with kidney disease, it should be taken by members of these groups only under the supervision of a doctor.

WHAT TO AVOID

Medication: Consult your doctor before talking milk thistle with drugs or other substances that are metabolized by the cytochrome P450 system in the liver, and with insulin or oral hypoglycemic agents. Milk thistle may reduce the effectiveness of oral contraceptives.

N-ACETYLCYSTEINE

N-ACETYLCYSTEINE (NAC) is an altered form of the amino acid cysteine that is found in high-protein foods. Also known as L-cysteine, acetylcysteine, and N-acetylcysteine, NAC has long been used in hospitals to treat acetaminophen poisoning.

NAC may also ease the symptoms of several respiratory conditions, including the chronic bronchitis of emphysema that often follows years of heavy smoking, or acute respiratory distress. NAC may show promise for a range of other conditions as well, from preventing heart disease to treating human immunodeficiency virus (HIV) infection.

WHAT IT DOES

NAC may be useful in treating respiratory illness because it helps break down mucus in the lungs, and may also ease symptoms and reduce the likelihood of acute attacks of chronic bronchitis. Although the results of studies have varied, evidence suggests that aside from improving the body's ability to clear itself of mucus, NAC may decrease cough severity and diaphragm fatigue (which is often associated with increased coughing from respiratory illness) in people with various respiratory conditions, such as cystic fibrosis and idiopathic pulmonary fibrosis.

NAC can also protect the kidneys from the contrast dye used in computed tomography (CT) imaging, help the liver to detoxify heavy metals such as mercury or lead, and help the body to synthesize glutathione—a powerful antioxidant that plays a major role in the body's detoxification mechanism.

For people with HIV who often have low levels of the antioxidant glutathione, NAC may prove useful for boosting levels of this antioxidant and strengthening the immune system's T cells, although additional research is needed to verify the role of NAC in HIV. However, preliminary studies suggest that NAC may play a role in preventing the progression from HIV infection to acquired immune deficiency syndrome (AIDS).

Some studies suggest that NAC may amplify the effects of the drug nitroglycerin in people who take this drug for heart disease, but severe headaches sometimes develop as a side effect of this combination.

Other small, preliminary studies suggest that NAC may reduce the levels of homocysteine, an amino acid that has been shown to be a risk factor for heart disease, perhaps suggesting that NAC may have a future role in preventing heart disease.

Research suggests that NAC may have protective effects against certain types of cancer including lung, skin, head and neck, mammary, and liver cancers, as well as protecting the body from the effects of chemotherapy for cancer. One recent study found that NAC may reduce cocaine-related withdrawal symptoms and cravings. Because NAC helps thin mucus, it may be a useful addition to the drugs used to treat *H. pylori,* the bacteria that cause stomach ulcers.

Other, early research suggests that NAC may have the potential to treat Sjogren's syndrome—an autoimmune condition of the salivary glands—hepatitis C, and degenerative conditions such as Alzheimer's disease, cataracts, some forms of Raynaud's syndrome, and amyotrophic lateral sclerosis (ALS; Lou Gehrig's disease). However, more research is needed to confirm these uses of NAC as safe and effective.

If you are an athlete, you may be interested to learn that a recent Australian study found that NAC improved endurance in well-trained individuals.

For additional information on specific health conditions and how you can treat them with supplements, see Part 3 of this book, beginning on page 309.

HOW IT WORKS

NAC helps clear mucus from the respiratory tract in two ways: It breaks down mucus and makes it less sticky. NAC also works as an expectorant by stimulating the action of cilia, the tiny, hairlike structures that line the airway and sweep mucus and foreign materials up the airway and away from the lungs.

In people with HIV infection, NAC may stimulate T cells, thus strengthening the immune system.

Early research shows that NAC may be a powerful antioxidant that fights the cell- and tissue-damaging effects of free radical molecules, which are associated with cancer, heart disease, and aging. Besides neutralizing free radicals, NAC works by helping the body to synthesize the antioxidant glutathione.

In terms of cancer prevention, NAC may prevent the transformation of certain compounds into others that carry the risk of causing cancer, while protecting healthy cells from the toxic effects of chemotherapy and radiation therapy. NAC may also slow the growth of certain cancer cells.

HOW TO TAKE IT

Generally healthy people don't need supplemental NAC. Typical dosages of NAC for respiratory conditions range from 600 to 1500 milligrams daily, divided into three doses. People with cancer or heart disease may be advised to take more—at a dosage as high as 2 to 4 grams a day—and people with HIV infection have been given 4 grams daily. A series of several doses of NAC are needed after an overdose of acetaminophen and must be started within 8 to 10 hours after the overdose.

Prescription NAC is available as a liquid medication or aerosol spray. You can buy L-cysteine powder and NAC tablets or capsules over the counter. Because NAC clears heavy metals from the body, it is important to take a multivitamin and mineral supplement that includes zinc, copper, and B vitamins when using NAC for any length of time.

LOOK OUT FOR THIS!

Acute respiratory distress and acetaminophen poisoning are medical emergencies that require immediate hospital care. Do not try to self-treat with NAC if you have either of these conditions—go directly to an emergency room.

NAC is generally well tolerated, although high oral doses can cause nausea and vomiting and are not advised for people with peptic ulcers. A few people are allergic to oral or intravenous NAC. Taking high doses of NAC alone, without other antioxidant supplements, may increase oxidative stress in the body.

No safety data exist about NAC for pregnant or lactating women, children, or people with serious kidney or liver disease.

WHAT TO AVOID

Medication: Consult your doctor before taking NAC if you are taking nitroglycerine for angina, angiotensin-converting enzyme (ACE) inhibitors for high blood pressure, or other heart medications, since

NAC may increase their effects. NAC may also change the effects of immunosuppressive medications (such as prednisone) and antifungal preparations, so consult your doctor if you're taking any of these.

NADH

YOUR BODY MAKES THE REDUCED or hydrogen-bearing form of the substance known as nicotinamide adenine dinucleotide (NADH) from vitamin B_3 and uses it to help enzymes perform a variety of functions in the body. NADH is known as a cofactor, or coenzyme, but is casually referred to as an "enzyme assistant." The name nicotinamide adenine dinucleotide indicates that NADH is made up of two nucleotides; the "H" is a chemical abbreviation indicating that the molecule of NADH is in a reduced (as opposed to a chemically oxidized) form (see How It Works, on the next page).

The most important role of NADH is to help cells produce energy. Claims for its therapeutic benefits range from help against relatively minor problems such as jet lag to improving the symptoms of several extremely debilitating illnesses characterized by a failure of the brain chemicals known as neurotransmitters to function properly. Some research on NADH as a supplement has been promising, but there are also studies suggesting that the body may have trouble utilizing NADH from both food sources and supplements.

WHAT IT DOES

Because of its role in cellular energy production, NADH has been suggested as a treatment for conditions characterized by low energy levels and tiredness. Chief among these are jet lag, chronic fatigue syndrome (CFS), and some forms of depression. In one study, 35 participants who had flown across four time zones overnight were given either an NADH supplement or a placebo and then tested for mental alertness; those who took NADH did significantly better in measures of wakefulness and alertness.

In another study, of 26 patients with CFS, 31 percent of those given NADH were reported to have alleviation of their symptoms, as compared to the effects of a placebo. One problem with this trial and others measuring the effectiveness of NADH in combating depression is that they were conducted by the developer of an NADH supplement; more objective evaluations would lend more credence to the findings about NADH.

NADH has also been evaluated as a symptom-reducing treatment for both Parkinson's disease and Alzheimer's disease (AD), with some promising but not definitive results. Both oral and injected NADH seemed to reduce physical impairment and the need for prescription medication in people with Parkinson's disease, but a more rigorous follow-up trial failed to support these findings. Research with AD patients also showed an improvement in mental function, but this was a so-called "open-label trial," meaning either the participants, the evaluators, or both knew who was getting the NADH, which could bias the study results. Follow-up double-blind trials have yet to be conducted.

Some recent research has investigated whether NADH might help lower blood pressure and reduce levels of LDL ("bad") cholesterol. NADH has also been touted by some as a sports supplement to enhance performance and boost energy levels, but there's little scientific support for these claims.

For additional information on specific health conditions and how you can treat them with supplements, see Part 3 of this book, beginning on page 309.

HOW IT WORKS

NADH resides in the mitochondria that are the energy-producing components of cells. It is involved in the process known as reversible reduction in which some of the electrons in the nicotinamide portion of the NADH molecule are "pulled away" and passed along the electron transport chain within the mitochondria—a process that leads to the creation of adenosine triphosphate (ATP), the chemical responsible for generating cellular energy.

The reason why some researchers think NADH may help treat CFS is that CFS is thought to result from a depletion of ATP caused by infection or stress.

In the brain, NADH plays a role in the production of neurotransmitters such as dopamine and norepinephrine, both of which help the brain function normally and keep the memory sharp. NADH also assists the enzyme tyrosine hydroxylase, which is involved in the synthesis of neurotransmitters. Parkinson's disease has been traced to insufficient dopamine, and this disease is often treated with the medication known as levodopa or "L-DOPA" (Larodopa), which the body turns into dopamine. NADH may facilitate the synthesis of L-DOPA, perhaps explaining why NADH has been observed to reduce the need for medication in people with Parkinson's disease.

HOW TO TAKE IT

Although NADH is present in the muscle tissue of fish, poultry, and beef, and in products containing yeast, tests suggest that it's broken down by the cooking process and by the body's own digestive processes.

NADH is available as a supplement in tablets of 2.5 and 5 milligrams. Dosage recommendations range from 2.5 milligrams to as much as 50 milligrams a day, but research results have been based on a dose of 10 milligrams a day, taken on an empty stomach, with water only.

Keep in mind that the value of NADH supplementation has not been confirmed, and some studies suggest that NADH may not be absorbed either from supplements or from food. One problem is that the outer membrane of mitochondria is impermeable to NADH, so that it probably can't be absorbed directly but must be synthesized within the mitochondria from vitamin B_3. However, it is not known whether increasing one's intake of vitamin B_3 actually helps raise NADH levels in the mitochondria.

Even if supplements of it do work, NADH decomposes rapidly, and although some manufacturers have taken steps to make it more stable, it is not clear which commercially available forms work best.

LOOK OUT FOR THIS!

Because the long-term safety of taking NADH supplements has not been established, supplementation is not recommended for children or for pregnant or nursing women.

NADH appears to have few side effects, although some people have reported mild nausea, loss of appetite, and increased nervousness when taking it.

Severe deficiency of vitamin B_3, which can cause a deficiency of NADH, is rare in Western societies, but is sometimes observed in people with alcoholism.

WHAT TO AVOID

NADH has no known interactions with other supplements, drugs, or herbs.

NIACIN

NIACIN, A FORM OF VITAMIN B$_3$, has been a rising star in the world of supplements. In the 1950s, scientists discovered that it could lower cholesterol levels in the blood, when taken in high doses. Since then, niacin has become one of the most closely scrutinized and studied vitamins. The evidence is now so strong for its cholesterol-lowering benefits that niacin has become a tool of mainstream medicine and is considered a relatively safe, inexpensive, and effective treatment for high cholesterol.

WHAT IT DOES

There are two main forms of niacin that have similar effects when taken in small doses: niacin (also known as nicotinic acid) and niacinamide (also called nicotinamide). Another form of niacin, called inositol hexaniacinate, may have additional health benefits of its own when taken at high doses, as do nicotinic acid and nicotinamide. Taking any type of niacin above the recommended dosage should be done only under medical supervision.

Several large clinical trials have confirmed that niacin can prevent or treat high cholesterol by lowering LDL ("bad") cholesterol and triglycerides, while raising HDL ("good") cholesterol. Preliminary studies suggest that niacin—when used in conjunction with other cholesterol-lowering agents, proper diet, and exercise—can slow the progress of atherosclerosis (in which cholesterol and other fats clog arteries, blocking the circulation of blood to organs). Studies also indicate that, when given to patients after a heart attack, niacin is a useful treatment for preventing a second heart attack. Niacin also reduces coronary heart disease morbidity and mortality when taken either alone or in combination with statins.

Certain people may need to take extra niacin, including those with a deficiency of this vitamin and people taking the drug isoniazid (Nydrazid), a treatment for tuberculosis, because this drug interferes with the body's ability to make niacin. Many antibiotics and estrogen medications also deplete levels of niacin in the body.

When taken in the form of niacinamide, niacin may improve strength, decrease fatigue, and increase mobility in people with osteoarthritis. It has also been used as part of a treatment program for schizophrenia. Niacin may also help regulate lipids in people taking medication for the treatment of HIV.

Preliminary studies suggest that supplementation with niacin may reduce symptoms of painful menstruation and hypoglycemia.

For additional information on specific health conditions and how to treat them with supplements, see Part 3 of this book, beginning on page 309.

HOW IT WORKS

Niacin plays an important role in many important processes in the body, including the production of hormones and blood cells, and the release of energy from fats, carbohydrates, and proteins. How niacin specifically lowers levels of cholesterol in the blood is not known.

HOW TO TAKE IT

The recommended daily intake (RDI) of niacin rises with age, and varies according to gender and condition. See the table below for the RDIs of niacin.

AGE/GENDER/CONDITION	RECOMMENDED DAILY INTAKE (RDI)*
Infants	
0–6 months	2 mg
7–12 months	4 mg
Children	
1–3 years	6 mg
4–8 years	8 mg
9–13 years	12 mg
Males	
14 years and older	16 mg
Females	
14 and older	14 mg
Pregnant Women	18 mg
Nursing Women	17 mg

For more information on RDIs, see Want to Know More About Intake? on page 8.

Niacin is a part of the B-complex vitamin group (a term given to a group of eight important B vitamins), and most general purpose multivitamin and mineral supplements contain the full range of B vitamins (be sure to check the label).

When taking niacin for a specific health condition (such as lowering cholesterol levels), a much higher dose than the RDI is often required. Typically, dosage schedules for niacin start low and increase weekly until positive results are noted or side effects develop (see below). Be aware that at high doses (over 100 milligrams per day), niacin is considered a drug and its use should be closely monitored by your doctor.

Niacin supplements are available in regular and slow-release forms. Although slow-release supplements are longer lasting, they can have greater side effects (see below).

LOOK OUT FOR THIS!

At high therapeutic doses, niacin can cause skin flushing (similar to hot flashes), headaches, hypotension (low blood pressure and lightheadedness), cramps, and nausea. It can also result in liver inflammation. People taking niacin at high doses should have their blood monitored regularly in order to make sure there is no damage to the liver.

When taken at recommended dosages, niacin is generally considered safe. Pregnant or nursing women should never take high doses of niacin. The maximum safe dosage is 35 milligrams per day (30 milligrams per day for people 18 years of age or younger).

Unless your doctor has advised it, do not take high doses of niacin if you have liver or gallbladder disease, diabetes, gout, arterial bleeding, glaucoma, or a peptic ulcer, or if you drink heavily.

WHAT TO AVOID

Medication: Although studies have shown that combining high-dose niacin with cholesterol-lowering drugs may further increase HDL ("good") cholesterol, always consult your doctor before combining niacin with any cholesterol-lowering medication.

OMEGA-3 FATTY ACIDS

IF THERE IS ONE SUPPLEMENT that appears to be a front runner, omega-3 fatty acids are a contender. Useful in the treatment of heart disease, pulmonary diseases, psychiatric

---

FOOD SOURCES

NIACIN

Because the body produces niacin, deficiencies of this vitamin are rare. Still, because niacin is involved in so many processes in the body, it's a good idea to get the recommended intake every day. Read on for some tasty ways to get this important nutrient through diet.

▶ Almonds, barley, bran, fish, lean meats, peanut butter, peanuts with skins, peas, poultry, seeds, whole wheat, wild and brown rice, and yeast.

disorders, inflammatory bowel disease, rheumatoid arthritis, and more, this is a supplement you will want to learn about.

We know that a high intake of certain dietary fats can lead to a variety of health conditions including obesity, coronary artery disease, diabetes, insulin resistance, and certain types of cancer. However, in the case of omega-3 fatty acids—polyunsaturated fats found in many cold-water fish and some other sources—fats can play a major role in preventing and treating a wide range of diseases.

Omega-3 fatty acids are necessary for a healthy life, particularly a healthy heart. However, even though they play an important role in maintaining optimum health, the human body does not produce omega-3 fatty acids on its own. Therefore, it is essential to get these fats from food sources, which is why omega-3 fatty acids are called "essential" fatty acids.

Given that seafood contains environmental toxins such as mercury, are fish and fish oil safe ways to increase my intake of omega-3 fatty acids?

Fish (as well as in milk and meat) contain environmental toxins. In a lifetime, everyone is exposed to some level of environmental toxins, and studies show that this exposure is escalating.

All fish contain environmental toxins, such as lead, dioxins, and mercury. Large fish consume higher amounts of environmental toxins than do small fish, and as a result, large fish contain higher levels of toxins than small fish. Fish oils, while rich in omega-3 fatty acids, can be dangerous if they also contain high levels of toxins. To avoid potential health risks of toxins, make sure to purchase a fish oil supplement that has been well purified and guarantees undetectable toxin levels.

Many people are particularly concerned about the toxic effects of mercury, a metal that is found in vaccines, dental fillings, and industrial pollution and has been linked to high cholesterol levels and the risk of heart attack. Exposure to high levels of mercury may also cause gastrointestinal problems or damage to the central nervous system and brain in children, triggering autism. Fish is one of the largest food sources of mercury. Young children and fetuses are especially vulnerable to the health risks of high levels of mercury, and the U.S. Food and Drug Administration (FDA) therefore advises that women who are pregnant, nursing, or expecting to become pregnant, as well as young children, should strictly avoid certain types of fish—including shark, swordfish, king mackerel, and tilefish—because they contain the highest levels of mercury. Some researchers believe that adults should steer clear of these fish as well. To reap the health benefits of the omega-3 fatty acids found in fish while avoiding the potential risks of mercury, the best and safest fish is wild Alaska salmon. Or, it may be necessary to take safe cod liver oil and omega-3 fatty acids.

WHAT IT DOES

Many studies have shown that people with a higher than average intake of omega-3 fatty acids have a decreased risk of developing heart disease. Studies indicate that omega-3 fatty acids contribute to cardiovascular health in a number of ways. For example, omega-3 fatty acids can reduce triglyceride levels as well as prevent blood platelets from clumping together to cause blood clots. Studies also suggest that omega-3 fatty acids may reduce the risk of having a heart attack and when taken after a heart attack may decrease the risk of death from cardiac causes. When taken prior to major heart surgery, omega-3 fatty acids help prevent postoperative complications and reduce the length of hospital stays.

Supplementation with omega-3 fatty acids may also reduce atherosclerotic deposits in people with atherosclerosis and improve the elasticity of the arteries—a measure often used to predict the chance of developing heart disease. Furthermore, omega-3 fatty acids may reduce the risk of sudden cardiac death, possibly by preventing dangerous irregularities in heart rhythm and by lowering blood pressure.

The powers of omega-3 fatty acids extend well beyond heart health. Several studies have found that these fatty acids may substantially ease depression and bipolar depression. Other preliminary studies indicate that omega-3 fatty acids may boost the effectiveness of certain antidepressant medications and may in some cases even replace the need for antidepressants. As a result, we may soon see antidepressants based on eicosapentaenoic acid (EPA; a main component of fish oil).

Omega-3 fatty acids may also have brain benefits. Studies show that either through supplementation or from the consumption of fish, these fatty acids may protect against Alzheimer's disease (AD), besides boosting cognition and mood. Further studies indicate that a deficiency of omega-3 fatty acids may increase the risk for developing AD. Researchers have also found a connection between a higher dietary intake of fish and a lower chance of developing dementia.

While several studies have found that omega-3 fatty acids may help treat the joint pain, stiffness, and inflammation associated with arthritis, new research suggests that they may also help to reduce cartilage degradation. As a result, supplementation with omega-3 fatty acids is often recommended for people taking medication for rheumatic conditions and may eventually allow the reduction or complete discontinuation of these medications.

Preliminary findings suggest that omega-3 fatty acids may play a role in treating attention deficit hyperactivity disorder (ADHD). Studies suggest that omega-3 fatty acids in the form of fish or fish oil may improve dyslexia, which often occurs in children with ADHD, as well as improving hyperactivity itself. One study has noted that boys with ADHD may not metabolize omega-3 fatty acids properly, which can lead to a deficiency of this nutrient. Test-taking anxiety also appears to be a alleviated by the use of omega-3 fatty acids.

When taken by people with advanced stages of certain types of cancer, fish oil supplements may prevent weight loss and loss of lean tissue, and may improve the overall quality of life. Preliminary studies suggest that omega-3 fatty acids also may suppress the growth of certain types of cancer, including colon and breast cancers. When taken prior to surgery, omega-3 fatty acids appear to improve the outcomes in people with cancer.

Chronic obstructive pulmonary disease is the fifth-leading cause of death throughout the world. Studies indicate that omega-3 fatty acids may be useful in alleviating some of the symptoms accociated with this disease. In terms of women's health, omega-3 fatty acids may decrease menstrual pain and although the findings for this are conflicting, may decrease migraine headaches in women, who often experience these headaches more than men. During pregnancy, omega-3 fatty acids may protect against preterm delivery and underweight babies, decrease the incidence of post partum depression and may prevent or ease pregnancy-induced high blood pressure. The children of women who take omega-3 while pregnant may have less asthma. (If you are pregnant or planning to become pregnant, be sure to speak with your doctor before taking omega-3 or any other supplement or herb.) For men, studies indicate that omega-3 fatty acids may lower the risk of prostate cancer and stroke. For both adults and children with inflammatory bowel disease, such as Crohn's and ulcerative colitis, omega-3 fatty acids may help to maintain remission after treatment with conventional medication.

Scientific trials suggest that omega-3 fatty acids may protect the kidneys of organ transplant patients who are taking the medication cyclosporine (Sandimmune).

Also under study are the effects of omega-3 fatty acids on lupus, multiple sclerosis, Huntington's chorea, and endometriosis; the role of these fatty acids in promoting bone growth and fighting osteoporosis; and their role in asthma and various skin conditions.

In fact, a recent study demonstrated that persons with exercised-induced asthma benefited from taking omega-3 fatty acid.

We may see more fish on the menu in hospitals soon: It appears that administration of omega-3 fatty acids may reduce mortality, antibiotic use, and length of hospital stay for a variety of illnesses.

For additional information on specific health conditions and how you can treat them with supplements, see Part 3 of this book, beginning on page 309.

HOW IT WORKS

Researchers speculate that the body metabolizes omega-3 fatty acids into prostaglandins and eicosanoids, which work similar to hormones. Although the exact functions of these substances are still unknown, eisosanoids may benefit the heart, and prostalandins may help regulate blood pressure and blood clotting and the dilation or relaxation of blood vessels—all of which is good news for cardiovascular health.

Omega-3 fatty acids also appear to function as blood-thinning agents by decreasing the adhesiveness of blood platelets to the walls of arteries so that they don't clog up with plaque.

Omega-3 fatty acids include two beneficial substances, known as docosahexaenoic acid (DHA) and eicosapentaenoic acid (EPA). These have been shown to lower "bad" cholesterol and raise "good cholesterol" levels. EPA also helps to lower blood pressure by relaxing and expanding blood vessels.

The body also uses omega-3 fatty acids to suppress hormone-like substances that cause inflammation; this may be why these fatty acids ease the pain associated with rheumatoid arthritis.

HOW TO TAKE IT

Foods rich in omega-3 fatty acids are the most effective sources of increasing your essential fatty acid intake. The American Heart Association recommends eating fish at least two times a week.

In supplement form, omega-3 fatty acids may be obtained from fish oil supplements, which provide two of these acids: EPA and DHA. Most fish oil supplements contain 18 percent EPA and 12 percent DHA or a total of 30 percent omega-3 fatty acids. The dosage of omega-3 fatty acids varies according to the condition being treated. In general, a total of 3 grams of EPA and DHA have

FOOD SOURCES

Several studies suggest that simply increasing your dietary intake of omega-3 fatty acids—especially in the form of fish—can substantially improve your health. Eicosapentaenoic acid (EPA) and docosahexaenoic acid (DHA), the omega-3 fatty acids found in fish oil, can also be acquired from a variety of foods. But if you like fish, you're in luck! Cold-water fish provides the most abundant source of these essential fatty acids. Read on for foods containing omega-3 fatty acids.

▶**Fish:** Anchovies, Atlantic halibut, bluefish, herring (both Atlantic and Pacific), sablefish (black cod), wild Alaska salmon, and sardines.

▶**Other Food Sources:** Canola oil, cod liver oil, English walnuts, flaxseed, mustard greens, soybeans, spinach, wheat germ oil, and wild game.

been recommended, which may require 10 grams of fish oil, since EPA constitutes 18 percent and DHA 12 percent of this dose.

LOOK OUT FOR THIS!

Omega-3 fatty acids are generally considered safe. People with bleeding disorders such as hemophilia or a tendency to hemorrhage should consult their doctor before taking omega-3 fatty acids. Individuals with diabetes should consult their doctor before taking omega-3 fatty acid supplements, because they may increase blood sugar levels.

Women who are pregnant or who are nursing should consult their doctors before taking any type of supplement, including omega-3 fatty acids.

WHAT TO AVOID

Medication: Consult your doctor before taking omega-3 fatty acids with blood-thinning drugs such as aspirin, anticoagulants such as warfarin, coumadin, or heparin, antiplatelet drugs such as clopidogrel, and nonsteroidal anti-inflammatory drugs (NSAIDs) such as ibuprofen.

The relationship between omega-3 fatty acids and drugs intended to affect cholesterol levels can be complex. Omega-3 fatty acids can lower triglyceride levels, but they may also marginally increase LDL ("bad") cholesterol levels. If you are taking triglyceride-lowering agents such as niacin/nicotinic acid, fibrates such as gemfibrozil, or resins such as cholestyramine, be aware that omega-3 fatty acids may intensify the effects of these medications. Omega-3 fatty acids may also work against the LDL-lowering effects of statin drugs such as atorvastatin and lovastatin.

PEPPERMINT

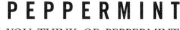

WHEN YOU THINK OF PEPPERMINT, mouthwash and mint jelly might come to mind. However, peppermint has been used for health purposes since the times of ancient Greece, Egypt, and Rome. The botanical name for peppermint, *Mentha piperita,* comes from the Greek name *Mintha,* a nymph in Greek mythology who turned herself into a plant, and from the Latin word *piper,* which means "pepper." Aside from its popularity as an ingredient in chewing gum, mouthwash, and toothpaste, peppermint also has a variety of medicinal uses. For centuries, peppermint has been valued for its use as a digestive aid, for symptomatic relief of cough, colds, and fever, and as a local anesthetic.

WHAT IT DOES

In modern medicine, peppermint is used for many of the same conditions as it was used in traditional medicine. Evidence suggests that peppermint can reduce excessive gas and nausea. And although the findings are mixed, some research indicates that peppermint oil may reduce the pain of intestinal spasms caused by irritable bowel syndrome (IBS). The oils found in peppermint have demonstrated in vitro antibiotic effects against *Streptococcus pneumoniae* and *Streptococcus pyogenes,* bacteria that commonly cause upper respiratory tract infections.

Limited evidence also suggests that peppermint oil, when applied to the forehead, may relieve tension headaches and temples. Peppermint has also been touted as an antiviral and a diuretic (promotes release of urine) agent, appetite stimulant, and mild sedative and has a cooling and pain-relieving effect on the skin when applied topically. When inhaled, the menthol in peppermint may also help temper a cough as well as relieve respiratory congestion when inhaled. Basic science research is finding that peppermint has antioxidant, anti-allergy, antiviral, antifungal, and antitumor qualities.

Preliminary studies also support the use of peppermint leaf for treating gallstones. While this use is approved by the German Commission E, it should be done only under close medical supervision. More research is needed to support the use of peppermint in treating gallstones.

One study found that peppermint oil was effective in treating the pain associated with neuralgia, and the German Commission E has approved the topical use of peppermint for this purpose. In an individual case report, a 76-year old woman with postherpetic neuralgia, who had not been responsive to traditional methods of treatment, was instructed to apply 2 to 3 drops of peppermint oil—containing 10 percent menthol—to affected areas of her skin three or four times daily. The result was an immediate and almost complete relief from pain that lasted 4 to 6 hours after the application of the oil. Although this evidence is highly preliminary, peppermint may prove to be a breakthrough treatment for this painful condition.

For additional information on specific health conditions and how to treat them with supplements, see Part 3 of this book, beginning on page 309.

HOW IT WORKS

When it comes to intestinal matters, peppermint works by relaxing the muscles of the small intestine, providing relief from gastrointestinal upset. Peppermint may also dissolve gallstones, via the menthol in its leaves. For sinus headaches, peppermint may reduce congestion, and many herbalists believe that inhaling the oil helps to clear the head and stimulate the brain, promoting clearer thinking.

HOW TO TAKE IT

Peppermint may be used in a variety of ways. For digestive and intestinal problems, peppermint oil is generally taken as enteric-coated capsules (to prevent stomach upset), dilute preparations, or suspensions. Peppermint oil (in methanol) may be applied topically as a linament or added to boiling water for use as an inhalant. However, pure peppermint oil should not be applied directly to the skin.

Few studies have been done of the safety, dosage, and effectiveness of peppermint leaf. In general, peppermint leaves may be used as an infusion (made by steeping the leaf in hot water) and drinking the resulting "tea." Peppermint leaves may also be taken in liquid preparations and in the form of dried herb extracts.

LOOK OUT FOR THIS!

Side effects of peppermint taken orally may include dizziness, nausea, loss of appetite, and heart problems. Topical use of peppermint may cause skin rash, hives, contact dermatitis, mouth sores, and eye irritation. High doses of peppermint oil can be dangerous, causing kidney failure, seizure, and even death.

Grow This!

Peppermint is not hard to grow at home. In fact, it's far too easy—you need to keep a close eye on peppermint or it will quickly take over your entire garden. Your best bet is to choose an isolated area in your garden and let the peppermint grow freely. Alternatively, you can plant the peppermint inside a barrel or pot.

Light: Full or partial sunlight.

Temperature: 75° to 80° F. If you experience cold winters, you might consider protecting the peppermint with a protective layer of mulch.

Potting: Using a rich, drained loam that will keep its water is the best way to pot peppermint. You may also want to consider using a sunken clay tile (if planting in an outdoor garden) to keep peppermint from spreading.

Regularly cut some leaves and stems of peppermint and use it fresh or dry. You can even freeze it for later use. Peppermint doesn't produce seeds, but is easily propagated by taking cuttings of the root or stem—if placed in water, the cuttings will produce roots quickly—or by dividing the plants in spring or autumn. Peppermint is a perennial plant, which means it will grow back every year.

Peppermint taken in small doses (as a tea, for example) is considered safe for adults. The use of peppermint oil or leaf is not suitable for children, pregnant or nursing women, or people with severe kidney or liver disease. Do not use the herb if you have gastrointestinal reflux, hiatal hernia, kidney stones, gallbladder or liver inflammation, or bile-duct problems without first consulting your doctor.

WHAT TO AVOID

Medication: Peppermint may increase blood levels of felodipine, simvastatin, and cyclosporine. It may also increase the absorption of 5-fluorouracil when the two are used together on the skin. Additionally, peppermint may interfere with drugs used to increase gastrointestinal motility, such as metoclopramide. If you are taking any of these medicines, do not use peppermint without consulting your doctor.

PHOSPHATIDYLSERINE

WHEN YOU END A LETTER OR NOTE with a PS, you're adding something you almost forgot. Perhaps that's a good way to remember that the chemical compound abbreviated as PS—its full name is phosphatidylserine—may be a legitimate memory enhancer. PS is one of a group of fatty-acid molecules called phospholipids, and it's an important constituent of the membranes of all our cells. It's found in the highest concentrations in the brain, but its concentrations may decline with age, which may explain the supposed ability of PS supplements to preserve or even improve memory in the elderly; some researchers believe that PS may have similar effects in younger people as well.

PS is also reputed to have other beneficial effects, however, the foods we eat contain only trace amounts of PS. Therefore, the only way to boost levels of this substance is with supplements, and the only PS supplements that have been studied in trials are those derived from the brains of cows. But because of concerns about Creutzfeld-Jakob or "mad cow" disease, which may be transmitted to humans who consume bovine brain tissue, bovine-based PS supplements are no longer available in the United States. The only kind of PS supplement you'll be able to get in the United States is derived from soy and other plants, and scientists are working to determine if soy-based PS works as well as animal-derived PS.

WHAT IT DOES

Several well-documented studies indicate that PS supplements may slow memory loss and improve cognitive function in people with Alzheimer's disease (AD), as well as those with the more benign condition known as age-related cognitive decline—the normal memory loss associated with aging. In one trial, patients with the early stages of AD who were given PS supplements did better on tests of mental functioning than those not taking PS. Researchers are quick to point out, however, that PS is far from a cure for memory decline. In fact, its benefits seemed to fade after 4 months of use, although steady improvements were seen before that. At best, PS may temporarily slow the rate of memory deterioration.

As noted above, PS has shown positive effects on memory in people with age-related cognitive decline, and it seemed to work best in cases in which memory loss was most severe. Another piece of encouraging evidence is that in cases of severe mental decline, PS was helpful regardless of whether the cause was AD, stroke, or another ailment that led to memory loss. These findings have suggested to some researchers that PS is just plain good for the brain, and that it may help combat the memory loss we all begin to experience past the age of 40.

Other studies indicate that PS may help relieve mild forms of depression in the elderly. Elderly women taking PS for 30 days reported a dramatic reduction in their symptoms of as much as 70 percent.

Levels of PS may be low in people with Parkinson's disease who are taking the prescription medication levodopa (Larodopa). In such cases, supplementation with PS may help improve both mood and mental function.

PS has also been claimed to help bodybuilders develop bigger and stronger muscles. Although the supporting evidence for this isn't as compelling as it is for conditions affecting memory, PS does appear to have effects that could lend credence to this claim. In fact, a recent small study demonstrated that 750 milligrams of soybean-derived phosphatidylserine, when taken daily for 10 days, improved exercise capacity in healthy males.

For additional information on specific health conditions and how you can treat them with supplements, see Part 3 of this book, beginning on page 309.

HOW IT WORKS

Cell membranes not only keep cells intact, but also serve as a conduit for nutrients from the outside to the inside of the cell and aid in the process of removing waste products from the interior of the cell. In its role as a major constituent of the cell membrane, PS is thought to keep cells healthy by supporting these functions.

PS may also help with the metabolism of neurotransmitters in the brain. Some theories speculate that AD is especially related to the poor functioning of the neurotransmitter called acetylcholine. In animal studies PS has been found to restore acetylcholine in the nervous system and to increase the supply of choline, the substance from which the body synthesizes acetylcholine.

A part of the brain called the hippocampus has structural features that are thought to be an important repository of information—in simplistic terms, "memory banks." We seem to lose some of these structures, known as dendritic spines, as we age, and they're also negatively affected by AD. In laboratory studies, PS has been found to reduce a loss of dendritic-spine density in aging animals.

Some studies have shown that PS slows the release of cortisol, which breaks down muscle tissue, potentially allowing weightlifters and other athletes to exercise longer and recover more quickly.

HOW TO TAKE IT

For treating AD and symptoms of age-related cognitive decline, researchers typically use a dosage of 300 milligrams a day of PS, divided into two or three doses for 3 to 6 months—after which point supplementation does not appear to provide any additional benefit. Some investigators have found that once the maximum effect is achieved, the dose of PS can be reduced to 100 milligrams a day. To treat mild depression in the elderly, doses of 300 milligrams a day of PS have been used.

Athletes who believe that PS supplements work to enhance performance typically take 800 milligrams a day, either right before or right after they work out. Some take as much as 1,000 to 2,000 milligrams.

LOOK OUT FOR THIS!

Keep in mind that only bovine-based PS supplements have shown definitive beneficial effects in clinical trials, and they are no longer available in the United States. If you're tempted to seek other sources of PS, you should think seriously about infection with "mad cow" disease as a real concern. You might want to keep watching the news, because tests of soy-based PS supplements are ongoing, and although they haven't yet had strong results, in theory they should work just as well as bovine-based PS. As with any supplement whose long-term safety hasn't been established, children and pregnant or nursing women are not advised to take PS.

WHAT TO AVOID

Medication: There's some indication that PS supplements may thin the blood. If you are taking a prescription blood-thinning drug such as warfarin or heparin, or if you take aspirin routinely, consult your doctor before taking a PS supplement.

POLICOSANOL

EVER WONDER ABOUT THE HEALTH benefits of wax? It's not as crazy as you might think. Policosanol is a supplement that comes from beeswax and sugarcane wax and has been studied since the early 1900s, mainly in Cuba, which is where the variety of sugarcane that is a source of policosanol is grown. Policosanol is most famous for its ability to lower cholesterol levels and may be a cost-effective alternative to prescription medications. In fact, in some studies policosanol performed as well as some of the most effective anticholesterol drugs on the market.

WHAT IT DOES

Several reliable studies have confirmed that supplementation with policosanol can reduce both overall cholesterol and LDL ("bad") cholesterol levels by 15 percent—a reduction similar to that achieved by popular cholesterol-lowering prescription medications such as simvastatin (Zocor). However, a recent large study performed in Germany did not reveal any benefit for lowering cholesterol with policosanol.

Policosanol may also be helpful for people with the condition known as intermittent claudication, which is caused by poor circulation in the legs as a result of hardening of the arteries, and may have effects similar to those of aspirin in reducing blood-clot formation in the arteries and improving overall bloodflow throughout the body. However, more research is needed to confirm these uses.

For additional information on specific health conditions and how to treat them with supplements, see Part 3 of this book, beginning on page 309.

HOW IT WORKS

It is not clear how policosanol works, but it may slow the body's production of cholesterol in the liver.

HOW TO TAKE IT

Policosanol is available in tablet and capsule form and taken in doses of 5 to 20 milligrams per day. Due to this low dose, policosanol is often combined with other cholesterol-lowering ingredients such as garlic, coenzyme Q10, fish oil, and other antioxidants for increased effect.

LOOK OUT FOR THIS!

Policosanol is generally well tolerated. Side effects include upset stomach, diarrhea, skin rash, headache, insomnia, excessive urination, and weight loss, although these effects are rare. People who have a food sensitivity to sugarcane or who are allergic to bee stings may experience side effects when taking policosanol.

Unless advised by a doctor, policosanol is not recommended for children and pregnant or nursing women since its long-term safety has not been studied. People with severe kidney or liver disease or blood clotting problems should also steer clear of policosanol.

WHAT TO AVOID

Medication: Because policosanol is a blood-thinning agent, it may cause excess bleeding when combined with medicines that have the same action, such as aspirin, warfarin, heparin, clopidogrel, ticlopidine, and pentoxifylline.

POTASSIUM

POTASSIUM IS AN ESSENTIAL MINERAL and one of the body's major electrolytes and is a vital part of many important processes in the body, from maintaining normal fluid balance to promoting cell and muscle growth. In pure, uncombined form, potassium can react in surprising ways—when combined with water, for example, it can burst into flames! But there is no cause for alarm; the potassium found in foods and supplements is always combined with other nonmetallic substances and is safe to take.

FOOD SOURCES

POTASSIUM

Eating potassium-rich foods—especially fruits—may be the best way to increase your intake of potassium. The potassium found in fruits does not irritate the stomach as supplements may do, and the amount of potassium in supplements (99 milligrams) is fairly low as compared to that found in fruit; a single banana can contain 500 milligrams of potassium! Read on for good food sources of potassium.

▶ Apples, apricots, avocados, bananas, cantaloupe, carrots, chicken, citrus fruits, cod, lima beans, milk, mushrooms, peas, potatoes (with the skin), salmon, spinach, and tomatoes. Adding even one potassium-rich serving of fruits or vegetables may decrease your risk of a stroke by 40 percent!

WHAT IT DOES

Potassium plays many different roles in the body. It plays an important role in the transmission of nerve impulses; contraction of cardiac, skeletal, and smooth muscle; production of energy; and maintenance of normal blood pressure. Potassium is also required for carbohydrate and protein metabolism.

Several studies have found that potassium supplementation can reduce blood pressure, particularly for people who may be lacking in potassium and for those who eat large amounts of salt. Potassium may also help prevent stroke and cardiovascular disease and reduce death caused by stroke. In fact, a recent long-term study of elderly Chinese veterans found that switching from regular to potassium-enriched salt prolonged life and reduced medical costs.

Some research suggests that people who have a high intake of potassium may be at a reduced risk for developing kidney stones. Some studies suggest that potassium in the form of potassium citrate may reduce both kidney stone formation and recurrence.

For additional information on specific health conditions and how to treat them with supplements, see Part 3 of this book, beginning on page 309.

HOW IT WORKS

How potassium lowers blood pressure is not clear, although this property may be associated with its ability to decrease the activity of renin, an enzyme produced by the kidney that can raise blood pressure.

The mechanism of potassium's role in stroke is also unknown but may be attributed to its ability to lower blood pressure, inhibit the formation of cell- and tissue-damaging free radical molecules, and prevent a condition known as arterial thrombosis, in which clots develop in the arteries.

HOW TO TAKE IT

A healthy daily requirement of potassium for children is 1,000 to 2,300 milligrams, while for adults it is 1,600 to 2,000 milligrams.

Most over-the-counter potassium supplements contain 99 milligrams of potassium per tablet. For people with high blood pressure, potassium citrate may be the best form in which to take potassium. It may be wise to take extra magnesium and vitamin B_{12} if you're taking extra potassium, in order to enhance the latter's positive effects.

Be sure to take potassium supplements with water; if they get caught in your throat, they can damage the esophagus that carries food and fluids from your mouth to your stomach.

Most people can get enough potassium just by eating a well-balanced diet. However, many people ingest twice as much sodium as they do potassium, despite the body's need for at least five times more potassium than sodium. Since sodium diminishes the effects of potassium, it's probably a good idea to take extra potassium to maintain a healthy balance of these two minerals.

Potassium depletion may be caused by excessive diarrhea or vomiting; excessive intake of alcohol, caffeine, salt or sugar; and stress. You may also require potassium supplements if you have certain medical conditions, such as severe diarrhea or diabetic ketoacidosis, or are taking medications such as certain diuretics that cause the body to lose too much potassium. Many antibi-otics, steroids, and blood pressure medications and aspirin deplete potassium.

LOOK OUT FOR THIS!

Even if you take a bit too much potassium, your body excretes any excess of this mineral through the urine (unless you have kidney disease). Common side effects of mild potassium overdosing include nausea, vomiting, abdominal discomfort, gas, and diarrhea. Taking the supplements with meals can help to reduce these effects. The most serious effect of excess potassium is hyperkalemia, a condition (involving too much potassium in the blood) that is often seen in people with kidney failure. Hyperkalemia can be lethal, but is rare among people whose kidneys are functioning normally.

Other rare side effects of potassium supplementation include rash, confusion, and irregular heartbeat.

Potassium is generally safe when taken at recommended doses, although it is not recommended for women who are pregnant or nursing without a doctor's advice.

WHAT TO AVOID

Be sure to tell your doctor if you plan to take potassium supplements, since your blood levels of this mineral may need to be monitored to ensure that you're not taking too much.

Medication: People taking potassium-sparing diuretic medications, such as spironolactone; angiotensin-converting enzyme (ACE) inhibitors, such as captopril; the antibiotic drug combination trimethoprim/sulfamethaxazole; or the oral contraceptive known as Yasmin, should consult their doctor before taking potassium supplements.

QUERCETIN

WE'VE KNOWN FOR SOME TIME that cultures that have diets with a high content of flavonoids—a group of substances found in plants—have less heart disease. Flavonoids are, therefore, bound to spur medical curiosity.

Quercetin, a flavonoid found in the rind and bark of various plants, is present in a wide range of foods and beverages, from apples and onions to red wine and green and black tea. (As if you needed another reason to have a glass of good red wine or be reminded that "an apple a day . . . "). As a supplement, quercetin is generally taken to reduce the risk of heart disease and protect cells from damage by free radicals.

WHAT IT DOES

Quercetin is a proven antioxidant that can protect cell structures from cell- and tissue-damaging free radical molecules. It is generally accepted as a vasodilator, which means that it could help to reduce blood pressure as well as protect the lining of blood vessels by its antioxidant action.

Quercetin may further boost heart health by helping to prevent the oxidation of LDL ("bad") cholesterol, a risk factor for cardiovascular disease. Some studies, however, have found no improvement in total cholesterol, LDL, HDL, or triglyceride levels in people taking 50 times the dietary intake of quercetin that's associated with a reduced risk of heart disease.

In one of the most promising human studies of quercetin, 67 percent of men with chronic prostatitis syndromes (including nonbacterial chronic prostatitis and prostadynia or prostate pain) had a reduction of their symptoms after taking quercetin, compared to only 20 percent of men taking a placebo. These findings are significant, since there are not many treatments available for these conditions.

Studies also indicate that people with interstitial cystitis—a condition marked by chronic inflammation of the bladder—may benefit from supplementation with quercetin, although more extensive research on this is needed.

Quercetin may also work as an anti-inflammatory agent, inhibiting the production of various inflammation-producing enzymes often associated with conditions such as asthma, hemorrhoids, and sprains and strains. Other laboratory research indicates that quercetin may have an antihistamine effect that could relieve symptoms of allergy, hay fever, and allergic conjunctivitis.

Preliminary studies suggest that quercetin may prevent cataracts. Quercetin may also help stomach ulcers caused by nonsteroidal anti-inflammatory drugs (NSAIDs), inhibit the human immunodeficiency virus (HIV), and boost the consumption of energy by the body and thermogenesis (heat production). However, more research is needed to support these possibilities.

Additionally, quercetin has been found to have an antiestrogen effect and in one study kept breast cancer cells from growing in a test tube.

Preliminary studies show that quercetin may have a chemopreventive role in colorectal cancer, as well as balance the immune system and fight viruses when taken with vitamin C.

Its use as a supplement to strengthen fragile capillaries and help prevent retinopathy and other complications of diabetes, while less documented, is promising.

For additional information on specific health conditions and how you can treat them with supplements, see Part 3 of this book, beginning on page 309.

HOW IT WORKS

Quercetin belongs to a group of plant pigments called flavonoids. Flavonoids work as antioxidants, and many of quercetin's therapeutic effects are due to its power as an antioxidant that destroys various tissue- and cell-damaging free radical molecules. Quercetin also inhibits the oxidation of LDL ("bad") cholesterol, and as an anti-inflammatory agent, it inhibits various inflammation-causing enzymes in the body.

Quercetin may prevent HIV from replicating by inhibiting HIV-protease, an enzyme that this virus needs to replicate itself and so make new viruses. This protease enzyme is also the target of many anti-HIV drugs (called "protease inhibitors").

FOOD SOURCES

Small amounts of quercetin can be found in a variety of foods. Although supplements are often necessary to provide therapeutic dosages of quercetin, the following foods can provide an added source of this nutrient.

▶Apples, beans, cabbage, garlic, grapefruit, grapes, green and black tea, green leafy vegetables, onions, pears, red wine, and spinach.

HOW TO TAKE IT

Quercetin comes in capsules of 250, 300, or 500 milligrams and in tablets of 50, 250, or 500 milligrams. A dosage of 400 to 500 milligrams taken three times daily is often recommended. The benefits of quercetin for men in the prostatitis study described earlier was achieved by taking 500 milligrams twice a day for 1 month. Eating quercetin-rich foods such as apples and onions is an excellent way to reap the quercetin bounty.

Some studies suggest that the proteolytic enzymes bromelain and papain may boost the power of quercetin.

LOOK OUT FOR THIS!

Quercetin is generally considered safe and easy to take. However, anyone at risk for low blood pressure or blood clotting problems should avoid taking high doses of quercetin since it exacerbates these conditions by dilating the vessels and inhibiting blood clotting.

Pregnant women and nursing mothers should avoid taking quercetin since there is no long-term safety information about its use in these groups.

WHAT TO AVOID

Medication: Quercetin may inhibit the efficacy of quinolone antibiotics. Quercetin should not be taken with cisplatin because of a theoretical risk of damage to the body's genetic material by this combination.

RED CLOVER

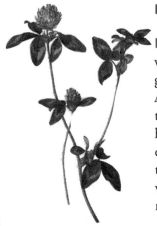

ITS RED FLOWERS ARE THE SOURCE of the many medicinal properties associated with red clover *(Trifolium pratense)*. In traditional medicine, red clover has been used internally to treat a variety of conditions including asthma, bronchitis, coughs, cancer, and gout. Topically, it is used to treat skin irritation. During the Middle Ages, red clover was used as a charm against witchcraft. In the nineteenth century it was popular as a blood purifier, at a time when many herbalists began to believe that several conditions—such as cancer, eczema, and venereal diseases—were caused by a buildup of toxins in the blood. Along with alfalfa, buckthorn, and prickly ash, red clover was a main ingredient in the famous Harry M. Hoxsey's cancer treatment formula in the early 1900s (see Did You Know? on page 240).

WHAT IT DOES

Today, scientists are exploring the hormonal effects of red clover. Red clover comes from the legume family—the same plant family as chickpeas and soybeans. Like soy, red clover contains phytoestrogens, compounds that can mimic estrogens in the body. Because red clover is one of the richest sources of phytoestrogens (also known as isoflavones), it has become a popular treatment for menopausal symptoms and is often used as an alternative to hormone replacement therapy.

One 12-week double-blind, placebo-controlled study found that a daily dose of 80 milligrams of red clover isoflavones significantly reduced hot flashes as compared to a placebo in women with menopause. While other studies did not reveal red clover to be as successful for this purpose, the most recent large study was able to document decreased menopause symptoms.

Preliminary research suggests that red clover may also help control blood pressure in postmenopausal women with type 2 diabetes.

Some researchers believe that red clover cream, when applied topically, may alleviate psoriasis and benefit bone growth and density; traditionally, red clover has been used topically to treat eczema and dermatitis.

Moreover, although red clover is an herb often associated with women's health, certain commercially available red clover products claim that they can prevent prostate cancer and prostate enlargement. Preliminary studies do suggest that red clover may be useful in treating early-stage prostate cancer, although further research on this is needed. Studies of red clover's effect on prostate enlargement have yielded less compelling results.

For additional information on specific health conditions and how you can treat them with supplements, see Part 3 of this book, beginning on page 309.

HOW IT WORKS

Scientists purport that through its phytoestrogen components, red clover may help maintain optimal levels of estrogen in women, particularly during menopause. Healthy estrogen levels also promote strong bones, clear skin, and a balanced mood.

Red clover contains more than 125 chemical compounds, but its isoflavone components—which act like estrogens—are thought to be responsible for most of its beneficial properties. These isoflavones may inhibit the imbalance of hormones that causes discomfort in menopause, such as hot flashes and mood swings.

The specifics of red clover's hormonal behavior in the body are still being investigated.

HOW TO TAKE IT

Red clover is commercially available as tablets, capsules, tinctures, liquid extracts, and teas. It can also be made into a topical ointment.

Based on trials, a dosage of 40 to 80 milligrams a day of red clover has reportedly been efficient for menopausal symptoms.

LOOK OUT FOR THIS!

Red clover is generally considered safe for adults. Children and pregnant or nursing women should not take red clover.

WHAT TO AVOID

Medication: Consult your doctor before taking red clover with agents metabolized through the cytochrome P450 3A4 enzyme system, as well as anticoagulant and antiplatelet agents, nonsteroidal anti-inflammatory drugs (NSAIDs), hormone replacement therapy, oral contraceptives, cancer treatment medications, or blood-thinning medications since these may interact negatively with the phytoestrogen properties of red clover.

Harry M. Hoxsey's Tonics

Did You Know?

Harry M. Hoxsey is known to the people he helped as a hero and by his opponents as a quack. Born in 1901, Hoxsey was a former coal miner who eventually gained recognition as a healer in the 1920s. He became known for his family recipe for cancer-treatment tonics, which often included red clover among other natural ingredients such as cascara, poke root, burdock root, barberry, buckthorn bark, stillingia root, and prickly ash bark. Hoxsey was labeled a charlatan by the American Medical Association (AMA) and the AMA Bureau of Investigation, which refused to look into the scientific merit of his claims at a time when alternative medicine was seen as sheer nonsense.

Although red clover has not been found to have any cancer-fighting abilities, many other studies of the herbs used in Hoxsey's tonics have provided preliminary evidence that they do have therapeutic properties. While many of Hoxsey's patients claim to have been cured under his treatment, Hoxsey's clinics were shut down in the 1950s. However, along with his long-time chief nurse Mildred Nelson, he set up a clinic in Tijuana, Mexico. This clinic, Hoxsey's Bio-Medical Center (often called The Hoxsey Clinic), was run by Mildred Nelson until her death in 1999, and was the first alternative cancer treatment facility in Mexico.

RED YEAST RICE

RED YEAST RICE *(MONASCUS PURPUREUS)* has a long history—the Chinese first used it medicinally during the Tang dynasty in 800 AD. Since then red yeast rice has become a common food staple in many Asian countries, where it's primarily used to flavor and color food. The name "red yeast rice" reflects how this rice is made—red yeast is grown on white rice and the product is fermented. After the yeast is inactivated, the mixture is powdered and made into a supplement.

WHAT IT DOES

Red yeast rice is most noted for its ability to significantly lower LDL ("bad") cholesterol levels and increase HDL ("good") cholesterol levels. Red yeast rice may also lower levels of the unhealthy fats known as triglycerides, which, like high cholesterol levels, can lead to heart disease.

Preliminary studies also suggest that red yeast may be of benefit in treating blood circulation problems, indigestion, and other stomach complaints, although more studies are needed to substantiate these potential uses.

For additional information on specific health conditions and how to treat them with supplements, see Part 3 of this book, beginning on page 309.

HOW IT WORKS

Red yeast rice contains compounds known as monacolins, which stop the liver from producing cholesterol by halting the activity of an important enzyme (called 3-hydroxy-3-methylglutaryl coenzyme A [HMG-CoA] reductase) that is responsible for the manufacture of cholesterol.

Lovastatin, a popular cholesterol-lowering drug, works in the same way as does red yeast rice to reduce cholesterol levels; however, lovastatin contains a higher level of monacolins than does red yeast rice.

Besides the monacolins, researchers believe that other components in red yeast rice, particularly sterols and fatty acids, may add to its cholesterol-lowering effects.

HOW TO TAKE IT

Caution: Red yeast rice should be used only under a doctor's supervision.

FRIENDS AND FOES

Cholesterol-lowering medicines of the statin type belong to the family of drugs known as HMG-CoA reductase inhibitors (see How It Works, alongside). Studies indicate that HMG-CoA reductase inhibitors interfere with the body's production of coenzyme Q10 (CoQ10), and use of these drugs should be therefore accompanied by supplementation with CoQ10. Consult your doctor about taking supplemental CoQ10 if you are taking a statin drug or red yeast rice (which contains the monacolins also found in some prescription cholesterol-lowering drugs). Consult your doctor immediately if you are taking a statin drug or red yeast rice and experience muscle weakness, numbness in your limbs, or pain.

Red yeast rice is available in tablet (including extended release) and capsule form. For adults, red yeast rice is usually taken orally in the form of capsules to lower cholesterol. The typically recommended dosage is 1,200 milligrams taken twice daily.

Since red yeast rice may interfere with CoQ10 production in the body, supplementation with CoQ10 is recommended when taking red yeast rice.

LOOK OUT FOR THIS!

Red yeast rice is not recommended for children, pregnant or nursing women, or people with liver disease.

Side effects of red yeast rice include mild headache, abdominal discomfort, heartburn, gas, bloating, muscle pain, dizziness, and kidney problems. There was one report of anaphylaxis (a severe and potentially life-threatening allergic reaction).

If you experience any muscle pain or weakness while taking red yeast rice, consult your doctor immediately.

WHAT TO AVOID

Medication: Few studies have been done on the interactions of red yeast rice with prescription drugs. However, interactions are possible with cyclosporine, ranitidine, antibiotics, drugs that inhibit the

Red Yeast Rice May Soon Be Classified as a Prescription Drug

Still In Debate

One of the monacolins in red yeast rice, called monacolin K, has been made into a prescription drug called lovastatin (Mevacor). As a result, the U.S. Food and Drug Administration (FDA) has argued that red yeast rice does not qualify as a dietary supplement under the Dietary Supplement Health and Education Act (DSHEA) of 1994 (see The ABCs of Supplements, page 3), but rather as an unapproved prescription drug. This decision was due largely to the close resemblance between the chemical composition of red yeast rice and that of the prescription drug lovastatin.

Pharmanex, the manufacturer of a product called Cholestin (whose main ingredient was red yeast rice), argued that red yeast rice has been used for centuries in China, and that Cholestin should therefore be classified as a dietary supplement.

After a 4-year battle with the FDA, Pharmanex lost its argument and the FDA prohibited Cholestin from being sold as a dietary supplement. As a result, Pharmanex created a new formulation of Cholestin that does not contain red yeast rice and which can be purchased on-line and from selected independent pharmacies. Many other products containing red yeast rice have also been pulled off the shelves of health food stores. Red yeast rice may require a prescription before it can be purchased, although it is still available in selected health food stores and on the Internet.

cytochrome P450 enzyme system, drugs that affect gamma-aminobutyric acid (such as neurotonin), aspirin, anticoagulants (such as warfarin), and nonsteroidal anti-inflammatory drugs (NSAIDs) such as ibuprofen. Consult your doctor before taking red yeast rice supplements with any drug or supplement that interacts with lovastatin.

Food: Alcohol should be avoided when taking red yeast rice. Also, regular consumption of grapefruit juice when taking red yeast rice may lead to muscle pain or weakness.

RHODIOLA

WHILE IT'S BEEN STUDIED IN SWEDEN, Norway, France, Germany, the Soviet Union, and Iceland for 45 years, rhodiola *(Rhodiola rosea)* is still relatively unknown to the United States. Also called arctic root, golden root, and roseroot, rhodiola is one of the most commonly used psychostimulants in Sweden. The herb has antistress, antifatigue, and performance-enhancing properties, and has been shown to increase alertness and well-being, relieve depression, and ease symptoms of stress such as poor work performance, irritability, and loss of concentration.

WHAT IT DOES

Like ginseng, rhodiola is an adaptogen, which means it increases the body's resistance to physical, environmental, and other stresses without upsetting normal physiology. It can both calm the body's stress response and protect the body from the damaging effects of stress. Rhodiola triggers a "nonspecific" resistance, working on a range of stressors, from cold and flu to intellectual exhaustion. Researchers believe that adaptogens work by changing the reactivity of the body's defense systems, including the immune, endocrine, and central nervous systems.

Studies of doctors on call, medical students, and employees taking moderate doses of rhodiola have shown rises in intellectual capacity, short-term memory, audiovisual perception, and concentration. Research with Olympic-level cross-country skiers and biathletes show improvements in maximum workload, endurance, coordination, and recovery time when they are taking rhodiola. In some studies, the performance boost was greater than with Siberian ginseng. No wonder the Vikings took rhodiola!

There is some evidence that rhodiola acts as an antioxidant for the nervous system, mobilizes fatty acids from fat tissue, improves weak erections and premature ejaculation, and stimulates menstruation. The herb's anticancer properties, studied in animals, appear promising. Researchers are also exploring the use of rhodiola for infertility, schizophrenia, bipolar disorder, thyroid dysfunction, and reducing the toxicity of cancer treatment. Rhodiola has demonstrated in vitro antibiotic properties against *Staphylococcus aureus*.

HOW IT WORKS

Stress affects the central nervous system and the hypothalamic–pituitary–adrenal–axis (HPA). Rhodiola appears to work directly on the central nervous system to increase levels of norepinephrine, dopamine, serotonin, and other neurotransmitters and speed their transport of messages and the reception of messages in the brain. This, in turn, stimulates two parts of the brain: the cerebral cortex (which controls the ability to think, analyze, and calculate) and the frontal cortex (which controls the ability to pay attention, remember, and learn). Rhodiola also appears to boost levels of acetylcholine, a neurotransmitter needed for memory retrieval, and could theoretically prevent memory loss that comes with age. This versatile herb also seems to positively affect the limbic system, which regulates emotion and mood.

Rhodiola, therefore, has a curious double benefit: emotional soothing and cognitive stimulation. The active ingredients identified so far in rhodiola are rosavins (a group of substances that includes rosavin, rosarin, and rosin) and salidroside.

HOW TO TAKE IT

A typical dose of rhodiola is from 100 to 150 milligrams of an extract, depending on the standardization. Clinical and research doses have gone as high as 600 milligrams a day. Look for extracts standardized to contain rosavins and salidroside.

To prepare for a stressful time, begin taking rhodiola a few weeks beforehand. For acute stress, take a single dose of three times the typical dose. Take the herb on an empty stomach 30 minutes before eating, and early in the day so that it won't disturb sleep.

At least 200 different species of rhodiola are known, but *R. rosea* has the most research behind its benefits, and only *R. rosea* has been certified as toxicologically safe. Read labels carefully to be sure a supplement contains "rhodiola rosea."

For additional information on specific health conditions and how to treat them with supplements, see Part 3 of this book, beginning on page 309.

LOOK OUT FOR THIS!

Side effects of rhodiola are rare, and include anxiety, nervousness, and overstimulation.

Rhodiola should be avoided by people with bipolar disorder since its antidepressant effect could potentially trigger a manic reaction.

WHAT TO AVOID

Medication: Rhodiola may enhance the effects of over-the-counter or prescription stimulants. In theory, rhodiola could change the absorption of pharmaceutical antidepressants.

RIBOFLAVIN

RIBOFLAVIN, ALSO KNOWS AS VITAMIN B_2, plays a key role in producing energy for your body. But that's not all—vitamin B_2 also activates vitamin B_6 and folic acid (vitamin B_9) so that they can work more effectively; assists in the production of red blood cells; and helps the nervous system function properly. Without enough riboflavin, you might experience some rather uncomfortable and unsightly conditions, from itching and peeling skin on the nose and scrotum to a sore tongue and burning eyes. Although diet is often the best source of riboflavin, supplements can be beneficial, especially since many people do not get sufficient amounts of this essential nutrient, particularly alcoholics, infants, and the elderly.

WHAT IT DOES

Taken in high doses, riboflavin may reduce the frequency of migraine headaches. At lower (nutritional) doses, this vitamin may also prevent the formation of cataracts.

Riboflavin may also combat atherosclerosis (in which cholesterol and other fats clog arteries, blocking the circulation of blood to organs), malaria, sickle cell anemia, and human immunodeficiency virus (HIV), and may additionally boost performance for athletes because of its involvement in muscle energy metabolism. Riboflavin may also prevent esophageal cancer, although more research on this and the other uses just named is necessary.

RESTORATIVE RECIPES

CARROT TOP SOUP

While it may seem strange, the tops of beets and carrots are actually edible! Not only can you eat them, but they are a good source of vitamins. Be sure to use organic products to ensure that your food has not been sprayed with pesticides.

Ingredients

3 tablespoons extra virgin olive oil
1 medium onion, minced
2 small carrots, diced
1 celery stalk, diced
3 cloves garlic, minced
1/2 teaspoon salt
1/2 teaspoon ground black pepper
6 cups vegetable broth
1/2 cup short grain rice
1 1/2 cups carrot tops, chopped
4 tablespoons fresh parmigiano/reggiano cheese, grated

Directions: Heat the olive oil in a large soup pot. Sauté the onion, carrots, celery, and garlic for 5 minutes over low heat until they become translucent. Add the salt and pepper, pour in the broth, and bring the mixture to a boil. When the mixture is boiling, add the rice and cook the broth for 15 minutes. Add the carrot tops and cook for an additional 5 minutes, making sure to mix the broth well. When the rice is done, sprinkle the broth with cheese and serve.

FOOD SOURCES

RIBOFLAVIN

Although little riboflavin is lost during ordinary cooking, healthy cooking techniques (such as steaming) are the best way to get the most of this and other vitamins into your body. Read on for some foods high in riboflavin that you can incorporate into your diet.

►Almonds, brewer's yeast, calf liver, eggs, milk, mushrooms, seafood, torula (nutritional) yeast, vegetables (especially leafy greens), wheat germ, and wild rice.

For additional information on specific health conditions and how you can treat them with supplements, see Part 3 of this book, beginning on page 309.

HOW IT WORKS

Most of riboflavin's purported benefits are thought to be associated with its antioxidant activity—the ability to neutralize the free radical molecules that damage cells and tissues—particularly in the lung, brain, and heart.

Riboflavin may help to prevent migraine headache by correcting small deficiencies in brain cells and may prevent esophageal cancer. Its benefits in helping to prevent atherosclerosis may be due to its role in breaking down the amino acid homocysteine, high levels of which are considered to increase the chances of heart disease and stroke.

HOW TO TAKE IT

Riboflavin may be sold as "riboflavin" or "vitamin B_2," depending on the brand and store. Be sure to check under both names.

The need for riboflavin increases as we age and is greatest for pregnant and nursing women. See the table below for the recommended daily intakes (RDIs) of riboflavin.

AGE/GENDER/ CONDITION	RECOMMENDED DAILY INTAKE (RDI)*
Infants and Children	
Birth–3 years	0.4–0.8 mg
4–6 years	1.1 mg
7–10 years	1.2 mg
Males	
Adolescents and adults	1.4–1.8 mg
Females	
Adolescents and adults	1.2–1.3 mg
Pregnant Women	1.6 mg
Nursing Women	1.7–1.8 mg

For more information on RDIs, see Want to Know More About Intake? on page 8.

The best way to get your RDI of riboflavin (see above) is to eat a well-balanced and varied diet.

Riboflavin is a part of the B-complex vitamin group (a term given to a group of eight important B vitamins), and most general-purpose multivitamin and mineral supplements contain the full range of B vitamins (be sure to check the label). A riboflavin-only supplement is usually not necessary. Taking your supplement with food improves the absorption of riboflavin.

LOOK OUT FOR THIS!

Riboflavin is a very safe supplement, and no side effects have been reported. If you consume too much of it, your body will excrete the excess in your urine—which will be bright yellow.

WHAT TO AVOID

Medication: Certain medications can interfere with the body's absorption of riboflavin, including cholestyramine, chlorpromazine, colestipol, doxorubicin, metoclopramide, probenecid, propantheline bromide, quinacrine, tricyclic antidepressants, and nucleoside reverse-transcriptase inhibitors such as those used against human immunodeficiency virus (HIV) including didanosine, lamivudine, stavudine, and zidovudine. Certain drugs, including antibiotics, estrogens, and antipsychotic medications, may deplete levels of riboflavin in the body.

S A M e

ACHING JOINTS? DEPRESSED? Problems with your liver? SAMe (S-adenosylmethionine) may be the answer. This compound occurs naturally in the body and is a form of methionine (an amino acid that contains sulfur) and adenosine triphosphate (the body's main energy molecule).

SAMe was first studied in Italy in the 1950s as a treatment for depression but was observed, accidentally, to improve osteoarthritis. It has been used as an antidepressant in Europe for the past 25 years. At present, SAMe may be expensive (up to $200 per month), but its benefits may be worth its cost.

WHAT IT DOES

SAMe has been documented in numerous studies to be as effective as conventional antidepressants, with fewer side effects and a more rapid onset of action. One recent pilot study found SAMe to be effective for the treatment of depression in people with AIDS/HIV.

Good evidence supports the use of SAMe for treating the symptoms of osteoarthritis. Studies have found SAMe to be as effective as nonsteroidal anti-inflammatory drugs (NSAIDs), including the cox-2 inhibitor Celebrex). SAMe may even slow the progression of the disease, although this is so far unproven. SAMe may also be helpful for certain liver diseases (such as cirrhosis and pregnancy-related jaundice), and to decrease the itching (pruritus) associated with liver disease. It may also be useful in the treatment of fibromyalgia (a painful muscle condition) and Parkinson's disease and for protecting the stomach from damage by alcohol. However, more research is needed to investigate these uses of SAMe.

For additional information on specific health conditions and how to treat them with supplements, see Part 3 of this book, beginning on page 309.

HOW IT WORKS

SAMe is a methyl donor, meaning that it provides the chemical entities known as methyl groups that are needed for many important processes in the body, including cell fluidity and function and the production of epinephrine (adrenaline), creatine, melatonin, glutathione, and other compounds vital for health. For depression, SAMe may also raise levels of serotonin and dopamine, neurotransmitters in the brain that are implicated in depression.

HOW TO TAKE IT

SAMe is not found in significant quantities in food; therefore, if you need more than your body produces (deficiencies in methionine, folate, or vitamin B_{12} can reduce SAMe levels), supplements are the only option.

SAMe is available in the form of capsules, enteric-coated tablets, and regular tablets. Enteric-coated tablets are better absorbed than the other forms. SAMe supplements are best taken on an empty stomach, between meals.

For people taking SAMe, a starting dosage of 800 milligrams taken twice a day is often recommended. It is important to try to take SAMe on an empty stomach for better absorption into the bloodstream. If improvements are noticed, the dosage may be lowered to 400 milligrams twice daily.

High doses of SAMe may theoretically lead to high levels of homocysteine, an amino acid that may increase the risk of heart disease and stroke, though human studies have not demonstrated this. However, it may be useful to take SAMe with supplemental folic acid and vitamin B_6 and B_{12} to prevent this effect.

LOOK OUT FOR THIS!

Side effects may occur uncommonly with SAMe. These include stomach pain, nausea, diarrhea, gas, anxiety, hyperactive muscle movements, insomnia, and hypomania (a highly excitable state). These side effects often go away with time or with lower doses of SAMe.

Children, pregnant or nursing women, and people with severe liver or kidney disease should consult their doctor before taking SAMe, since safety guidelines in these groups have not been established.

SAMe, like any antidepressant medication, may trigger manic episodes in people with bipolar disorder or unmask mania in people with depression.

WHAT TO AVOID

Medication: SAMe can interact with antidepressants including monoamine oxidase (MAO) inhibitors, selective serotonin reuptake inhibitors (SSRIs), and tricyclic antidepressant medications (though several studies have found that it is useful to add SAMe to a regimen of conventional antidepressants to increase their efficacy and speed the onset of action.

It can also interact with levodopa (used to treat Parkinson's disease), and although SAMe may relieve the side effects of levodopa, its continued use may reduce levodopa's effectiveness. Consult your doctor before taking SAMe with levodopa or with antidepressant medication.

SAW PALMETTO

THE RIPE, BLACK, OLIVE-LIKE BERRIES of the saw palmetto *(Serenoa repens)* bush were a staple food and medicine for Native Americans in the southeastern United States. These people would make an infusion from the berries to treat stomach ailments and dysentery, and used the fruit itself as a diuretic and a sexual tonic. In the 19th century, natural healers began using saw palmetto to treat a range of genitourinary and endocrine-related conditions, including sexual dysfunction. Saw palmetto has recently seen a resurgence in the United States as a treatment for male-pattern disorders such as impotence and hair loss and also for loss of libido.

WHAT IT DOES

The only scientifically proven use of saw palmetto berries is to reduce the symptoms associated with an enlarged prostate gland, a common condition in older men. Curiously, however, a recent study published in the *New England Journal of Medicine* found that saw palmetto was not effective for treating this condition. In Europe, saw palmetto extract is the most common treatment for this condition, and the effectiveness of new prescription medications for prostate enlargement is often measured against that of saw palmetto. Studies also suggest that saw palmetto relieves symptoms associated with an enlarged prostate—including difficulty in urinating, frequent urination, waking in the middle of the night to urinate, and a weak urine stream. Saw palmetto may also delay the onset of the symptoms of bladder outlet obstruction, which is common as men age. However, studies have not shown it to be helpful for prostatitis or pelvic pain.

Saw palmetto has also been used to treat other genitourinary problems, including low sperm count and lack of libido. Research also indicates that saw palmetto may inhibit the production of various inflammatory factors.

For additional information on specific health conditions and how you can treat them with supplements, see Part 3 of this book, beginning on page 309.

HOW IT WORKS

Studies have suggested that saw palmetto acts on the prostate by curbing the metabolism and action of male steroid hormones that are responsible for excessive growth of the prostate. Saw palmetto berries contain polysaccharides, which are usually associated with anti-inflammatory or immune-stimulating effects and which may help decrease inflammation in the prostate. Other active ingredients of saw palmetto include fatty acids, plant sterols, and flavanoids, although scientists suspect that these latter substances do not affect the steroid hormones that cause prostate enlargement. More study is needed to understand exactly how saw palmetto works.

HOW TO TAKE IT

As a supplement, saw palmetto comes in many forms—dried berries, tea, powdered capsules, tablets, liquid tinctures, and lipo-sterolic extracts. Many saw palmetto products are not standardized, and it is therefore necessary to be sure the product you purchase contains at least 85 to 95 percent fatty acids and sterols. Although dosages vary depending on the form of saw palmetto you are taking, the usual total daily dose is 320 milligrams. Take it with meals if you experience digestive upset.

Note: It may take from 4 to 6 weeks to experience the therapeutic effects of saw palmetto.

LOOK OUT FOR THIS!

Saw palmetto is generally considered safe, with few side effects. Occasionally, mild stomach and digestion problems and minor headaches have been reported.

Saw palmetto is not recommended for children, pregnant or nursing women, or people with liver or kidney disease.

WHAT TO AVOID

Medication: Because saw palmetto may work similarly to finasteride—a prescription medication used to treat an enlarged prostate—people taking finasteride should consult their doctor before taking saw palmetto.

SCHISANDRA

ANCIENT CHINESE DOCTORS were the first to discover that the bright red berries of the schisandra vine *(Schisandra chinensis)*—a member of the magnolia family—have beneficial properties. The vine grows throughout northern China, Russia, and Korea, where the leaves are cooked and eaten as a vegetable and the bright red berries are considered a snack food. The berries have a complex flavor, sometimes described as sour, sweet, salty, hot, or bitter. This explains the Chinese name for schisandra, *wu-wei-zi*, which means "five-flavored seed."

WHAT IT DOES

In China and Russia, traditional medicine has touted schisandra as a useful herb for tempering a host of conditions, from coughs and asthma to diarrhea and kidney problems, as well as impotence and insomnia. However, its efficacy for these claims has not yet been proven.

Recent studies conducted on animals suggest that schisandra may have liver-protective properties and may stimulate healthy cell reproduction in the liver. In China, schisandra is frequently used to improve liver function in people with hepatitis. Schisandra also aids in the body's detoxification process by stimulating the first phase of detoxification (see Detoxification, page 406). More extensive human trials are needed to confirm these findings.

Schisandra may be able to boost energy (particularly sexual vitality), relieve stress, and promote better mental functioning. Some herbal practitioners consider schisandra to be an adaptogenic herb, somewhat like ginseng. An adaptogenic herb is an herb that does not have a specific action, but helps to maintain normal body function and improves the body's response to stress.

Other preliminary studies suggest that schisandra may protect the heart during a heart attack, as well as reduce stress-induced heart palpitations. However, more study is needed to support these claims.

For additional information on specific health conditions and how to treat them with supplements, see Part 3 of this book, beginning on page 309.

HOW IT WORKS

Scientific studies of schisandra are limited, and researchers are not completely sure how or even whether schisandra is effective. However, some studies have confirmed schisandra's traditional uses and have found that the herb may have liver-protective, adaptogenic, and antioxidant properties. Schisandra seeds do contain many chemicals that might be medicinally beneficial. Among them are lignans—compounds that researchers suspect could stimulate the immune system, help protect the liver, potentially increase the body's ability to cope with stress, and even act as mild sedatives.

HOW TO TAKE IT

Schisandra is commercially available as dried berries and in tablet, capsule, and tincture form. It is often combined with other supplements in preparations advertised to boost energy, bolster the immune system, and reduce stress. There is no standardized dosage for schisandra, but a common dosage is from 1.5 grams to 6 grams daily. Consult your doctor about determining an appropriate dosage of this herb for you.

Side effects of schisandra appear to be rare, but may include mild stomach upset and skin rash.

The use of schisandra appears to be safe, but human studies are limited. Children and women who are pregnant or nursing should not take schisandra.

People with liver or kidney disease should consult their doctor before using schisandra.

WHAT TO AVOID

Medication: Use schisandra with caution if you are taking barbiturates or similar medications, since it may increase the sedating effects of these drugs. Schisandra should not be combined with methylphenidate, other amphetamine medications, or caffeine since it may decrease the stimulating effects of these drugs.

SELENIUM

SELENIUM IS ONE OF THE MOST POWERFUL safeguards for long-term health. This trace mineral plays a direct role in helping the body protect itself from cell- and tissue-damaging free radical molecules. Although selenium can be obtained from food, supplements are a great way to capitalize on the wide-ranging benefits this mineral has to offer.

WHAT IT DOES

While selenium was once feared because researchers believed industrial forms were carcinogenic, new evidence suggests that supplements of this mineral may actually help prevent some forms of cancer (including prostate, colorectal, and lung cancer). The National Cancer Institute is currently sponsoring a large study to determine selenium's role in cancer prevention. Selenium may be particularly useful in preventing colorectal cancer in people who smoke.

Some research has shown that selenium may help the body fight the human immunodeficiency virus (HIV) and hepatitis virus and may increase fertility in men. Other uses of selenium include prevention of cataracts and macular degeneration, boosting the immune system, and combating a number of skin conditions including dandruff, eczema, and warts, as well as promoting overall skin health. However, recent studies have not confirmed a beneficial effect of supplemental selenium

SELENIUM

The amount of selenium in food depends on how much of it was in the soil in which the food was grown. Today, farm land has become increasingly depleted of selenium. However, most people in the United States do get enough selenium from their diets. If you're looking for a powerful dose of selenium, eat some Brazil nuts. One ounce of Brazil nuts, dried, unblanched, contains about 550 micrograms of selenium, more than enough for a daily dose.

►Meat, seafood, dairy foods, wheat germ, nuts, oats, whole-wheat bread, bran, brown rice, turnips, garlic, barley, and orange juice.

on cardiovascular disease. And, while some studies indicated that selenium might be useful to benefit mood and quality of life in elderly people, recent studies have not been able to confirm this.

Research shows that a deficiency of selenium may lead to cervical dysplasia.

For additional information on specific health conditions and how to treat them with supplements, see Part 3 of this book, beginning on page 309.

HOW IT WORKS

Selenium is part of an antioxidant enzyme called glutathione peroxidase, which helps reduce the effect of cell- and tissue-damaging free radical molecules. It also strengthens the immune system, has anti-inflammatory properties, and maintains the viability of sperm cells.

HOW TO TAKE IT

The need for selenium rises with age, and is greatest for pregnant and nursing women. See the table below for the recommended daily intakes (RDIs) of this important nutrient.

AGE/GENDER/ CONDITION	RECOMMENDED DAILY INTAKE (RDI)*
Infants	
0–6 months	15 mcg
7–12 months	20 mcg
Children	
1–3 years	20 mcg
4–8 years	30 mcg
9–13 years	40 mcg
Males and Females	
14 years and older	55 mcg
Pregnant Women	60 mcg
Nursing Women	70 mcg

For more information on RDIs, see Want to Know More About Intake? on page 8.

You may need extra selenium if you have certain digestive conditions (such as Crohn's disease and ulcerative colitis).

Selenium supplements come in two forms: organic (selenite) and inorganic (selenomethinone and high-selenium yeast). Some studies suggest that the organic form may be easier for the body to absorb. Selenium supplements are available as capsules, extended-release tablets, and regular tablets. Taking vitamin E along with selenium can enhance the benefits of both nutrients. Be aware that most mulitvitamins/minerals include selenium.

LOOK OUT FOR THIS!

Selenium is considered safe when taken at recommended doses. High doses of selenium (900 micrograms or more) can cause depression, nervousness, irritability, skin rashes, nausea, vomiting, and brittleness or loss of hair and fingernails.

Never exceed the maximum safe doses (see below) for selenium without first consulting your doctor.

AGE/GENDER/ CONDITION	MAXIMUM SAFE DOSAGE
Infants	
0–6 months	45 mcg
7–12 months	60 mcg
Children	
1–3 years	90 mcg
4–8 years	150 mcg
9–13 years	280 mcg
Males and Females	
14 years and older	400 mcg
Pregnant and Nursing Women	400 mcg

Note: Maximum safe doses of selenium have not been set for people with severe kidney or liver disease.

WHAT TO AVOID

Medication: Selenium may interfere with the absorption of certain prescription medications, including proton-pump inhibitors and histamine blockers.

SLIPPERY ELM

NATIVE AMERICANS WERE THE FIRST to discover that the inner reddish bark of the slippery elm tree *(Ulmus rubra, Ulmus fulva)*—also called red elm or sweet elm—had medicinal uses. When in contact with liquid, this part of the tree forms a slippery, soothing coating that the Native Americans used to dress injuries such as burns, infected wounds, and skin irritations. Because it also coats and soothes the mucous membranes in the throat that are irritated by common cold and cough, slippery elm later became a popular cough and cold remedy.

WHAT IT DOES

Although slippery elm has had little scientific scrutiny, the U.S. Food and Drug Administration (FDA) has approved it as an over-the-counter drug. Slippery elm is often used in lozenge form to suppress coughs. It may also be recommended for treating burns, canker sores, and heartburn because of its ability to soothe mucus membranes. It is used in part of the Edgar Cayces treatment for psoriasis, which also includes dietary suggestions such as avoiding red meat and eating fresh fruits and vegetables.

Besides these uses, slippery elm also contains astringent tannins that may help alleviate diarrhea. It may also be useful for inflammatory bowel disease and irritable bowel syndrome (IBS).

For additional information on specific health conditions and how to treat them with supplements, see Part 3 of this book, beginning on page 309.

HOW IT WORKS

The way in which slippery elm works is simple, and is due mainly to the texture of the herb when combined with water. Exposure to water activates the gelatinous mucilage in slippery elm bark that can soothe and coat mucous membranes in the throat and lining of the intestines.

HOW TO TAKE IT

Slippery elm is commercially available as tablets, capsules, lozenges, finely powdered bark for use in drinks, and coarsely powdered bark for poultices. It is often sold in combination with zinc, vitamin C, and other supplements that may prevent or alleviate symptoms of the common cold.

Slippery elm is similar to oatmeal in texture and can be made into a porridge. Because it's gentle and easily digested, it is beneficial for people with gastritis and other intestinal problems.

A general dosage of slippery elm ranges from 500 to 1,000 milligrams taken three times a day. However, dosages vary depending on the form in which this herb is taken; be sure to carefully read individual product labels for dosage information.

LOOK OUT FOR THIS!

While the safety of slippery elm has not been formally studied, it is a very safe supplement when taken in recommended dosages. Occasional allergic reactions may occur.

WHAT TO AVOID

Medication: Theoretically, slippery elm may delay the absorption of certain drugs, however, more research is needed to test this theory.

SOY

IF YOU LIKE JAPANESE FOOD, then you probably already know about the multitude of ways the Japanese include soybeans in their diet—as whole soybeans (edamame), tofu, miso, natto, tempeh, soy oil, and, of course, soy sauce. Numerous studies have pointed to the nutritional and potential health benefits of soy, particularly its protective effects on the human heart, although some of the health claims for soy are now subject to controversy (see Still in Debate, page 259).

WHAT IT DOES

Studies have suggested that soy can help lower blood cholesterol and triglyceride levels and improve the ratio of HDL ("good") cholesterol to LDL ("bad") cholesterol. Studies suggest that when taken at an average dosage of 47 grams a day, soy may reduce total cholesterol by 9 percent, LDL cholesterol by 13 percent, and triglycerides by 10 percent.

Other studies suggest that soy can help suppress the hot flashes associated with menopause without the problems that often accompany estrogen therapy. A recent study found that postmenopausal women who drank two glasses of soy milk per day had decreased osteoporosis of the lumbar spine (but not if it was used simultaneously with progesterone).

Preliminary studies have also suggested that soy may play a role in preventing uterine, breast, and prostate cancer, although more research is needed to sustain these uses.

For additional information on specific health conditions and how to treat them with supplements, see Part 3 of this book, beginning on page 309.

HOW IT WORKS

Among the phytoestrogens, or plant estrogens, found in soy—which are also found in certain herbs, grains, and seeds, notably flaxseed—are substances called isoflavones. The chemical structure of isoflavones is similar enough to that of the reproductive hormone estrogen to allow them to bind to the estrogen receptors on cells in the body. Yet at the same time, the structure of isoflavones is different enough from that of estrogen as to weaken the latter's hormonal effects.

In theory, isoflavones extracted from soy are associated with a variety of beneficial health effects, particularly in menopausal and postmenopausal women. Among these effects are replenishing the body's declining estrogen levels and relieving menopausal symptoms, as well as decreasing the risk of heart disease and osteoporosis. Scientific research is under way to determine if soy isoflavone supplements have many of the same health effects as soy foods. While not all studies are finding benefit, at least one recent study found that soy isoflavones had a similar effect as conjugated estrogen on lowering fasting blood glucose and insulin levels in postmenopausal women. Other studies have found that soy isoflavones reduce the hot flashes and vaginal dryness associated with menopause and improve serum lipid profiles. One long-term study found increased endometrial hyperplasia at the end of 5 years of treatment with soy isoflavones.

HOW TO TAKE IT

The best way to get the nutritional and health benefits of soy is by enjoying a diet rich in soy products. Miso, tempeh, natto, and tamari are all excellent food sources of soy. You can also boost your intake of soy by using soy powder. Soy supplements are also available in the form of capsules and tablets. The recommended dosages differ

continues on page 260

The Soy Controversy

Still in Debate

The U.S. Food and Drug Administration (FDA) recently gave approval to manufacturers of soy foods to label products having a high content of soy protein with the statement that these products may help reduce heart disease risk. Even in the wake of the FDA's recent acknowledgement of soy's heart benefits, scientists at the FDA recognize that concerns have surfaced about certain soy-product components, as discussed below. Although evidence suggests that soy products may not be as healthy as was first imagined, the FDA emphasizes that all health claims have some amount of controversy. Although soy is synonymous to many people with "low carb," "high protein," "low fat," and "low cholesterol," this popular bean, often touted for its health benefits, is more complicated than it might at first appear.

Antinutrients. Certain substances found in soy known as "antinutrients"—including soy protein isolate, phytic acid, protease inhibitors, and lecithins—interfere with the body's ability to utilize and absorb key nutrients, including calcium, magnesium, copper, iron, and zinc. These antinutrients can cause gastric distress as well as inhibit the digestion of protein. Furthermore, diets high in phytates—substances that come from the phytic acid found in soy—have been found to cause growth problems in children.

Although the process of fermentation destroys the antinutrients found in soy, as well as increasing the availability of various minerals, these harmful substances remain present in unfermented soy products. Fermented soy products include miso, tempeh, and tamari; unfermented soy products include tofu, soy beverages (including soy-based infant formulas), soy nuts, soy cheese, and soy burgers.

Incomplete protein. Although fermented soy products contain protein, vitamins, fatty acids, and anticarcinogenic substances, they are still considered to be incomplete proteins. What is missing from soy are a number of important amino acids (including cystine and methionine), and as a result, soy should not be thought of as a substitute for animal products or milk. Moreover, studies suggest that soy products actually increase the body's need for certain fat-soluble vitamins such as vitamins A and D.

Toxins. When soy is processed, various toxins are often added or formed. These toxins include aluminum, which is toxic to the nervous system and kidneys; nitrates, which are carcinogens; and free glutamic acid or monosodium glutamate (MSG), which are neurotoxins or toxins that act specifically on the nervous system.

Phytoestrogens. The phytoestrogens—or hormone-like plant chemicals found naturally in soy—may adversely affect the endocrine system, the system of glands that produce hormones that control metabolic activity. The potential problems that can result from such disruption include reproductive problems, infertility, and breast cancer in women. The phytoestrogens found in soy may also cause hypothyroidsism and thyroid cancer. Furthermore, infants given soy-based formulas may be at risk for developing thyroid disease.

New studies are under way to resolve the confusion surrounding the harms and benefits of soy. Keep in mind that when soy is prepared according to traditional fermentation methods, it does have some health benefits, although it should not be used as a replacement for animal foods. In the meantime, you should be able to enjoy a heart-friendly diet without completely eliminating soy, but you may want to stick to fermented soy products. For example, try replacing a tofu burger with a tempeh burger.

GRILLED TEMPEH BURGERS

Although the consumption of unfermented soy products may be controversial, try sinking your teeth into some grilled tempeh, a fermented soy product that is delicious when marinated with lemon juice.

Ingredients

1/4 cup lemon juice
1/8 cup olive oil
2 cloves garlic, minced
1/8 teaspoon black pepper
16 ounces tempeh
1 onion, sliced
4 hamburger rolls (whole wheat)

Directions: Make a marinade by combining the lemon juice, olive oil, garlic, and black pepper in a bowl and mixing. Cut the tempeh into pieces and steam it in a steamer or metal sieve for 15 minutes. Place the steamed tempeh in a casserole dish and cover it with the marinade and onions. Refrigerate for 4 hours to marinate. After the tempeh has marinated, cook it over a grill until it is heated through, making sure to baste it with the marinade. Once the tempeh is cooked, garnish it with lettuce and sliced tomatoes and serve.

according to the form of supplement used, so be sure to read and carefully follow the label directions.

LOOK OUT FOR THIS!

Side effects of soy include mild nausea, headache, and stomach upset.

Soy supplements are generally considered safe for adults. The use of soy supplements is not suitable for children or women who are pregnant or nursing, since the estrogen-like effects of soy are not yet fully understood. However, one long-term study (5 years) in post-menopausal women found increased endometrial hyperplasia (abnormal growth of the lining of the uterus). Women should be sure to continue with regular checkups and examinations with their gynecologists when taking soy supplements for long periods of time.

People with liver or kidney disease or prostate cancer should consult their doctor before taking soy supplements, since these supplements have a high phosphorus and potassium content.

Food sources of soy are appropriate and considered safe for adults and children. However, some research indicates the soy formulas for infants may contain various toxins. Consult your doctor about this matter before using such formulas.

People with impaired thyroid function should consult their doctor before consuming soy or taking any type of soy supplement, since soy may have various potentially harmful effects on the thyroid gland.

WHAT TO AVOID

Medication: Women taking any of the estrogen-receptor modulator class of drugs should consult their doctor before taking soy supplements or consuming soy in amounts greater than usually found in a normal diet. Since soy contains phytoestrogens, it is recommended that women using hormone therapy consult their doctor about their soy intake. Women taking oral contraceptives that contain estrogen should also consult their doctor before consuming large amounts of soy or soy supplements.

SPIRULINA

O JUMP IN THE LAKE" is an old expression, but as it happens, it just might be good for you. The lake is where you'll find spirulina—also known as blue-green algae—one of the most nutritious substances on earth. Because it's microscopic, you're not likely to see it, but spirulina grows naturally in warm, alkaline waters, especially in Central and South America and in Africa.

WHAT IT DOES

Spirulina contains many important nutrients, including all the essential amino acids and essential fatty acids. It contains chlorophyll and carotenoids, both of which are important antioxidants. It's a rich source of other nutrients, including B-complex vitamins, beta-carotene, vitamin E, manganese, zinc, copper, iron, selenium, and gamma-linoleic acid (GLA).

Evidence indicates that spirulina stimulates the immune system, improves liver function, and may have antiviral properties against herpes virus, cytomegalovirus, influenza virus, and HIV. In fact, a compound extracted from spirulina and other blue-green algae, cyanovirin-N, may be a potent tool in the fight against HIV and influenza. Recent scientific studies have suggested that spirulina may play a role in preventing and even tempering the symptoms accompanying certain types of cancer. Specifically, in a study in India, scientists reported that patients with oral cancer exhibited complete regression of oral lesions when given spirulina. Spirulina plus zinc may help protect against chronic arsenic poisoning, which occurs in Bangladesh, Taiwan, and Chile as a result of high concentrations of arsenic in drinking water.

In a controlled human study, spirulina appeared to lower cholesterol levels, but more research is needed to confirm these findings. Preliminary studies suggest that spirulina may be useful for treating diabetes, allergic rhinitis, and suppressing the appetite. It has been shown to be a useful supplement for children in Africa.

For additional information on specific health conditions and how you can treat them with supplements, see Part 3 of this book, beginning on page 309.

HOW IT WORKS

In controlled studies, spirulina seemed to increase the production of antibodies, cytokines (proteins made by the immune system that fight infections and perform other roles), and cells of the immune system.

Furthermore, in studies performed on rats, spirulina lowered triglyceride levels and boosted lipid and plasma production.

SUPPLEMENTAL TRIVIA

Since ancient times, the Aztecs, Mayans, and people of Africa and Asia have used spirulina as a health supplement. The Aztecs called it "blue mud." Dwellers in the Sahara Desert near Lake Chad called it "dihe." Today, spirulina is commercially grown and harvested in outdoor tanks in California, Hawaii, and Asia.

A component of spirulina—a polysaccharide known as calcium spirulan (Ca-SP)—has been identified as an antiviral agent. Researchers believe that this component may enable spirulina to suppress viruses in the body.

Spirulina is also a rich source of GLA, which may promote the loss of body fat, and Ca-SP, which may play a role in counteracting blood clotting.

HOW TO TAKE IT

Spirulina is available in tablet and capsule form, as well as a powder made from these algae. Although there is no recommended dosage of spirulina, the manufacturers often recommend an intake of 2,000 to 3,000 milligrams daily, divided into several doses. Studies are still being performed to verify the best dosages of spirulina for specific ailments. Consult your doctor about determining the appropriate dosages to suit your individual needs.

LOOK OUT FOR THIS!

The most important safety concern with spirulina supplementation is heavy metal contamination from the soil. Make sure to choose a manufacturer who screens for this kind of contamination.

Few side effects are associated with spirulina, but some individuals have reported headaches, muscle pain, flushing of the face, sweating, and difficulty in concentrating while taking it.

Spirulina is generally considered safe for adults. Its use is not suitable for children or for women who are pregnant or nursing, because no scientific studies of it have been performed in these groups. People with liver or kidney disease should consult their doctor before taking spirulina.

WHAT TO AVOID

Herbs and Dietary Supplements: Continuous ingestion of spirulina at high doses may elevate levels of calcium in the body.

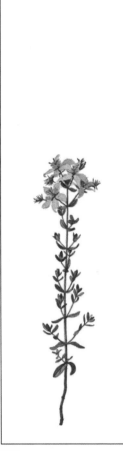

ST. JOHN'S WORT

THE ANCIENT GREEKS WERE AMONG the first to discover the health benefits of St. John's wort *(Hypericum perforatum)*, and at the time, it was also known as a protector against evil spirits. In the Middle Ages St. John's wort was considered a remedy for mental disorders, and by the 19th century it was being used to treat, among other things, a "nervous disposition" and "hysteria." The yellow, five-petaled flower of St. John's wort grows all over northern California and southern Oregon.

WHAT IT DOES

Although its mood-elevating properties were previously recognized in Europe, St. John's wort has only recently become a popular herb in the United States for elevating the mood of people with mild to moderate depression. Today it is one of the most popular herbal products in the United States and Europe. Numerous studies show that St. John's wort is often as effective in tempering mild and moderate depression as are certain prescription antidepressant medications, such as tricyclic antidepressants and selective serotonin reuptake inhibitors (SSRIs). St. John's wort may be especially helpful for the elderly, who often cannot tolerate the side effects of prescription antidepressants. St. John's wort may also be effective for the treatment of somatoform disorders (physical symptoms that can't be traced to a physical cause).

A recent German study found St. John's wort to be effective for more serious depression, but St. John's wort is not recommended for treating severe depression with symptoms including extreme fatigue, suicidal thoughts, severe anxiety, and an inability to cope with daily life. These symptoms can be life-threatening and should be treated by a psychiatrist.

St. John's wort may be sometimes applied as an external topical solution (as an oil). Oily extracts containing hyperforin have demonstrated antibacterial and anti-inflammatory effects, and several recent studies suggest that it may be effective for treating eczema when applied topically. The German Commission E has approved external use of oily preparations of St. John's wort for treatment of bruises, muscle aches, and first-degree burns. Herbalists use the oil topically as a treatment for neuralgia and nerve pain, although this use has not received scientific study.

St. John's wort taken orally may also have antibacterial and antiviral properties, possibly easing symptoms of several viral infections, including herpes simplex and mononucleosis.

St. John's wort may also help to temper symptoms of seasonal affective disorder (SAD), obsessive-compulsive disorder (OCD), menopause, premenstrual syndrome (PMS), temporomandibular joint disorder (TMJ) and fibromyalgia, but more studies are needed to confirm these findings.

For additional information on specific health conditions and how to treat them with supplements, see Part 3 of this book, beginning on page 309.

HOW IT WORKS

Although the exact effects of St. John's wort are not yet determined, scientists believe that it helps alleviate depression, mainly by boosting levels of a neurotransmitter in the brain called serotonin, which is needed to maintain emotional balance. St. John's wort may also affect other brain chemicals such as noradrenaline and dopamine.

HOW TO TAKE IT

St. John's wort comes in many forms, including capsules, tablets, tinctures, drops, teas, oil-based skin lotions, and even snack chips. Chopped or powdered forms of the dried herb are also available.

All St. John's wort products should contain at least 0.3 percent hypericin, the major medicinal substance in this herb, or 3 to 5 percent hyperforin, another medicinal component. It's important to note that when various St. John's wort products have been studied, large differences in both hypericin and hyperforin content have been found, and significant variations have even been discovered within batches of the same brand.

As with prescription antidepressants, it may take about 4 to 6 weeks to notice the effects of St. John's wort.

LOOK OUT FOR THIS!

Side effects of St. John's wort may include stomach upset, hives or other skin rashes, fatigue, bloating, weight gain, constipation, restlessness, headache, dry mouth, dizziness, and mental confusion. However, a German study found that St. John's wort caused less severe and fewer side effects than the prescription antidepressant fluoxetine (Prozac).

Although an uncommon effect, St. John's wort can make the skin overly sensitive to sunlight. Light-skinned people taking this herb for a prolonged time should be careful about sun exposure and should avoid sunlamps, as well as tanning beds and booths.

St. John's wort is generally considered safe for adults. However, it is not suitable for children, women who are pregnant or nursing, or people with severe kidney or liver disease. Use of St. John's wort should be stopped 1 week before surgery and for several weeks after surgery.

WHAT TO AVOID

Medication: Studies show that St. John's wort may interfere with many types of prescription drugs. Consult your doctor before taking St. John's wort if you are already taking any prescription medications, particularly antidepressants, cyclosporine, digoxin, immuno-suppressive medications, indinavir and other protease inhibitors, loperamide, oral contraceptives, reserpine, theophylline, and warfarin. Also, do not take St. John's wort if you are undergoing chemotherapy.

TEA TREE OIL

FRAGRANT *AND* EFFECTIVE? These two factors don't often go hand in hand, but when it comes to tea tree oil, that is precisely what happens—and perhaps why this fragrant oil is one of the most popular herbal exports of its native Australia. Tea tree (Melaleuca alternifolia) oil is extracted from the leaves of the tea tree through a process called steam distillation. The oil is a potent antiseptic that helps in the fight against many bacteria and fungi, even those resistant to antibiotic treatment.

WHAT IT DOES

Studies suggest that tea tree oil may be effective for stopping fungal infections of the skin and nails, including athlete's foot. A number of randomized, controlled human trials have indicated that tea tree oil may be effective against dandruff and various parasites including scabies and head lice. As a result, tea tree oil is included in many shampoos.

Because of its antiseptic properties, tea tree oil may also be useful for treating acne when applied topically, and with fewer side effects than other topically used medications.

Additionally, preliminary studies have suggested that diluted preparations of tea tree oil may be useful in combating the oral candida yeast infection known as thrush, the sores of herpes simplex (cold sores), and gum disease. It may also work as a deodorant. However, more studies are needed to confirm these effects.

For additional information on specific health conditions and how to treat them with supplements, see Part 3 of this book, beginning on page 309.

SUPPLEMENTAL TRIVIA

The tea tree was named by the famous explorer Captain James T. Cook when he discovered that its leaves made a suitable substitute for tea. More than a century later, an Australian chemist discovered the strong antiseptic properties of tea tree oil, and beginning in the 1920s it became a standard preparation for preventing and treating wound infections. The tea tree became so important that during World War II it was classified as an essential commodity and its harvesters and farmers were excused from military service. With the advent of antibiotics, however, tea tree oil lost its popularity as an antiseptic.

HOW IT WORKS

Tea tree oil has received a substantial amount of acclaim when it comes to fighting fungi and bacteria. It has been found to stop the growth of several kinds of bacteria and also seems to curb inflammation. The oil blends with the skin's own oils, creating an inhospitable environment for bacteria and fungi and promoting the rapid healing of cuts or bruises.

HOW TO TAKE IT

Tea tree oil is available as an oil, gel, cream, shampoo, and mouthwash. It should only be used topically, and the undiluted oil should never be taken orally or internally. When using tea tree oil as a mouthwash for oral disorders such as thrush or gingivitis, be sure to use a diluted preparation containing 0.4 to 2 percent tea tree oil. Such diluted preparations of tea tree oil should not be swallowed.

For topical use, choose a tea tree oil product containing oil from the species *Melaleuca alternifolia,* with 10 percent cineole and at least 30 percent terpinen-4-ol.

Shampoos containing 2 to 5 percent tea tree oil are available for treating dandruff, head lice, and scabies.

LOOK OUT FOR THIS!

Side effects of topically applied tea tree oil include a severe allergic reaction that can affect the entire body, as well as dry skin and skin

Tea Tree Oil May Help Kill Staph Infection

Did You Know?

Tea tree oil may be an effective agent for killing various species of the common bacteria called *Staphylococcus aureus*—more simply known as "staph." For the most part, these bacteria live harmlessly on the human skin surface, especially around the nose, mouth, genitals, and rectum. It is only when the skin is punctured or broken that these staph bacteria enter the wound that they may cause an infection. If left untreated,

staph infection can become a dangerous illness.

Although some kinds of staph bacteria have become resistant to antibiotic medication, researchers have found that some of these resistant strains of staph may be destroyed with large dosages of tea tree oil.

Although studies of the use of tea tree oil as an antiseptic in hospitals (a common place where staph infection occurs) have shown promising results, more research is needed to determine its value.

irritation, especially in the vaginal area and in people with highly sensitive skin. As a safety precaution, dab a small amount of tea tree oil on your inner arm with a cotton swab before using it. If you are allergic, your arm will quickly become red or inflamed, in which case you should not use tea tree oil.

Tea tree oil can be poisonous if ingested in large doses, causing drowsiness, confusion, weakness, inability to sit, stand, or walk, diarrhea, abdominal pain, and a severe rash. When using tea tree oil orally (such as for gingivitis and thrush), be sure to use it as a diluted mouthwash, and do not swallow any of it.

Tea tree oil is considered safe for adults when applied topically. Its use is not suitable for children or pregnant or nursing women, since its long-term safety effects have not yet been studied. Additionally, people with severe kidney or liver disease should avoid tea tree oil.

WHAT TO AVOID

Medication: Tea tree oil may increase the effects of other agents used topically on the skin, such as tretinoin.

THIAMINE

OF ALL THE B VITAMINS, thiamine (Vitamin B_1) was the first to be discovered in 1911, when the German chemist Casimir Funk isolated it from rice bran extracts. This was a momentous step in nutrition science, not only because of the discovery, but also because Funk coined the term "vitamin" to reflect the "vital" role of thiamine. So vital is thiamine that every part of your body, especially your heart, needs it to make energy in order to function day in and day out.

WHAT IT DOES

Evidence suggests that supplementation with thiamine may help to ease the symptoms of congestive heart failure, in which the pumping ability of the heart diminishes and fluids build up in the lungs and legs.

Supplementation with thiamine may also slow the progression of the disease human immunodeficiency virus (HIV) to acquired immune deficiency syndrome (AIDS) and improve the chances of survival in AIDS according to observational studies. Supplemental thiamine may also be needed by people with alcoholism, mood disorders, Alzheimer's disease, epilepsy, mouth sores, fibromyalgia,

FOOD SOURCES

THIAMINE

Not only is it important to incorporate foods containing thiamine into your diet, but it is equally as important to know how to retain the thiamine in your food when you cook it. Thiamine is often lost in cooking, but using whole-grain pasta without rinsing it after cooking; cooking vegetables in a minimal amount of water; and cooking meat until it's done without overcooking are all ways to retain this important nutrient in your food.

And if you're looking for a good dose of thiamine, 2 tablespoons of brewer's yeast has 2.3 milligrams of this vitamin. Read on for other thiamine-rich foods.

▶ Black beans and navy beans, brewer's yeast, cashews, green peas, organ meats, pork, potatoes, soy nuts, sunflower seeds, torula (nutritional) yeast, whole grains, and whole-grain pasta.

and glaucoma. In people with diabetes, thiamine may prevent or delay the progress of atherosclerosis. Ongoing research is being done to support these uses of thiamine.

For additional information on specific health conditions and how to treat them with supplements, see Part 3 of this book, beginning on page 309.

HOW IT WORKS

Thiamine plays a key role in the breakdown of carbohydrates to produce energy. It works to maintain the nervous system and heart muscle, and may have antioxidant activity, reducing the effect of cell- and tissue-damaging free radical molecules. Thiamine also helps to break down glucose (blood sugar) and may reduce the build-up of smooth-muscle cells in the arteries in diabetes—which may prevent or delay the cardiovascular effects of this disease.

HOW TO TAKE IT

See the table below for the recommended daily intakes (RDIs) of thiamine.

AGE/GENDER/ CONDITION	RECOMMENDED DAILY INTAKE (RDI)*
Infants	
0–6 months	0.2 mg
7–12 months	0.3 mg
Children	
1–3 years	0.5 mg
4–8 years	0.6 mg
9–13 years	0.9 mg
Males	
14 years and older	1.2 mg
Females	
14–18 years	1.0 mg
19 years and older	1.1 mg
Pregnant and Nursing Women	1.4 mg

For more information on RDIs, see Want to Know More About Intake? on page 8.

Thiamine is a part of the B-complex vitamin group—a term given to a group of eight important B vitamins—and most general purpose multivitamin and mineral supplements contain the full range of B vitamins. Most, if not all, mutivitamin/mineral supplements contain enough thiamine to meet the RDI for this vitamin. Thiamine-only supplements are generally unnecessary.

You may need extra thiamine if you have certain medical conditions (such as alcoholism, anorexia, Crohn's disease, and folate deficiency), if you require kidney dialysis or are taking certain medications such as loop diuretics or antibiotics, or theophylline for asthma, or if you regularly eat certain foods that can interfere with the absorption of thiamine (such as fish, shrimp, clams, and mussels). In addition, people who have a high intake of calories (for example, athletes) may need more thiamine to help process them into energy.

In the United States, thiamine deficiency is most commonly seen in elderly people and malnourished infants. People with alcoholism may also develop a thiamine deficiency because large amounts of alcohol can diminish the body's absorption of this important vitamin.

Symptoms of thiamine deficiency include depression, irritability, memory loss, confusion, indigestion, weight loss, edema, muscle weakness, fatigue, heart palpitations, rapid heart rate, decreased muscular coordination, and soreness of the calves. Severe thiamine deficiency may result in a condition known as beriberi, which can damage the heart and nervous system.

LOOK OUT FOR THIS!

Even when taken in very high doses, oral thiamine appears to be safe, and no side effects of this vitamin have been reported.

WHAT TO AVOID

Food: Thiamine may be inactivated when taken with foods and beverages containing sulfites, including wine, beer, wine coolers, and most distilled liquors; drinks containing sugar or corn syrup; canned, bottled, and frozen fruit juices and vegetables; dehydrated fruits; Maraschino cherries; products made with dough conditioners, such as cookies, crackers, crepes, soft pretzels, and tortillas; many condiments, including horseradish and pickled foods; wine vinegar; puddings; and frostings. Tea, coffee, and decaffeinated coffee may also inactivate thiamine.

UVA URSI

THE UVA URSI PLANT *(Arctostaphylos uva-ursi)* is a low, woody, flowering plant that has berries resembling cranberries. Bears tend to be fond of these bitter, astringent berries; in fact, uva ursi is often called bearberry. The leaves of the uva ursi plant (not the berries) have a long history of medicinal use as an astringent, tonic, and diuretic. Native Americans used uva ursi leaves to treat urinary tract infections. European and American medicine has embraced the plant as well. Until the discovery of sulfa drugs and antibiotics, arbutin—the principal medicinal ingredient in uva ursi leaves—was a standard treatment for bladder infections.

WHAT IT DOES

The German Commission E (see page 16) approves the use of uva ursi for treating urinary tract infections. Some researchers suspect that uva ursi can be used for other urological problems, including cystitis (bladder inflammation) and kidney stones. Laboratory and animal tests have shown that uva ursi may have antimicrobial properties. One study found that uva ursi significantly reduced the amount of antibiotic needed to treat infection with the very dangerous bacteria known as methicillin-resistant *Staphylococcus aureus.* Uva ursi may also fight various bacteria that cause prostatitis. More research is needed to explore these uses of uva ursi.

Some healthcare practitioners also consider uva ursi to have mild diuretic properties, but there is no scientific evidence to back this claim. Preliminary studies with animals suggest that uva ursi may enhance the anti-inflammatory and antiallergenic effects of corticosteroid medications.

For additional information on specific health conditions and how you can treat them with supplements, see Part 3 of this book, beginning on page 309.

HOW IT WORKS

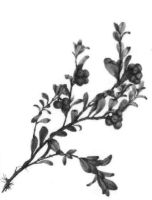

Uva ursi leaves contain several compounds that appear to have medicinal properties, including arbutin, which has antimicrobial effects; tannins, which act as astringents; and phenol glucososides, which have antibacterial effects. These compounds are absorbed in the gastrointestinal tract and then transported to the kidneys and excreted through the urine. As they pass through the urinary tract they work together to fight infection and soothe irritation in the mucus membranes.

HOW TO TAKE IT

Uva ursi is commercially available in a variety of forms, including dried leaf powder, capsules, tea, and tincture. The recommended dosage of uva ursi varies depending on the form taken. Uva ursi should be taken as a supplement standardized to contain 400 to 800 milligrams of arbutin per dose, with two to four doses taken daily.

Uva ursi should not be taken for more than 14 consecutive days or more than five times a year unless otherwise directed by a doctor. Uva ursi should be taken with meals to minimize gastrointestinal upset.

LOOK OUT FOR THIS!

Uva ursi is generally considered safe when taken for short periods of time. Side effects may include nausea, vomiting, irritability, insomnia, and an increased heart rate. When taken in excess, uva ursi may cause inflammation and irritation of the bladder and urinary tract. It may also cause liver damage when taken for extended periods.

The use of uva ursi is not safe for children or for women who are pregnant or nursing. Also, because of concerns that it may have toxic effects on the liver, people with liver or kidney disease should not take uva ursi.

WHAT TO AVOID

Medication: Consult your doctor before taking uva ursi with nonsteroidal anti-inflammatory drugs (NSAIDs), corticosteroids, or any medication that causes acidic urine.

Herbs and Dietary Supplements: Uva ursi works best in alkaline urine, and cranberry juice and vitamin C may therefore interfere with its antimicrobial effects.

Food: Because uva ursi works as an antimicrobial agent only when the urine is alkaline, individuals taking it should avoid eating acidic foods like citrus fruits, pineapple, or tomato.

Note: To keep your urine alkaline, mix 1½ teaspoons (6 to 8 grams) of baking soda in a glass of water and drink this, or take an over-the-counter antacid preparation.

VALERIAN

THE DRIED ROOTS OF THE VALERIAN plant *(Valeriana of-ficinalis)* have been used as a gentle tranquillizer and seda-tive since the time of the Greek physician Hippocrates in the 4th century BC. In the 2nd century AD, Galen, the most famous physician in the Roman Empire, recommended valerian as a treat-ment for insomnia. Valerian began to be widely used in Europe in the 17th century, and continued to be popular until it was replaced in modern times by prescription sedatives. In fact, valerian is often referred to as "the Valium of the 18th century" because of its wide-spread use in the mid-1800s.

WHAT IT DOES

Taken before bedtime, valerian is a gentle treatment for insomnia and other sleep disorders, as well as for restlessness and anxiety. Studies show that it reduces the time needed to fall asleep, although it is unclear whether valerian has an effect on the quality of sleep it-self. Moreover, valerian does not adversely affect the critical rapid eye movement (REM) phase of sleep and does not cause morning drowsiness. Valerian is often considered an excellent alternative to many prescription sedative drugs because of its lack of side effects.

Preliminary studies suggest that when taken in conjunction with St. John's wort, valerian may be helpful in treating depression associ-ated with anxiety. And because of its ability to promote relaxation, valerian is often recommended for treating headaches and various other ailments that may be caused by stress.

Valerian is often combined with other herbs—such as hops, pas-sionflower, lemon balm, lavender, skullcap, and chamomile—for use as a relaxant.

For additional information on specific health conditions and how to treat them with supplements, see Part 3 of this book, beginning on page 309.

HOW IT WORKS

It is unclear which compounds in valerian are active, but they seem to affect the brain in a manner similar to the prescription tranquiliz-ers diazepam (Valium) and triazolam (Halcion). Researchers are continuing to isolate various compounds from valerian in an effort to determine which ones are most effective.

Note: The prescription tranquilizer diazepam is not extracted from valerian. Diazepam, sold under the trade name of Valium, has no relationship to valerian.

HOW TO TAKE IT

Valerian root powder and valerian extract are the most commonly available forms of this herb. Commercially, they come in tinctures, infusions, and dried extracts sold in capsules and tablets. Valerian is also sold as a tea. Valerian products are standardized to contain 0.8 percent valerenic or valeric acid.

A general dosage of valerian ranges from 250 to 500 milligrams daily, although dosages vary according to the condition being treated. For insomnia, take only at bedtime.

LOOK OUT FOR THIS!

Valerian is generally considered safe, with few side effects. Mild headaches and digestive problems have occasionally been reported.

Pregnant or nursing women and children under the age of 3 years should not take valerian. Because valerian may interact or intensify the effects of anesthesia, some physicians recommend that its use be stopped 24 hours before surgery.

While it does not seem to cause morning sleepiness, valerian may impair judgment and driving ability for a few hours after you take it. There have also been reports of a "paradoxical reaction" to valerian—in which some people instead of feeling calmer, feel anxious and restless and may experience a rapid heartbeat after taking it. There have also been reports of "valerian withdrawal" if this herb is discontinued suddenly after the chronic use of high doses. The symptoms of this withdrawal include confusion and rapid heartbeat.

WHAT TO AVOID

Medication: Valerian should not be combined with barbiturates and should be used with caution by people taking the benzodiazepine class of drugs and other sedatives, including antihistamines, selective serotonion reuptake inhibitors (SSRIs), beta blockers, antiseizure medications, and alcoholic beverages. If you are taking any of these medications, consult your doctor before taking valerian.

VITAMIN A

EVERY TISSUE IN THE BODY needs vitamin A for growth and repair. Vitamin A is especially important for healthy skin, hair, and vision; the formation of bones; healing of wounds; reproduction; and the functioning of the immune system. Vitamin A is a fat-soluble vitamin that is part of a family of compounds that includes retinol, retinal, and beta-carotene. Beta-carotene is known as "pro-vitamin A" because the body can convert it into vitamin A when needed. Supplementation with beta-carotene may be safer than taking vitamin A as a supplement, since experts believe that the body converts beta-carotene only when it requires vitamin A, reducing chances of overdosage with this vitamin.

WHAT IT DOES

Since vitamin A is an integral part of so many functions in the body, a bevy of health claims are associated with its supplemental use.

Experts believe that vitamin A promotes healthy skin, prevents infections, and helps fight cancer and aging. After a burn injury, the body's level of vitamin A becomes depleted and more is needed to form new skin and tissue. Vitamin A is also linked to good vision—in fact, the first sign of vitamin A deficiency is often night blindness.

Vitamin A may help boost the immune system and the body's resistance to infection by stimulating white blood cells and increasing the activity of antibodies. Some animal studies have suggested that vitamin A can protect cells from dioxins, a family of toxic chemicals released into the air by combustion and air pollution. Dioxins are also a component of cigarette smoke.

Topical vitamin A is used in prescription medications, can help clear up acne and psoriasis, and may also help in healing other skin disorders such as rosacea, premature aging marks, and warts. Vitamin A derivatives are widely used in cosmetics and skin products designed to combat skin aging and treat acne. Vitamin A has been used for decades as a treatment for various vision-related conditions, including night blindness, cataracts, conjunctivitis, retinopathy, and macular degeneration. It may also help prevent or treat Crohn's disease, diarrhea, heavy menstruation, peptic ulcers, and premenstrual syndrome.

Vitamin A deficiency is common among children in developing countries and is associated with a high risk of infection, including human immunodeficiency virus (HIV) infection. Preliminary research suggests that vitamin A may also be useful for preventing anemia and cervical dysplasia and for treating lupus, alcoholism, and fibrocystic breast disease.

For additional information on specific health conditions and how to treat them with supplements, see Part 3 of this book, beginning on page 309.

HOW IT WORKS

Vitamin A has a variety of functions in the body: It helps the body to properly reproduce cells, thus reducing the likelihood of cells replicating improperly, which can lead to cancer; it protects eyesight by promoting the health of various cells in the eye and it helps the eyes to process light; and it appears to promote healthy reproduction by maintaining the health and function of sperm cells, egg cells, the ovaries, and the placenta.

HOW TO TAKE IT

See the table below for the recommended daily intakes (RDIs) of vitamin A.

AGE/GENDER/CONDITION	RECOMMENDED DAILY INTAKE (RDI)*
Infants	
0–6 months	1,330 IU
7–12 months	1,665 IU
Children	
1–3 years	1,000 IU
4–8 years	1,333 IU
9–13 years	2,000 IU
Males	
14 years and over	3,000 IU
Females	
14 years and over	2,330 IU
Pregnant Women	2,565 IU (2,500 IU if under 18 years)
Nursing Women	4,335 IU (4,000 IU if under 18 years)

For more information on RDIs, see Want to Know More About Intake? on page 8.

Healthy people can usually get sufficient vitamin A by eating a well-balanced diet containing foods rich in vitamin A (see Food Sources, alongside). Most general-purpose multivitamin/mineral supplements also contain vitamin A (be sure to check the label). Vitamin A can be depleted by the antibiotic neomycin and by bile acid sequestrant medications such as cholestyramine.

Vitamin A deficiency is rare in the United States. Vitamin A supplementation is recommended for strict vegetarians (those who do not eat meat, fish, eggs, milk, or milk products) and people who have had stomach surgery or other digestive conditions that may affect the body's absorption of vitamin A, such as pancreatic disorders or cystic fibrosis.

As a supplement, vitamin A is available either as retinol or retinyl palmitate in the form of tablets, capsules, and topical creams. Vitamin A cream (Retin-A) is available as a prescription drug.

LOOK OUT FOR THIS!

Note that as a fat-soluble vitamin, vitamin A can be stored in the body for a long time, allowing its levels to build up. In fact, the liver can store up to a year's supply of vitamin A, although this becomes depleted if you are sick or have an infection.

People taking high doses of vitamin A may be at risk for toxicity, with potential side effects such as headache, fatigue, muscle and joint pain, dry skin and lips, dry or irritated eyes, nausea, vomiting or diarrhea, and hair loss. Too much vitamin A can also contribute to bone loss and increase triglyceride levels in the blood, which can increase the risk of heart disease.

As noted earlier, taking beta-carotene can be safer than taking vitamin A, since beta-carotene, unlike vitamin A, does not build up in the body and is therefore safer to take in larger amounts. Children, people with liver or kidney disease, and pregnant women should take beta-carotene instead of supplemental vitamin A.

WHAT TO AVOID

Medication: Consult your doctor before taking vitamin A with any vitamin A-derived drugs such as isotretinoin and tretinoin, antacids, birth-control medications, blood-thinning medications, cholesterol-lowering medications, doxorubicin, neomycin, omeprazole, or weight loss products such as orlistat or olestra.

Food: Alcohol can intensify the effects of vitamin A and have harmful effects on the liver. Do not take more than 5,000 IUs of vitamin A if you drink regularly.

VITAMIN B₅

ITAMIN B₅ IS FOUND IN ABUNDANCE in many foods—a fact reflected in its other name, pantothenic acid, which comes from the Greek words "pantos" and "thenos," meaning "everywhere." This vitamin is so commonly found in foods that its deficiency in people is rare. Still, vitamin B₅ shouldn't be discounted since it's vital for health, can aid in treatment for various ailments, particularly cardiovascular, and can offer life-saving benefits.

WHAT IT DOES

Vitamin B₅ is converted to pantethine in the body. Many small studies suggest that pantethine can lower triglyceride levels and to a lesser extent can reduce cholesterol levels in the blood. This benefit may be particularly helpful for people who have high levels of triglycerides and for those with type 2 diabetes.

Vitamin B₅ may also help in treating rheumatoid arthritis, help the body to better cope with stress, and perhaps boost athletic performance, although more research is needed to confirm its value in these conditions.

For additional information on specific health conditions and how to treat them with supplements, see Part 3 of this book, beginning on page 309.

HOW IT WORKS

Vitamin B₅ is used by the body to make proteins, including enzymes and other important substances needed for breaking down fats and carbohydrates, and to make hormones, red blood cells, and acetylcholine—an important neurotransmitter that carries signals between nerve cells in the brain. Additionally, vitamin B₅ is believed to have antioxidant, anti-inflammatory, antiviral, and wound-healing properties.

HOW TO TAKE IT

The need for vitamin B₅ increases with age and is greatest for pregnant and nursing women. See the table on page 278 for the recommended daily intakes (RDIs) of vitamin B₅.

FOOD SOURCES

VITAMIN B₅

Vitamin B₅ is available in a variety of foods, making it easy for even the choosiest of eaters to find a healthy source of this important nutrient.

▶Avocados, brewer's yeast, buckwheat, cashews, egg yolks, fish, lean meat, mushrooms, nuts, oatmeal, organ meats (liver, kidney), poultry, red chili peppers, rye flour, soybeans, split peas, sunflower seeds, torula (nutritional) yeast, and whole grains.

AGE/GENDER/ CONDITION	RECOMMENDED DAILY INTAKE (RDI)*
Infants	
0–6 months	1.7 mg
7–12 months	1.8 mg
Children	
1–3 years	2 mg
4–8 years	3 mg
9–13 years	4 mg
Males and Females	
14 years and older	5 mg
Pregnant Women	6 mg
Nursing Women	7 mg

For more information on RDIs, see Want to Know More About Intake? on page 8.

Vitamin B_5 is a part of the B-complex vitamin group (a term given to a group of 8 important B vitamins), and most general-purpose multivitamin/mineral supplements contain the full range of B vitamins (be sure to check the label).

Vitamin B_5 supplements are available as capsules, extended-release capsules, oral liquid, tablets, and extended-release tablets. Vitamin B_5 is often sold as "calcium pantothenate."

If you are seeking to reduce your levels of triglycerides and cholesterol, be aware that you need to take a supplement of pantethine—a metabolic product of vitamin B_5—since regular pantothenic acid does not appear to provide these benefits. The therapeutic dosage of pantethine for lowering cholesterol is 300 milligrams taken three times daily. Be sure to consult your doctor before using these supplements.

LOOK OUT FOR THIS!

Vitamin B_5 (both as pantothenic acid and pantethine) does not appear to cause any significant side effects.

Vitamin B_5 supplements should be used with caution in young children, pregnant or nursing women, or people with severe kidney or liver disease, since maximum safe dosages in these groups have not been set.

WHAT TO AVOID

There are no known interactions of vitamin B$_5$ with drugs or with herbs or other supplements.

VITAMIN B$_6$

LIKE OTHER MEMBERS OF THE VITAMIN B family, vitamin B$_6$—also known as pyroxidine—serves many important functions, including the making of proteins, hormones, and the neurotransmitter substances that carry signals between nerve cells in the brain.

Unfortunately, a mild deficiency of this vitamin is extremely common—a 1990 survey found that 71 percent of men and 90 percent of women had too little vitamin B$_6$ in their diets. Vitamin B$_6$ is also the most commonly deficient water-soluble vitamin in the elderly population.

WHAT IT DOES

Strong evidence indicates that vitamin B$_6$ supplementation can significantly lower the chances of developing heart disease and can reduce the nausea of morning sickness in pregnancy.

Other proposed uses of vitamin B$_6$ include treatment for carpal tunnel syndrome, premenstrual syndrome (PMS), diabetic neuropathy, childhood asthma, gestational diabetes (diabetes that develops during pregnancy), human immunodeficiency virus (HIV), tardive dyskinesia, Parkinson's disease, Alzheimer's disease, and seborrheic dermatitis (when used topically). Vitamin B$_6$ may also reduce the side effects of theophylline (an asthma drug), such as hand tremor.

Additionally, when combined with magnesium, vitamin B$_6$ may be helpful for improving autistic behaviors in children and for reducing oxalate excretion, thereby helping to decrease the risk of kidney stones.

For additional information on specific health conditions and how you can treat them with supplements, see Part 3 of this book, beginning on page 309.

HOW IT WORKS

It is unclear how vitamin B$_6$ reduces the risk of heart disease. It may do so directly, by reducing clot formation and lowering blood pressure, or indirectly, by combining with folic acid and vitamin B_{12} to reduce the level of homocysteine in the blood. (High levels of homocysteine are believed to increase the chances of developing heart disease.)

Vitamin B_6 is needed to make the neurotransmitters serotonin and dopamine, which may explain its potential for treating neurologic conditions such as Alzheimer's and Parkinson's diseases. It is also involved in making prostaglandins, hormone-like fatty acids that help to regulate blood pressure, maintain heart and muscle function, and control pain.

HOW TO TAKE IT

The need for vitamin B_6 increases with age and is greatest for pregnant and nursing women. The table below shows the recommended daily intakes (RDIs) of vitamin B_6, but note that many experts believe these intakes should be increased to achieve optimum benefit.

AGE/GENDER/ CONDITION	RECOMMENDED DAILY INTAKE (RDI)*
Infants	
0–6 months	0.1 mg
7–12 months	0.3 mg
Children	
1–3 years	0.5 mg
4–8 years	0.6 mg
9–13 years	1.0 mg
Males	
14–50 years	1.3 mg
51 years and older	1.7 mg
Females	
14–18 years	1.2 mg
19–50 years	1.3 mg
51 years and older	1.5 mg
Pregnant Women	1.9 mg
Nursing Women	2.0 mg

*For more information on RDIs, see Want to Know More About Intake? on page 8.

Vitamin B$_6$ is a part of the B-complex vitamin group (a term given to a group of 8 important B vitamins), and most general-purpose multivitamin/mineral supplements contain the full range of B vitamins (be sure to check the label).

Vitamin B$_6$ is also available by itself in tablet (including extended-release tablet) and capsule form.

Supplemental vitamin B$_6$ is needed by people who consume a high-protein diet or who have a poor quality diet, as well as by women taking birth control pills, people with alcoholism, and the elderly. It is also needed by people who take certain medications that reduce vitamin B$_6$ levels in the blood (see What to Avoid, below).

LOOK OUT FOR THIS!

Vitamin B$_6$ is generally safe when taken as a supplement in recommended doses. However, very large doses (over 2,000 mg per day) can cause reversible nerve damage in the arms and legs, resulting in loss of sensation, and may worsen acne.

Always avoid taking excessive amounts of vitamin B$_6$. See the table below for the maximum safe daily dosages of vitamin B$_6$.

AGE/GENDER/ CONDITION	MAXIMUM SAFE DOSAGE
Children	
1–3 years	30 mg
4–8 years	40 mg
Males and Females	
9–13 years	60 mg
14–18 years	80 mg
19 years and older	100 mg
Pregnant and Nursing Women	100 mg (80 mg if 18 years or younger)

Note: Maximum safe dosages have not been set for people with severe liver or kidney disease.

WHAT TO AVOID

Medication: Large doses of vitamin B$_6$ (more than 5 milligrams per day) may interfere with the effects of the drug levodopa. Vitamin B$_6$ may also reduce the level of certain medications in the blood,

FOOD SOURCES

VITAMIN B$_6$

Because deficiencies in vitamin B$_6$ are common, eating foods rich in this important nutrient may help to increase your daily intake of it. Read on for foods high in vitamin B$_6$.

▶Avocados, bananas, baked potato (with skin), brewer's yeast, buckwheat flour, fish, garbanzo beans, lentils, lima beans, poultry, soybeans, sunflower seeds, and torula (nutritional) yeast.

including theophylline, isoniazid, penicillamine, hydralazine, and monoamine oxidase (MAO) inhibitors. Antibiotics, estrogen, some cardiac medications, and diuretics may deplete levels of vitamin B_6 in the body.

VITAMIN B$_{12}$

IF YOU'RE A STRICT VEGETARIAN, over age 50, or taking medication that reduces the body's production of stomach acid, you may be among those people who need an extra dose of vitamin B_{12}. This essential nutrient—also called cobalamin because it contains the metal cobalt—comes from the food you eat (primarily from animal products), and is essential for maintaining healthy nerve cells and red blood cells, and for producing deoxyribonucleic acid (DNA), the genetic material in all cells.

WHAT IT DOES

Supplementation with vitamin B_{12} is important for treating a deficiency of this vitamin, which can cause pernicious (persistent) anemia, nerve damage, and brain damage. It may also boost the number of sperm cells in men with abnormal sperm production and, when combined with folic acid, may reduce the risk of cardiovascular disease.

Weak or preliminary evidence suggests a role for vitamin B_{12} in treating Alzheimer's disease, multiple sclerosis, and tinnitus. Preliminary evidence also suggests that vitamin B_{12} may play a role in the treatment of cataracts. Low B_{12} levels have been found in people with recurrent canker sores (aphthous ulcers).

For additional information on specific health conditions and how to treat them with supplements, see Part 3 of this book, beginning on page 309.

HOW IT WORKS

Vitamin B_{12} is attached to proteins in your food. During digestion, stomach acid releases the vitamin so that it can combine with a substance called intrinsic factor, which allows the vitamin to be absorbed and used by the body.

Vitamin B_{12} helps nerve cells to function properly and works with folate (vitamin B_9) to reduce levels of homocysteine in the blood (high levels of homocysteine are believed to increase the chances of developing heart disease and stroke). Vitamin B$_{12}$ is also involved in the body's production of DNA and S-adenosylmethionine (SAMe; see page 247).

HOW TO TAKE IT

The recommended daily intake (RDI) of vitamin B$_{12}$ increases with age. It is highest among pregnant and nursing women. See the table below for the RDIs for vitamin B$_6$.

AGE/GENDER/ CONDITION	RECOMMENDED DAILY INTAKE (RDI)*
Infants	
0–6 months	0.4 mcg
7–12 months	0.5 mcg
Children	
1–3 years	0.9 mcg
4–8 years	1.2 mcg
9–13 years	1.8 mcg
Males and Females	
14 years and older	2.4 mcg
Pregnant Women	2.6 mcg
Nursing Women	2.8 mcg

For more information on RDIs, see Want to Know More About Intake? on page 8.

Vitamin B$_{12}$ is a part of the B-complex vitamin group (a term given to a group of eight important B vitamins), and most general purpose multivitamin/mineral supplements contain the full range of B vitamins (be sure to check the label).

Vitamin B$_{12}$ supplementation is recommended for strict vegetarians (vegans, who do not eat meat, fish, eggs, milk, or milk products), elderly people with reduced absorption of this vitamin, and people who have had stomach surgery or other digestive conditions that can cause a vitamin B$_{12}$ deficiency. Supplementation is also recommended for people who take certain medications that may interfere with the absorption of vitamin B$_{12}$ or reduce its blood levels (see What to Avoid, on page 284).

FOOD SOURCES

VITAMIN B$_{12}$

While vitamin B$_{12}$ is found naturally in high quantities in many foods, no plant sources provide people with a safe and healthy dose of this important vitamin, which is why vitamin B$_{12}$ supplementation is especially important for vegetarians. Read on for some good food sources of vitamin B$_{12}$.

▶Beef, beef kidney, brewer's yeast, cheese, calf and chicken liver, clams, eggs, lamb, liver, salmon, sardines, trout, tuna, and whey.

FRIENDS AND FOES

If you take the diabetes medication metformin (Glucophage), vitamin C may help improve the absorption of vitamin B_{12} when the two vitamins are taken together.

Vitamin B_{12} supplements are available in three forms—cyanocobalamin, hydrocobalamin, and methylcobalamin. Although the first is the most widely available and least expensive of the three, the latter two forms may be more effective.

It can be beneficial to take vitamin B_{12} with other B vitamins since they usually work most effectively when taken together.

LOOK OUT FOR THIS!

Vitamin B_{12} is a safe supplement, and no adverse health effects have been reported even when too much is taken. High doses may, however, worsen acne.

WHAT TO AVOID

Medication: Medicines that reduce stomach acid, and colchicine, metformin and phenformin, zidovudine, and nitrous oxide may reduce the body's ability to absorb vitamin B_{12}. Antibiotics, hormone replacement therapy (HRT), oral contraceptives, histamine blockers, some cholesterol-lowering medication and oral hypoglycemic agents, antiseizure medications, and some HIV medications may deplete levels of vitamin B_{12}.

Herbs and Dietary Supplements: Slow-release potassium supplements may reduce the body's ability to absorb vitamin B_{12}.

VITAMIN C

VITAMIN C, ALSO CALLED ASCORBIC ACID, is the most popular dietary supplement in the world, taken by more people than any other vitamin, mineral, or herbal product. Two-time Nobel Prize winning biochemist Linus Pauling spent a great deal of his life researching the benefits of vitamin C. He believed that a deficiency of this vitamin was a main cause of cardiovascular disease and that it could cure a variety of ailments ranging from the common cold to cancer. While the health benefits of vitamin C are still somewhat controversial, many people swear by their daily dose of this water-soluble vitamin, which performs a range of functions in the body from manufacturing collagen to being a powerful antioxidant.

WHAT IT DOES

Vitamin C is a general term used to describe substances containing two compounds: L-ascorbic acid (also known simply as ascorbic acid), which is the dietary form of vitamin C, and L-dehydroascorbic acid, which is the oxidation product of ascorbic acid.

Vitamin C is probably best known as a defense against the common cold. A number of studies have shown that while vitamin C may not prevent colds, taking vitamin C on a regular basis reduces the duration of colds when they do occur, as well as easing the symptoms that accompany colds. Thus, in most cases, taking vitamin C when a cold starts will probably not work as effectively as taking the vitamin on a regular basis. However, studies do show that people who have a deficiency of vitamin C, as well as those who experience exercise-endurance-related colds, may benefit from taking vitamin C preventively.

Vitamin C may be one of the most powerful water-soluble antioxidants in living nature and can protect the body from the cell and tissue damage caused by free radical molecules. It works together with various enzymes in the manufacture of collagen, an important protein in connective tissue such as tendons and ligaments, as well as in skin, scar tissue, and blood vessels. This is why vitamin C is often recommended to help treat wounds and is a main ingredient in many skin-care products and supplements. Early research suggests that creams containing vitamin C may help improve the overall quality of aging skin and reduce skin damage caused by the sun. And for people who tend to bruise easily—especially those with a deficiency of this nutrient—vitamin C may reduce the tendency to bruise. Because of its role in producing the connective tissue for tendons and ligaments, vitamin C is also recommended for conditions that damage these structures, such as bursitis and tendonitis.

Vitamin C may also help prevent the buildup of atherosclerotic plaque in the arteries. People with low levels of vitamin C may be at greater risk for heart attack, stroke, and peripheral artery disease. When taken in conjunction with vitamin E, vitamin C may keep LDL ("bad") cholesterol from oxidizing, although research indicates that vitamin C may also have this same effect when taken alone. Some studies have suggested that vitamin C may also reduce blood levels of total cholesterol, although this requires more research.

Vitamin C is widely hailed as a treatment for cancer, but this is highly controversial. While some studies show that some people with cancer may benefit from high doses of vitamin C (for example 10,000 milligrams daily) in terms of surviving for longer periods, other studies do not find any benefits of this vitamin in cancer patients. Some population-based studies have shown that people who

FOOD SOURCES

VITAMIN C

While animals can synthesize their own vitamin C, the human body cannot make or store vitamin C on its own, for which reason it is important to eat foods that contain plenty of this vitamin and to take vitamin C supplements as well. Although vitamin C may be synonymous with citrus-derived products, it can be found in more food sources than orange juice. Because vitamin C is sensitive to light, heat, and air, its health benefits are strongest when it is consumed in fruits and vegetables that are eaten raw or lightly cooked. Read on for the best food sources of vitamin C.

▶ Broccoli, brussels sprouts, cantaloupe, citrus fruits, collard greens, guava, kiwi, kale, parsley, red chili peppers, red and green bell peppers, strawberries (and other red berries), tomatoes, and turnip greens.

eat foods rich in vitamin C are less likely to develop cancer. Further research is needed to ascertain the connection between vitamin C and cancer prevention and treatment.

Small studies have shown that vitamin C may have a modest blood pressure–lowering effect. One double-blind study conducted of people taking hypertension medication showed that they had a 10 percent reduction in blood pressure when they were also given vitamin C. Other population-based studies have shown that people who consume a diet rich in antioxidants, including vitamin C, are less prone to develop high blood pressure than those who do not have such a diet.

A number of studies show that people taking nitrate drugs (often prescribed for angina) may benefit from vitamin C supplementation, since this has been found to increase the effectiveness of nitrate medications over time when it would otherwise tend to diminish. Vitamin C may also aid the body in its detoxification of heavy metals, including mercury, lead, cadmium, and nickel.

Vitamin C also has numerous other potential uses, including the prevention of cataracts, glaucoma, cervical dysplasia, pre-eclampsia, gum disease, gallstones, and Alzheimer's disease, and the prevention and treatment of constipation, sexual dysfunction, infertility, herpes simplex, human immunodeficiency virus (HIV), lupus, and of asthma and allergy symptoms; however, further research is needed to verify its benefit for these uses.

For additional information on specific health conditions and how to treat them with supplements, see Part 3 of this book, beginning on page 309.

HOW IT WORKS

Vitamin C protects fat-soluble vitamins (such as vitamins A and E) from oxidation. It also strengthens connective tissue by producing collagen. Vitamin C works within the cells to provide hydrogen and oxygen to the amino acids lysine and proline—a process that helps to form procollagen, a substance that is later turned into collagen. As an antioxidant, vitamin C "rounds up" and destroys free radicals before they have a chance to harm the body. Vitamin C may also reduce the effect of many heavy metals (such as lead) in the body, perhaps by stimulating enzymes in the liver that aid in detoxifying these metals.

In terms of cardiovascular health, vitamin C not only protects tissues from cell- and tissue-damaging free radical molecules but also helps the body metabolize fat. As noted earlier, vitamin C may also prevent the buildup of plaque in blood vessels by curbing LDL ("bad") cholesterol. In addition, vitamin C may combat plaque build-up by preventing platelets from gathering on blood vessel walls and forming blood clots.

HOW TO TAKE IT

See the table below for the recommended daily intakes (RDIs) of vitamin C.

Note: Smokers in all of the groups in this table should increase their intake of vitamin C by a minimum of 35 milligrams, since smoking depletes the body of vitamin C.

AGE/GENDER/ CONDITION	RECOMMENDED DAILY INTAKE (RDI)*
Infants	
0–6 months	40 mg
7–12 months	50 mg
Children	
1–3 years	15 mg
4–8 years	25 mg
9–13 years	45 mg
Males	
14–18 years	75 mg
19 years and older	90 mg
Females	
14–18 years	65 mg
19 years and older	75 mg
Pregnant Women	85 mg
Nursing Women	120 mg

For more information on RDIs, see Want to Know More About Intake? on page 8.

Researchers have studied this vitamin very thoroughly and it is well established that higher dosages can be beneficial. An expert panel recently called for increasing the recommended daily allowance (RDA) for vitamin C as a result of current scientific research. The

National Institutes of Health (NIH) recommends a dosage of 100 to 200 milligrams daily of vitamin C for healthy adults.

Note: Vitamin C should be taken in several small doses throughout the day in order to achieve optimal absorption.

While scurvy—a condition caused by vitamin C deficiency and characterized by weakness, anemia, bruising, bleeding gums, and loose teeth—is extremely rare in the developed world, studies indicate that about 40 percent of Americans have slight vitamin C deficiencies.

Vitamin C is commercially available in a number of forms, including tablets and capsules, and in chewable form. It also comes in powdered crystalline, effervescent (which is a combination of ascorbic acid and sodium bicarbonate), and liquid forms. Note that because of its high acid content, chewable vitamin C can erode tooth enamel.

Vitamin C seems to come in so many forms—how do I distinguish between various products?

You may see a variety of vitamin C combination products on the shelf at your local pharmacy or health food store. Since all of these forms are good sources of vitamin C, you can choose a product that best suits your particular preferences. Read on for a guide to help clear up some of the confusion.

Vitamin C with Bioflavonoids: Vitamin C is often sold with bioflavonoids, which are antioxidant compounds derived from the rinds and pulp of lemons, oranges, and grapefruit. Flavonoids enhance the action of vitamin C and improve the body's absorption of this important nutrient. The best blend of vitamin C should have a 1:1 ratio of vitamin to flavonoids (for example, 100 milligrams of vitamin C to 100 milligrams of bioflavonoids).

Acerola Vitamin C: This form of vitamin C is derived from the acerola fruit, one of the richest sources of vitamin C. Acerola also contains flavonoids and other vitamins, including thiamine, riboflavin, niacin, pantothenic acid, and beta carotene, and minerals such as magnesium and potassium.

Vitamin C with Rose Hips: Rose hips are the fruit of the rose, which remains on the bush after the petals of the flower have fallen off. They have a high content of vitamin C, and rose hips from one species, *Rosa rugosa,* have the highest content of vitamin C of any natural source in the world! Aside from their vitamin C content, rose hips contain various carotenoids, flavonoids, catechins, polyphenols, and pectins.

Reduced-Acidity Vitamin C: This buffered form of vitamin C is a combination of ascorbic acid (50 percent) and sodium ascorbate, and is often recommended for people who have sensitive stomachs or ulcers.

Ascorbate and Vitamin C Metabolites: Perhaps the best-known member of this category is Ester-C, a readily absorbed chemical derivative of vitamin C. Metabolites are compounds produced by the body from nutrients, but which can also be created synthetically. Research shows that several vitamin C metabolites are well absorbed and retained in the body.

If regular ascorbic acid upsets your stomach, you can get vitamin C in buffered form, which is usually better tolerated.

LOOK OUT FOR THIS!

Vitamin C is generally considered safe, even at relatively high doses, since most of any excess taken as a supplement is excreted through the urine. Extremely high doses can occasionally lead to stomach cramps, nausea, and diarrhea.

Vitamin C increases the amount of iron absorbed from food. People with hemochromatosis, a condition marked by excess iron in the body's tissues, should consult their doctor before taking vitamin C.

WHAT TO AVOID

Medication: Consult your doctor before taking vitamin C with warfarin.

VITAMIN D

FOR YEARS, THE MANTRA OF SKIN and cancer doctors has been to avoid unnecessary exposure to the harmful rays of the sun. Yet even though we get most of the vitamin D we need from the food we eat, regular exposure to the sun helps our bodies supplement that by making their own vitamin D from its precursor substances consumed in foods. Vitamin D is essential for developing and maintaining healthy bones, preventing osteoporosis, and keeping the immune and nervous systems functioning normally. Without enough vitamin D, we are vulnerable to the childhood disease known as rickets and the adult disease called osteomalacia, both of which produce weakened bones.

WHAT IT DOES

The main job of vitamin D is to maintain healthy levels of calcium and phosphorus in the blood. Vitamin D promotes both the absorption of calcium from the intestines into the blood and the removal of calcium from the bones into the blood in order to balance the body's content of this vital mineral. Vitamin D also reduces the loss of calcium that takes place during urination. When taken in combination with calcium, it can slow bone loss and reduce the number of bone fractures. As a result, vitamin D—along with calcium—is an important vitamin for preventing osteoporosis.

Preliminary research suggests that vitamin D may help prevent various forms of cancer, including breast, prostate, and colon cancers.

Research also suggests that when combined with calcium, vitamin D may help strengthen teeth and prevent tooth loss. In addition to this, maintaining adequate levels of vitamin D may help prevent cataracts, and vitamin D may act to prevent osteoarthritis, multiple sclerosis, and seasonal affective disorder (SAD), although more research is needed to support these actions of the vitamin.

HOW IT WORKS

Vitamin D is a fat-soluble vitamin that the body makes in the skin as a result of exposure to sunlight. Here's how it works: Ultraviolet rays convert a precursor of vitamin D into an inactive form of vitamin D. This inactive form is then converted to the active form of vitamin D in the liver and kidneys.

Vitamin D functions as both a hormone and a vitamin—it is a vitamin because it's essential for the absorption of calcium, and its active form functions as a hormone in promoting the absorption of calcium and phosphorus from the intestine.

HOW TO TAKE IT

See the table below for the recommended daily intakes (RDIs) for vitamin D.

AGE/GENDER/ CONDITION	RECOMMENDED DAILY INTAKE (RDI)*
Infants	
0–12 months	200 IU (5 mcg)
Males and Females	
1–50 years	200 IU (5 mcg)
51–70 years	400 IU (10 mcg)
71 years and over	600 IU (15 mcg)
Pregnant Women	200 IU (5 mcg)
Nursing Women	200 IU (5 mcg)

For more information on RDIs, see Want to Know More About Intake? on page 8.

Vitamin D is a standard ingredient in most multivitamins. It can also be found as softgel capsules, tablets, and liquids.

Healthy, young people who are often outdoors in sunlight (for about 15 minutes a day) do not need vitamin D supplements. That's not the case for people living in northern climates where little or no vitamin synthesis takes place during the winter months. This also holds true for people who don't drink milk, who have dark skin, who live in a cloudy climate, or who rarely go outside.

The elderly should also consider taking vitamin D supplements, since the skin loses its ability to synthesize vitamin D with age.

Keep in mind that sunscreen can reduce the skin's ability to produce vitamin D, so if you regularly slather it on, you may not be getting all the vitamin D you need.

People with epilepsy, heart or blood vessel disease, chronic diarrhea, any disease of the kidney, liver, or pancreas, intestinal problems, sarcoidosis, or high blood calcium or phosphorus levels should consult their doctor before taking vitamin D.

LOOK OUT FOR THIS!

Because vitamin D is stored in the body, it can potentially reach toxic levels if taken in high doses for a long time. The symptoms of too much vitamin D include nausea, diarrhea or constipation, skin rash, headaches, excessive thirst, metallic taste, poor appetite, weight loss, bone pain, fatigue, sore eyes, itchy skin, headache, vomiting, excessive urination, kidney stones or kidney damage, high blood pressure, and muscle problems.

Note: It's impossible to get too much vitamin D from the sun, since the body regulates this form of the vitamin's production.

FOOD SOURCES

VITAMIN D

Looking to get a healthy dose of vitamin D? Although very few foods naturally contain this important vitamin (the best source being coldwater fish), many foods are fortified with vitamin D. And don't forget to get some sunlight! Remember, ultraviolet rays from the sun trigger vitamin D synthesis in the skin. Try spending 5 to 15 minutes (depending on your skin type—people with darker skin can tolerate longer sun exposure) in the sun before you apply sunscreen. Read on for healthy ways to eat your vitamin D!

▶ Beef, butter, cheese, cod-liver oil, cream, egg yolks, fish liver oils, fortified milk, liver, mackerel, oysters, salmon, and sardines.

Treating SAD with Vitamin D

Did You Know?

Seasonal affective disorder (SAD) is a type of depression that occurs during the winter months. It is caused by a biochemical imbalance in the hypothalamus that results from the short daylight hours and lack of sunlight during winter. People with SAD often have sleep problems, lethargy, overeating, depression, social problems, anxiety, lack of libido, and mood swings.

Although people with SAD are often helped by light therapy, some studies suggest that they also improve when they take vitamin D supplements. Consult your doctor to see whether vitamin D supplementation is right for you.

WHAT TO AVOID

Medication: People who are taking estrogen, isoniazid (a medication to treat tuberculosis), or thiazide (a diuretic) may be getting vitamin D from the effects of these medications and should consult a doctor before taking supplemental vitamin D. People taking antacids, calcium channel blockers, cholestyramine, anticonvulsant medications, or mineral oil may be getting too little vitamin D and may need to take additional supplements of this vitamin. Vitamin D may intensify the effects of the cancer-treatment drug doxorubicin. People taking digoxin or weight-loss products should consult their doctor before taking vitamin D. Antiseizure medicines, oral steroids, ulcer medications, and antituberculosis medications may deplete the body's store of vitamin D.

VITAMIN E

VITAMIN E IS ONE OF THE BODY'S main defenses against the condition called "oxidative stress"—the ongoing assault by cell- and tissue-damaging free radical molecules that our cells undergo every day. Vitamin E is also a fat-soluble vitamin, which means that the body absorbs it along with the fatty components of food. Because of this fat solubility, it makes sense that most of the vitamin E in our diet can be found in high-fat foods such as oils and spreads, nuts, and seeds.

WHAT IT DOES

Vitamin E is actually a family of related compounds called tocopherols and tocotrienols. As an antioxidant, it helps block the damage caused by cell- and tissue-damaging free radical molecules and may prevent heart disease, cancers, and other diseases. Vitamin E may be especially useful for reducing the free radical damage to blood and tissues caused by strenuous exercise and may decrease the occurrence of exercise-induced muscle damage. It also boosts the immune system, protects red blood cells, and plays an important role in reproduction.

Although the ability of vitamin E to reduce the risk of cancer is not substantiated, studies have shown that people with cancer often have lower levels of vitamin E in their bodies. Moreover, a large study suggested that diets rich in antioxidants, including vitamin E, may be linked to a reduced risk of some cancers, such as colon, breast, prostate, rectal, cervical, pancreatic, oral, liver, and lung cancers.

Additionally, vitamin E may help prevent cataracts and protect vision in people with macular degeneration.

Preliminary research suggests that vitamin E may prevent breast pain, a symptoms often seen in women with premenstrual syndrome (PMS).

Some research indicates that vitamin E may slow the progression of Parkinson's and Alzheimer's diseases and enhance immunity in elderly people. However, studies have given mixed results for these effects, and more research is needed to support them.

People with rheumatoid arthritis are often more susceptible than healthy people to cell and tissue damage by free-radical molecules. As a result, supplementation with vitamin E may help reduce this damage in addition to reducing the pain associated with rheumatoid arthritis. Supplementation with vitamin E may also be useful in people with hypo- and hyperthyroidism, who are also more susceptible to free radical damage.

As a liquid applied to the skin, vitamin E oil can moisturize dry, chapped skin. However, its reputation as an aid to healing scars may be undeserved. One recent study of the effectiveness of vitamin E in improving surgical scars found that compared to an antibiotic ointment, it had no added benefit. However, vitamin E oil may help heal inflamed gums when applied topically to the skin and may also be useful in relieving eruptions of herpes simplex virus and shingles.

Among the other conditions for which vitamin E may be helpful are asthma, hypertension, poor circulation, high cholesterol, diabetes, restless legs syndrome, gallstones, and gout. More research is needed to ascertain the benefits of vitamin E in a number of chronic health conditions.

For additional information on specific health conditions and how to treat them with supplements, see Part 3 of this book, beginning on page 309.

HOW IT WORKS

As an antioxidant, vitamin E binds to free radicals, turning the hostile compounds into harmless substances.

Vitamin E reduces the risk of cardiovascular disease in two ways. The first is by attaching directly to low-density lipoprotein (LDL) cholesterol—the "bad" cholesterol that circulates in the blood—and helping to prevent it from forming obstructions that block the arteries and cause heart attacks and strokes. The second way in which vitamin

E reduces the risk of cardiovascular disease is by thinning the blood and thereby allowing it to flow more easily through the arteries.

HOW TO TAKE IT

See the table below for the recommended daily intakes (RDIs) of vitamin E. Vitamin E dosages are often measured in international units (IUs). In order to convert milligrams of vitamin E to IUs, you must first determine whether the vitamin E you are taking is natural or synthetic. One IU of natural vitamin E is equal to 0.67 milligrams of alpha-tocopherol. One synthetic IU of vitamin E is equal to 0.45 milligrams of alpha-tocopherol. For example, if you want to meet the 15-milligram RDI of vitamin E, you would take 22 IU of natural vitamin E or 33 IU of synthetic vitamin E.

AGE/GENDER/ CONDITION	RECOMMENDED DAILY INTAKE (RDI)*
Infants	
0–6 months	4 mg
7–12 months	5 mg
Children	
1–3 years	6 mg
4–8 years	7 mg
9–13 years	11 mg
Males and Females	
14 years and older	15 mg
Pregnant Women	15 mg
Nursing Women	19 mg

For more information on RDIs, see Want to Know More About Intake? on page 8.

As a supplement, vitamin E is available in softgels, tablets and capsules, and topical oils. It comes in both natural and synthetic forms—the natural form, d-alpha tocopherol, is preferred because it is absorbed and retained in the body better than the synthetic form, dl-alpha tocopherol. Ideally, vitamin E should be taken with selenium, another important antioxidant.

Vitamin E is also sold as a topical oil. It should not be exposed to direct sunlight, which can destroy it, and with time, the oil can turn rancid.

Vitamin E deficiency is rare, but it can occur is certain situations. Premature or low-birth-weight infants, people with a rare disorder in which the body cannot properly metabolize fat, people with cystic fibrosis, and those with malabsorption problems such as Crohn's disease may be at an increased risk for having a vitamin E deficiency. Signs of vitamin E deficiency include dry skin, eczema, dull dry hair, easy bruising, poor wound healing, hot flashes, and muscle weakness.

LOOK OUT FOR THIS!

Low-dose vitamin E supplements are generally considered safe, with few side effects. One exception is in people with bleeding disorders, or people about to undergo surgery or labor and delivery, since vitamin E may contribute to blood thinning and thus increase the risk of abnormal bleeding. Recently published reports suggest that a daily dose of vitamin E greater than 400 IU might be harmful. Therefore, it's best not to exceed this dosage.

Also, there is some indication that a prolonged diet rich in fish oil may create a deficiency of vitamin E. People whose diet contains a lot of fish or who take fish oil supplements may therefore also want to take vitamin E.

WHAT TO AVOID

Medication: Vitamin E may increase the blood-thinning effects of certain medications such as warfarin, heparin, clopidogrel, ticlopidine, pentoxifylline, and aspirin. When taken in high doses, vitamin E may also affect insulin levels in people taking oral hypoglycemic medications. Cholesterol-lowering medications may deplete the body's levels of vitamin E. If you are taking any of these medications, consult your doctor before taking vitamin E.

VITAMIN K

VITAMIN K, ALSO KNOWN AS phytonadione, is the least known member of the vitamin family but is absolutely necessary for normal blood clotting. In fact, the "K" in the name of this vitamin comes from the German word "koagulation," meaning "clotting" (see Supplemental Trivia, page 297). Vitamin K also plays an important role in maintaining healthy bones. While we get most of the vitamin K we need from our diets, a certain amount of this nutrient is produced by bacteria in our intestines.

WHAT IT DOES

Vitamin K is often recommended for elderly people with low bone density and a high risk of osteoporosis. Studies show that people with osteoporosis often have low levels of vitamin K and that a higher intake of this vitamin may reduce the risk of developing this condition. Other research indicates that vitamin K helps the body to incorporate calcium into bones and decreases the amount of calcium lost in urine.

Some research shows that vitamin K supplements can increase bone formation and slow the loss of bone mass in postmenopausal women. Special, prescribed forms of vitamin K are often used to counter the effects of blood-thinning drugs like warfarin (Coumadin). Vitamin K deficiency in newborn babies can lead to bleeding problems, which is why newborns are often given injections of vitamin K. One curious study performed in China and Italy found that injecting vitamin K into certain acupuncture points was a useful treatment for severely painful menses.

For additional information on specific health conditions and how to treat them with supplements, see Part 3 of this book, beginning on page 309.

HOW IT WORKS

Vitamin K is needed for the proper function of certain proteins (such as osteocalcin and matrix G1a) in bone. It also plays a key role in the synthesis of prothrombin, the precursor to thrombin, a substance integral to healthy blood clotting.

HOW TO TAKE IT

See the table below for the recommended daily intakes (RDIs) of vitamin K.

AGE/GENDER/ CONDITION	RECOMMENDED DAILY INTAKE (RDI)*
Infants	
0–6 months	2 mcg
7–12 months	2.5 mcg

AGE/GENDER CONDITION	RECOMMENDED DAILY INTAKE (RDI)*
Children	
1–3 years	30 mcg
4–8 years	55 mcg
9–13 years	60 mcg
14–18 years	75 mcg
Males	
19 years and older	120 mcg
Females	
14–18 years	400 mg
19 years and older	425 mg
Pregnant Women	450 mg
Nursing Women	550 mg

For more information on RDIs, see Want to Know More About Intake? on page 8.

Although vitamin K plays a critical role in both blood clotting and bone metabolism, the body requires only a very small amount of this vitamin. Vitamin K is available as an isolated supplement without a prescription in dosages of up to 100 micrograms. Dosages above 100 micrograms require a prescription from a doctor. Small amounts of vitamin K are often included in multivitamin complexes, bone-health formulas, and calcium supplements.

Vitamin K is available over the counter in tablet form and by prescription in tablet and injection forms.

There are three main types of vitamin K:

- Vitamin K_1 (also called phylloquinone) is the main source of this vitamin in plants (see Food Sources, on page 298).
- Vitamin K_2 (also called menaquinone) is produced by bacteria in the intestinal tract.
- Vitamin K_3 (also called menaphthone or menadione) is a synthetic form of vitamin K that can be converted to vitamin K_2 by the body.

Note: Since vitamin K is fat soluble, it is best absorbed in the body if taken with a fatty food. For instance, someone eating spinach might want to put salad dressing on it for maximum absorption of the vitamin K in the spinach.

Deficiency of vitamin K is rare. Vitamin K supplementation may be recommended for pregnant and premenopausal women, children born to women taking anticonvulsant medication during pregnancy and other people taking such medication, people taking long-term antibiotic therapy, and people with digestive disorders such as diarrhea, celiac sprue, ulcerative colitis, or Crohn's disease.

Note that certain antibiotics may destroy the beneficial bacteria in the intestinal tract that produce vitamin K. Individuals taking antibiotics, sedatives, or cholestyramine may want to increase their intake of foods with vitamin K.

LOOK OUT FOR THIS!

Vitamin K is considered safe when taken at recommended dosages. People with liver or kidney disease should consult their doctor before taking vitamin K.

WHAT TO AVOID

Medication: People taking warfarin should not take vitamin K supplements or eat foods rich in vitamin K without the approval and supervision of a doctor and may need to have specific dosages. Many antibiotic, sedative, and cholestyramine resin-type drugs reduce the body's levels of vitamin K.

Herbs and Dietary Supplements: High doses of vitamin A or vitamin E may decrease the body's ability to absorb vitamin K.

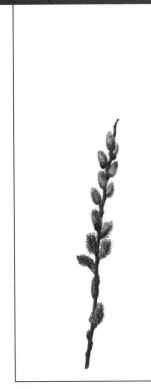

WILLOW BARK

NATIVE AMERICANS WERE FAMILIAR with the medicinal benefits of white willow tree *(Salix alba)* bark, which they steeped in water and drank as a tea. But the use of different species of willows (including black willow, pussy willow, purple willow, weeping willow, European willow, and crack willow), which have similar benefits, dates back to ancient Greece, when people would chew on the bark to alleviate pain and reduce fever and inflammation.

In the early 19th century, scientists discovered a substance in willow bark, called salicin, which they purified to create salicylic acid. Years later, chemists modified salicylic acid to create acetylsalicylic acid, which is commonly known as aspirin.

WHAT IT DOES

Willow bark is a natural and effective alternative to aspirin. Aside from alleviating headaches and other aches and pains, as well as reducing fever, willow bark has been found effective in reducing back pain and the pain of osteoarthritis and may be useful in alleviating the pain associated with bursitis, tension and migraine headaches, rheumatoid arthritis, and tendinitis.

One study comparing the effectiveness of a willow bark extract to the pharmaceutical medication rofecoxib (Vioxx)—a medication used to treat osteoarthritis, rheumatoid arthritis, and acute pain—found that the herb and the prescription drug were equally effective and that their side effects were similar. However, willow bark was 40 percent less expensive than rofecoxib.

For additional information on specific health conditions and how to treat them with supplements, see Part 3 of this book, beginning on page 309.

HOW IT WORKS

The active ingredient in willow bark is salicin, a compound that the body converts into salicylic acid, a powerful pain reliever and anti-inflammatory agent.

It is interesting to note that the body also converts the synthetic compound acetylsalicylic acid (aspirin) to salicylic acid. However, the recommended dose of willow bark contains much less salicylic acid than the recommended dose of aspirin. Researchers have thus speculated that willow bark may contain other, yet-unknown compounds that add to its therapeutic effects.

Other components in willow bark have antioxidant, fever reducing, antiseptic, antibiotic, and immune-boosting properties.

HOW TO TAKE IT

Willow bark is commercially available in the form of tablets, dried or powdered herb, tincture, or tea leaves. Willow is milder than its synthetic cousin aspirin, and research indicates that an extract that provides 120 to 240 milligrams of salicin a day is equivalent to 50 milligrams of aspirin daily.

LOOK OUT FOR THIS!

Willow bark is generally considered safe, with few side effects. Prolonged high doses of willow bark can cause the same side effects as

FRIENDS AND FOES

Studies indicate that people taking willow bark may combine it with devil's claw or evening primrose oil for an increased anti-inflammatory effect.

aspirin, including gastrointestinal problems such as ulcers, nausea, and diarrhea. In general, however, the body can tolerate willow bark better than aspirin.

Although willow bark can increase the risk of bleeding, studies have found that the blood-thinning effect of willow bark is substantially weaker than that of acetylsalicylate (aspirin).

People with asthma, diabetes, gout, gastritis, hemophilia, or stomach ulcers should consult a doctor before taking willow bark. People who are sensitive or allergic to salicylates should not take willow bark or aspirin since they are converted to salicylic acid in the body. Serious allergic reactions to willow bark have occurred in people allergic to aspirin.

Pregnant or nursing women should not take willow bark. Consult your doctor before giving willow bark to young children.

WHAT TO AVOID

Medication: Consult your doctor before taking willow bark with aspirin, blood-thinning agents such as warfarin, anticoagulants or antiplatelet medications, other anti-inflammatory agents, sulfonamide drugs, methotrexate, metoclopramide, phenytoin, pro-benecid, spironolactone and other potassium-sparing diuretics, and valproate.

XYLITOL

A LOW-CALORIE SWEETENER that can actually prevent cavities may seem too good to be true, but xylitol can do just that. A natural sugar found in plants and fruits, xylitol was approved by the U.S. Food and Drug Administration (FDA) as a food sweetener in 1986. Since then it has been used in sugar-free gums, candies, toothpastes, and mouthwashes, providing the same sweetening power as sugar but with one-third fewer calories.

WHAT IT DOES

Several double-blind, placebo-controlled studies have confirmed that xylitol gum, toothpaste, and candy can significantly reduce the development of cavities. In one study of 1,677 children, those using a toothpaste containing 10 percent xylitol over a 3-year period had substantially fewer cavities than children using a standard toothpaste containing fluoride. Another study found that xylitol improved the dental health of a group of frail elderly people in nursing homes.

Xylitol may also reduce the acid damage on the teeth of people with bulimia—a common effect of this eating disorder. Additionally, preliminary research suggests that xylitol may be useful in preventing gum disease, although proof of this requires more research.

Other studies indicate that xylitol may prevent middle ear infections (also called otitis media). But it should be kept in mind that xylitol won't stop such infections once they have started and needs to be taken in fairly high doses to prevent ear infections.

For additional information on specific health conditions and how you can treat them with supplements, see Part 3 of this book, beginning on page 309.

HOW IT WORKS

It is believed that xylitol helps to prevent cavities by stopping the growth of *Streptococcus mutans*, a species of bacteria that causes cavities by interfering with the ability of these bacteria to adhere to the teeth.

Xylitol's action on other bacteria—including *Streptococcus pneumoniae*, which cause ear infections—may explain its ability to stop middle ear infections.

HOW TO TAKE IT

Xylitol is available as a gum, candy, toothpaste, and mouthwash. It also comes in a concentrated syrup form.

Dosages vary according to the specific condition for which it is being used and range from 4 to 10 grams daily. Be sure to read individual product labels for dosage information and consult your doctor regarding your specific condition.

LOOK OUT FOR THIS!

Xylitol appears to be safe when used at its recommended dosage of 4 to 10 grams daily. When taken at higher doses (more than 30 grams per day) it may cause stomach upset and diarrhea. These side effects occur more often in children taking xylitol syrup, which has a higher concentration of xylitol.

WHAT TO AVOID

Xylitol does not appear to interact with other drugs, herbs, or supplements.

YOHIMBE

AN EXTREMELY POPULAR COMMERCIAL supplement in the United States, an extract of the bark of the yohimbe tree *(Pausinystalia yohimbe)* is promoted as a remedy for one of the most distressing human problems—sexual dysfunction. Because of its reputation for this purpose, yohimbe has earned the nickname "herbal Viagra."

The yohimbe tree is an evergreen tree native to West Africa, where indigenous people have used its bark for many years as a stimulant and aphrodisiac. In traditional African medicine, yohimbe is also considered a remedy for high blood pressure and angina and is smoked as a mild hallucinogenic agent. Some people claim that yohimbe also enhances athletic performance by increasing muscle mass, promoting weight loss, and boosting energy.

WHAT IT DOES

The active component in yohimbe—called yohimbine—is sold as a prescription drug in the United States to treat male impotence. Laboratory studies have demonstrated the effectiveness of yohimbine in dilating blood vessels and increasing blood flow to the genital organs.

Some herbalists believe that yohimbe is more effective than its prescription component yohimbine, perhaps because the whole herb contains active ingredients that are still unknown. However, yohimbe bark extract often contains only low concentrations of yohimbine; one study of 26 commercial yohimbe products found that most contained almost no yohimbine.

The German Commission E (see page 16) lists the treatment of sexual disorders as an unofficial use of yohimbe, but because the claims made for it in this application have not been substantially backed by scientific research, it is categorized as an unapproved herb for this purpose. Many experts believe that the benefits of yohimbe do not outweigh its risks (see Look Out for This! page 303).

While yohimbe has also been used to increase female libido and to ease dryness of the mouth, scientific studies do not support these uses. In fact, most of the claims associated with yohimbe are not conclusively supported.

For additional information on specific health conditions and how you can treat them with supplements, see Part 3 of this book, beginning on page 309.

HOW IT WORKS

Yohimbine, the active ingredient in yohimbe, is the same agent found in a South African herb called quebracho. Besides dilating blood vessels, yohimbine blocks a specific type of neurotransmitter receptor in the sympathetic nervous system, and scientific studies suggest that yohimbine also works as a monoamine oxidase (MAO) inhibitor to stimulate levels of the neurotransmitter norepinephrine in the brain—which can make it effective in treating mild depression. However, St. John's wort is considered safer and more effective than yohimbe for alleviating depression.

HOW TO TAKE IT

Caution: Yohimbe should be used only under a doctor's supervision.

Yohimbe can be taken as a tea or in tablet, capsule, or liquid form. Dosages of yohimbe range from 15 to 30 milligrams of a standardized extract daily.

A problem in taking yohimbe is that most commercial yohimbe bark extracts do not state their yohimbine alkaloid content. The pharmaceutical drug yohimbine is the only form of yohimbe that states exactly how much yohimbine it contains.

Herbal products that do not list their content of yohimbine are not recommended.

LOOK OUT FOR THIS!

Yohimbe has been linked to numerous adverse side effects, including dizziness, headaches, loss of coordination, hallucinations, irritability, anxiety and tension, high blood pressure, increased heart rate, heart palpitations, skin flushing, piloeretion (in which the hairs of the body stand up), painful urination, genital pain, reduced appetite, agitation, tremors, and insomnia.

Yohimbe should not be taken by pregnant or nursing women, people with kidney, liver, or ulcer disease, or people with high blood pressure.

Men with enlarged prostates or individuals with psychiatric problems should avoid yohimbe supplements.

WHAT TO AVOID

Medication: People taking antidepressant medications, nasal decongestants, or diet aids should consult a doctor before taking yohimbe.

Also use caution when taking yohimbe with blood pressure–lowering medications or any medication that stimulates the central nervous system. Yohimbe may enhance the effects of monoamine oxidase (MAO) inhibitor drugs.

Herbs and Supplements: People taking antidepressant supplements should consult a doctor before taking yohimbe. It is also important to be aware that yohimbe may interfere with herbs or supplements that lower blood sugar levels or that affect the liver's enzyme system.

Food: Be careful when taking yohimbe together with foods containing the substance tyramine, such as red wine, liver, aged cheeses, or caffeinated products, since its combination with them may trigger cluster headaches or increased blood pressure.

ZINC

ZINC IS AN ESSENTIAL TRACE MINERAL that plays an indispensable role in human health. It is present in every organ, tissue, and fluid in the body, but mainly in muscles and bones, and is required by about 300 different enzymes to do their work. Zinc is essential for normal human growth, development, and reproduction. Because the body does not make zinc naturally, we must get what we need of this mineral from the food we eat or from supplements.

WHAT IT DOES

Zinc plays an important role in the body's immune system, which is why it may be helpful in treating the common cold. Double-blind trials have shown that zinc lozenges may reduce the duration and severity of colds in adults. Furthermore, studies have suggested that people with a deficiency of zinc may be more susceptible to infection. Zinc is most effective when taken at the first sign of a cold. However, no benefit of zinc has been observed for colds in children.

Although the results of studies have been mixed, some research indicates that oral supplementation with zinc may be useful for treating acne. Zinc is often combined with topical antibiotics used to treat acne, but it is unknown exactly how much of the effectiveness of this treatment technique can be attributed to zinc versus the antibiotic.

When applied topically, zinc may be effective in preventing canker sores and cold sores and relieving their accompanying pain.

Other studies suggest that a deficiency of zinc may cause recurrent canker sores.

Zinc is also an important element for healthy eyes, because some of the enzymes in the retina that are needed for proper vision require zinc. While studies have given varying results, some studies suggest that supplementation with zinc may delay the loss of vision in people with macular degeneration.

Zinc also helps to regulate the appetite, and some studies suggest that people with anorexia or bulimia may be especially deficient in this important nutrient. Zinc deficiency may also be common in people with diabetes, and supplementation with zinc is often recommended for people with diabetes since this vital mineral plays a role in the production and storage of insulin. Preliminary studies suggest that low levels of zinc in men—and especially in men who smoke—may contribute to infertility by reducing the sperm-cell count and sperm motility. Zinc deficiency may also play a role in causing tinnitus, although it is unclear whether supplementation with zinc will help against tinnitus in people who do not already have a deficiency of this mineral. Zinc deficiency is common in people with Crohn's disease, and using zinc supplements may be useful for decreasing the intestinal permeability associated with the condition.

Additionally, zinc is found in a number of antidandruff shampoos and may help kill the fungus that causes dandruff. Zinc may also be useful for treating psoriasis.

As further possible benefits, zinc may be helpful for people with alcoholism, benign prostatic hyperplasia, and for preventing warts.

For additional information on specific health conditions and how you can treat them with supplements, see Part 3 of this book, beginning on page 309.

HOW IT WORKS

Zinc has a variety of important functions in the body. It plays a role in the activities of various enzymes; is required for the synthesis of deoxyribonucleic acid (DNA) and ribonucleic acid (RNA) and for immune function, promotes wound healing and fertility, and has antiviral activity.

Although recent studies have shown that zinc can have a beneficial effect on the body's immune system, the exact way in which it

FRIENDS AND FOES

ZINC AND COPPER

When taking zinc for a prolonged period, it is advisable to also take 1 to 3 milligrams of copper daily, because zinc supplements by themselves can cause a copper deficiency.

does this is unknown. Some test-tube studies have shown that zinc can block the viruses from replicating. What is clear is that zinc lozenges help kill cold viruses in the mouth and throat, but only if taken soon after symptoms begin.

For some people with diabetes, high doses of zinc can mimic the effects of insulin in reducing blood sugar and promoting the healing of wounds.

HOW TO TAKE IT

See the table below for the recommended daily intakes (RDIs) of zinc.

AGE/GENDER/ CONDITION	RECOMMENDED DAILY INTAKE (RDI)*
Infants	
0–6 months	2 mg
7–12 months	3 mg
Children	
1–3 years	3 mg
4–8 years	5 mg
Males and Females	
9–13 years	8 mg
Males	
14 years and over	11 mg
Females	
14–18 years	9 mg
19 years and over	8 mg
Pregnant Women	11 mg (13 mg if 18 years old or younger)
Nursing Women	12 mg (14 mg if 18 years old or younger)

For more information on RDIs, see Want to Know More About Intake? on page 8.

Although only a small amount of zinc is required from food in order to maintain a healthy level of this important mineral in the body, most people do not get enough zinc. In fact, many people have a mild form of zinc deficiency, and as a result, supplementation with this mineral may be a good idea.

Signs of zinc deficiency include loss of appetite and taste and disturbances in the sense of smell; poor wound healing; diminished immune function; night blindness; problems with skin, hair, or nails; poor sensitivity to light; and joint problems.

The most common zinc supplement is zinc sulfate. Although it's the least expensive zinc supplement, it is also the least easily absorbed form of zinc and can upset the stomach. Preferred forms are zinc picolinate, zinc citrate, zinc acetate, zinc glycerate, and zinc monomethionine, all of which are more easily absorbed. When choosing zinc lozenges to treat common colds, look for those that don't contain the sweeteners sorbitol or mannitol or citric acid as a flavoring, since they can reduce the effectiveness of zinc. Zinc-based nasal gels and sprays may reduce nasal and sinus congestion.

Zinc supplements should be taken with water or juice. If this causes an upset stomach, then take zinc supplements with meals. Zinc should not be taken together with iron or calcium supplements.

LOOK OUT FOR THIS!

Zinc can be toxic when taken in high doses. See the table below for the maximum safe dosages of zinc.

AGE/CONDITION	MAXIMUM SAFE DOSAGE
Infants	
0–6 months	4 mg
7–12 months	5 mg
Children	
1–3 years	7 mg
4–8 years	12 mg
9–13 years	23 mg
Males and Females	
14–18 years	34 mg
19 years and older	40 mg
Pregnant or Nursing Women	40 mg (34 mg if 18 years or younger)

FOOD SOURCES

ZINC

Although zinc may be found in a variety of foods, it is most abundant in oysters, with six medium oysters containing 16 milligrams of this important nutrient. Zinc is also abundant in other shellfish and in red meats, and poultry and is least abundant in plant foods. Read on for other sources of foods that are high in zinc.

▶Cashews, crab (and other shellfish), eggs, green peas, lamb (and other red meat), liver, oatmeal, oysters, pork, turkey, walnuts, wheat germ, and whole grains. Sources from which zinc is somewhat less easily absorbed by the body include black-eyed peas and other legumes—especially lima beans, pinto beans, and soybeans.

Caution: Maximum safe dosages have not been established for people with liver or kidney disease.

Although zinc supplements are generally considered safe at recommended doses, do not take high doses for more than 2 weeks. Some side effects of zinc include upset stomach, nausea, vomiting, and a metallic aftertaste in the mouth.

Taking more than 150 milligrams of zinc a day may interfere with the body's ability to make use of other minerals. Some symptoms of excessive zinc supplementation are a weakened immune system, copper deficiency, higher LDL ("bad") cholesterol, anemia and neutropenia, and a decrease in the number of white blood cells.

Pregnant and nursing women should not take zinc supplements in dosages higher than the RDI (see page 307).

WHAT TO AVOID

Medication: Consult your doctor before taking zinc with bisphosphonates, angiotensin-converting enzyme (ACE) inhibitors, and other blood pressure medications, hormone replacement therapy, thiazide diuretics, medications that reduce stomach acid (such as omeprazole or ranitidine), hydralazine, immunosuppressant medications, nonsteroidal anti-inflammatory drugs (NSAIDs), pencillamine, quinolones, and tetracycline and other antibiotics.

Herbs and Dietary Supplements: Separate the time of your intake of zinc from that of calcium, copper, iron, or soy, since zinc may interfere with the absorption of these nutrients.

Food: Certain foods, when taken with zinc, inhibit the body's ability to absorb zinc. They include coffee or other caffeinated beverages; foods rich in oxalic acid, such as spinach, sweet potatoes, and rhubarb; foods rich in phytic acid, such as unleavened bread, raw beans, seeds, nuts and grains; and teas containing tannin. Some foods that are rich in cysteine-containing proteins, such as animal muscle tissue may increase the body's absorption of zinc if taken together with zinc.

PART THREE

···

Using Supplements
to Manage Health

ACNE

ACNE IS OFTEN THOUGHT OF AS the bane of teenage existence. The truth? Acne is not limited to those between the ages of 10 and 20; adults up to age 40 and beyond experience this condition as well. While not a major health threat, acne can be upsetting, unsightly, and downright inconvenient. With so many myths about the causes and treatment of acne, it's enough to make you throw a towel over your head and vow to stay home forever. It's time to set the record straight.

WHAT IS IT?

Acne is a common skin condition that affects nearly 17 million people in the United States. It is characterized by pimples on the face, chest, or back and occurs when pores become clogged with oil, called *sebum,* released from the skin's sebaceous glands. Experts believe that male hormones, particularly a derivative of testosterone called dihydrotestosterone (DHT), induce these glands to produce extra oil, which forms a plug in the pore where bacteria (*Propionic bacterium*) grow and inflame the skin. The result of this inflammation—a pimple—is often a pus-filled whitehead or a dark plug of dried oil known as a blackhead. In some cases, a cyst can form under the skin. If left untreated, acne can lead to permanent scarring.

Keep in mind that washing alone is not an effective treatment for acne and can lead to further inflammation if done too often or too vigorously.

The Chocolate-Acne Connection

Still in Debate

Chances are you've heard the rumor that chocolate causes acne. Despite this widespread and long-lasting myth, there is no scientific evidence that eating chocolate either causes or worsens acne. Still, experts don't all agree on the relationship. Studies suggest that no direct correlation exists between consumption of chocolate and acne flare-ups. One famous study, conducted more than 20 years ago at the University of Pennsylvania, included a group of 20 students without acne. Ten of the students were given a dense chocolate bar, and the other 10 students were given a candy bar that contained no cocoa. *The findings?* No difference in the number of new flare-ups in either group. Yet many people with acne report that certain foods—including chocolate—aggravate their acne. This may be because certain chemicals in chocolate trigger hormones that set off the blemishes of this condition.

While researchers continue to sort this out, it is probably best to identify your personal acne triggers. And, of course, it is important to follow a common-sense diet and steer clear of foods and behaviors that worsen your complexion.

WHAT SHOULD I USE?

Boswellia essential oil • Calendula • Guggul
Lavender • Tea Tree Oil • Vitamin A • Zinc

Boswellia is often found in topical herbal treatments for acne. While no specific studies have been performed using as an acne treatment, it does have known antibiotic properties against a variety of common bacteria. (For more information on boswellia, see page 52.)

Calendula is a time-honored herbal treatment for inflamed skin. No specific studies have been conducted on its use for acne, but it might help reduce the redness and inflammation. Be aware that there have been some reports of allergic reaction to the topical use of this herb. (For more information on calendula, see page 61.)

While clinical trials of **guggul** for acne have been somewhat inconclusive, one study that compared tetracycline (a general antibiotic commonly prescribed for people with acne) with guggul found more improvement in patients treated with guggul than in those treated with tetracycline. Guggul especially helped patients with oily skin and was found to have far fewer side effects than tetracycline. (For more information on guggul, see page 162.)

Lavender is well known for its wonderful scent and the beautiful flowers and plant. Less well known, however, is that lavender has documented antibiotic properties. While documentation of lavender's antbacterial properties against *Propionic bacterium* is scarce, herbalists have used lavender topically as an acne treatment for some time. (For more information on lavender, see page 184.)

The antibacterial, antifungal, and antiviral properties of **tea tree oil** make it a wonderful antiseptic, killing the bacteria that can cause acne flare-ups. Tea tree oil has been shown to be as effective as benzoyl peroxide (Triaz) for treating acne and often to have fewer side effects. (For more information on tea tree oil, see page 265.)

Studies suggest that **vitamin A**, when taken orally in extremely high doses (300,000 IU daily), may temporarily treat acne, but high-dose vitamin A is not recommended, since the benefit it provides does not outweigh the risk. However, Retin-A—a prescription medication derived from vitamin A—is an effective topical treatment for acne. (For more information on vitamin A, see page 274.)

Several studies indicate that **zinc** may be beneficial for reducing the inflammation accompanying acne. However, the recommended dose of zinc for treating acne is high and should be taken only under the supervision of a doctor. (For more information on zinc, see page 304.)

MY SUPPLEMENT LIST—ACNE	
SUPPLEMENT	**RECOMMENDED DOSAGE**
Boswellia	*Topical—Lotions containing boswellian essential oil:* Apply topically one to two times per day.
Calendula	*Topical—Lotion/Cream:* Apply a lotion or cream product containing calendula two or three times each day to the affected area. Follow the individual product label for application instructions
Guggul	*Oral—Capsule:* Take 1,000 mg of an extract standardized to contain 2.5% guggulsterones three times daily.
Lavender	*Topical—Lotion/Cream:* Apply a lotion or cream product containing lavender two or three times each day to the affected area. Follow the individual product label for application instructions. Or, use the essential oil and apply sparingly to the affected area two to three times per day.
Tea Tree Oil	*Topical—Gel/Oil:* Apply 5% tea tree oil gel to affected skin daily. You may also use pure tea tree oil, which can be diluted with water—usually at a ratio of about 1 part oil to 20 parts water—to avoid sensitivity reactions. Full-strength tea tree oil (undiluted) may also be applied to affected areas with a cotton swab.
	Note: Some people are sensitive to some or all of tea tree oil's components, especially when used in too strong a dosage. Tea tree oil products should be tested on a small patch of skin in an unobtrusive area to make sure no allergic reaction occurs.
Vitamin A	*Topical:* Consult your doctor to determine if Retin-A is appropriate for you.
Zinc	*Tablet:* Take 30 mg daily.
	Note: It may take up to 12 weeks to notice any effect. Take zinc with 1–2 mg of copper, since zinc taken in high doses may deplete levels of copper in the body.

AGING

I N 1930, THE LIFE EXPECTANCY in the U.S. was 59.7 years. Now it's 77.2 years. But what kind of *health* can you expect in those years? Even though genetics plays a huge role, supplements can help stave off signs of aging, even when your genes aren't perfect.

WHAT SHOULD I TAKE?

Calcium and Vitamin D (for osteoporosis) • *DHEA* (for general aging) • *Garlic* (for cardiovascular health) • *Ginkgo Biloba* (for memory) • *Glucosamine and Chondroitin* (for osteoarthritis) *Lutein* (for cataracts and macular degeneration) • *Melatonin* (for general aging) • *Multivitamins* (for general aging) • *Saw Palmetto* (for prostate health) • *Vitamins C and E* (for glaucoma)

Calcium supplements help protect against the bone-weakening disease known as osteoporosis. Since **vitamin D** is essential to the body's absorption of calcium, these two supplements, when taken together, may slow the progression of this disease and may actually reverse this condition to a certain extent. Keep in mind that you must take calcium and vitamin D, along with other important nutrients, on a constant basis in order to reap their health benefits; studies show that improvements cease once supplementation with them is discontinued. Ask your doctor to check your DHEA-S level. If it is low, then your doctor may have you take supplemental DHEA under supervision. (For more information on calcium and vitamin D, see pages 57 and 289.)

DHEA is the most abundant steroid hormone produced by the adrenal glands. Unlike those of other adrenal steroids, levels of DHEA in the body decline with age, and some research suggests that higher levels of DHEA may be correlated with increased longevity. As a result, researchers have speculated that a deficiency in DHEA may speed the aging process. Animal studies indicate that supplementation with DHEA may prevent obesity, diabetes, certain types of cancer, and heart disease, as well as strengthen the immune system, prolong life, and improve sexual function. However, DHEA should only be used under a doctor's supervision. Ask your doctor to check your DHEA-S level. If it is low, then your doctor may have you take supplemental DHEA under supervision. (For more information on DHEA, see page 100.)

Garlic has strong antioxidant properties, and preliminary research shows that it may help to promote cardiovascular health. Small studies

You May No Longer Need to Count Glasses of Water

Did You Know?

How many glasses of water do you need to drink each day to stay properly hydrated? Eight, right? Maybe not! A recent report issued by the Institute of Medicine of the U.S. National Academy of Sciences says there is no need to drink eight glasses of water daily to maintain hydration.

According to the report, women appear to be well hydrated when drinking 91 ounces of fluids a day, and men about 125 ounces. While this amount is actually more than the 64 ounces you would get from eight glasses of water, only about 80 percent of fluids must be obtained from drinking water. The remaining intake of fluid can be achieved through food or by drinking other beverages such as juice, milk, or even caffeinated drinks including tea and coffee. Despite common conception, caffeinated beverages *do not* lead to dehydration. So don't lose hope if you have trouble consuming pure water. The key to staying hydrated is not counting glasses of water, but rather drinking your favorite beverages whenever you feel thirsty.

show that garlic may reduce the incidence of a second heart attack as well as reduce death rates from heart disease. Other research has found that garlic may be useful in reducing the total amount of cholesterol in the body, although more studies are needed to determine whether it is best used whole or in supplements. Early evidence also suggests that garlic may help prevent atherosclerosis (hardening of the arteries), a common cause of heart attack and stroke. In addition to its heart-protective effects, garlic may strengthen the immune system and prevent cancer. (For more information on garlic, see page 134.)

Ginkgo improves blood flow in the brain and contains components that act as antioxidants. It may improve memory and thinking and help delay the initial symptoms of Alzheimer's disease. Other studies show that ginkgo may improve mental function in people with age-related memory loss. (For more information on ginkgo, see page 138.)

Research shows that **glucosamine**, which stimulates cartilage growth, may work as well as nonsteroidal anti-inflammatory drugs (NSAIDs) in reducing pain from osteoarthritis and may produce fewer side effects than these drugs. It may also cause better mobility and slow or prevent joint damage. Glucosamine is often taken with **chondroitin**, which has been found to reduce swelling and fluid in the joints, as well as to increase mobility and slow the onset of arthritis. (For more information on glucosamine and chondroitin, see pages 144 and 74.)

Lutein supplements may help to prevent the development of cataracts and macular degeneration, the two most common causes of vision loss in older people. One study found that people who ate a diet high in lutein and zeaxanthin, another carotenoid, had less than half the risk of developing macular degeneration than those who did not. (For more information on lutein, see page 195.)

While researchers aren't exactly sure how **melatonin** works, one thing they know is that levels of melatonin in the body decrease with age. Many researchers suspect that this decrease in melatonin may lead to premature aging, cancer, and cardiovascular disease. In some animal studies, melatonin increased lifespan, although other studies did not show any benefit from melatonin supplementation. (For more information on melatonin, see page 208.)

Taking a daily **multivitamin** may be your best bet for insuring that you receive adequate amounts of important vitamins and minerals. Antioxidants, including vitamins A, C, D, E, and selenium, work to protect cells from damage caused by free radical molecules. Several studies indicate that free-radical damage is the primary cause of aging. Other research suggests that certain nutrients—such as folic acid (vitamin B_9), vitamin B_{12}, niacin, and zinc—may help prevent spontaneous damage to chromosomes, another factor that contributes to the aging process. (For more information on multivitamins, see page 9.)

Studies have shown that not only does **saw palmetto** relieve symptoms of benign prostatic hyperplasia (BPH), a very common condition characterized by enlargement of the prostate gland in aging men, but it may even reverse prostate enlargement. Studies suggest that saw palmetto may be as effective (if not more effective) than prescription medications often used to treat BPH, while causing fewer side effects. (For more information on saw palmetto, see page 249.)

A number of studies have shown that taking **vitamin C** reduces pressure inside the eye, which may make it useful for preventing glaucoma, a condition marked by increased pressure from fluid buildup in the eye. Other studies have shown that when taking **vitamin E** along with regular glaucoma medication, people with glaucoma experienced an increase in their field of vision. (For more information on vitamins C and E, see pages 284 and 292.)

MY SUPPLEMENT LIST—AGING

SUPPLEMENT	RECOMMENDED DOSAGE
Calcium	*Capsule or Tablet (Adults under 50 years):* Take 500 mg twice daily. *(Adults 50 years and over):* Take 1,200 mg daily divided into three doses.
Chondroitin	*Capsule or Tablet:* Take 400 mg three times daily with meals, or 1,200 mcg with dinner. Chondroitin products are often sold in combination with glucosamine (see next top of page). *Note:* It may take several weeks before you notice any effect.
DHEA	DHEA should be taken only under the supervision of a doctor. The ideal dose and long-term effects of this supplement are unknown.
Garlic	*Capsule or Tablet:* Take 600 to 900 mg daily of a garlic extract standardized to contain 1.3% allicin, providing about 12,000 mcg of allicin daily or 6,000 mcg of allicin potential. *Fresh:* Take one fresh clove per day, which is a better source of allicin since this compound is decreased when the garlic is dried. The garlic can be minced and swallowed together with a bit of yogurt or applesauce.
Ginkgo	*Capsule or Tablet:* For the treatment of dementia and to improve cognitive ability, take 240 mg daily divided into two or three doses. Make sure to buy a product

MY SUPPLEMENT LIST—AGING	
SUPPLEMENT	**RECOMMENDED DOSAGE**
	standardized to contain 24% ginkgo flavone glycosides and 6% terpene lactones, since these are the effective ingredients used in clinical trials.
Glucosamine	*Capsule or Tablet:* Take 500 mg three times daily with food, or 1,500 mg with dinner. Glucosamine products are often sold in combination with chondroitin (see previous page). *Note:* It may take several weeks before you notice the effects of glucosamine.
Lutein	*Capsule or Tablet:* Take 6 mg of lutein as two "divided" doses of 3 mg each for protection against macular degeneration. If you have cataracts in an early stage, studies suggest that 15 mg daily may be useful. *Note:* Take lutein with fatty food to increase the body's absorption of this nutrient.
Melatonin	The ideal dosage of melatonin for general aging is unknown. Consult your doctor before taking melatonin supplements to determine an appropriate dosage.
Multivitamin	Take a multivitamin/mineral supplement every day. Follow the individual product label for dosage information.
Saw Palmetto	*Capsule:* Take 160 mg twice a day of an extract standardized to contain 85% to 95% fatty acids and sterols. Studies also indicate that taking a single dose of 320 mg of such an extract may be equally as effective.
Vitamin C	*Capsule or Tablet:* Take up to 500 mg three times daily. *Note:* Be sure to use a buffered form of vitamin C. If taking vitamin C causes loose stools, decrease the dosage and then gradually increase the dosage as tolerated.
Vitamin D	*Capsule or Tablet:* Take 800 IU daily, along with calcium (see previous page) for preventing osteoporosis. Ask your doctor to check your vitamin D to see if this dose is sufficient.
Vitamin E	*Capsule:* Take 400 to 800 IU daily of a natural product containing mixed tocopherols.

ALCOHOLISM

THERE IS A FINE LINE BETWEEN healthy enjoyment and addiction. For many people, moderate drinking of alcoholic beverages—up to two drinks per day for men and one drink per day for women—is not harmful and may even provide some health benefits. But for the estimated 14 million Americans—one in every 13 adults—who have an addiction to alcohol, drinking has dangerous and sometimes fatal consequences. Heavy drinking can take a major toll on health, with effects that include an increased risk of developing certain types of cancer, liver cirrhosis, immune system problems, and brain damage. Aside from its deleterious effects on health, alcoholism can be devastating to family members and loved ones—not to mention the dangers associated with drinking and driving. The only effective cure for alcoholism is to stop drinking immediately.

WHAT IS IT?

Alcohol dependence is marked by a strong urge to drink, an inability to control the intake of alcohol once drinking has started, an increased tolerance of the effects of alcohol, and a strong physical reaction to the withdrawal of alcohol or abrupt cessation of its use, including anxiety, nausea, sweating, and shakiness. *Alcohol intolerance* occurs when the body lacks an enzyme (called aldehyde dehydrogenase-2) that is needed to digest alcohol. People with alcohol intolerance do not have to consume a large quantity of alcohol in order to feel its effects; their drinking is often accompanied by facial flushing, muscle weakness, and nausea when they ingest alcohol. The upshot? Quantity is not the sole factor in determining whether you or someone you know has an alcohol problem.

Since alcohol leaches key vitamins and minerals from the body, the first step in recovery is to replenish the stores of these vital nutrients. By improving their overall nutritional condition, people with an alcohol dependency may prevent many of the diseases associated with alcoholism. Additionally, some studies show that the symptoms of craving for and withdrawal from alcohol may be reduced through diet changes and nutritional supplementation. Unfortunately, alcohol diminishes the body's ability to absorb, disperse, and eliminate many vitamins and minerals; it is therefore important to start supplementation gradually and not take high doses of fat-soluble vitamins such as vitamins A and D. Check with

Alcoholism and Your Genes

Did You Know?

A growing body of evidence suggests that there may be a genetic link to alcoholism, although the exact genes have not yet been identified. Studies in both animals and humans show that genetic factors may play a role in a person's development of alcoholism, although just how much of a role it plays is unknown. According to the American Academy of Child and Adolescent Psychiatry (AACAP), children of alcoholic parents are four times more likely to become alcoholics than are children from nonalcoholic families. The possibility of controlling this disease before passing it down to your children is just one more reason to seek help if you think you may have an alcohol problem.

an integrative medicine specialist or a naturopathic doctor to establish a supplement plan that's right for you.

WHAT SHOULD I TAKE?
Betaine • Choline • Magnesium • Milk Thistle • Vitamin A
Vitamin B Complex • Vitamin C • Vitamin E • Zinc

Betaine, in the form of betaine citrate or betaine aspartate, may protect the liver from alcohol-induced fatty liver disease. Studies indicate that because of its ability to help the liver process fats, betaine may reduce the amount of fat that accumulates in the liver in first-stage liver damage resulting from alcohol intake. (For more information on betaine, see page 42.)

Studies indicate that **choline**—in the form of phosphatidyl-choline—may reduce inflammation to the liver caused by excess alcohol intake. (For more information on choline, see page 71.)

Magnesium is believed to decrease withdrawal symptoms and reduce the incidence of osteoporosis and cardiovascular disease in people with chronic alcoholism. (For more information on magnesium, see page 203.)

Studies from Europe have shown that in experiments lasting up to 5 years, **milk thistle** improved liver function and decreased the number of deaths resulting from cirrhosis. (For more information on milk thistle, see page 210.)

Vitamin A deficiencies in alcoholics have been known to cause night blindness, cirrhosis, and impaired immune function. However, heavy drinkers should use vitamin A with caution, since this supplement may hasten liver disease when used in conjunction with alcohol. (For more information on vitamin A, see page 274.)

Vitamins belonging to the **B-complex** group are often deficient in people with alcoholism because of an inadequate intake of these vitamins coupled with the body's inability to absorb them. Preliminary animal studies also show that a deficiency of these vitamins may cause a craving for alcohol. (For more information on vitamin B complex, see pages 277, 279, and 282.)

Experimental studies show that **vitamin C** supplementation may reduce the effects of alcohol toxicity by improving the body's ability to eliminate alcohol. (For more information on vitamin C, see page 284.)

Heavy alcohol intake reduces the levels of **vitamin E** in the body. Supplementation with vitamin E will help the body maintain adequate levels of this important nutrient. (For more information on vitamin E, see page 292.)

Low levels of **zinc** impair the body's ability to metabolize alcohol, which increases the risk of liver damage. Zinc supplementation aids the metabolism of alcohol and may also prevent seizures caused by alcohol withdrawal and alcohol-related brain dysfunction. (For more information on zinc, see page 304.)

MY SUPPLEMENT LIST—ALCOHOLISM

Consult your doctor before taking any of the supplements named below. Certain supplements may be harmful or you may need careful medical monitoring if you have alcohol-induced liver or pancreas disease.

SUPPLEMENT	RECOMMENDED DOSAGE
Betaine	*Capsule or Tablet:* Take 1 to 2 g of betaine citrate or betaine aspartate three times per day.
Choline	*Capsule or Tablet:* Take 450 mg of phosphatidylcholine daily, divided into three doses, with meals.
Magnesium	*Tablet:* Take 200 to 300 mg two or three times daily. *Note:* Take magnesium in the form of magnesium glycinate to avoid loose stools. Large amounts of magnesium can cause diarrhea; if this becomes a problem for you, reduce your dosage.
Milk Thistle	*Capsule or Tablet:* Take 140 to 200 mg of an extract standardized to contain 70% silymarin three times a day. After 6 weeks, decrease the dosage to 90 mg taken three times a day. When formulated with phosphatidylcholine (see choline, above)—a preparation of milk thistle that some studies suggests is better absorbed—take 100 to 200 mg twice daily.
Vitamin A	Heavy drinkers should consult with a doctor before taking vitamin A supplements to avoid damage to the liver. The doctor will check blood levels in order to determine an appropriate dose of this vitamin.
Vitamin B Complex	*Tablet:* Take vitamin B complex in a dose of 50 to 100 mg daily. Read the individual product label for dosage information.
Vitamin C	*Capsule:* Take 250 to 500 mg two times a day. *Note:* Be sure to use a buffered form of vitamin C. If taking vitamin C causes loose stools, decrease the dosage and then gradually increase the dosage as tolerated.
Vitamin E	*Capsule:* Take 400 IU once a day of a natural product containing mixed tocopherols.
Zinc	*Tablet:* Take 15 mg once a day.

ALZHEIMER'S DISEASE AND MEMORY PROBLEMS

GIVEN THE FAST PACE OF MODERN LIFE, coupled with the vast amount of knowledge that a person acquires over a lifetime, it's no wonder that we forget things from time to time. *Where did I leave those keys? What is the name of my new neighbor? Which grandchild's birthday is approaching?* Forgetting things now and then is perfectly normal. And it's also normal if the perfect sense of recall you had as a youngster begins to dwindle with age, particularly after age 50. On the other hand, frequent forgetfulness may be a sign of Alzheimer's disease (AD), a brain disorder that affects an estimated 4 million Americans, most often over the age of 65.

WHAT IS IT?

It is important to make a distinction between normal memory loss and AD. As we age, it is natural that some of the millions of brain cells we are born with die, without being replaced. Furthermore, with age, our bodies produce less of the chemicals necessary to help brain cells work.

Memory may be divided into three main categories: short-term, recent, and long-term; eventually, AD affects all three. *Short-term memory* stores information for anywhere from seconds to hours (for example, a phone number recently dialed), whereas *recent memory* stores information from the recent past (for example, what you ate for breakfast this morning). *Long-term memory* stores information for days, years, and even a lifetime (for example, childhood memories). Various factors can cause memory loss or dementia, including certain medications, stroke, head injury, or hearing and vision problems.

The most common form of dementia—AD—is a progressive disease affecting the memory. Although the cause of AD is unknown, experts do know that this condition is marked by abnormal clusters of proteins in the brain. Since the presence of these clusters can only be seen in an autopsy, doctors can only definitively diagnose AD after a patient has died. While it is often hard to diagnose, certain common symptoms can help doctors make a *likely* diagnosis of AD. Symptoms include the inability to do familiar tasks; difficulty in communicating; changes in personality, mood, and behavior; disorientation; and problems with speech and writing.

While there is no cure for AD, early detection is the key to properly managing this condition. Some medications may help slow the progression of AD and improve the quality of life for AD patients. Many supplements are available to improve memory as well as to prevent memory problems from occurring.

WHAT SHOULD I TAKE?

Alzheimer's disease is a serious condition. Make sure to consult your doctor before taking any type of supplement especially if you have been diagnosed with AD or think you may have AD.

Choline • Folic Acid • Ginkgo Biloba (Ginkgo)
Huperzine A • Magnesium • Omega-3 Fatty Acids
Phosphatidylserine • Vitamin B$_{12}$ • Vitamin C • Vitamin E

Choline is a main ingredient of acetylcholine, a chemical in the brain that is needed to transmit nerve signals and help the brain to function. A 6-month double-blind study involving 261 people with AD showed that those who took a specific form of choline, called choline alfoscerate, experienced marked improvement in their cognitive function. (For more information on choline, see page 71.)

Preliminary studies show that elevated levels of homocysteine, a harmful amino acid that is frequently associated with an increased risk of heart disease and stroke, may also cause an increased risk of AD. Since a deficiency in **folic acid** (vitamin B$_9$) may cause increased levels of homocysteine, supplementation with this vitamin may prevent the risk of AD, especially in people with a low intake of folic acid. (For more information on folic acid, see page 130.)

Ginkgo is the best-established herbal remedy for AD and memory problems. Various double-blind, placebo-controlled studies indicate that ginkgo has a positive effect on many forms of dementia.

Brain-Boosting Tips

Healthy Hints

You can help keep your memory sharp in a variety of ways. Read on for tips to boost your memory.

■ **Get a new hobby.** Various activities can help give your brain a workout. Try doing crossword puzzles, playing Scrabble, reading, learning a foreign language, or starting a new hobby such as painting or gardening.

■ **Become part of a system.** If you feel you are experiencing information overload, take some steps to create triggers for your memory. Writing things down, creating routines, and setting up cues are all ways to help prompt your memory.

■ **Relax!** One thing that won't help your memory is stress. Make sure to relax so that you can stay focused, and don't become panicked if you can't remember things. Feeling stressed will only interfere with your concentration, making it even harder to remember.

Ginkgo appears to increase memory capacity and per- formance, may slow the age-related loss of choline in the brain, and helps certain areas of the brain absorb choline. Ginkgo is also thought to work by improving blood flow in the brain and neutralizing the cell-damaging free radicals that may play a role in AD by damaging the brain. (For more information on ginkgo, see page 138.)

Huperzine A is a strong alkaloid (a substance found naturally in plants) that can be compared to caffeine and cocaine in terms of natural potency. Huperzine A appears to exert its effect in AD by preventing the breakdown of acetylcholine in the brain. In clinical trials, huperzine A has been shown to be more effective than certain prescription medications for AD, and it also caused fewer side effects. In a multi-center, prospective, double-blind, parallel, placebo-controlled study involving 103 AD patients, 58 percent of patients taking huperzine A had an improvement in memory, cognitive, and behavioral function without any side effects. This powerful alkaloid, available over-the-counter in most health food stores, seems to have a promising future in the world of dementia. (For more information on huperzine A, see page 171.)

Magnesium deficiency is associated with an increased risk of AD. While it remains unclear whether magnesium supplements will decrease symptoms of AD once they occur, magnesium supplements are safe, relatively inexpensive, non-toxic, and useful for a variety of other conditions. (For more information on magnesium, see page 203.)

The **omega-3 fatty acids** found in certain types of fish may reduce the risk of AD. One study conducted in 2003 at the Rush-Presbyterian-St. Luke's Medical Center in Chicago and involving people over the age of 65 found that those who ate fish at least once a week had a 60 percent less chance of developing AD during the study period than those who rarely ate fish. (For more information on omega-3 fatty acids, see page 221.)

Numerous studies indicate that **phosphatidylserine** is helpful in improving memory, learning, concentration, and word choice, as well as mood and the ability to deal with stress. Phosphatidylserine is very well tolerated, with few side effects, and is compatible with many prescription medications. (For more information on phosphatidylserine, see page 229.)

Vitamin B$_{12}$ deficiency is often associated with an increased risk of AD as well as a decline in mental function. While it is unclear whether supplementation with vitamin B_{12} is effective in slowing the effects of AD, this vitamin may be useful in preventing AD in the first place. (For more information on vitamin B_{12}, see page 282.)

Vitamin C and **vitamin E** are antioxidants that may play a role in preventing and treating AD by neutralizing rogue free radicals before they inflict damage. One large study conducted in the Netherlands in 2002 found that eating a diet with a high content of these vitamins was associated with a lower risk of AD. Other studies suggest that when taken in high doses, vitamin E may slow the progression of AD. (For more information on vitamins C and E, see pages 284 and 292.)

MY SUPPLEMENT LIST—ALZHEIMER'S DISEASE AND MEMORY PROBLEMS

SUPPLEMENT	RECOMMENDED DOSAGE
Choline	*Tablet:* Take 400 mg of choline alfoscerate three times daily.
	Note: Choline alfoscerate may also be sold as "Alpha GPC." It may take up to 6 months for this supplement to be effective.
Folic Acid	*Tablet:* Take 400 to 800 mcg daily divided into two or three doses.
Ginkgo	*Capsule or Tablet:* Take a concentrated leaf extract, standardized to contain 24% flavonoid glycosides and 6% terpenoids, 120 to 240 mg daily in two to three divided doses.
Huperzine A	*Tablet:* Take 30 to 200 mcg twice daily.
	Caution: Huperzine A should be taken only under a doctor's supervision.
Magnesium	*Tablet:* Take 300 to 600 mg daily.
	Note: Take magnesium in the form of magnesium glycinate to avoid loose stools. Large amounts of magnesium can cause diarrhea; if this becomes a problem for you, reduce your dosage. Do not take if you have diabetes or kidney disease.
Omega-3 Fatty Acids	*Oral:* Take 1–2 g of omega-3 fatty acids per day, in divided doses, with meals. The amount of omega-3 fatty acid will vary by manufacturer, so be sure to check the product label carefully.
Phosphatidyl-serine	*Capsule:* Studies show that effective intakes of phosphatidylserine range from 100 to 900 mg daily. For memory, take 300 mg daily; for mood enhancement, up to 600 mg daily is recommended. Take this supplement with meals in divided doses. Follow individual product labels for specific dosage information.

MY SUPPLEMENT LIST—ALZHEIMER'S DISEASE AND MEMORY PROBLEMS	
SUPPLEMENT	**RECOMMENDED DOSAGE**
Vitamin B$_{12}$	*Tablet:* Take 500 mcg a day, or take a sublingual formulation for better absorption. *Injection:* If you have AD, your doctor may prescribe weekly injections of 1,000 mcg of vitamin B$_{12}$.
Vitamin C	*Capsule or Tablet:* Take 500 to 1,000 mg of vitamin C daily, divided into 250-mg doses. *Note:* Be sure to use a buffered form of vitamin C. If taking vitamin C causes loose stools, decrease the dosage and then gradually increase the dosage as tolerated.
Vitamin E	*Capsule:* Take 100 to 1,000 IU of natural vitamin E with mixed tocopherols daily. For people with AD, consult your doctor to determine an appropriate dosage for you. Studies using up to 2,000 IU daily have slowed the progression of AD, but these doses are high and should be taken only under a doctor's supervision.

ANEMIA

THE TERM "ANEMIC" HAS WORKED its way into our common vocabulary as an adjective to describe something that's weak, tired, and just kind of blah, such as an actor's poor performance in a movie. While that use of the word is uncomplimentary, it gives an accurate sense of how the disease known as anemia can make someone feel. More than 3 million Americans have this condition, which may make them feel weak, fatigued, and easily winded because their blood isn't able to properly carry life-giving oxygen throughout their bodies.

WHAT IS IT?

Anemia occurs when the body either doesn't have enough red blood cells or has too little hemoglobin—the protein in red blood cells that carries oxygen molecules. The most common cause of anemia is iron deficiency (see Iron, page 175). Iron is an essential element in hemoglobin and allows the proper transport of oxygen in the blood. Menstruation and pregnancy can cause iron deficiency, and because of this, anemia is more common in women than in men. Abnormal bleeding in the digestive system can cause anemia in either sex.

Anemia may also be caused by a deficiency of folic acid (vitamin B$_9$) or vitamin B$_{12}$ (see pages 130 and 282), two nutrients that are crucial for the growth and maintenance of red blood cells. *Pernicious*

FRIENDS AND FOES

If your doctor has recommended taking **iron** supplements to treat anemia, be sure to also take from 100 to 400 milligrams of **vitamin C**, since it helps the body to better absorb iron.

anemia is a type of anemia caused by a lack of intrinsic factor in the body, a substance that the body normally produces and requires in order to absorb vitamin B_{12}. *Sickle-cell anemia* is a serious, and often fatal, form of anemia in which inherited, genetic factors create red blood cells that are crescent-shaped instead of round. Rather than flowing smoothly through the bloodstream, these abnormal red blood cells clog blood vessels, causing pain and damage to areas deprived of oxygen. This form of anemia is most common in African Americans.

If you have anemia, your doctor should investigate its cause and supervise your treatment closely. If your anemia is caused by nutritional deficiencies, taking the proper supplements should help solve the problem. Be sure to discuss supplemental treatment of anemia with your doctor before starting a supplement program.

WHAT SHOULD I TAKE?
Folic Acid • Iron • Vitamin A • Vitamin B Complex
Vitamin B_2 • Vitamin B_{12}

Supplements of **folic acid** (vitamin B_9), are used to treat anemia caused by a deficiency of this nutrient. (For more information on folic acid, see page 130.)

Not surprisingly, in view of the vital role of **iron** in the body's production of hemoglobin, iron supplements are a common treatment for types of anemia caused by iron deficiency. People who are deficient in iron often need to take iron supplements for about 6 months to 1 year until their blood tests are normal. Some people with recurrent iron deficiency, particularly post-menopausal women, need to continue to take small amounts of iron as supplements, which can usually be obtained from a multivitamin. Keep in mind,

The Anemia-Malaria Connection

Did You Know?

Being a carrier of the genetic anomaly that causes sickle-cell anemia was once a blessing in disguise. Thousands of years ago in parts of Africa, the Mediterranean, and the Middle East, children who carried a defective gene that causes sickle-cell anemia were resistant to the mosquito-borne parasite that causes malaria. Thus, they survived malaria epidemics in the area and passed their genetic defect down to another generation.

Inheriting the defective gene from only one parent doesn't cause the disease, but inheriting it from both parents does. Since malaria isn't a widespread problem in the United States, carrying sickle-cell anemia genes is no longer a plus.

however, that iron or iron-containing supplements should only be used if specifically directed by your physician to correct an iron deficiency. (For more information on iron, see page 175.)

Surveys show that populations with a high prevalence of anemia tend to have **vitamin A** deficiency. When intakes of vitamin A were increased to healthy levels in people with such anemia, the risk of anemia was reduced as well. (For more information on vitamin A, see page 274.)

Since so many of the B vitamins are important for preventing and treating a variety of types of anemia, it may be best to take a daily dose of **vitamin B complex**. Studies indicate that the B vitamins work most effectively when taken together. (For more information on vitamin B complex, see pages 277, 279, and 282.)

Low intakes of **riboflavin** (vitamin B_2) may interfere with the body's ability to properly absorb and utilize iron. A deficiency of vitamin B_2 may also reduce the body's ability to metabolize folic acid, vitamin B_6, and other important B vitamins. (For more information on riboflavin, see page 238.)

Supplemental **vitamin B_{12}** is given for anemia caused by a vitamin B_{12} deficiency. In North America, this type of anemia occurs mainly in vegetarians. Many doctors recommend that all strict vegetarians supplement their diets with vitamin B_{12} to avoid a deficiency of this vitamin. Vitamin B_{12} is also important for people with sickle-cell anemia or pernicious anemia (which results from the body's inability to absorb vitamin B_{12}), who tend to have a deficiency in this vitamin. (For more information on vitamin B_{12}, see page 282.)

MY SUPPLEMENT LIST—ANEMIA

SUPPLEMENT	RECOMMENDED DOSAGE
Folic Acid	*Tablet:* General dosages range from 400 to 800 mcg daily. Consult your doctor to determine an appropriate dosage of this nutrient for you.
Iron	*Tablet:* Doses as high as 100 mg daily in the form of ferrous fumerate, ferrous glycinate, or ferrous glycerate may be recommended by your doctor for 3 months to 1 year to correct iron-deficiency anemia. *Note:* This is a high dose of iron and should be taken only under a doctor's supervision. Men and post-menopausal women should be extra careful with supplemental

(continued)

MY SUPPLEMENT LIST—ANEMIA (continued)	
SUPPLEMENT	**RECOMMENDED DOSAGE**
	iron, since they don't lose iron through menstruation and it may accumulate in their bodies. Iron overload may cause liver disease, intestinal bleeding, and even death. If you are advised to take iron supplements, keep in mind that even safe doses can cause digestive upset. To keep this side-effect to a minimum, take your supplement with food, and consider starting with a smaller dose of iron and working your way up to a full dose.
Vitamin A	*Capsule (Adults 14 years and older):* Take 5,000 IU daily.
Vitamin B Complex	*Capsule or Tablet:* Take vitamin B complex in a dose of 50 to 100 mg once daily. Read the individual product label for dosage information.
Vitamin B_2	*Capsule or Tablet:* Take 50 mg daily, an amount which can be found in most B-complex-50 supplements.
Vitamin B_{12}	*Injection:* Some studies show that regular injections of vitamin B_{12} are the only effective treatment for people with anemia caused by a deficiency of this vitamin. Consult your doctor to determine if this form of treatment is appropriate for you. *Tablet:* If your anemia is caused by a diet that doesn't provide enough vitamin B_{12}, you may be able to correct the problem by taking supplements and eating certain foods. Consult your doctor in order to determine an appropriate dosage of vitamin B_{12} for you.

ANXIETY

MOST PEOPLE CAN AGREE THAT it is impossible to live a life completely free from worry, and the anticipation that something terrible is going to happen is a major cause of anxiety. On the other hand, feeling apprehensive can sometimes be a great motivator. After all, that deadline at work may never have been achieved without a constant reminder in the form of a racing heartbeat and stomach pains!

WHAT IS IT?

Anxiety can include physical symptoms such as muscle tension, a rapid heartbeat; irritability; trouble with sleeping, breathing, or concentrating; and racing thoughts. Anxiety can last from a few minutes to months and varies in severity. The National Institutes of Health (NIH) characterizes generalized anxiety disorder (GAD) as 6 months or more of chronic, exaggerated worry and tension that is unfounded or is much more severe than the normal anxiety that most people experience. GAD often starts in childhood or adolescence, although it can begin in adulthood as well, and it is more prevalent in women than in men.

WHAT SHOULD I TAKE?

While anxiety can be a long-term problem, some of these supplements may also help transitory anxiety.

Kava • Lavender • Lemon Balm • Magnesium
Melatonin • Valerian • Vitamin B Complex

Several European studies have shown that **kava** (also called kava kava) is helpful in alleviating anxiety and stress-related problems. Preliminary evidence suggests that kava may be as effective as benzodiazepine drugs, such as diazepam (Valium), in the treatment of anxiety. Kava is also helpful in relieving short-term anxiety. However, because of its potential health risks, kava should be taken only under a doctor's supervision. (For more information on kava, see page 178.)

The German Commission E (see page 16) recommends **lavender** for a number of nervous disorders including "nervous stomach irritation" and "nervous intestinal discomfort," which often accompany anxiety. Studies suggest that lavender may promote sleep and relieve anxiety when used in the form of aromatherapy. (For more information on lavender, see page 184.)

The German Commission E (see page 16) recommends **lemon balm** for nervous sleeping disorders (see also Insomnia, page 516). Preliminary studies suggest that lemon balm may increase feelings of calm and reduce mental alertness. (For more information on lemon balm, see page 190.)

Both **magnesium** and **vitamin B complex** are believed to relieve anxiety, tension, and muscle spasms. (For more information on

FRIENDS AND FOES

Kava is well known around the world for its use as an anti-anxiety supplement. However, in 2002 the FDA issued a warning stating that kava-containing supplements have been associated with liver injury, including hepatitis, cirrhosis, and liver failure. It is important that people who have liver disease or who are taking drugs that can affect the liver consult with their doctor before taking any kava-containing supplements.

Aromatherapy May Help Snuff Out Stress

Did You Know?

Fragrant oils have been used for thousands of years for a variety of reasons. The modern use of aromatherapy—the practice of using fragrant substances to promote health, prevent illness, and affect mood—began in 1930 when the French chemist René Maurice Gattefossé began studying the healing effects of essential oils. How does aromatherapy work? Scientific studies of this practice, although limited, have shown that breathing in certain scents stimulates nerves in the nose, which then send messages to the limbic system, a part of our brain responsible for processing emotion. Some stress-busting scents that aromatherapists use are lavender, lemon balm, chamomile, rose, and jasmine.

vitamin B complex and magnesium, see pages 279 and 203.) Two studies indicate that *melatonin* maybe useful in alleviating anxiety prior to undergoing surgery. Ask your doctor if this might be right for you. (For more information on melatonin, see page 208).

Human studies show that taking **valerian** before bedtime helps reduce the amount of time it takes to fall asleep. Valerian is usually characterized as a mild tranquilizer and is deemed safe by the German Commission E (see page 16) for use against restlessness associated with sleep disorders or nervous conditions. Additionally, smaller studies suggest that valerian is helpful in reducing symptoms of non-specific anxiety and short-term anxiety. (For more information on valerian, see page 272.)

MY SUPPLEMENT LIST—ANXIETY

SUPPLEMENT	RECOMMENDED DOSAGE
Kava	Take 200 mg extract (standardized to contain 60 mg kavalactones), two capsules, two-three times per day, between meals. *Note:* Consult your doctor before taking kava. Kava may cause liver damage when taken in high dosages. Kava may also enhance the effects of alcohol, antidepressant medications, and sedative medications.
Lavender	*Inhalant:* Put 2 to 4 drops of essential lavender oil in 3 cups of boiling water and inhale the vapors daily, during times of stress. *Tea:* Steep 2 tsp of dried lavender flowers in 1 cup of boiling water for 15 minutes; drink up to three times a day.
Lemon Balm	*Tea:* Pour 1 cup of hot water over 1 to 3 tsp of dried herb and strain after 10 minutes. Drink up to three times daily.
Magnesium	*Capsule:* Take 200 to 300 mg in the form of magnesium glycinate twice daily with meals.
Melatonin	Ask your doctor if taking melatonin to decrease anxiety prior to surgery may be right for you.
Valerian	*Capsule or Tablet:* Take a morning dose of 150 to 300 mg and an evening dose of 300 to 600 mg daily. Be sure to use a product standardized to contain 3.3% valpotriates. *Note:* The strength of valerian products may vary greatly. Be sure to choose a standardized product and carefully follow the instructions on the label. Valerian may also be found in commercially prepared teas, usually in combination with other herbs, to mask the unusual taste.
Vitamin B Complex	*Tablet:* Take vitamin B complex in a dose of 50 to 100 mg once daily. Read the individual product label for dosage information.

APPETITE LOSS

MEALTIME COMES AND GOES, but you just don't feel like eating anything at all. Wafting smells from your favorite foods cooking in the kitchen or nearby restaurants are no longer enticing. While many people often wouldn't mind eating a little *less* to decrease their waist size, unwanted appetite loss can be disturbing, affect your health, and be a warning signal of a more serious condition.

WHAT IS IT?

Appetite loss can be caused by a variety of problems, including stress, anxiety, and depression; changes in taste sensitivity; digestive upset; viral infection; cancer; underactive thyroid gland; alcohol consumption; and hormonal changes due to pregnancy and menopause.

Certain prescription medicines, such as amphetamines and antibiotics, can also dull the appetite. Oftentimes, appetite loss is a significant concern for people with acquired immune deficiency syndrome (AIDS), cancer patients receiving chemotherapy, and the elderly. Luckily, several herbs can help restore a taste for eating again.

If you experience sudden appetite loss accompanied by weight loss, it is important to consult your doctor immediately to make sure you have no other serious health conditions.

Household Foods and Spices May Stimulate More Than Just Taste Buds

Did You Know?

A number of common foods and spices have traditionally been used to stimulate appetite. Not only are these spices tasty, but they can get your eating habits back on track if you have been experiencing a loss of appetite.

If you don't mind the tears that come along with chopping them, onions are approved by the German Commission E (see page 16) as an appetite stimulant. Try cutting an onion and putting it in your favorite salad to help increase your appetite.

Although you may be more familiar with cinnamon as a tasty addition to pastries, rice pudding, and apple cider, the German Commission E has approved its use for stimulating appetite as well. Try making a tea with cut or ground cinnamon bark, or sprinkling it on your favorite foods to wake up tired taste buds.

Coriander has also been approved by the German Commission E for treating appetite loss. Moreover, coriander seed, aside from stimulating appetite, may be useful for relieving various stomach ailments including cramps, excessive gas, and digestive complaints.

Last but certainly not least, chocolate lovers everywhere can rejoice. While eating an excess of chocolate is not recommended, a small piece of chocolate may stimulate appetite as well.

WHAT SHOULD I TAKE?

Cranberry • Dandelion • Devil's Claw • Fenugreek
Ginger • Ginseng • Lavender • Peppermint

Cranberry—one of three fruits originating in North America—has a long history of use as an appetite stimulant. One reason why cranberries can help restore the appetite is that they are extremely tart and are more flavorful than other, blander foods, thus stimulating the taste buds and appetite. (For more information on cranberry, see page 90.)

One of the main uses of **dandelion** root is for appetite stimulation, and this herb may have an added effect by aiding in digestion. The German Commission E (see page 16) recommends dandelion for people experiencing appetite loss. (For more information on dandelion, see page 96.)

The German Commission E (see page 16) recommends the root of **devil's claw**, a plant native to southern Africa, for people experiencing a loss of appetite. (For more information on devil's claw, see page 98.)

Fenugreek, a very popular food and spice in many parts of the world, is approved by the German Commission E (see page 16) for treating appetite loss. (For more information on fenugreek, see page 116.)

Ginger may be especially helpful for people with appetite loss caused by nausea, since this powerful herb is famous for its nausea-fighting abilities. (For more information on ginger, see page 136.)

Ginseng has a long tradition of use in Asia as an appetite stimulant. Siberian ginseng, a distant relative of American and Asian ginseng, is particularly useful for stimulating the appetite. The German Commission E (see page 16) has approved the use of Siberian ginseng to help boost the recovery from illness, and this herb may also be helpful for treating appetite loss resulting from fatigue or illness. (For more information on ginseng, see page 141.)

Peppermint and **lavender** teas are soothing to the digestive system and may help to increase appetite. (For more information on peppermint and lavender, see pages 226 and 184.)

MY SUPPLEMENT LIST—APPETITE LOSS

SUPPLEMENT	RECOMMENDED DOSAGE
Cranberry	*Fresh:* Cook fresh, organic cranberries and use as a condiment with one meal a day. *Juice:* Drink 8 to 16 oz daily. You want the tartness of cranberry to stimulate the digestive enzymes in your mouth, but if the juice is too tart, dilute it with water

SUPPLEMENT	RECOMMENDED DOSAGE
	and use stevia, instead of sugar, to sweeten it slightly. Pure cranberry juice (not sugary juices or cranberry juice cocktails) should be used for the best effect.
Dandelion	*Fresh:* You may purchase dandelion greens at selected health food supermarkets and other specialty stores. Sauté or braise the greens to stimulate appetite. *Capsule:* Take 200 to 500 mg of powdered 4:1 extract of dandelion root daily in divided doses. *Juice:* Take 1 or 2 tsp of fresh dandelion leaf juice daily. *Tea:* Steep 1 to 2 tsp of dried dandelion root in 1 cup of water for 15 minutes, and drink daily.
Devil's Claw	*Capsule:* Take up to 1,000 mg three times daily of a preparation standardized to contain 3% iridoid glycosides or 50 mg harpogoside. *Tea:* Take ¼ teaspoon of dried tuber and steep in boiling water for 15 minutes.
Fenugreek	*Fresh:* Eat 6 g of crushed or cut fenugreek seeds or sprouts daily. Beware that the seeds may be bitter, and some people prefer fenugreek in capsule form. *Capsule:* Take 1,200 mg three times a day.
Ginger	*Fresh:* Eat 2 to 4 g of fresh root daily to treat nausea and indigestion. Or chew a one quarter-of-an-ounce piece of fresh ginger to alleviate nausea and stimulate appetite. *Ale:* Drink ginger ale as needed to calm a queasy stomach and stimulate appetite. Be sure to buy a natural ginger ale product as most varieties of ginger ale do not contain any ginger. Another way to take ginger is to press out the juice using a garlic press. Take 1–2 tbsp as needed. Be careful because the juice will be very strong. It might be necessary to dilute it in water.
Ginseng	*Capsule:* Take 100 to 200 mg of solid Asian or American ginseng extract, standardized to contain eleutherosides B and E, three times daily. Or simmer 3–9 g of dried root in 2 cups of water for 30–45 minutes, strain and drink. Discard the boiled root.
Lavender	*Tea:* Steep 1–2 tsp of dried flowers or one teabag in 1 cup of boiling water for 5–10 minutes. Drink up to 3 cups daily.
Peppermint	*Tea:* Steep 1 or 2 tsp or teabags of dried peppermint leaf in 8 oz of hot water for 5 minutes. Drink as needed.

ASTHMA

THE AVERAGE PERSON TAKES 20,000 breaths each day. Just imagine taking a majority of those breaths through a drinking straw, and you will have some idea of how an asthma attack feels. Although most people don't give much thought to breathing, a person with asthma may find this simple act difficult, frightening, and in some cases even impossible. The number of people with asthma in the United States has doubled in the past 15 years, accounting for 1.8 million emergency-room visits annually.

WHAT IS IT?

Asthma is a chronic lung disease that may be caused by a number of different factors. Some people have asthma attacks because of a reaction to allergens, including pollen, animal dander, and debris left from cockroaches and dust mites. In other cases, irritants such as cold air, physical exertion, emotional stress, tobacco smoke, chemical fumes, and weather changes may trigger an asthma attack.

No matter what the irritants, bronchial tubes become inflamed and constricted, causing an overproduction of mucus. This reduces the airflow through the lungs, making breathing difficult. Symptoms of an asthma attack include coughing, wheezing, shortness of breath, and chest pain.

The best way to prevent asthma attacks is to find their causes, or "asthma triggers," and to either avoid them or ask your doctor how you can best manage them. Quitting cigarette smoking is an important way to prevent and reduce asthma attacks. Many prescription medications are available for treating and managing asthma, and certain nutritional supplements may reduce the severity of asthma attacks and make breathing easier. Under no circumstances, however, should anyone who is taking a prescription medication for asthma ever replace it with a supplement.

WHAT SHOULD I TAKE?

Asthma is a potentially life-threatening disease. Make sure to consult your doctor before taking any type of supplement, especially if you have been diagnosed with asthma or think you may have asthma.

The Asthma-Melatonin Connection

A recent study published in *The Journal of Allergy and Clinical Immunology* suggests that an increase in melatonin levels in the body may have a role in creating nighttime or nocturnal asthma.

Many people with nocturnal asthma experience increased airway inflammation during sleep. Melatonin was suspected as a possible culprit in this problem, since the levels of this sleep-inducing chemical increase at night. The study described in

The Journal of Allergy and Clinical Immunology compared the lung function of various patients with nocturnal asthma with that of healthy patients and people with non-nocturnal asthma. The study found that peak melatonin levels were higher in the patients with nocturnal asthma than in the healthy control group. Furthermore, as levels of melatonin rose, lung function fell.

Although more research is needed about this issue, it may be wise to steer clear of melatonin supplements if you have nocturnal asthma.

Boswellia • Coenzyme Q10 • Cordyceps • Eucalyptus
Magnesium • Omega-3 Fatty Acids • Quercetin • Selenium
Vitamin C • Vitamin E

Because of its anti-inflammatory properties, **boswellia** may help to relieve symptoms of asthma. In a small study involving 80 people with mild asthma symptoms, boswellia helped to reduce the frequency of asthma attacks and also increased breathing capacity. In a double-blind, placebo-controlled, crossover study, 70 percent of patients with asthma showed improvement with a boswellia supplement, experiencing less difficulty in breathing, reduced wheezing, and a reduced number of asthma attacks. (For more information on boswellia, see page 52.)

Two small studies found that **Coenzyme Q10** levels are decreased in persons with asthma. While no study has yet been performed to see if supplemental COQ10 will help treat asthma, there is no harm in using this supplement while taking conventional asthma medication. (For more information on Coenzyme Q10, see page 80.)

Cordyceps—a wild mushroom that is now grown primarily on soybeans and other nutrient sources—has been used for centuries in traditional Chinese medicine to protect the lungs and treat asthma. Although cordyceps has not been well studied in the United States, one small study showed that a supplement containing cordyceps (CordyMax, by Pharmanex) significantly increased oxygen intake. (For more information on cordyceps, see page 88.)

Eucalyptol—the active ingredient in **eucalyptus**—may work as an anti-inflammatory agent to help reduce symptoms of asthma. One preliminary study, conducted on people who had asthma that required steroid drug treatment, showed that those who were given eucalyptol were able to considerably reduce their dosage of steroid medication. (For more information on eucalyptus, see page 111.)

Studies show that people with asthma who have adequate intakes of **magnesium** may experience better lung function as well as a reduction in overall wheezing than those who do not get adequate amounts of this mineral. Not only may magnesium prevent asthma, but animal studies have indicated that magnesium may block the release of histamine in the body, thus causing fewer allergic reactions. (For more information on magnesium, see page 203.)

While studies have shown that people with asthma may benefit from diets with a low content of omega-6 fatty acids, supplementation with **omega-3 fatty acids** may help reduce inflamed airways and thus reduce the overall number of asthma attacks. (For more information on omega-3 fatty acids, see page 221.)

Quercetin is a flavonoid that may limit the amount of inflammatory chemicals (such as histamine) unleashed in the body during an allergic reaction. As a result, quercetin may reduce allergy-related inflammation in the airways and may be beneficial to people with asthma. (For more information on quercetin, see page 236.)

Studies indicate that a deficiency in the mineral **selenium** may increase the risk of inflammatory processes in asthma. Several studies indicate that selenium supplementation may enable people with steroid-dependent asthma to reduce their dosage of steroid medication. (For more information on selenium, see page 253.)

Antioxidants may have a positive effect in reducing the symptoms and occurrence of asthma. In Britain, population-based studies have been conducted to see whether a declining intake of antioxidants in the British population was a cause of an increase in asthma frequency.

Results revealed that a decreased intake specifically of the antioxidants **vitamins C** and **vitamin E** was a possible cause for the prevalence of asthma and asthma-related symptoms such as wheezing; however, a recent U.S. study did not find a correlation between people with asthma and antioxidant deficiency.

Other studies have shown that vitamins C and E may be particularly helpful in decreasing symptoms of asthma caused by environmental pollutants. (For more information on vitamins C and E, see pages 284 and 292.)

MY SUPPLEMENT LIST—ASTHMA

SUPPLEMENT	RECOMMENDED DOSAGE
Boswellia	*Tablet:* Take 300 to 400 mg three times a day of a standardized extract that contain 37.5% boswellic acids.
Coenzyme Q10	Take 50 mg per day, with meals.
Cordyceps	*Capsule:* Take 5 to 10 g daily to increase the body's ability to use oxygen. This amount may be taken in decoction, pill, or powder form.

	MY SUPPLEMENT LIST—ASTHMA
SUPPLEMENT	**RECOMMENDED DOSAGE**
Eucalyptus	*Inhalant:* Add 2 or 3 drops of eucalyptus oil to hot water or the water in a vaporizer. Deeply inhale the steam or vapor. *Topical—Oil:* Rub several drops of essential eucalyptus oil onto the chest daily.
Magenesium	*Capsule or Tablet:* Take 300 mg two or three times daily. *Note:* Take magnesium in the form of magnesium glycinate to avoid loose stools. Large amounts of magnesium can cause diarrhea; if this becomes a problem for you, reduce your dosage.
Omega-3 Fatty Acids	*Fish Oil—Capsule:* Studies conducted on children with asthma found that dosages of 300 mg daily of a fish oil supplement containing 84 mg eicosapentaenoic acid (EPA) and 36 mg docosahexaenoic acid (DHA) yielded positive results. Consult your doctor before taking fish oil supplements to determine an appropriate dosage for you.
Quercetin	*Capsule:* Take 200 to 500 mg two or three times daily.
Selenium	*Tablet:* Take 200 mcg daily.
Vitamin C	*Capsule or Tablet:* Take 250 to 500 mg twice a day. *Note:* Be sure to use a buffered form of vitamin C. If taking vitamin C causes loose stools, decrease the dosage and then gradually increase the dosage as tolerated.
Vitamin E	*Capsule:* Take 400 IU daily of a natural formulation that contains d-alpha tocopherol and mixed tocopherols.

ATTENTION DEFICIT HYPERACTIVITY DISORDER

LOOK AROUND A TYPICAL SCHOOL classroom and you'll find plenty of energetic kids: Class clowns pulling a prank, fidgety playground athletes itching to get outside, and chatterboxes passing scribbled notes. But according to the National Institutes of Health (NIH), odds are good that in an average classroom in America, at least one child has the condition called attention deficit hyperactivity disorder (ADHD).

WHAT IS IT?

ADHD is the most commonly diagnosed disorder of childhood, and the U.S. government estimates that nearly 2 million American children have this disorder. It is three times more common in boys than in girls. Moreover, from one-third to two-thirds of all children with ADHD continue to show symptoms of this condition well into adult life, although ADHD is traditionally underrecognized and undertreated in adults.

ADHD is marked by three main characteristics: *inattention*, or trouble staying focused on the task at hand; *hyperactivity*, typified by extreme restlessness and trouble with sitting still; and *impulsivity*, or difficulty in curbing the urge to immediately say or do things that come to mind, however inappropriate. While the cause of ADHD is unknown, evidence suggests that genetics and neurological factors may play a role in its occurrence.

WHAT SHOULD I TAKE?
Ginkgo Biloba (Ginkgo) • Ginseng
Magnesium • Omega-3 Fatty Acids • Valerian

Ginkgo and **ginseng** were shown in a 2001 study to have some promise in treating ADHD. The researchers who conducted this study gave a supplement that combined extracts of American ginseng and ginkgo to 36 children with ADHD. After a month of treatment, the results were impressive enough to warrant the researchers to recommend further exploration into the use of these herbs for treating ADHD. (For more information on ginkgo and ginseng, see pages 138 and 141.)

Critics Object to Large Number of Medicated Kids with ADHD

Did You Know?

According to the National Institute of Mental Health, doctors wrote 6 million prescriptions for stimulant medications (often used to treat Attention Deficit Hyperactivity Disorder [ADHD]) for children and teenagers in 1996, including Ritalin (methyl-phenidate), a medication commonly prescribed for ADHD.

Critics argue that doctors are too quick to diagnose ADHD in children and to hastily prescribe medications for them even though the long-term effects of these medications are still unknown. Aside from its being habit forming, Ritalin has side effects that include nervousness, insomnia, and headaches. There are ways to treat ADHD other than with Ritalin. Many people find that psychotherapy, in which a psychologist or therapist works with an affected child and his or her family so that they can learn to recognize and change troublesome behaviors, is a safe, prescription-free alternative to dealing with ADHD.

Experts often advise that treatment for ADHD should include structured classroom management, parent education (to address discipline and behavior limits), and tutoring and/or behavioral therapy. Some studies show that children with ADHD have allergies to milk, wheat, and sugar. Avoiding these foods and replacing them with other, high-quality organic foods may help children with ADHD to perform better in school and at home.

Be sure to discuss your treatment plans with your child's doctor so as to integrate and coordinate all aspects of his or her treatment.

Magnesium is often in short supply in many children's diets, and a deficiency of this mineral may play a role in some cases of ADHD. One study of this possible connection found that nearly all of the children in the study group were deficient in magnesium. Other research has found that children with ADHD who took supplemental magnesium for 6 months showed more improvement in their behavior than those who didn't take the supplement. (For more information on magnesium, see page 203.)

A deficiency of **omega-3 fatty acids** may play a role in some children's behavioral problems. One study found that boys who had less omega-3 fatty acids in their bodies demonstrated more problems with their behavior and didn't process information as well as boys with normal levels of these nutrients. (For more information on omega-3 fatty acids, see page 221.)

People have been using **valerian** for centuries to ease jitteriness and help induce sleepiness. Valerian may also be useful in reducing hyperactivity in children with ADHD. (For more information on valerian, see page 272.)

MY SUPPLEMENT LIST—ATTENTION DEFICIT HYPERACTIVITY DISORDER

SUPPLEMENT	RECOMMENDED DOSAGE
Ginkgo and Ginseng	*Capsule:* Take a combination product containing 50 mg of standardized ginkgo extract and 200 mg of Asian or American ginseng extract twice daily.
Magnesium	*Capsule (Children under age 3):* Take 40 to 80 mg. *(Children ages 4 to 6):* Take 120 mg daily. *(Children ages 7 to 10):* Take 170 mg daily. *(Adolescent boys):* Take 270 mg daily. *(Adolescent girls):* Take 280 mg daily.
Omega-3 Fatty Acids	*Flaxseed Oil:* Add 1 tsp of flaxseed oil to your child's food each day. The oil can be mixed into oatmeal, drizzled over a salad, or hidden creatively in other foods. *Fish Oil:* Take 300 to 600 mg daily of a supplement containing more docosahexaenoic acid (DHA) than eicosapentaenoic acid (EPA) divided into three doses with meals.
Valerian	*Capsule or Tablet:* The dose of valerian is calculated from the standard dose for a 150-lb adult. The adult daily dosage is 150 to 300 mg of valerian extract or one-half to 1 tsp of fluid extract. A 50-pound child would get one-third of that amount. *Note:* The strength of valerian products may vary greatly. Choose a standardized product and carefully follow the instructions. Valerian may also be found in prepared teas with other herbs, which mask the unusual taste.

AUTOIMMUNE DISORDERS

YOUR IMMUNE SYSTEM NORMALLY attacks unfriendly invaders such as viruses and bacteria and cancer cells that develop within the body itself, destroying them or limiting the harm that they can cause. Sometimes, however, the cells of your immune system get confused and attack parts of your own body. The outcome may be a disorder, known as an *autoimmune disorder,* that can destroy tissues and even organs, resulting in serious illness. Exactly why this happens remains a mystery. You might have particular genes that increase your risk of developing an autoimmune disorder, which then begins after you're exposed to something in your environment, such as a virus, drug, or chemical. Sometimes even pregnancy triggers an autoimmune disorder.

WHAT IS IT?

A number of autoimmune disorders are discussed in separate chapters in this book. These include rheumatoid arthritis (see page 574), type 1 diabetes (see page 410), psoriasis (see page 569), and multiple sclerosis (see page 538), all of which are well-known diseases.

Lupus is another well-known autoimmune disorder. The most common form of lupus is called *systemic lupus erythematosus* (SLE) and affects different people differently, striking the brain, joints, kidneys, lungs, heart, or skin, depending on the path the disease takes. Common symptoms of SLE include a distinctive butterfly-shaped rash across the nose and cheeks, sensitivity to sunlight, sores on the skin or inside the mouth, and painful joints. Symptoms of lupus can appear periodically throughout life, often causing fatigue and aching. Although the cause of lupus is unknown, doctors believe that heredity, hormones, and environmental factors may play a role.

Scleroderma is probably best known for causing tightness and hardening of the skin, but it can also damage internal organs. This condition occurs when the body produces an excess amount of collagen, although doctors are still unsure about why this happens. Scleroderma is a progressive disease, often beginning with dry patches of skin and resulting in eventual scarring of the skin and connective tissue. Other symptoms of this condition include Raynaud's phenomenon, pain in the joints, stiffness, and swollen hands and feet. Scleroderma can also cause digestive problems, specifically in the esophagus and intestines, making it hard for the body to properly absorb nutrients. People with scleroderma should consult a doctor about taking a multivitamin in order to provide the body with nutrients that might otherwise be hard to obtain from foods because of absorption problems.

Supplements are not recommended as a first line of treatment in autoimmune disorders. They may prove helpful, however, if used in conjunction with your treatment and with your doctor's advice.

WHAT SHOULD I TAKE?

Autoimmune disorders are serious conditions. Make sure to consult your doctor before taking any type of supplement, especially if you have been diagnosed with an autoimmune disorder or think you may have an autoimmune disorder.

Cordyceps (for lupus) • *Dehydroepiandrosterone* (DHEA; for lupus)
Gotu Kola (for scleroderma) • *Omega-3 Fatty Acids* (for lupus)
Selenium (for lupus and scleroderma)
Vitamin A (for lupus) • *Vitamin B$_{12}$* (for lupus)
Vitamin C (for lupus and scleroderma)

Preliminary studies suggest that **cordyceps**—a Chinese mushroom grown on soybeans—may prevent the recurrence of lupus nephritis, a condition caused by SLE. Studies also indicate that cordyceps may protect kidney function, which is helpful for lupus nephritis, because the condition causes kidney inflammation. (For more information on cordyceps, see page 88.)

DHEA is a hormone produced by the adrenal glands. In research conducted at the Stanford University Medical Center, 28 women with SLE took either DHEA or a placebo for 3 months. Those who took the hormone showed improvements on a standard scale used for assessing SLE and also in their own and physician assessments of their condition. Several other studies have shown that DHEA reduces the symptoms and frequency of lupus flare-ups. DHEA may also be useful in reducing the side effects of the corticosteroid medications that are often prescribed to people with SLE. (For more information on DHEA, see page 100.)

Supplements containing **gotu kola** are typically used for disorders involving connective-tissue damage, such as scleroderma and some types of arthritis. Several studies have tested gotu kola's effects on scleroderma. In some people this herbal supplement has reduced skin hardness, eased joint pain, and improved the ability to move the fingers. (For more information on gotu kola, see page 153.)

Although **omega-3 fatty acids** are often recommended to people with rheumatoid arthritis, early studies suggest that fish oil containing omega-3 fatty acids may be useful for SLE because of the anti-inflammatory effects of this supplement. It is not, however, useful for people with lupus nephritis. (For more information on omega-3 fatty acids, see page 221.)

Damage by the wayward cell- and tissue-damaging molecules known as free radicals plays a significant role in lupus. Several studies suggest that supplementation with antioxidants such as **vitamin C** (see also below), **vitamin E**, and **selenium** may help speed healing of the rashes and other effects that occur in lupus, in addition to protecting the heart, blood vessels, joints, skin, and other areas that can be damaged by the inflammatory process of this disease. Other studies show that the body's content of selenium may be low in scleroderma. (For more information on vitamins C and E and selenium, see pages 284, 292, and 253.)

Studies comparing blood samples from people in whom SLE was diagnosed with those of healthy people found that levels of **vitamin A** and beta carotene were significantly lower in those with SLE. In a study in which women with SLE were given high doses of vitamin A (100,000 IU daily for 2 weeks), the results showed an increased immune response, with no significant side effects and good tolerance of these doses of vitamin A. Although a vitamin A deficiency may worsen symptoms of SLE, high doses of this vitamin can be dangerous and are not recommended unless taken under the close supervision of a doctor. (For more information on vitamin A, see page 274.)

I've heard that hair dye treatments can cause flare-ups of lupus. Should I stop dyeing my hair if I have lupus?

There is a common belief that hair dye can aggravate lupus, causing flare-ups, but a small amount of research discounts this as a myth. A study at Harvard Medical School found that hair dye was not related to the risk of SLE; and a 2-year study of 91 women with SLE and 22 with cutaneous lupus (CL), conducted in Spain, found no significant differences in the severity of lupus symptoms between those who did not use hair dyes, used permanent hair dyes, or used non-permanent hair dyes.

Although definitive conclusions cannot be drawn from such small sample groups, keep in mind that foreign chemicals and toxins (such as hair dye) may put an additional burden on an already compromised immune system. And look out for additional studies that may shed more light on the effects of hair dye on lupus.

Vitamin B$_{12}$ may need to be added in people with lupus, since studies have found much lower levels of this important nutrient in patients with SLE than in healthy individuals. (For more information on vitamin B$_{12}$, see page 282.)

A 4-year study of female patients with SLE showed that **vitamin C** may prevent flare-ups of the disease, thus keeping it in remission. Other studies show that people with scleroderma have low levels of vitamin C and may benefit from supplementation with this vitamin. (For more information on vitamin C, see page 284.)

MY SUPPLEMENT LIST—AUTOIMMUNE DISORDERS

SUPPLEMENT	RECOMMENDED DOSAGE
Cordyceps	*Capsule:* Take 5 to 10 g daily. This amount may be taken in decoction, pill, or powder form.
DHEA	DHEA should be taken only under the supervision of a doctor. The ideal dose and long-term effects of this supplement are unknown.
Gotu Kola	*Capsule:* Standardized extract containing up to 100% total saponins (triterpenoids), 60 mg once or twice per day. Take a 2-week break from the herb after using it for a 6-week period. *Tea:* Make a tea by steeping 1 teaspoon or teabag of dried herb in a cup of boiling water for 10 minutes, and drink. Drink a half cup three times daily.
Omega-3 Fatty Acids	*Oral:* Take 3–5 g of omega-3 fatty acids per day, in divided doses, with meals. The amount of omega-3 fatty acid will vary by manufacturer, so be sure to check the product label carefully.
Selenium	*Tablet:* Take 100 to 200 mcg daily.
Vitamin A	*Tablet:* Take 15,000 to 25,000 IU daily.
Vitamin B$_{12}$	*Tablet:* Take 10 to 25 mcg daily.
Vitamin C	*Capsule or Tablet:* Take 500 to 1,000 mg daily. *Note:* Be sure to use a buffered form of vitamin C. If taking vitamin C causes loose stools, decrease the dosage and then gradually increase the dosage as tolerated.

BACK PAIN

IF YOU HAVE A BACK, odds are *very* good that it will someday be hurting. The back is the second most common site of pain in the body, and back pain is the second most common reason that people visit a doctor. Eight of 10 adults will have back pain at some point in their lives, most likely in their lower back.

Sometimes the pain will flare up for no apparent reason. At other times, back pain may occur after periods of stress, a day of heavy lifting, vigorous exercising, or simply sitting in an office chair for one hour too many.

WHAT IS IT?

The back is a highly intricate structure, containing a stack of bony vertebra interspersed with soft discs that offer cushioning and flexibility. These parts are held together by a collection of muscles, ligaments, and tendons. Considering its complexity (there are also many pain-sensing nerves in the back), it's not surprising that plenty can go wrong with the back.

Back pain may range from a nagging ache to a sharp pain that makes it hard to move around. Frequently, back pain is caused by a muscle spasm or strained ligament. Another cause is that the disc between vertebrae ruptures and presses on nerves. Other potential causes of back pain include obesity (which puts extra strain on the back); habitually using improper posture while sitting and walking; lifting heavy objects improperly; and sustaining injuries during exercise or sports. And according to doctors at New York University Medical Center, as many as 90 percent of chronic back pain cases are caused by anxiety, anger, or internalized stress.

Getting Off Your Back!

Healthy Hints

The best way to prevent recurring back pain is to strengthen the muscles in and around your back. Tempting as it may be to lie in bed, the reality is that exercise and stretching are probably your best tools in the battle against back pain.

■ **Don't slouch.** Good posture not only makes for a good impression, it could also lead to a pain-free back. Do as your mother told you: sit and stand tall, and hold your shoulders back and your head up.

■ **Reach for the sky.** Stretching is a quick and easy way to prevent back pain. Always stretch your back before doing any type of strenuous activity, and if you sit at a desk or in your car for extended periods, stand up and stretch your spine once each hour. This movement will pump fluid back into your spinal disks, easing discomfort.

■ **Get a six-pack.** Your abdomen supports your back, so if your stomach muscles are weak, your back will feel strained and sore. Daily exercises to improve the strength in your abdomen will promote a stronger, healthier back.

■ **Ask and you shall receive.** Your doctor or physical therapist can recommend the best type of back-strengthening exercises for you. In a study published in the medical journal *Spine,* Finnish researchers determined that regular exercise to increase back flexibility and mobility, such as swimming, walking, and yoga, was very beneficial to those experiencing mild back pain.

Thus, managing stress and anxiety can be an important aspect of reducing chronic back pain.

In addition to these causes, pain in the lower back, also known as "spinal arthritis," can be caused by arthritis in the facet joints (parts of the bony vertebrae of the spine that both limit and allow motion). If you have back pain caused by spinal arthritis, refer to the section of this book on osteoarthritis (page 547).

WHAT SHOULD I TAKE?
Bromelain • Calcium • Devil's Claw
Magnesium • Valerian • Willow Bark

Bromelain contains enzymes derived from pineapples, and is a supplement often used for treating injured, inflamed muscles and ligaments. It reduces swelling and inflammation and has been shown in research studies to work as well as aspirin for strains, specifically in people recovering from exercise-induced injuries and surgery. (For more information on bromelain, see page 54.)

Calcium is a mineral that works in conjunction with magnesium (see page 203) to ensure that your muscles work properly, without cramping. Calcium is also important for maintaining strong bones and preventing osteoporosis, another common cause of back pain. (For more information on calcium, see page 57.)

Devil's claw may reduce the pain and inflammation associated with back problems, specifically in the lower back. A recent study comparing an extract of devil's claw with the prescription non-steroidal anti-inflammatory (NSAID) medication rofecoxib (Vioxx) found that devil's claw was equal in effect to the prescription NSAID. (For more information on devil's claw, see page 98.)

Magnesium in adequate amounts helps ensure that your muscles—including those in your back—contract and relax properly, without developing painful cramps. (For more information on magnesium, see page 203.)

Valerian is a supplement well known for promoting relaxation and thus may be helpful for reducing back pain caused by stress or anxiety. (For more information on valerian, see page 272.)

Willow bark contains an ingredient called salicylic acid that's very similar to the active ingredient in aspirin. One study found that people who took willow bark for lower back pain had more pain relief than people who took a placebo (an inactive substance). (For more information on willow bark, see page 298.)

FRIENDS AND FOES

Avoid combining **willow bark** with medications that reduce blood clotting, such as aspirin, nonsteroidal anti-inflammatories such as Celebrex, ibuprofen (Motrin, Advil), and naproxen (Aleve, Naprosyn), clopidogrel (Plavix), heparin, pentoxifylline (Trental), ticlodipine (Ticlid), or warfarin (Coumadin), since it may contribute to the anticlotting effects of these medications and increase the risk of potentially dangerous bleeding.

MY SUPPLEMENT LIST—BACK PAIN

SUPPLEMENT	RECOMMENDED DOSAGE
Bromelain	*Tablet:* Take 300 to 600 mg three times daily between meals. Look for a product containing 2,400 gelatin-dissolving units (GDU) or 3,600 milk-clotting units (MCU) per gram.
Calcium	*Capsule or Tablet:* Take 1,500 to 2,000 mg daily in the form of calcium citrate in 500-mg doses.
Devil's Claw	*Capsule:* Take 800 to 1,000 mg up to three times daily of an extract standardized to contain 3% iridoid glycosides or 50 mg of harpagoside total.
Magnesium	*Tablet:* Take 400 mg twice daily. *Note:* Take magnesium in the form of magnesium glycinate to avoid loose stools. Large amounts of magnesium can cause diarrhea; if this becomes a problem for you, reduce your dosage.
Valerian	*Capsule or Tablet:* Take an extract containing the equivalent of 2–3 g of crude herb, up to three times per day, as needed. A slighty higher dose may be taken at night, if the low back pain causes difficulty sleeping. *Note:* The strength of valerian products may vary greatly. Be sure to choose a standardized product and carefully follow the instructions on the label.
Willow Bark	*Capsule:* Take an extract standardized to contain 60 to 240 mg of salicin daily. *Caution:* Do not use willow bark if you have an aspirin allergy, bleeding disorder, diabetes, or a peptic ulcer.

BRONCHITIS

THINK OF ACUTE BRONCHITIS as a Hollywood movie entitled The Cold Virus, Part II. Like a sequel you didn't really want to see, a common cold can sometimes progress to acute bronchitis. Chronic bronchitis, on the other hand, most often strikes smokers, although it is also common in people who work around areas of heavy dust and fumes. Whatever the cause, bronchitis can make breathing painful and difficult, and make you feel as though there is a heavy weight resting on top of your chest.

WHAT IS IT?

Bronchitis occurs when the walls lining your bronchial tubes (the main passageways of air through your lungs) become inflamed, often as the result of a virus. Swelling and fluid accumulation usually occur as your body fights the virus.

The two types of bronchitis are *acute bronchitis* and *chronic bronchitis*. Bouts of acute bronchitis often last for a few days without having any damaging effects. Since the cause is usually viral, antibiotics will not help; rather, the illness must run its course naturally. A cough resulting in yellow-gray or green mucus is one of the most common signs of bronchitis. Other symptoms include wheezing, shortness of breath, and soreness or constriction in the chest.

Chronic bronchitis results from long-term irritation in the bronchial tubes. The tubes become thick and mucus-filled, setting the stage for frequent infection and constant, persistent coughing.

WHAT SHOULD I TAKE?

Astragalus • Bromelain • Coenyme Q10 • Echinacea • Garlic Goldenseal • L-Carnitine • Licorice N-Acetylcysteine (NAC) • Slippery Elm • Vitamin C

Studies show that because of its numerous components, which include flavanoids, polysaccharides, triterpene glycosides, amino acids, and trace minerals, **astragalus** may be useful in strengthening and enhancing the immune system. As a result, astragalus may benefit people with bronchitis. (For more information on astragalus, see page 35.)

Bromelain—an enzyme derived from pineapples—is useful for a variety of upper respiratory infections. It decreases bronchial secretions and acts as a cough suppressant, possibly by decreasing inflammation in the airways. (For more information on bromelain, see page 54.)

Coenzyme Q10 may be useful in the treatment of chronic bronchitis and chronic obstructive pulmonary disease (COPD) because of its effects on muscular energy metabolism. (For more information of this enzyme, see page 80.)

Echinacea is a popular herb for reducing the symptoms and length of upper respiratory tract infections. It may also help stimulate the immune system and fight off viruses. (For more information on echinacea, see page 107.)

Garlic may help speed up recovery time from bronchitis because of its antibiotic properties. (For more information on garlic, see page 135.)

Goldenseal has traditionally been used to treat bronchitis and more recently has become a popular cold remedy. It has earned the nickname "king of the mucous membranes" because of its ability to reduce inflammation in the lungs and soothe mucous membranes. (For more information on goldenseal, see page 151.)

KITCHEN TIPS

STEAM FOR EASY BREATHING

If you're having trouble breathing, try a steam inhalant. Boil water in a pot on the stove, remove the pot from the stove, and inhale the steam with a towel draped both over your head and the pot in order to direct the steam into your nose and mouth. (Be extremely careful not to get burned.) The steam will help open your bronchial tubes, making it easier to breathe. For extra relief, add a little eucalyptus or peppermint oil to the water, since these herbs act as expectorants, helping to break up the mucus in the lungs.

Studies show that **L-carnitine** may improve the ability to exercise of people with chronic bronchitis, by improving the efficiency of the muscles that control the lungs and other muscles. (For more information on L-carnitine, see page 256.)

The German Commission E (see page 16) recommends **licorice** for inflammation of mucous membranes, including those in the nose and throat, which often occurs in bronchitis. The World Health Organization (WHO) has also recognized the traditional use of licorice for sore throat, cough, and bronchitis. (For more information on licorice, see page 192.)

NAC is a derivative of the amino acid cysteine. It helps minimize the symptoms of chronic bronchitis by breaking up mucus and protecting lung tissue. (For more information on NAC, see page 213.)

Slippery elm is an herb derived from the inner bark of the sweet elm tree. While there have been no scientific studies on the use of this herb for cough, it is often found in herbal lozenges and other cough medicines. (For more information on slippery elm, see page 256.)

Although many large studies of the effects of **vitamin C** on the common cold show no benefit, several small studies indicate that vitamin C may prevent illness in people who are deficient in or have low dietary intakes of this vitamin. Other research shows that a low intake of vitamin C may lead to chronic bronchitis. (For more information on vitamin C, see page 284.)

MY SUPPLEMENT LIST—BRONCHITIS

SUPPLEMENT	RECOMMENDED DOSAGE
Astragalus	*Capsule:* Take a 400-mg capsule six to eight times daily in divided doses.
Bromelain	*Tablet:* Take 250 to 500 mg daily between meals. Look for a product containing 2,400 gelatin-dissolving units (GDU) or 3,600 milk-clotting units (MCU) per gram.
Coenzyme Q10	Take 50 mg per day, with food. Increase as per the direction of your physician.
Echinacea	*Capsule:* Take up to 1,200 mg daily of an extract standardized to contain 125 mg of *E. augustfolia* root and at least 3.2% to 4.8% of echinacoside. Other echinacea species, such as *E. purpurea* and *E. pallida* are also used. *Tea:* Make a tea by steeping 1 tsp (1 g) or a teabag of powdered echinacea root in a cup of hot water for 10 minutes; drink up to three times daily.
Garlic	*Fresh:* An easy way to get an effective dose of garlic is to eat one-half to 2 raw garlic cloves up to four times a day. Try chopping up the garlic and mixing it into foods, or mix it with olive oil and dip bread into it. *Capsule:* Take 900 mg of a garlic powder extract standardized to contain 1.3% allicin divided into two or three doses.

MY SUPPLEMENT LIST—BRONCHITIS	
SUPPLEMENT	**RECOMMENDED DOSAGE**
Goldenseal	*Capsule or Tablet:* Take 500 mg of a standardized extract two to three times daily. *Tea:* Make a tea by steeping one-quarter to one-half tsp or a teabag of powdered goldenseal root in a cup of hot water for 10 minutes; drink up to three times daily.
L-Carnitine	*Capsule:* Take 2 g two times daily.
Licorice	*Capsule:* Take 200 mg of a licorice-root extract standardized to contain 50 mg of glycyrrhizinic acid daily. Do not take the glycyrrhiznic acid product for longer than 1 month. *Note:* Licorice candy is made with artificial flavorings or anise and has no medicinal properties.
NAC	*Capsule:* Take 1,800 mg daily for chronic bronchitis divided into two to three doses.
Slippery Elm	*Tea:* Take 1 teaspoon of the bark powder in 8 ounces of water, allow to steep for 1 hour, drink two to three times per day.
Vitamin C	*Capsule or Tablet:* Take 500 to 1,000 mg one to two times daily. *Note:* Be sure to use a buffered form of vitamin C. If taking vitamin C causes loose stools, decrease the dosage and then gradually increase the dosage as tolerated.

BRUISES

BRUISES MAY SERVE AS REMINDERS of a wayward fastball, bumped noggin, clumsy fall, or recent blood test or surgery. Bruises may look scarey, in most cases they are no cause for alarm.

WHAT IS IT?

A bruise is a sign that tiny blood vessels have been broken, allowing blood to leak out. A fresh bruise may look black, blue, purple, or red. As your body reabsorbs the red blood cells causing the discoloration, the bruise may turn brown, green, and yellow as it fades.

As you age, you may bruise more easily from minor injuries because the protective fat layer under your skin diminishes and blood vessels become increasingly delicate. Medications and supplements that reduce blood clotting, such as aspirin and vitamin E, can also make you bruise more readily. In rare cases, bruising may signify a serious health condition such as a blood-clotting problem or blood-related disease.

WHAT SHOULD I TAKE?
Arnica • Bilberry • Bromelain • Calendula • Gotu Kola Grape Seed Extract • St. John's Wort • Tea Tree Oil • Vitamin C

Arnica may be beneficial when used topically to treat minor bruising and may speed the healing of bruises incurred from surgery. (For more information on arnica, see page 33.)

Bilberries are rich in anthocyanidins, which may strengthen the tiny blood vessels known as capillaries. In one study, patients with varicose veins and other vein problems reported decreased bruising after 2 months of taking bilberry. (For more information on bilberry, see page 44.)

Bromelain—an enzyme derived from pineapples—has been shown in studies to help bruises disappear more quickly and reduce swelling and bruising in people recovering from surgery. (For more information on bromelain, see page 54.)

Calendula (also known as marigold) is believed to have wound-healing properties (by repairing damaged tissue, in part by stimulating the production of new blood vessels). While the research is preliminary, calendula is a time-honored herbal remedy for bruises that is safe for children and the elderly when used topically. (For more information on calendula, see page 61.)

Gotu kola is more commonly used to treat varicose veins but may also play a useful role in helping heal wounds, including bruises. Gotu kola may strengthen veins and connective tissues in the body, as well as improve the blood supply to inflamed skin. (For more information on gotu kola, see page 153.)

Research indicates that **grape seed extract** (GSE)—a member of a group of flavanoids called proanthocyanidins—maintains collagen and elastin, two important proteins that help strengthen connective tissue. Studies indicate that doses of GSE as low as 100 milligrams per day may strengthen capillaries and thus minimize bruising. (For more information on grape seed extract, see page 155.)

Tea tree oil has potent antiseptic properties. Used topically, it can be helpful in healing cuts and bruises. Be careful not to apply too much undiluted oil directly to skin, since it can cause a burning sensation. (For more information on tea tree oil, see page 265.)

St. John's wort has been used for a variety of skin ailments including cuts, wounds, burns, and allergic skin conditions. Early studies show if used topically, St. John's wort may have anti-inflammatory properties. (For more information on St. John's wort, see page 262.)

Back when people didn't know much about vitamins, seafarers were plagued by a condition that resulted in weakness, bad gums, and bruising. We now call this condition "scurvy," and **vitamin C** both prevents and treats it. Even if you're not prone to hitting the high seas, you may benefit from extra vitamin C with bioflavonoids to reduce bruising. It strengthens connective tissue and helps keep blood-carrying capillaries from growing fragile. (For more information on vitamin C, see page 284.)

MY SUPPLEMENT LIST—BRUISES

SUPPLEMENT	RECOMMENDED DOSAGE
Arnica	*Topical—Tincture:* Combine 1 tbsp of arnica tincture with 1 cup of water. Soak a washcloth or piece of gauze in the mixture and apply it to bruises for 15 minutes four or five times daily.
Bilberry	*Capsule or Tablet:* Take 150 to 600 mg daily between meals of an extract standardized to contain 25% anthocyanosides, divided into two or three doses.
Bromelain	*Tablet:* Take 250 to 500 mg daily between meals. Look for a product containing 2,400 gelatin-dissolving units (GDU) or 3,600 milk-clotting units (MCU) per gram.
Calendula	*Topical—Lotion/Cream:* Apply a lotion or cream product containing calendula two or three times each day to the affected area. Follow the individual product label for application instructions.
Gotu Kola	*Oral—Capsule:* Standardized extract containing up to 100% total saponins (triterpenoids), 60 mg once or twice per day. Take a 2-week break from the herb after using it for a 6-week period. *Topical:* Gotu kola is also available in topical form to apply to your skin. Follow the product label for dosage instructions.
	Caution: Avoid taking gotu kola if you have precancerous skin changes or a history of skin cancer.
Grape Seed Extract	*Capsule:* Take 200 to 500 mg daily of an extract standardized to contain 92% to 95% oligomeric proanthocyanidins (OPCs) in divided doses between meals.
St. John's Wort	*Topical—Ointment:* Apply St. John's wort oil topically as needed. Follow individual package instructions for dosage information.
Tea Tree Oil	*Topical—Gel/Oil:* Apply 5% tea tree oil gel to affected skin daily. You may also use pure tea tree oil, which can be diluted with water—usually at a ratio of about 1 part oil to 20 parts water—to avoid sensitivity reactions. Full-strength tea tree oil (undiluted) may also be applied to affected areas with a cotton swab.
	Note: Some people are sensitive to some or all of tea tree oil's components, especially when used in too strong a dosage. Tea tree oil products should be tested on a small patch of skin in an unobtrusive area to make sure no allergic reaction occurs.
Vitamin C	*Capsule or Tablet:* Take 250 to 500 mg a day of buffered vitamin C with bioflavonoids to prevent and treat bruising. Decrease the dose if loose stools or diarrhea occurs.

BURNS

BURNS CAN RANGE IN SEVERITY from causing aggravating pain that lasts a few days to an injury that is disfiguring and perhaps life-threatening. You are probably familiar with the searing pain from a hot oven or piece of metal cookware, a steaming clothes iron, or a little too much time spent out in the sun.

WHAT IS IT?

The skin acts as a large thermometer, sensing various temperatures and protecting our internal organs from outside damage by heat and other factors. A burn is damage to the skin caused by heat or the sun or by chemicals, electrical shock, and radiation. Burns are classified into three levels of severity.

First-degree burns occur to the outermost layer of the skin. In a first-degree burn, the skin turns red and painful, and thin pieces of skin may peel off a few days after the burn occurs. Most sunburns can be categorized as first-degree burns. *Second-degree* burns penetrate the skin more deeply, causing it to blister and turn a mottled reddish-white color. *Third-degree* burns are the most severe types of burns. They damage the entire thickness of skin and may extend to the tissue below the skin.

The following supplements are intended for mild burns and sunburn, or to use on more serious burns with your doctor's approval. A word of caution: nothing should be applied topically to skin that is broken or appears infected.

WHAT SHOULD I USE?

Aloe • Bromelain • Calendula • Chamomile • Green Tea
Slippery Elm • Vitamin A • Vitamin C • Vitamin E

Its benefit in treating burns has made **aloe** (also called aloe vera) a household staple. Its thick, spiky leaves can be cut and squeezed to obtain a clear gel that may be applied directly to a burn. The gel contains components that relieve pain, inflammation, and itching, and which also improve blood circulation to the site of in-jury and discourage infection. (For more information on aloe, see page 27.)

When applied topically, **bromelain** may speed the healing process by separating burn-damaged skin from healthy skin and making dead skin easier to remove. Additionally, using bromelain cream to treat burns often prevents scar tissue from forming. (For more information on bromelain, see page 54.)

Laboratory and animal tests suggest that products containing **calendula** can help reduce inflammation and skin damage. You can find numerous skin products containing calendula at most health food stores. (For more information on calendula, see page 61.)

Studies indicate that **chamomile**, when applied topically, may work as both an anti-inflammatory and antiseptic agent. Cham-omile's apparent ability to treat wounds, burns, and skin infection is due to an ingredient called chamauzulene, which can be found in both German and Roman chamomile but is more concentrated in German chamomile. (For more information on chamomile, see page 67.)

Green tea, whether taken orally or applied topically, may have some burn-preventing benefits. Studies have found that a potent antioxidant in green tea, called epigallocatechin gallate, reduces skin inflammation and protects against damage caused by ultraviolet light, whether green tea is ingested or applied topically. (For more information on green tea, see page 157.)

Often used in herbal medicine, powdered bark from the **slippery elm** tree, when mixed with water, forms a paste that is soothing to burned skin. (For more information on slippery elm, see page 256.)

Antioxidants may play an important role in preventing burns by protecting the skin against ultraviolet rays when applied topically or taken orally. Research suggests that in addition to applying sunscreen, oral supplementation with **vitamins A**, **C**, and **E** may help reduce the risk of sunburn. The topical application of vitamins C and E may also prevent sunburn. (For more information on vitamins A, C, and E, see pages 274, 284, and 292.)

KITCHEN TIPS

HONEY MAY TAKE THE STING OUT!

While honey may not be the first line of treatment for burns—especially if other options are available—applying it to raw blisters on a burn may be a good way to keep the injury clean until you can get medical treatment. Raw, unfiltered honey may contain components that fight bacteria, and health professionals have reported its usefulness in treating burns. Preliminary research on honey's effect on burns is extremely promising. One study found that honey healed 100 percent of burns in 50 people within 15 days!

MY SUPPLEMENT LIST—BURNS

SUPPLEMENT	RECOMMENDED DOSAGE
Aloe	*Topical—Gel:* After cleaning a burn, cut an aloe leaf, squeeze out its contents, and apply them to the injured area as needed. You can also use commercially bottled aloe gel. If you use a commercially produced aloe product other than pure aloe gel, be sure that aloe gel is one of its main ingredients.
Bromelain	*Topical—Cream:* Apply a cream containing 35% bromelain in an oil base to burns as needed. Follow the individual product label for application instructions.
Calendula	*Topical—Lotion/Cream:* Apply a lotion or cream product containing calendula two or three times each day to the affected area. Follow the individual product label for application instructions.

(continued)

MY SUPPLEMENT LIST—BURNS (continued)	
SUPPLEMENT	**RECOMMENDED DOSAGE**
Chamomile	*Topical—Lotion/Cream:* Apply a lotion or cream product containing chamomile two or three times daily to the affected area. Follow the individual product label for application instructions.
Green Tea	*Oral—Capsule:* Take 125 to 150 mg three times daily. *Topical:* Use cold green tea as a wash for mild burns. *Topical—Cream:* An over-the-counter cream containing green tea extract may be useful as a sunscreen.
	Note: Do not use green tea as your only form of sunscreen, since its effectiveness has not yet been widely demonstrated.
Slippery Elm	*Topical—Paste:* Mix enough hot water with powdered slippery elm bark to make a thin paste. Let cool and apply to the affected area as needed.
Vitamin A	*Oral—Capsule:* Take 20,000 IU daily until the burn subsides.
Vitamins C and E	*Oral—Capsule or Tablet:* Taking 2 to 3 g of vitamin C and 400 IU of vitamin E daily has been shown to help reduce sunburn severity. *Topical—Cream:* Look for a sunscreen containing vitamins C and E. Follow the individual product label for application instructions.
	Note: Be sure to use a buffered form of vitamin C. If taking vitamin C causes loose stools, decrease the dosage and then gradually increase the dosage as tolerated.

BURSITIS AND TENDONITIS

SOMETIMES, THE ACTIVITIES WE LOVE the most cause us the most pain. If gardening is your passion, you may be all too familiar with the pains associated with a day of raking, squatting, or bending to plant new seedlings. And any tennis or golf enthusiast can attest to the reminder of a game well played in the form of shooting pains in the elbow.

Although in terms of exercise, the musculoskeletal system, in the form of our bones and muscles, gets most of our attention, our bursae and tendons—two members of this system that normally stay behind the scenes—become *much* more noticeable when inflammation strikes.

WHAT IS IT?

Bursitis occurs when the bursae—fluid-containing sacs that encapsulate our joints and cushion the area between bones, tendons, and muscles in the joint—become inflamed. The joints most commonly affected by bursitis are the shoulders, elbows, and hips.

Bursitis occurs when a joint is overused, directly injured, or exposed to prolonged, repeated pressure. Once treated, bursitis-related pain often goes away, although many people experience recurrent flare-ups.

Tendonitis occurs when the tendons—the connective tissue "cords" that attach muscles to bone—become inflamed. Tendonitis most often affects the shoulders, elbows, heels, and knees. It often results from the overuse, aging, or injury to these joints, although it may also be associated with certain inflammatory conditions such as rheumatoid arthritis (see page 567).

Because they frequently occur when the body's joints are overworked or stressed, both bursitis and tendonitis can be referred to as "overuse injuries." Certain repetitive movements, such as raking leaves, may cause a flare-up of these conditions.

Common symptoms of both bursitis and tendonitis include stiffness, pain, and tenderness in the affected area. Sometimes simply resting and covering the affected joint with a cloth-enclosed ice pack can help reduce the pain and inflammation of bursitis and tendonitis. The following supplements may also help to ease the pain.

WHAT SHOULD I TAKE?

Boswellia • Bromelain • Devil's Claw • Digestive Enzymes
Evening Primrose Oil • Glucosamine and Chondroitin
Omega-3 Fatty Acids • Vitamin C • Willow Bark

Pressure May Relieve Pain

Did You Know?

Since 2000 BC, acupressure has been used as a noninvasive healing practice in Asia to promote healing and ease pain. It can be considered as acupuncture without the needles: Acupressure practitioners apply pressure with their hands and fingers to specific points throughout the body. According to the philosophy of acupressure, pressing on specific pressure points on the body surface can release blocked energy and tension that is considered to cause pain, such as the pain of bursitis or tendonitis. It is also proposed that acupressure may improve blood circulation, release endorphins, and release restrictions in the connective tissue.

Acupressure uses the same pressure points as acupuncture, and the best part about acupressure is that once you learn the proper points, you can perform it on yourself!

Boswellia, which hails from India's Ayurvedic health tradition, is a supplement derived from a tree of the same name. It contains ingredients called boswellic acids that can reduce pain and inflammation in joint injuries. (For more information on boswellia, see page 52.)

Bromelain may be useful in treating sports injuries in general, including bursitis and tendonitis. A protein-digesting enzyme derived from pineapple, bromelain seems to play a role in decreasing inflammation throughout the body. (For more information on bromelain, see page 54.)

A number of **digestive enzymes** (also called proteolytic or "protein digesting" enzymes) may be useful in bursitis and tendonitis for their anti-inflammatory, pain-relieving, and water-reducing properties. Various studies comparing digestive enzymes to nonsteroidal anti-inflammatory drugs (NSAIDs), such as aspirin, have found that digestive enzymes (when taken on an empty stomach) may be equally useful for relieving pain. (For more information on digestive enzymes, see page 102.)

Germany's Commission E has approved **Devil's claw** (a plant from Africa) for the treatment of tendonitis. Two recent studies found that a daily dose of Devil's claw, standardized to 50 mg or 100 mg harpagoside, was better than placebo for short-term improvements in low back pain. (For more information of Devil's claw, see page 98.)

Several clinical studies show that **evening primrose oil** and **omega-3 fatty acids** may have anti-inflammatory properties, making them useful in the treatment of bursitis and tendonitis. (For more information on evening primrose oil and omega-3 fatty acids, see pages 115 and 221.)

Although **glucosamine** has been studied most extensively for its effects on osteoarthritis, it also has some popular use for treating bursitis and tendonitis, based on its beneficial effects on connective tissue and joint health. Animal studies suggest that glucosamine is more effective when taken together with **chondroitin**, a substance that is a component of connective tissue. While human studies have not yet confirmed this, many glucosamine/chondroitin combination supplements are sold at local health food stores. (For more information on glucosamine and chondroitin, see pages 144 and 74.)

Among its many uses, **vitamin C** is crucial for your body's production of collagen, which is an important component in strengthening connective tissue. This makes vitamin C potentially useful for treating bursitis and tendonitis. (For more information on vitamin C, see page 284.)

Willow bark has a long history as a pain reliever, and studies confirm its usefulness in relieving pain from musculoskeletal problems. Supplements made from willow bark contain ingredients similar to aspirin but don't irritate the stomach as aspirin does. (For more information on willow bark, see page 298.)

MY SUPPLEMENT LIST—BURSITIS AND TENDONITIS

SUPPLEMENT	RECOMMENDED DOSAGE
Boswellia	*Oral—Tablet:* Take 450 to 1,200 mg a day of standardized boswellia extract divided into two to three doses daily.
Bromelain	*Oral—Tablet:* Take 250 to 500 mg daily between meals. Look for a product containing 2,400 gelatin-dissolving units (GDU) or 3,600 milk-clotting units (MCU) per gram.
Devil's Claw	*Oral—Capsule:* Take up to 1,000 mg three times daily of a preparation standardized to contain 3% iridoid glycosides. *Tea:* Take 1/4 teaspoon of dried tuber and steep in boiling water for 15 minutes.
Digestive Enzymes	*Oral—Capsule:* Take 3 to 4 g of "4X pancreatin"—which contains protease, lipase, and amylase enzymes—daily divided into three doses, between meals.
Evening Primrose Oil	*Oral—Capsule:* Take 3,000 to 6,000 mg daily of an extract standardized to contain 8% to 12% gamma linoleic acid.
Glucosamine and Chondroitin	*Oral—Tablet:* Take a combination supplement containing 500 mg of glucosamine and 400 mg of chondroitin 3 times daily with meals, or take the total amount at night with dinner.
Omega-3 Fatty Acids	*Oral—Capsule:* Take 3–5 g of omega-3 fatty acids per day, in divided doses, with meals. Theamount of omega-3 fatty acid will vary by manufacturer, so be sure to check the product label carefully.
Vitamin C	*Oral—Capsule or Tablet:* Take 500 to 1,000 mg twice daily with food. *Note:* Be sure to use a buffered form of vitamin C. If taking vitamin C causes loose stools, decrease the dosage and then gradually increase the dosage as tolerated.
Willow Bark	*Capsule:* Take a standardized extract containing 120 to 240 mg of salicin daily as needed. *Caution:* Do not take willow bark if you have an aspirin allergy, bleeding disorder, diabetes, or a peptic ulcer.

CANCER PREVENTION

THE CHANCES ARE THAT YOU KNOW someone whose life has been affected by cancer. Cancer is the second leading cause of death in the United States, and one-third of all women and half of all men will battle some type of cancer in their lifetime. While we can't do much about some of the risk factors that increase our chances of getting cancer, such as genes inherited from parents, we can change many factors that increase our risk. As many as 75 percent of all cancer cases in America are caused by some environmental factor, such as smoking, diet, or sun exposure. Furthermore, about one-third of all cancer deaths are related to poor diet and poor exercise habits. With the right information, you can make lifestyle choices that will greatly increase your protection against cancer.

WHAT IS IT?

Cancer occurs when cells in a particular area of the body begin to grow in an "out-of-control" manner instead of growing normally, dividing, and then dying off, as they are supposed to do. Instead of dying, cancerous cells outlive normal cells and produce new ab-

The Fluoride Controversy

Still in Debate

In most places in the United States, drinking water is fortified with fluoride, based on the premise that fluoride improves dental health. However, over the years there has been much concern and debate about the possibility of fluoride being associated with an increased risk of cancer.

In 1991, a report released by the U.S. Public Health Service (PHS), based on a survey of more than 50 human studies conducted over a 40-year period, concluded that drinking water with fluoride does not pose any kind of detectable cancer risk to humans. The Centers for Disease Control and Prevention (CDC) released a similar report, stating that there is "no credible evidence" of an association between fluoride and the risk of cancer.

However, a recent study suggests a more complicated correlation between fluoride intake and cancer risk. In this study, which included more than 21 million people in the United States who lived in areas with fluoridated drinking water, investigators found that the association of fluoride with cancer may be specific to certain types of cancer. Although fluoride did not seem to be associated with lip cancer, melanoma, skin cancer, thyroid cancer, or prostate cancer, the prevalence of other cancers, including cancers of the colon, rectum, urinary organs, and pharynx, did seem to be linked to the presence of fluoride in drinking water.

The same researchers who conducted this study also noted that a study of rats found an association between fluoride intake and an increased risk of brain cancer, leukemia, Hodgkin's disease, and non-Hodgkin's lymphoma. This animal study concluded that the results illustrate the complicated ways fluoride acts in the body and recommended further research to determine the role of fluoride in cancer risk.

normal cells. This abnormal growth is caused by damage to the genetic material—deoxyribonucleic acid (DNA)—in the cells, which is either inherited in damaged form or damaged by environmental factors.

Cancer cells can spread from their original growths (tumors) and travel around the body (metastasize), where they form tumors in sites other than where they originated. Certain types of cancer, such as leukemia, affect the blood or other parts of the body and are not associated with tumor development. Symptoms of different types of cancer vary, but in general may include fever, fatigue, weight loss, yellowing or reddening of the skin, or itchy skin.

Various practices can help you to prevent cancer from developing in your body. Avoiding tobacco and excessive sun exposure are two ways to reduce your risk. Avoiding excessive drinking will help reduce the risk of prostate and colon cancer. Eating a healthy diet that's rich in fruits and vegetables (over 100 studies have shown that eating cruciferous vegetables, such as broccoli and brussels sprouts, will decrease your risk of cancer) and has a low content of fatty foods, meat, salt, and refined sugar can also help reduce your risk of cancer. While eating these foods is preferable to taking nutritional supplements in isolation, the following supplements may help to even further cut your risk of getting cancer.

WHAT SHOULD I TAKE?

*The following supplements should be taken to reduce the risk of developing cancer. Cancer is a life-threatening disease. Make sure to see your doctor before taking any type of supplement, especially if you have been diagnosed with cancer or think you may have cancer. **The recommendations below are not a substitute for the medical treatment of cancer.***

Calcium · Coenzyme Q10 (CoQ10) · Folic Acid
Garlic · Green Tea · Lycopene · Magnesium · Melatonin
Omega-3 Fatty Acids · Selenium · Vitamin A
Vitamin C · Vitamin D · Vitamin E

Not only may **calcium** reduce the risk of stomach cancer, but studies have found that it may have protective effects against rectal and colon cancers as well. Researchers have speculated that calcium may work to prevent cancer by binding to various acids in the bowel and preventing them from irritating the colon. However, people with prostate cancer should consider avoiding high doses of calcium supplements.

Some studies indicate that calcium may worsen prostate cancer by reducing the amount of vitamin D in the kidneys, which researchers believe may increase the risk of prostate cancer progression. (For more information on calcium, see page 57.)

Early research suggests that **CoQ10** may have a role in treating advanced breast cancer and other studies suggest that it may have a positive effect on prostate tumors. (For more information on CoQ10, see page 80.)

Studies have found that a low intake of folate and high alcohol consumption may increase the risk of colon cancer. One study found that **folic acid** (vitamin B_9) may be especially helpful for reducing cancer risk in people who have a family history of colon cancer. Another study found that women who took a multivitamin containing folic acid every day had a 75 percent decrease in their risk of developing colon cancer over a 15-year period. Other large, population-based studies have found that a low intake of folic acid may increase the risk of cervical, lung, esophageal, brain, breast, pancreatic, and especially colon cancers. (For more information on folic acid, see page 130.)

Preliminary evidence suggests that eating **garlic** may reduce the risk of cancer, particularly in the colon and stomach. In the Iowa Women's Study, women who ate significant amounts of garlic had a 30 percent less chance of developing colon cancer than those who did not. Garlic may work by inhibiting cancer growth and helping

Cartilage May Help Beat Cancer

Did You Know?

Cartilage is a type of connective tissue found in many parts of the body, including the nose, ears, and joints. The use of cow (bovine) cartilage and shark cartilage has been studied for many years for its medicinal value, including its potential as a treatment for cancer. In preliminary studies, shark cartilage has shown promise as an effective anti-cancer agent, mainly because of its ability to fight tumors. Researchers believe that shark cartilage may stage a three-pronged attack against cancer, by boosting the immune system, killing cancer cells, and preventing new blood vessels from forming, and thereby, preventing the growth of tumors.

Although a growing number of studies are testing the effectiveness of shark cartilage in treating cancer, they include only a handful of human studies, and these have had conflicting results. While cartilage may be easy to find at your local health food store—with over 40 different brand-name products available—there is no proof that the cartilage supplements currently sold have any therapeutic value. It may be best to wait until results from human studies have been established before spending money on cartilage supplements.

the immune system to tackle and destroy cancer cells. (For more information on garlic, see page 135.)

The ability of **green tea** to reduce the risk of cancer may stem from its powerful antioxidant effect, which comes from the polyphenols in the tea. Green tea may also kill cancerous cells. Preliminary studies suggest that green tea may prevent a variety of cancers from forming, including cancers of the stomach, lung, esophagus, duodenum, pancreas, liver, breast, and colon. (For more information on green tea, see page 157.)

Lycopene is the antioxidant that gives the red color to fruits such as tomatoes, watermelon, and ruby grapefruit. Research has found that eating foods with tomato sauce, such as pizza and spaghetti, may reduce the risk of prostate cancer. However, the effectiveness of taking lycopene-containing supplements is unknown, since other factors in the foods that contain this red antioxidant could play a role in its cancer-preventing effects. (For more information on lycopene, see page 197.)

Various studies have looked at the role of **magnesium** in cancer prevention. One study, of different concentrations of magnesium in drinking water, suggests that this important mineral may have protective effects against prostate and stomach cancers. Another study, of the role of diet in kidney cancer, found that a low intake of magnesium may be associated with a higher risk of this cancer. A study prompted by the finding of low rates or oral cancer in Greece found that aside from an increased intake of olive oil and fruits, magnesium may have protective effects against oral cancers. (For more information on magnesium, see page 203.)

Researchers believe that there is a connection between **melatonin** levels and the progression of cancer. Changes in melatonin levels in the body may cause stress and depression, which may in turn weaken the body's immune system, allowing cancers to progress. Early research suggests that melatonin may increase the survival rate in people with certain types of cancer. (For more information on melatonin, see page 208.)

Omega-3 fatty acids may help prevent cancer of the colon, breast, and prostate. Animal and laboratory studies have associated these fatty acids with smaller tumors and less invasive cancer cells. Human research has shown that populations that eat larger quantities of fish rich in omega-3 fatty acids have lower rates of colorectal and prostate cancer. Studies also suggest that increasing your intake of omega-3s may be especially helpful if you have recently undergone surgery for stomach cancer. (For more information on omega-3 fatty acids, see page 221.)

Studies have found an inverse relationship between **selenium** and certain types of cancers, including those of the stomach, lung, and prostate. Researchers are still trying to determine how selenium may work to prevent cancer, as well as whether taking selenium supplements is effective for this. Most of the studies so far conducted have obtained the best results with organic selenium derived from yeast. Until more research is done, it's best to take a multivita-min/mineral supplement that will supply you with the amounts of selenium your body needs. (For more information on selenium, see page 253.)

Studies indicate that a deficiency of **vitamin A** may increase the risk of precancerous changes in the body, a condition known as *metaplasia*. Maintaining adequate levels of vitamin A may be an important way to prevent this condition and thus to prevent cancer. (For more information on vitamin A, see page 274.)

A large number of studies have found that **vitamin C** may help protect against cancer, particularly of the mouth, esophagus, stomach, and pancreas. In one 13-year-long study, men with cancer had lower levels of vitamin C in their system than did healthy subjects; men with stomach cancer had the lowest levels and had eaten below-average amounts of citrus fruits. Other observational studies have shown positive results with vitamin C in reducing the risk of many other types of cancer, including cervical, colon, esophageal, rectal, breast, and lung cancer. (For more information on vitamin C, see page 284.)

Preliminary laboratory and animal studies suggest that **vitamin D** may slow the growth of tumors in the breast, prostate, and colon. One study of men with prostate cancer found that they had low levels of vitamin D. After supplementation with 2,000 International Units of vitamin D, study participants experienced a reduction in painful symptoms as well as an improved overall quality of life. (For more information on vitamin D, see page 289.)

Studies have indicated that a high intake of **vitamin E** may help prevent certain cancers, particularly breast and prostate cancer. Research involving large numbers of people suggests that diets providing high levels of antioxidants, including vitamin E, may help reduce the risk of cancer. Other studies indicate that vitamin E may protect against colon, lung, rectal, cervical, pancreatic, liver, and oral cancers. (For more information on vitamin E, see page 292.)

MY SUPPLEMENT LIST—CANCER PREVENTION

SUPPLEMENT	RECOMMENDED DOSAGE
Calcium	*Capsule or Tablet:* Take 1,200 mg of calcium citrate daily divided into two or three doses. *Note:* Do not take calcium supplements if you have prostate cancer.
CoQ10	*Softgel:* Dosages may range from 30 to 150 mg daily. If you have cancer, consult your doctor about taking higher dosages of CoQ10.
Folic Acid	*Tablet:* Take 400 mcg daily. This dosage of folic acid can be found in most multivitamins.
Garlic	*Fresh:* Eat up to 2 to 4 cloves of fresh, raw, chopped garlic daily. Mincing the garlic and swallowing it with applesauce or yogurt may make it more palatable.
Green Tea	*Tea:* Steep 1 tsp or a teabag in 1 cup of boiling water for 20 minutes. Drink 3 cups daily. *Capsule:* Take 300–400 mg of standardized green tea extract daily.
Lycopene	*Diet:* Eat five or more servings each week of foods containing tomatoes, such as tomato sauce or juice or cooked tomatoes. Cooked tomatoes appear to be more effective than raw ones for providing lycopene.
Magnesium	*Tablet:* Take 250 to 500 mg daily. This dosage can be found in most multi-vitamin/mineral supplements.
Melatonin	*Tablet:* Studies of people with cancer have used melatonin in dosages of 10 mg per day. Consult your doctor to determine whether supplementation with melatonin is appropriate for you.
Omega-3 Fatty Acids	*Diet:* Eat 2 or 3 servings of fatty fish, such as salmon and mackerel, each week. Beware of larger fish that may have an excess accumulation of mercury, such as tuna and swordfish. *Capsule:* Take 2–3 g of omega-3 fatty acids per day, in divided doses, with meals. The amount of omega-3 fatty acid will vary by manufacturer, so be sure to check the product label carefully.
Selenium	*Tablet:* Take 100 to 200 mcg of selenium daily. This dosage can be found in most multivitamin/mineral supplements.
Vitamin A	*Capsule or Tablet: (Adults 14 years and older): Male:* Take 3,000 IU daily. *Female:* Take 2,300 IU daily to meet the daily RDI. These dosages may be found in most multivitamin supplements.
Vitamin C	*Capsule or Tablet:* Take 250 to 500 mg twice daily. *Note:* Be sure to use a buffered form of vitamin C. If taking vitamin C causes loose stools, decrease the dosage and then gradually increase the dosage as tolerated.
Vitamin D	*Tablet:* Take 200 to 600 IU of vitamin D daily. Ask your doctor to perform a blood test to determine if you have a deficiency of vitamin D. If so, you may need a higher dose to correct it.
Vitamin E	*Capsule:* Take 400 IU daily of a natural product containing mixed tocopherols.

CANKER SORES

JUST BECAUSE A SORE IS SMALL doesn't mean it can't be extremely painful. While a canker sore, also known as anaphthous ulcer, won't kill you, you may be amazed at how painful such a small sore can be, especially when you're drinking orange juice or eating marinara sauce. Even though canker sores may disappear on their own, after staking a 2-week claim to your mouth, anyone suffering with this pesky sore knows that 2 weeks is just not soon enough!

WHAT IS IT?

A canker sore occurs inside the mouth, or on the on the inner lining of the lips, cheeks, tongue, or palate. It is typically either white or red and differs from cold sores, which are contagious and generally occur on the external surface of the lips.

Exactly why canker sores occur isn't completely understood, but stress, anxiety, food sensitivity, and certain acidic foods (such as citrus fruits and tomatoes) may cause them. Another cause may be injuries, such as irritating your mouth with your toothbrush while brushing, accidentally biting the inside of the mouth, or chafing caused by dentures. Many toothpastes contain a detergent called sodium lauryl sulfate. Several studies indicate that this may cause or aggrevate canker sores. So try to choose a toothpaste that does not contain this chemical. Although canker sores should be gone completely within 2 weeks, some people have worse problems with them

Keep a Journal

Healthy Hints

Although doctors haven't named a specific cause for canker sores, you may be able to figure out the source of your own "triggers" that cause canker sore outbreaks. If you experience recurring canker sores, read on for information on how to keep a diary to identify these triggers:

■ **Detail dental hygiene.** Record any changes in toothbrush, toothpaste, dental floss, or mouthwash, since changes in any of these may cause canker sores. Try using a detergent-free toothpaste that does not contain sodium lauryl sulfate (SLS) to prevent recurring canker sores.

■ **Make note of trigger foods.** It is especially smart to make note of foods likely to instigate a canker sore such as citrus or acidic foods, like oranges or tomatoes, and salty foods, like potato chips or pickles.

■ **Track your stress.** Some researchers believe that stress and anxiety may contribute to canker sores. If your life has recently taken a hectic or emotional turn, you may be at risk for canker sores.

■ **Keep a record of your sore "cycle."** For some women, it seems, canker sores may be connected to their menstrual cycle. Keeping track of your menstrual cycle may alert you as to when a canker sore will occur.

than others; in extreme cases the sores are more than one-third of an inch in size and recur often.

WHAT SHOULD I TAKE?

Goldenseal · Lactobacillus Acidophilus · Licorice
Multivitamin · Slippery Elm · Vitamin B Complex · Zinc

During the 1960s, several articles appeared in medical literature that mention using Lactobacillus acidophilus as a treatment for canker sores. Since that time, it appears little follow-up research has been done on this topic. However, if you have recurrent canker sores, this supplement is certainly worth a try. (For more information on Lactobacillus acidophilus, see page 180.)

A **licorice** product called deglycyrrhizinated licorice (DGL) may help heal canker sores. In one study, 15 of 20 people who used DGL had as much as a 75 percent improvement in their canker sore pain in a single day, with the sores disappearing by the third day. Other studies suggest that using a licorice-containing mouthwash may help against canker sores because of its anti-inflammatory properties. (For more information on licorice, see page 192.)

Herbalists use goldenseal as an oral rinse for canker sores, and recent research demonstrates that berberine found in goldenseal has antibiotic properties against several common pathogenic bacteria found in the mouth. (For more information on goldenseal, see page 151.)

A number of nutrient deficiencies may contribute to the development of canker sores, particularly deficiencies of vitamins B_1, B_2, B_6, B_{12}, and C, as well as of calcium and folic acid. Thus, a **multivitamin** supplement may be useful in treating and preventing canker sores by ensuring that your body has adequate levels of these important nutrients. (For more information on multivitamins, see page 9.)

Because its inner bark has a high content of mucilage—which turns to "goo" when mixed with water—**slippery elm** acts as a "demulcent." This means it soothes mucous membranes, which is why it may help bring relief from painful canker sores. (For more information on slippery elm, see page 256.)

Since many of the nutritional deficiencies reported in people with canker sores are from B-vitamin deficiencies, additional supplementation with **vitamin B complex** may be a smart move for people with canker sores. (For more information on vitamin B complex, see pages 277, 279, and 282.)

A study of the effect of **zinc** supplementation, conducted on 40 people with recurring canker sores, found that not only were zinc levels low in these people, but that supplementation with zinc caused recurring canker sores to disappear for 3 months. (For more information on zinc, see page 304.)

MY SUPPLEMENT LIST—CANKER SORES

SUPPLEMENT	RECOMMENDED DOSAGE
Goldenseal	Take ½–1 tsp of the powdered root in 1 cup boiling water. Let cool, and use three to four times per day as oral rinse.
Lactobacillus Acidophilus	Take 1- to 2-billion colony forming units (CFUs) per day, with meals.
Licorice	*Tablet:* Take 1 or 2 chewable DGL tablets 20 minutes before meals. Allow the tablets to mix well with your saliva to ensure maximum effectiveness. *Mouthwash:* Make licorice mouthwash by combining one-half teaspoonful of liquid extract with one-fourth of a cup of water. Use mouthwash up to four times daily. *Note:* Licorice candy is made with artificial flavorings and has no healing properties.
Multivitamin	*Tablet:* Take a multivitamin/mineral supplement every day. Follow the individual product label for dosage information.
Slippery Elm	*Lozenge:* You can find lozenges containing slippery elm in health food stores. Follow the directions on the product label.
Vitamin B Complex	*Tablet:* Take 25 to 50 mg of B-complex vitamin twice daily to prevent canker sores from recurring. Be sure that the formula you purchase has all of the essential B vitamins, including B_1, B_2, niacin, B_6, folic acid, B_{12}, and biotin.
Zinc	*Tablet:* Take 10 to 50 mg daily for one month. *Note:* When taking zinc supplements at high doses or for prolonged periods, be sure to take 2 mg daily of a copper supplement, since zinc may deplete levels of copper in the body.

CARPAL TUNNEL SYNDROME

REPETITION MAY CAUSE MORE than just boredom; if it involves your wrists and hands it may cause sharp, recurring pain in your carpal tunnels—conduits of bone and connective tissue in each wrist that enclose the "bundles" of nerves and tendons entering the hand. For many people, repeated manual tasks, including typing, gardening, carpentry, and knitting, lead to this painful syndrome. If you spend day after day using a computer or painting, you may have noticed numbness or pain shooting from your wrists all the way through your fingers—pain that may sometimes become severe enough to prevent sleep. Fortunately, proper ergonomic corrections, exercises, and supplements, can usually alleviate or prevent carpal tunnel syndrome.

WHAT IS IT?

Carpal tunnel syndrome occurs when the tendons and ligaments in the wrist become inflamed, often from overuse. The narrowed "tunnel" of bones and ligaments in the wrist begins to pinch the nerves that extend to the fingers and surrounding muscles. This can cause numbness and tingling in the hand, specifically in the pad of the thumb, index, and middle fingers, and the palm. These problems may feel worse at night.

As carpal tunnel syndrome progresses, it may weaken the grip and over time may cause muscles in the thumb to wither. If you think you have these symptoms, ask your doctor to send you to a specialist (either a Physical Medicine and Rehabilitation [Physiatrist] or a Neurologist) for an electrodiagnostic study (EMG). This is the only definitive way to know whether or not you have the condition.

People who regularly make repeated hand motions, such as those who knit as a hobby or who work on an assembly line, are at greater risk for carpal tunnel syndrome. Obesity also raises the risk for this condition, as do the hormonal changes that occur during pregnancy and menopause.

Splints for Carpal Tunnel Syndrome

Did You Know?

While the best defense against carpal tunnel syndrome is preventive action, a little extra care and some rest may help aching wrists to heal quickly. Wrists tend to twist and bend frequently during the day and night, aggravating symptoms of carpal tunnel syndrome.

An excellent first line of treatment for carpal tunnel syndrome is to immobilize the wrist with a splint. The splint is worn for several weeks to keep the hand from moving, particularly at night, when the pain of carpal tunnel syndrome is often worse. By keeping the wrist still, splints may not only ward off pain and numbness, but may also prevent further damage. You do not need a prescription or visits to a physical therapist to receive a splint; you can purchase one at your local drugstore. Most models have Velcro fasteners and are therefore easy to adjust and easy to remove before taking a bath or shower. Ask your doctor if this is the right option for you.

WHAT SHOULD I TAKE?

*Arnica • Boswellia • Bromelain • Cat's Claw • Devil's Claw
Digestive Enzymes • Glucosamine and Chondroitin • Vitamin B$_6$*

Topical **arnica** may be useful at alleviating the pain associated with carpal tunnel syndrome and also, should a corrective surgery be performed, be useful at diminishing the postoperative pain. (For more information on arnica, see page 33.)

Boswellia works as an anti-inflammatory agent and may be helpful in treating carpal tunnel syndrome. Studies have shown that boswellia has similar anti-inflammatory potency to that of non-steroidal inflammatory drugs (NSAIDs), which are prescribed for many inflammatory conditions including carpal tunnel syndrome. (For more information on boswellia, see page 52.)

Some evidence suggests that **bromelain**—an enzyme derived from pineapples—can be useful in treating carpal tunnel syndrome. In research, bromelain has reduced swelling and inflammation in injured tissues by inhibiting hormones that can cause inflammation. (For more information on bromelain, see page 54.)

Cat's claw, because of its power as an anti-inflammatory agent, may help in easing the pain associated with carpal tunnel syndrome. (For more information on cat's claw, see page 63.)

Another "claw," this time not a cat's but **Devil's claw**, may also be helpful in alleviating the inflammation of carpal tunnel. One study found Devil's claw equally as effective as Vioxx for relieving pain. (For more information on Devil's claw, see page 98.)

Digestive enzymes, when taken on an empty stomach, appear to have activity as anti-inflammatory agents. (For more information of digestive enzymes, see page 102.)

Glucosamine and **chondroitin**, when taken together, can be helpful for easing carpal tunnel syndrome as well as for alleviating arthritis in the hands. Not only do glucosamine and chondroitin work as anti-inflammatory agents, but when taken together, they may have a stronger effect than either does when taken alone. (For more information on glucosamine and chondroitin, see pages 144 and 73.)

Vitamin B$_6$ is the most commonly recommended supplement for treating carpal tunnel syndrome, but the evidence supporting it is controversial. One long-held reason for its use is that people with carpal tunnel syndrome have a deficiency of this vitamin. However, recent research indicates that there is no link between the syndrome and a B$_6$ deficiency. Complicating the issue is that taking too much of the vitamin can cause nerve damage, which might cause the hands to go numb—the very problem you're trying to stop. Yet many people have given B$_6$ a try, and a number have reported experiencing relief from carpal tunnel syndrome. Talk to your doctor to see whether this vitamin may work for you. (For more information on vitamin B$_6$, see page 279.)

MY SUPPLEMENT LIST—CARPAL TUNNEL SYNDROME

SUPPLEMENT	RECOMMENDED DOSAGE
Arnica	*Topical—Tincture:* Combine 1 tbsp of arnica tincture with 1 cup of water. Soak a washcloth or piece of gauze in the mixture and apply it the palmar surface of the wrist several times per day.
Boswellia	*Tablet:* Take 300 to 400 mg three times daily of an extract standardized to contain 70% boswellic acids between meals.
Bromelain	*Tablet:* Take 250 to 500 mg daily between meals. Look for a product containing 2,400 gelatin-dissolving units (GDU) or 3,600 milk-clotting units (MCU) per gram.
Cat's Claw	*Tea:* Add one-fourth teaspoon of cat's claw root bark to 1 cup of boiling water. Strain and drink up to twice daily. *Capsule:* Take a standard extract in the form of *Uncaria tomentosa* or *Uncaria guyanensis* one to three times daily according to the manufacturers directions.
Digestive Enzymes	*Capsule or Tablet:* Take 3–4 g in the form of 4x pancreatin daily between meals.
Glucosamine and Chondroitin	*Tablet:* Take a combination supplement containing 500 mg of glucosamine and 400 mg of chondroitin from one to three times daily, with meals or take the entire amount with dinner.
Vitamin B$_6$	*Tablet:* The usual recommended dose for treating carpal tunnel syndrome is 50 to 200 mg daily for up to 3 months.
	Note: Consult your doctor before exceeding a dosage of 100 mg of vitamin B$_6$ daily.

CATARACTS

IF YOU HAVE EVER TRIED TO LOOK through a foggy window, what you saw through it was probably very blurry. That resembles what it's like to have cataracts. In Latin, *cataracta* means waterfall—an appropriate description for a condition that may make you feel as though you're looking through a sheet of cascading water. Many people over age 65 begin to experience some level of clouding of the lens of the eye, and depending on its severity, it may interfere with daily living. However, cataracts are not an inevitable part of the aging process, and you can take many actions to reduce the risk of developing them.

WHAT IS IT?

A common misconception about cataracts is that they occur when a layer of film forms on the eye. Cataracts actually occur *inside* the eye, when the lens (the part of the eye responsible for focusing light and producing clear, sharp images) becomes cloudy. Age-related cataracts, which are the most common form of cataracts, can occur for two main reasons. Think of the lens of the eye as being contained in a sealed bag. As cells in the eye die, which is a normal part of the aging process, they become trapped within the bag. As the cells build up in the eye, they cause the lens to cloud, which in turn blurs images. Another form of cataract may affect the way in which color is perceived. Over the course of aging, the lens of the eye begins to color, and things may begin to take on a brownish hue. Over time, this tinting may lead to vision problems, making it difficult to read or see properly.

Once a cataract develops in the eye, the only real solution is surgery to replace the clouded lens with a clear lens implant. However, there are many ways to prevent cataracts from occurring in the first place. Lifestyle changes and certain dietary supplements may help to maintain clear, healthy vision for many years to come.

WHAT SHOULD I TAKE?

Alpha Lipoic Acid • Bilberry • Folic Acid • Gingko Biloba Lutein • Multivitamin • Quercetan • Selenium • Vitamin A Vitamin B₁₂ • Vitamin C • Vitamin D • Vitamin E

Preliminary research indicates that **alpha lipoic acid** (ALA), because of its power as an antioxidant, may be useful in preventing cataracts. (For more information on alpha lipoic acid, see page 29.)

Some experts believe that taking **bilberry** will help strengthen blood vessels in the eye and reduce the risk of developing cataracts. In one study of 50 people with age-related cataracts, their formation halted in 97 percent of people taking bilberry extract with vitamin E. (For more information on bilberry, see page 44.)

When the body contains inadequate levels of glutathione—one of the substances known as amino acids from which proteins are constructed—the "antioxidant defense system" in the eye can be compromised. Certain nutrients, such as **vitamin C**, **vitamin E**, and **selenium** can help increase and activate levels of glutathione in the body. Several studies have linked low levels of vitamin E to an increased risk of developing cataracts. One study showed a decreased risk when a multivitamin including vitamin C was taken for a 10-year period. Also, preliminary research suggests that levels of glutathione are low and levels of free radicals are high in populations that are deficient in selenium. (For more information on vitamins C, E, and selenium, see pages 284, 292, and 253.)

Several animal studies indicate that the antioxidant properties of **Ginkgo biloba** appear to help in the prevention of cataracts. (For more information on Ginkgo biloba, see page 138.)

Additional studies show that **folic acid** (vitamin B$_9$) and **vitamin B$_{12}$** may have protective effects against cataracts. (For more information on folic acid and vitamin B$_{12}$, see pages 130 and 282.)

Lutein is a carotenoid that can be found in abundant supply in the back of the eye, where the retina is located. Lutein may protect the eye by damage to it from free radicals, as well as absorbing and reflecting harmful UV rays that can injure the eye. (For more information on lutein, see page 195.)

Multivitamins have been shown to reduce the risk of cataracts by 20 to 60 percent. They include a host of important nutrients that may help prevent cataracts, including vitamin B$_{12}$, folate, niacin (vitamin B$_3$), and riboflavin (vitamin B$_2$). However, make sure to carefully monitor your riboflavin intake, since studies suggest that doses above 10 mg a day may actually generate free radicals that can cause cataracts. (For more information on multivitamins, see page 9.)

The antioxidant effects of **quercetan** may help prevent cataracts, although the research is still preliminary. However, eating quercetan-rich food is a great part of a healthy diet. (For more information about quercetan, see page 236.)

Studies show a reduction in cataracts in people who have adequate intakes of **vitamin A.** One study of more than 500,000 nurses showed a 39 percent reduction in cataract formation in those who had adequate intakes of vitamin A over an 8-year period. (For more information on vitamin A, see page 274.)

Along with vitamin C and selenium, studies suggest that people with healthy levels of **vitamin D** may be less likely to develop cataracts. (For more information on vitamin D, see page 289.)

MY SUPPLEMENT LIST—CATARACTS

SUPPLEMENT	RECOMMENDED DOSAGE
Alpha Lipoic Acid	*Capsule:* Take 150 mg daily.
Bilberry	*Tablet:* Take 80 mg of an extract containing 25% anthocyanidins three times daily.
Folic Acid	*Tablet:* Take 400 mcg daily. This amount of folic acid can be found in most multivitamins.
Ginkgo Biloba	Take 120–160 mg once daily of an extract standardized to contain 24% ginkgo flavone glycosides and 6% terpene lactones.
Lutein	*Capsule:* Take 6 mg of lutein per day, divided into two doses. If you have a cataract in its early stages, studies suggest that taking 15 mg daily may be useful. Note: Take lutein with fatty food to increase the body's absorption of this nutrient.
Multivitamin	Take a multivitamin/mineral supplement every day that does not contain iron. Follow the individual product label for dosage information.
Selenium	*Tablet:* Take 200 mcg of selenium daily. This amount of selenium can be found in most multivitamins.
Vitamin A	*Capsule (Adults 14 years and older):* Take 5,000 IU daily. This can be found in most multivitamins.
Vitamin B$_{12}$	*Tablet (Ages 14 and over):* Take 50 mcg daily. This can be found in most 50 mg B-complex supplements.
Vitamin C	*Capsule or Tablet:* Take 1,000 mg of vitamin C daily, divided into two doses. *Note:* Be sure to use a buffered form of vitamin C. If taking vitamin C causes loose stools, decrease the dosage and then gradually increase the dosage as tolerated.
Vitamin D	*Tablet:* Take 800 IU daily. Ask your doctor to check your vitamin D level. If you are deficient in vitamin D, a higher dose may be required.
Vitamin E	*Capsule:* Take 400 IU daily of a natural product containing mixed tocopherols.

CERVICAL DYSPLASIA

THERE AREN'T TOO MANY INSTANCES in which a cotton swab can save your life, but cervical dysplasia is definitely one of them. If you're a woman past your teenage years, you're probably familiar with the Pap smear, in which a gynecologist takes a sampling of cells from your cervix with a cotton swab or small spatula or brush. A specially trained doctor or technologist then examines those cells under a microscope. If abnormal cells are found, you should take the proper steps to keep them from becoming cancerous. These steps include letting the doctor examine your cervix with a lighted scope and perhaps removing samples of potentially troublesome tissue for further testing.

WHAT IS IT?

Cervical dysplasia refers to precancerous changes in the cervix. This diagnosis doesn't mean that dysplasia (or abnormal cells) will necessarily become cancerous, but it does warrant future attention. Furthermore, cervical cancer is one type of cancer that can be prevented through early detection, since the dysplasia that precedes this cancer is identifiable before actually reaching dangerous levels. Most mild dysplasias go away on their own within a few months or years. However, doctors may remove abnormal cells by freezing them, burning them off with a laser, or cutting them off with a heated wire loop.

In most cases, cervical cancer is the result of infection by a human papillomavirus (HPV). Having a high number of sexual partners and becoming sexually active at age 18 or younger increases your risk. Smoking increases the risk of cervical dysplasia.

The American Cancer Society recommends that all women be screened regularly for cervical cancer beginning 3 years after they start having vaginal intercourse and no later than at the age of 21 years. These screenings should take place annually or bi-annually until the age of 30, when it may be possible to have screenings every 3 years, depending on prior test results. The supplements described

What is HPV? Will condoms protect me against the transmission of this virus?

HPV, or human papillomavirus, refers to a group of more than 100 types of viruses. Many of these viruses cause warts or noncancerous tumors called papillomas. (Warts that grow on the hands or feet are also caused by a type of HPV.) Thirty types of HPV are sexually transmitted, making HPV infection one of the most common sexually transmitted diseases. Some human papillomaviruses cause visible genital warts or abnormal, flat growths in the genital area and on the cervix. Often, however, there are no symptoms of HPV infection. Because HPV is now recognized as the leading cause of cervical dysplasia, it is important that sexually active women be screened for HPV annually.

Unfortunately, condoms are not a sure defense against HPV infection. In a study published in the journal *Sexually Transmitted Diseases* in 2002, researchers reported a lack of consistent evidence that condoms, even when used properly, reduce the risk of HPV transmission.

in the following section may be useful additions to monitoring and medical treatment for preventing cervical cancer.

WHAT SHOULD I TAKE?

Cervical dysplasia can develop into a life-threatening condition. Consult your doctor before taking any supplement, especially if you have been diagnosed with cervical dysplasia or think you may have cervical dysplasia.

Folic Acid • Lycopene • Selenium • Vitamin A
Vitamin B_2 • Vitamin C • Vitamin E

For women with a high intake of alcohol, increasing **folic acid** in the diet may help prevent cervical cancer. (For more information about folic acid, see page 130.)

Research indicates that **lycopene**—abundant in tomatoes—may offer some protection against cervical dysplasia. Some studies show that lycopene has an inverse relationship to cervical dysplasia: a greater intake of lycopene may decrease your chances for developing the condition. (For more information on lycopene, see page 197.)

Research has shown that women with cervical dysplasia were deficient in the mineral **selenium**, and low levels of this mineral have been associated with a number of cancers. (For more information on selenium, see page 253.)

Studies suggest that a low intake of **vitamin A** and **vitamin B_2** (riboflavin) may put women at an increased risk for cervical dysplasia. Furthermore, preliminary evidence suggests that women who have been diagnosed with cervical dysplasia have a lower risk of developing cervical cancer if their intakes of vitamin A are adequate. (For more information on vitamins A and B_2, see pages 274 and 245.)

As antioxidants, **vitamin C** and **vitamin E** have been shown to decrease the risk of precancerous cervical changes. Besides reducing this risk, vitamins C and E may strengthen and help keep the cells lining the cervix in a normal state. (For more information on vitamins C and E, see pages 284 and 292.)

MY SUPPLEMENT LIST—CERVICAL DYSPLASIA

SUPPLEMENT	RECOMMENDED DOSAGE
Folic Acid	If you have a high alcohol intake, it may be important to eat more foods that contain folic acid. These foods include beans and legumes, citrus fruits, eggs, whole grains, dark green leafy vegetables, poultry, pork, shellfish, and liver.

MY SUPPLEMENT LIST—CERVICAL DYSPLASIA	
SUPPLEMENT	**RECOMMENDED DOSAGE**
Lycopene	*Diet:* Eat five or more servings each week of foods containing processed tomatoes, such as tomato sauce or juice, or cooked tomatoes. Cooked tomatoes appear to be more effective than raw ones for providing lycopene.
Selenium	*Tablet:* Take 100 to 200 mcg daily. This dosage can be found in most multivitamin/mineral supplements.
Vitamin A	*Capsule or Tablet:* Take 20,000 IU daily.
Vitamin B$_2$	*Tablet:* Take a B-complex vitamin with a label dose of 25 to 50 mg twice daily.
Vitamin C	*Capsule or Tablet:* Take 1,000 mg daily, divided into four doses. *Note:* Be sure to use a buffered form of vitamin C. If taking vitamin C causes loose stools, decrease the dosage and then gradually increase the dosage as tolerated.
Vitamin E	*Capsule:* Take 400 IU daily of a natural product containing mixed tocopherols.

CHRONIC FATIGUE SYNDROME AND GENERAL FATIGUE

EVEN THOUGH THE CLOCK SAYS 3 PM, your sleepy eyes and tired body insist that it's bedtime. Most of us are no strangers to this kind of fatigue. It can result from too much stress, too little sleep, lack of exercise, or poor eating habits. Fixing these problems may bring your pep and energy back in no time. The condition called chronic fatigue syndrome (CFS), however, is a much tougher nut to crack.

WHAT IS IT?

CFS is marked by profound, unrelenting fatigue that can last for many months or years. It is a poorly understood condition that can be difficult to diagnose because it shares symptoms with many other ailments. Aside from fatigue, people with CFS often report digestive complaints, depression, and a sense of being in a "mental fog."

CFS is generally believed to exist in someone who experiences at least four of the following symptoms: memory or concentration problems, sore throat, tenderness in the neck or armpits, muscle or joint pain, unsatisfying sleep, extreme tiredness that lasts for more than a full day after exercise, and unexpected severe or persistent headaches.

Although the cause of CFS is unknown, it may be linked to viral infection, immune or nervous system problems, or hormonal abnormalities. Doctors may try to help solve the condition with antidepressant medications. Gentle exercise programs are another standard recommendation for people with CFS. The following supplements may help as well.

WHAT SHOULD I TAKE?

Astragalus • Beta-Carotene • Cordyceps • Ginseng
Lactobacillus Acidophilus • L-Carnitine • Magnesium
Melatonin • Nicotinamide Adenine • Dinucleotide (NADH)
Omega-3 Fatty Acids • Rhodiola • Siberian Ginseng
Vitamin B Complex • Vitamin C

Astragalus is a well-known "Qi" tonic in traditional Chinese herbal medicine, and is typically included in formulas designed to treat fatigue. Since Chinese herbal medicine is a complex system, it might be best to seek out a qualified practitioner to aid you in selecting the proper formula to take. (For more information on astragalus, see page 35.)

Preliminary research conducted on people with reduced natural killer cells (immune-system cells that kill viruses and cancer cells) found that a majority of those who took **beta-carotene** supplements had an increase in their natural killer cells. These people also noted less fatigue. (For more information on beta carotene, see vitamin A, page 274.)

Cordyceps, another Chinese herb, was once reserved only for the elite of Chinese society, as it was very rare and expensive to produce (it is a fungus grown on a caterpillar). In modern times it has become more widely available, and ordinary people can avail them-

Positive Thinking May Help to Alleviate Chronic Fatigue

Did You Know?

A report appearing in the January 2004 issue of *The Journal of Psychosomatic Medicine* suggests that CFS may be tempered by improving mental health. To evaluate factors that might influence how individuals cope with chronic fatigue, researchers followed 100 patients with CFS for 18 months. After 18 months, about one-fifth of the patients in the study appeared to have experienced such a marked improvement that they no longer met the criteria for a diagnosis of CFS.

The difference between the patients in the foregoing study who recovered and those who did not may have been in their state of mind. The researchers found that patients who felt that their symptoms were primarily due to non-physical or emotional problems (such as stress) and who tried to make lifestyle changes to improve their overall health fared much better than those who took sedatives or muscle relaxants to alleviate symptoms. Although more research is needed to determine the exact role of mental health in CFS, studies show promise for the future treatment of this condition.

selves of the famous tonic properties attributed to cordyceps. Clincal studies have not documented these historical uses. (For more information on Cordyceps, see page 88.)

Yet a third Chinese herb, **Ginseng**, is renowned as a tonic to alleviate fatigue. A recent study indicated that ginseng might improve performance and subjective feelings of mental fatigue during sustained mental activity. (For more information about ginseng, see page 141.)

People with CFS often have low levels of "good" bacteria in their intestines. **Lactobacillus acidophilus** are a species of such "good" bacteria, and taking supplements that provide these bacteria may boost the immune system of people with CFS. (For more information on Lactobacillus acidophilus, see page 180.)

L-carnitine is an amino acid used in producing energy for muscles, and a deficiency of it can cause you to become weak and fatigued. Research has shown that some people with CFS have significantly low carnitine levels and may benefit from supplementation with this compound. (For more information on L-carnitine, see page 186.)

Magnesium is also useful for combating both chronic and general fatigue. In fact, fatigue is one of the main symptoms of a long-term magnesium deficiency. In a study of 32 CFS patients, most of those who received magnesium injections had more energy, a better emotional state, and less pain than those who did not. But you don't have to get your magnesium through injections; your body can put orally taken magnesium to work quite well, and taking it in the form of magnesium aspartate has an even better fatigue-fighting effect than taking it in other forms. (For more information on magnesium, see page 203.)

Certain persons with CFS may benefit from **melatonin**. However, not all studies have demonstated this. Ask your doctor about melatonin if you have CFS, but don't try taking it on your own. (For more information about melatonin, see page 208.)

A study conducted on 26 people with CFS who were experiencing fatigue, flu-like symptoms, weakness, and sleep disturbances, showed that those who were given **NADH**—an active coenzyme form of vitamin B_3—had improvements in fatigue as well as a decrease in other symptoms. More research is needed to determine the role of NADH in treating CFS. (For more information on NADH, see page 216.)

Studies suggest that people with CFS may have low levels of essential fatty acids. Thus, supplementation with **omega-3 fatty**

acids may be helpful for people with CFS. (For more information on omega-3 fatty acids, see page 221.)

Rhodiola is another herb that may be helpful in alleviating fatigue. Among its traditional uses are increasing physical endurance and productivity. It has been used for centuries in Scandinavia and Russia. (For more information about Rhodiola, see page 243.)

The effects of **Siberian ginseng** on the immune system and adrenal glands make it a potentially useful herb for treating CFS. Healthy people who have taken Siberian ginseng have shown increased activity of their natural killer cells and an increased number of T cells both of which are important cells of the immune system and helpful in easing CFS. Siberian ginseng is also useful for counteracting general fatigue. (For more information on Siberian ginseng, see page 141.)

B vitamins are used to turn the carbohydrates you eat into glucose, which is the fuel your body uses for energy. Being deficient in a number of the B vitamins, such as folic acid (vitamin B_9), pantothenic acid (vitamin B_5), thiamine (vitamin B_1), and cobalamin (vitamin B_{12}), will cause fatigue. Taking a **B-complex** vitamin can correct deficiencies, and experts often recommend extra pantothenic acid for CFS. (For more information on vitamin B complex, see pages 277, 279, and 282.)

A deficiency of **vitamin C** may actually cause fatigue, and some evidence indicates that supplementation with this vitamin may make you more energetic, even if you've only been mildly depleted for a long time. (For more information on vitamin C, see page 284.)

MY SUPPLEMENT LIST—CHRONIC FATIGUE SYNDROME AND GENERAL FATIGUE

SUPPLEMENT	RECOMMENDED DOSAGE
Astragalus	*Tea:* Take 9–15 g sliced root, slowly boiled in 2 to 3 cups of water for 1 hour. Divide into two doses each day.
Beta-Carotene	*Capsule:* Take 10,000 to 35,000 IU daily of vitamin A, which contains beta-carotene.
Cordyceps	Take 3–9 g twice daily as a liquid extract, as food, or as powdered extract.
American or Asian Ginseng	*Capsule:* Take 100–200 mg of *Panax ginseng,* standardized to contain about 5% to 7% ginsenosides, once a day.
Lactobacillus Acidophilus	*Capsule:* Take 1- to 2-billion colony forming units (CFU) per day.

MY SUPPLEMENT LIST—CHRONIC FATIGUE SYNDROME AND GENERAL FATIGUE	
SUPPLEMENT	**RECOMMENDED DOSAGE**
L-Carnitine	*Capsule:* Take 2 g daily of proprionyl–L-carnitine divided into two doses, between meals.
Magnesium	*Tablet:* Take 400 to 1,000 mg of magnesium aspartate daily, divided into two or three doses.
	Caution: Consult your doctor before taking magnesium at this dosage, since it is considered a high dosage.
Melatonin	Ask your doctor if taking melatonin would be appropriate for you if you have this condition.
NADH	*Tablet:* Take 10 mg daily with water, on an empty stomach.
Omega-3 Fatty Acids	Take a 2–3 g of omega-3 fatty acids per day, in divided doses, with meals. The amount of omega-3 fatty acid will vary by manufacturer, so be sure to check the product label carefully.
Rhodiola	*Capsule:* Take 100 mg of standardized extract, twice daily, with meals.
Siberian Ginseng	*Capsule:* Take 300 to 400 mg daily of a solid extract of *Eleutherococcus senticosus* standardized to contain more than 1% eleutheroside E between meals.
Vitamin B Complex	*Tablet:* Take a B-50, B-75, or B-100 supplement daily, along with an extra 250 mg of pantothenic acid.
Vitamin C	*Capsule or Tablet:* Take 1,000 mg daily, divided into four doses.

CIRCULATORY HEALTH

IMAGINE WHAT WOULD happen if some type of "gunk" started building up on the insides of the pipes in your home. It's a dry, scorching summer, so you set up a sprinkler to water your lawn, but alas, the "gunk" has also built up in the garden hose leading to your sprinkler, and only a trickle of water makes it through. Eventually the grass withers from lack of water. The same thing can happen in your body when you have problems with your circulatory system.

WHAT IS IT?

The circulatory system consists of a complex network of blood vessels—arteries, veins, and capillaries—that work to distribute blood and oxygen around the body. When certain factors interfere with this healthy distribution process, the result may be pain, discomfort, and in some cases a serious health problem. Peripheral arterial disease (PAD) and Raynaud's disease are two conditions stemming from circulatory problems in the veins and arteries (see also Varicose Veins, page 608, and Heart Disease, page 470).

PAD affects your arteries—muscular-walled blood vessels that carry oxygen-rich blood from the heart to all parts of the body—primarily the ones going down your legs. PAD occurs when the arteries that supply blood to your legs narrow and harden, leading to an inadequate blood flow to the legs. PAD often manifests itself as cramp-like pain in the leg muscles, a condition referred to as *intermittent claudication.* This occurs when fatty deposits build up in the walls of arteries that supply the legs with blood—a condition called *atherosclerosis.* The pain that results from this is often triggered by exercise, since exercise increases the tissues' need for oxygen, which the constricted arteries cannot adequately supply. PAD can occur for the same reasons that blockages occur in arteries in other areas of the body (such as the heart and brain), and can be an important sign of this disease. Risk factors for PAD include high blood pressure, smoking, diabetes, and high cholesterol. *If you are having new onset symptoms of leg pains when walking, it's crucial to see your doctor to obtain a proper diagnosis.*

Raynaud's occurs when arteries have a spasm in response to cold or stress, causing them to narrow and thus blocking the flow of blood to the skin. As a result, fingers, toes, the tip of the nose, and the ears become cold and numb and may turn white or blue. When Raynaud's occurs on its own and not because of another disease, it is known as *Raynaud's disease.* When Raynaud's results from an underlying disease—such as scleroderma (SLE) (see page 584), systemic lupus erythematosus (see page 340), or rheumatoid

You May Be Able to Walk Off PAD

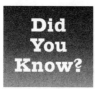
Did You Know?

If you have PAD, you had better start walking! Walking—specifically on a treadmill—can help alleviate symptoms of PAD. Walking on a treadmill may be better than walking around the block because on a treadmill you can monitor your time and speed. Also, you can feel secure by knowing that you won't find yourself far away from home, too tired or too sore to return.

Walking daily on a treadmill will help improve your circulation by developing collateral (new, small) blood vessels. Start at your own pace; a slow pace of even 1 mile an hour will do. Also, don't be worried if at first you can't walk for very long. When beginning, 5 minutes a day may be your limit, but if you stick with the treadmill, your time will improve. A 6-month study of patients with intermittent claudication found that many of them, simply by keeping up a routine, were able to greatly increase their walking distance over a 2-month period.

No matter how far or how fast you are able to walk, making the treadmill your best friend can improve your circulatory health.

arthritis (see page 574)—it is known as *Raynaud's phenomenon* or *secondary Raynaud's.*

Lifestyle changes, proper nutrition, and the addition of certain supplements to the diet can play a key role in aiding circulation. The best measure you can take if you have PAD or Raynaud's syndrome is to quit smoking immediately. Walking every day, preferably on a treadmill, is another important way to treat these conditions (see also Did You Know? on previous page). Some prescription medications can also help ease circulation problems, so again, if this is the first time you are experiencing pain in the legs with walking, allow your doctor to do a thorough investigation.

WHAT SHOULD I TAKE?
*Garlic • Ginkgo Biloba (Ginkgo) • L-Carnitine
Magnesium • Omega-3 Fatty Acids • Vitamin B Complex
Vitamin C • Vitamin E*

Garlic has been shown to have some effectiveness in treating intermittent claudication. People taking tablets of garlic powder in one study had greater improvements in their walking distances than those who took a placebo. (For more information on garlic, see page 135.)

Ginkgo may help ease intermittent claudication by improving blood flow. Although the results were modest, in one study of 111 patients, those who were given ginkgo for 6 months could walk an average of approximately one-fiftieth of a mile farther on a treadmill and without pain than those who were given a placebo. A number of other studies have also shown improved pain-free walking distances with ginkgo. (For more information on ginkgo, see page 138.)

Several studies have found that **L-carnitine** supplements may be useful in helping people with intermittent claudication. In one study, people who took L-carnitine daily for 3 weeks could walk 75 percent farther than those who did not. Another study, of 12 people with Raynaud's disease, showed that 1 gram of L-carnitine taken three times daily helped reduce blood-vessel spasms in the fingers that were caused by exposure to cold weather. L-carnitine probably helps to ease claudication by improving energy production in the leg muscles, rather than by improving bloodflow. (For more information on L-carnitine, see page 186.)

Many experts have noted poor **magnesium** metabolism in people with Raynaud's disease. The same symptoms also occur in people with magnesium deficiency, probably because a deficiency in this important mineral can cause blood vessel spasms. Consult your doctor about taking magnesium supplements if you have Raynaud's disease. (For more information on magnesium, see page 203.)

Preliminary research suggest that **omega-3 fatty acids** in the form of fish oil may be helpful for people with artherosclerosis and PAD. Fish oil may also work to prevent blood clotting and reduce blood vessel spasms in people with Raynaud's disease. Note, however, that fish oil supplementation was not helpful in cases in which Raynaud's phenomenon was the result of another dis-ease or condition. (For more information on omega-3 fatty acids, see page 221.)

Vitamin B complex—specifically, folic acid (vitamin B_9) and vitamin B_6—may be useful in treating PAD and intermittent claudication by reducing the content in the blood of the amino acid known as homocysteine. This harmful amino acid has been linked to atherosclerosis, and may account for 60 percent of cases of peripheral vascular disease. Vitamins in the B complex help break down homocysteine. A special component of niacin (vitamin B_3)—called inositol hexaniacinate—may also be useful against intermittent claudication and Raynaud's disease. (For more information on vitamin B complex, see pages 277, 279, and 282.)

Vitamin C deficiency has been theorized to play a role in atherosclerosis, and an increased intake of this vitamin may reduce the risk of PAD. Some evidence supports using vitamin C supplementation to improve circulation in the peripheral arteries. (For more information on vitamin C, see page 284.)

Vitamin E has also been associated with a lower risk of peripheral vascular disease. Additionally, several studies have found that people taking supplemental vitamin E could walk farther and with less leg pain. Vitamin E helps prevent abnormal clotting of the blood, helping it to flow better, and helps prevent plaque buildup on blood-vessel walls. (For more information on vitamin E, see page 292.)

MY SUPPLEMENT LIST—CIRCULATORY HEALTH

SUPPLEMENT	RECOMMENDED DOSAGE
Garlic	*Fresh:* Eat 1 or 2 raw cloves daily. *Capsule:* Take 600 to 900 mg daily of a garlic extract standardized to contain 1.3% alliin, providing about 12,000 mcg of alliin daily, or 6,000 mcg of allicin potential.
Ginkgo Biloba	Take 120 to 160 mg once daily of an extract standardized to contain 24% ginkgo flavone glycosides and 6% terpene lactones.

MY SUPPLEMENT LIST—CIRCULARTORY HEALTH	
SUPPLEMENT	**RECOMMENDED DOSAGE**
L-Carnitine	*Capsule or Tablet:* Take 2 g of proprionyl–L-carnitine daily in divided doses.
Magnesium	*Tablet:* Take 200 to 300 mg twice daily. *Note:* Take magnesium in the form of magnesium glycinate to avoid loose stools. Large amounts of magnesium can cause diarrhea; if this becomes a problem for you, reduce your dosage.
Omega-3 Fatty Acids	*Capsule:* Take 2–3 g of omega-3 fatty acids per day, in divided doses, with meals. The amount of omega-3 fatty acid will vary by manufacturer, so be sure to check the product label carefully.
Vitamin B Complex	*Tablet:* Take a B-50, B-75, or B-100 supplement daily. Read individual product labels for dosage information.
Vitamin C	*Capsule or Tablet:* Take 250 to 500 mg twice daily. *Note:* Be sure to use a buffered form of vitamin C. If taking vitamin C causes loose stools, decrease the dosage and then gradually increase the dosage as tolerated.
Vitamin E	*Capsule:* Take 400 IU daily of a natural product containing mixed tocopherols.

COLDS AND FLU

COLDS AND INFLUENZA (FLU) are unavoidable. And these pesky viral illnesses aren't likely to be leaving anytime soon, since scientists have not managed to find a cure for either one. The U.S. National Institute of Allergy and Infectious Diseases estimates that Americans catch *one billion* colds each year. That's a lot of runny noses, sore throats, congestion, and sneezing. Adults, on average, may experience up to four colds per year. The number is even higher for children whom—given their underdeveloped immune systems and the close quarters of classrooms and daycare—may experience up to one cold every month.

WHAT IS IT?

While scientists have created a number of vaccines to prevent a host of various illnesses, many people are often left wondering, "Why is there no cure for the common cold?" The common cold is a viral illness that is characterized by a sore throat, runny nose, and sneezing. Over 200 viruses may cause the common cold, which is why we haven't seen a vaccine to prevent this illness and probably won't. When your immune system is weak, you are even more apt to attract one of these many viruses, and the result can be an unpleasant cold. (See also Immune-System Support, page 507.)

KITCHEN TIPS

ROOT TEA FOR THE COMMON COLD

Thinly sliced, unpeeled fresh ginger root (a piece about the size of your thumb) in combination with a bundle of coarsely chopped scallions (using the white part, including the rootlets) can be boiled to make a very effective traditional Chinese herbal remedy for the common cold. Bring the roots to a boil in 2 cups of water. When half the water has boiled off, the remainder is your cup of tea. Strain and drink your preparation, adding honey if desired, and drink as often as necessary to cause mild sweating. Be sure to keep warm and get plenty of rest. The tea works best when used at the first onset of symptoms.

The flu can be a more serious problem than a cold. While researchers have developed a vaccination for the flu, the viruses that cause this illness still manage to sweep across the country from the late fall through the winter every year, striking up to a quarter of all Americans annually. This is because there are several types of flu viruses and because the vaccination does not cover all of these strains (especially new ones) of the virus (see also Q&A: Flu Shots, page 376). The flu is more likely than a cold to cause fever, achiness, and severe fatigue. Furthermore, the flu can lead to serious complications such as pneumonia.

Avian influenza A (H5N1), which has been the topic of significant coverage in the news media, does not yet appear to spread readily from person to person. It is unknown whether any of the following recommendations will have any effect on a person infected with the avian flu. Since influenza may be a potentially life-threatening illness, particularly in the elderly, immuncompromised, or chronically ill, it's important to see your doctor if you think that you have a case of influenza.

Symptoms of both colds and the flu usually develop from 2 to 4 days after infection and can last for up to 2 weeks. Symptoms of a cold include a runny nose, sneezing, sore throat, headache, and swelling of the sinuses. Symptoms of the flu include fever, chills and sweats, a dry cough, achiness, headache, weakness and fatigue, loss of appetite, and nasal congestion.

You can catch either of these ailments if someone around you sneezes or coughs, or if someone has spread the virus to a surface that you touch and you then touch your face, thus transferring the virus to your nose or mouth. One way to avoid infection by a cold or flu virus is to make sure your immune system is in tip-top shape. Supplements may help you find relief from the symptoms if you do become ill.

WHAT SHOULD I TAKE?

Astragalus • Bilberry • Chamomile • Echinacea • Elderberry Garlic • Ginger • Ginseng • Goldenseal • Peppermint Selenium • Siberian Ginseng • Spirulina • Vitamin C • Zinc

Astragalus may strengthen your immune system, especially if you're prone to frequent bouts of the common cold or upper respiratory infection. Keep in mind, however, that astragalus will probably not help you if you develop an acute illness such as bronchitis or pneumonia. (For more information on astragalus, see page 35.)

While **bilberry** may be a supplement more commonly associated with eye health, its anti-inflammatory properties make it useful for colds accompanied by a sore throat. Try gargling with bilberry mouthwash to soothe the inflamed mucous membranes of a sore throat. (For more information on bilberry, see page 44.)

Chamomile has antibacterial and anti-inflammatory properties. As with bilberry, you may gargle with a chamomile mouthwash to soothe an irritated throat. Furthermore, inhaling chamomile in a steam vapor may help to soothe the respiratory tract. (For more information on chamomile, see page 67.)

Echinacea has racked up fairly impressive research backing its effectiveness in reducing the severity of respiratory tract infections such as colds and flu, although evidence for its usefulness in *preventing* these conditions is lacking. By stimulating your immune system, it may make symptoms of a cold or flu resolve up to 4 days more quickly than they otherwise would. (For more information on echinacea, see page 107.)

It seems that increasing numbers of people are getting flu shots every year. How do I know whether getting a flu shot is appropriate for me?

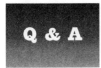

Each fall, the U.S. Centers for Disease Control and Prevention (CDC) urges Americans to immunize themselves against the flu. The flu shot, or influenza vaccine, contains a small amount of inactive viruses that prepare the immune system to fight against active flu viruses. However, the vaccination is ineffective against many other viruses that cause flu-like symptoms.

Although anyone can get flu vaccine from a physician or at a health care center, certain people are at a greater risk for developing the flu and should especially consider immunization. In most areas, flu shots are free, especially for people in groups at risk for the flu, such as the elderly population.

High Risk

- People with chronic conditions such as diabetes, HIV infection or AIDS, kidney disease, asthma, or a weakened immune system
- Anyone over 65 years old
- Pregnant women past their first trimester
- Healthcare providers
- People who spend significant amounts of time with those in a high-risk group

Caution: People who are allergic to eggs should not receive a flu shot.

The flu shot does, however, contain a mercury preservative as well as aluminum and other toxins and as a result, healthcare practitioners often recommend boosting the immune system rather than receiving a flu shot. Before the next flu season arrives, talk to your doctor about this vaccination to determine if it's appropriate for you.

Preliminary studies show that **elderberry** may be an effective immune stimulant, in addition to inhibiting the growth of viruses. In one double-blind study, elderberry decreased the recovery time of patients with the flu. While more research is necessary, taking elderberry may also provide some prevention against colds and the flu. (For more information on elderberry, see page 109.)

Garlic has been used traditionally to prevent and treat colds. In a recent double-blind, placebo-controlled study, patients were given either a placebo or a garlic extract once daily between November and February. Those who received the garlic extract were almost two-thirds less likely to catch colds than those who took the placebo, showing how powerful garlic may be as a cold preventive. Garlic has also been shown to kill viruses in laboratory experiments. (For more information on garlic, see page 135.)

Preliminary laboratory studies show that **ginger** may have antibacterial, antifungal, and antirhinoviral (the viruses known as *rhinoviruses* cause the common cold) properties. In traditional Chinese medicine, ginger is said to "warm the interior and dispel cold." (For more information on ginger, see page 136.)

Ginseng may increase the immune system's response to flu vaccine when the two are taken together. One study of 227 volunteers found that those who took ginseng for a 12-week period and received flu vaccination during week 4 developed the flu or common colds less frequently than those who had the flu vaccination without taking ginseng supplements. Other studies indicate that supplementation with American ginseng *(Panax ginseng)* may work to enhance the immune system overall. (For more information on ginseng, see page 141.)

Goldenseal has been used for thousands of years for its antibacterial and antiviral activity. Studies indicate that this herb is significantly effective against an array of viruses, bacteria, and fungi and that it may directly kill the viruses that cause colds. (For more information on goldenseal, see page 151.)

Peppermint, a common ingredient in many over-the-counter cold lozenges, has a long history of traditional use for soothing sore throats and colds. Taking peppermint in the form of lozenges or tea and applying peppermint ointment topically to the nose may help sooth a sore throat and clear nasal congestion. (For more information on peppermint, see page 229.)

Siberian ginseng, like ginseng, may also stimulate the immune system and have antiviral properties, and may therefore help in the prevention and treatment of colds and flu. (For more information of Siberian ginseng, see page 141.)

Spirulina stimulates the immune system and may have antiviral activity against influenza. (For more information on spirulina, see page 260.)

Vitamin C helps strengthen the immune system and makes cells more resistant to viral attacks. Thus, vitamin C is good for preventing colds and flu and for reducing their severity if they have already occurred. Although there is some debate about the optimal dosage of vitamin C, supplementation with this important vitamin will help temper the severity of a cold. (For more information on vitamin C, see page 284.)

Research indicates that low-dose supplementation with **selenium** and **zinc** (see also below) may be useful in reducing the duration of infection and even in thwarting respiratory infection in elderly people, especially if levels of these minerals are low. A randomized, double-blind, placebo-controlled study found that institutionalized seniors who received supplements of selenium and zinc had a significant decrease in the average number of infections after a 2-year period of supplementation. (For more information on selenium and zinc, see pages 253 and 304.)

Zinc lozenges may hinder the viruses that cause many colds. Most studies have shown that lozenges containing zinc acetate or zinc gluconate reduce the severity and duration of cold symptoms. However, a recent study found that when taken in the form of a nasal spray, zinc reduced the duration of the common cold by 75 percent. In order to work most effectively, zinc should be taken at the first sign of cold. (For more information on zinc, see page 304.)

MY SUPPLEMENT LIST—COLDS AND FLU

SUPPLEMENT	RECOMMENDED DOSAGE
Astragalus	*Capsule:* Take 2,400 to 4,000 mg daily, divided into three or four doses, between meals.
Bilberry	*Mouthwash:* Gargle with a mouthwash containing 10% bilberry as needed.
Chamomile	*Tea:* Prepare a chamomile tea by adding from 3 to 10 g of fresh flower to 1 cup of boiling water. Steep for 5 to 10 minutes and drink up to three times daily. *Mouthwash:* Follow the same procedure as for preparing chamomile tea, and once cool, use as a gargle three or more times daily. *Inhalation:* Combine 3 to 10 g of

(continued)

SUPPLEMENT	RECOMMENDED DOSAGE
	dried herb with 1 cup of boiling water and inhale the vapor from one to three times daily.
Echinacea	*Capsule or Tablet:* At the first sign of symptoms, take 300 mg every 2 hours for the first day. Follow this with 300 mg three times a day for the next 7 to 10 days.
Elderberry	*Tea:* Steep 3 to 5 g (one-half to 1 tsp) of dried flowers in 1 cup of boiling water for 10 to 15 minutes. Drink three times daily. *Syrup:* Take from 2 tsp to 2 tbsp twice daily. *Note:* Elderberry syrup dosages may vary for different products. Be sure to read the individual product label for dosage information.
Garlic	*Fresh:* Eat 2 to 4 raw cloves daily. *Capsule or Tablet:* Take 600 to 900 mg daily, delivering 5,000 to 6,000 mcg of allicin potential, divided into two or three doses.
Ginger	*Capsule:* Take 1 to 4 g daily divided into two to four doses. *Tea:* Steep 2 tsp or teabags in 1 cup of boiling water for 10 minutes. Drink up to four times daily.
Ginseng	*Capsule:* Take 100 to 200 mg of *Panax ginseng,* standardized to contain about 5% to 7% ginsenosides, once a day. *Note:* After 2 to 3 weeks of continuous use, it may be useful to discontinue ginseng supplementation for 1 to 2 weeks before starting again.
Goldenseal	*Capsule:* Take 200 to 500 mg of an extract standardized to contain 8% to 12% of goldenseal alkaloids three times a day. *Liquid Extract:* Take 2 to 4 ml three times daily. *Note:* After taking goldenseal for 3 weeks, it may be useful to discontinue use for 2 weeks before taking goldenseal again.
Peppermint	*Oral—Tea:* Combine 1.5 g or 1 teabag of dried peppermint leaf with 1 cup of boiling water. Steep for 5 to 10 minutes and drink up to five times a day. *Inhalant:* Add 3 to 4 drops of peppermint oil to hot water. Deeply inhale the steam vapor to treat nasal congestion. *Topical—Nasal Ointment:* Apply a nasal ointment, containing 1% to 5% of peppermint oil to the nose to soothe inflammation and treat congestion.
Selenium and Zinc (for seniors)	*Tablet:* Take 100 mcg of selenium daily, along with 20 mg of zinc.
Siberian Ginseng	*Capsule:* Take 300–400 mg daily of a solid extract of *Eleutherococcus senticosus* standardized to contain more than 1% eleutheroside E between meals.
Spirulina	*Capsule:* Take 3–5 g daily, divided into three doses.
Vitamin C	*Capsule or Tablet:* Some doctors recommend taking 500 to 1,000 mg of vitamin C divided into two or four doses. Other experts recommend taking dosages as high as 1 g a day for treating the common cold.

MY SUPPLEMENT LIST—COLDS AND FLU (continued)	
SUPPLEMENT	**RECOMMENDED DOSAGE**
	Note: Be sure to use a buffered form of vitamin C. If taking vitamin C causes loose stools, decrease the dosage and then gradually increase the dosage as tolerated.
Zinc	*Lozenges:* Take a lozenge that contains from 13 to 25 mg of zinc acetate or zinc gluconate every 2 hours at the first sign of a cold. Continue this treatment for 2 to 3 days. *Nasal Spray:* Zinc nasal spray is available in many health food stores. Follow the individual product label for dosage information.
	Caution: Chronic over-supplementation of zinc can cause stomach upset as well as serious health problems, including anemia and irregular heartbeat.

CONCEPTION AND PREGNANCY

IN 2002, JUST OVER 4 MILLION women had babies in the United States. For nine long months, these mothers-to-be needed to deliver the proper nutrients to their growing fetuses for healthy development. In addition to the strange cravings, long nights, and overall excitement of being pregnant, getting the proper amounts of nutrients will help ensure that both mother and child are happy, healthy, and in the best physical condition possible in order to embark on a new life together.

WHAT IS IT?

You can do many things to ensure that you are in optimal health if you are thinking of conceiving. Quitting alcohol consumption and smoking, reducing stress levels, cutting down on caffeine, and exercising are all ways to increase your chances of becoming pregnant, as well as to set up healthy habits for when you do become pregnant.

An integral part of any conception and pregnancy plan is making sure your body receives adequate amounts of nutrients. During pregnancy, the body requires an additional 300 calories a day. If a woman is pregnant and her fetus doesn't receive proper nutrients, it may take them from the mother's personal stores, compromising her health. Although some nutrients are crucial for normal development, others including various vitamins, minerals, and herbs can also help pregnant women avoid many of the common and unpleasant aspects of pregnancy, such as nausea and leg cramps.

Under no circumstances should pregnant women take any vitamins, minerals, or herbs without first consulting a doctor. However, many doctors will recommend a variety of safe, effective supplements and other measures that may aid in conception, encourage healthy pregnancy, and reduce some of the negative effects of pregnancy on the body. And remember, if you want to give your baby the best start in life, it's important to think about your health status even before you become pregnant.

WHAT SHOULD I TAKE?

If you are pregnant or think you may be pregnant, consult your doctor before taking any type of supplement.

Calcium • Choline • Folic Acid • Iron
Magnesium • Multivitamin • Omega-3 • Vitamin C

Growing babies need **calcium** to aid in the development of bones and other vital structures. Pregnant women who do not get enough calcium can be at greater risk for developing the bone-weakening condition known as osteoporosis, because the fetus will draw on the mother for its own supply of calcium. Supplemental calcium may also reduce the risk of high blood pressure during pregnancy. (For more information on calcium, see page 57.)

Animal studies suggest that an adequate intake of **choline** may help promote proper cellular brain development of the fetus during pregnancy, theoretically improving later learning and memory and

Breastfeeding Bonuses

Did You Know?

Sometimes the best nutrients cannot be bought in the store. Breastfeeding provides babies with an abundance of benefits aside from a special experience shared by mother and newborn child. The American Academy of Family Physicians recommends that all babies be either breastfed and/or fed with expressed human milk until at least 6 months of age. Read on for just a few of the health benefits both moms and babies can procure from breastfeeding:

Immune System Benefits: Breastfed babies have a lower risk of a variety of health conditions in infancy, including allergies, respiratory and urinary tract infections, and gastroenteritis. They also have a reduced risk of developing type 1 and type 2 diabetes, asthma, and inflammatory bowel disease later in life.

Brain Benefits: Children who are breastfed have higher IQs and higher developmental scores than children who are not breastfed.

Benefits to Mom: Women who breastfeed have lower rates of anemia as well as less postpartum bleeding and a more rapid recovery from vaginal delivery. Women who have breastfed for a significant amount of time over the course of a lifetime have lower rates of ovarian, endometrial, and breast cancer. Breastfeeding may also decrease the risk of developing postmenopausal osteoporosis. And it burns a huge number of calories, making it easier to get rid of those pregnancy-induced pounds!

decreasing vulnerability to toxins. (For more information on choline, see page 71.)

Folic acid (vitamin B$_9$) is probably the most well-known nutrient recommended for pregnant women. It is crucial to fetal health, yet often hard to get in adequate amounts from dietary sources. Research has found that women who take folic acid supplements before becoming pregnant and in the first trimester of pregnancy can reduce the risk of their baby's having neural tube defects (incomplete development of the neural tube, which develops the brain and spinal cord) in their child by up to 100 percent, as well as decrease their chances of miscarriage. (For more information on folic acid, see page 130.)

Pregnant women have a greater need for **iron**, since their bodies are producing an increased number of red blood cells in order to carry oxygen to the fetus, and iron is needed to make the oxygen-carrying hemoglobin in those cells. Additionally, low iron levels in the placenta have been associated with low birth weight in babies. However, some studies suggest that only women who are iron deficient should take additional iron during pregnancy. Be sure to consult your doctor before taking any iron-containing vitamins or supplements during pregnancy. (For more information on iron, see page 175.)

Magnesium supplements may be useful for reducing the leg cramps associated with pregnancy, reducing pregnancy-related high blood pressure, and helping to prevent premature birth and complications during delivery. Research also indicates that women who take magnesium supplements have healthier babies and lower rates of complications after pregnancy, including birth defects. (For more information on magnesium, see page 203.)

Perhaps the best insurance that you are receiving adequate amounts of the nutrients you require during pregnancy is taking a **multivitamin**. Many multivitamin formulas are developed specifically for pregnant women or women planning to become pregnant. Ask your doctor to recommend a multivitamin as well as additional supplements to make sure you are receiving the proper nutrients before pregnancy, during pregnancy, and while breastfeeding. (For more information on multivitamins, see page 9.)

Omega-3 fatty acids in the form of fish oil aid pregnant women in a variety of ways: by decreasing post-partum depression, decreasing asthma occurrence in the offspring, and providing longer gestation periods. (For more information on omega-3 and pregnancy, see page 221.)

Studies show that pregnant women with low intakes of **vitamin C** are at a greater risk for premature delivery. Taking a vitamin C supplement may be a sensible way of making sure you have a healthy intake of this important nutrient. (For more information on vitamin C, see page 284.)

MY SUPPLEMENT LIST—CONCEPTION AND PREGNANCY

SUPPLEMENT	RECOMMENDED DOSAGE
Calcium	*Capsule or Tablet:* During pregnancy, take 1,200 to 1,500 mg of calcium daily in two or three divided doses.
Choline	*Tablet:* Be sure to take a multivitamin/mineral supplement that contains choline. The recommended daily intake for choline in pregnant women is 450 mg daily.
Folic Acid	*Tablet:* For women trying to conceive, take 400 to 800 mcg daily; during pregnancy take 600 mcg daily; for breastfeeding women, take 500 mcg daily. *Note:* It is a good idea to get your supplemental folic acid in a multivitamin that also provides other B vitamins needed for the folic acid to be used properly.
Iron	*Tablet:* Pregnant women need 27 mg of iron daily. Begin adding iron to your diet in your first trimester, and continue throughout your pregnancy.
Magnesium	*Tablet:* For pregnant women under 18 years of age, take 400 mg daily; for women ages 19 to 30, take 350 mg daily; and for women ages 31 to 50, take 360 mg daily.
Multivitamin	*Tablet:* Take a multivitamin/mineral supplement daily. Be sure to follow the individual package label for dosage information.
Omega-3 Fatty Acids	Ask your obstetrician to help you decide the correct dose of omega-3 supplement to help while pregnant. Be sure to avoid eating fish such as tuna and swordfish that contain high levels of mercury.
Vitamin C	*Capsule or Tablet:* Take 250 mg daily.

CONJUNCTIVITIS

HAVE YOU EVER WOKEN UP in the morning only to feel like someone has glued your eyes shut? While you may think that someone has pulled a prank on you, chances are much more likely that you have a case of conjunctivitis, or "pink eye." This malady often occurs in children, since they are prone to touching their eyes without first washing their hands. However, pink eye can occur for a variety of reasons, and whatever the cause, it often leaves eyes feeling itchy and sticky, and with an extremely pink color.

WHAT IS IT?

The conjunctiva is a layer of tissue that covers the eyeball and inner surface of the eyelids. It contains glands that keep the eyeball lubricated. Conjunctivitis occurs when the conjunctival tissue becomes inflamed or infected, often because of allergies or viral or bacterial infections.

Conjunctivitis is often marked by redness in one or both eyes, excessive itching of the eyelids, sensitivity to light, a discharge from the eyes that often becomes crusty at night (hence the "glued-eye" feeling), and the impression that you have something stuck in your eye. Both viral and bacterial conjunctivitis are extremely contagious; these infections may be spread from one eye to the other as well as from one infected person to another. At times it may seem impossible to keep the infection from spreading, especially if you are caring for a small child with conjunctivitis.

Viral conjunctivitis often accompanies a cold, respiratory infection, or sore throat, and much like a bad cold, it often has to run its course. Allergic conjunctivitis may be triggered when an allergic person is exposed to pollen, mold, certain animals, or dust mites, and it often occurs in both eyes. In cases of allergic conjunctivitis, your doctor may prescribe an antihistamine and advise you to stay away from allergens. Bacterial conjunctivitis is often caused by the bacteria known as *staphylococcus* and *streptococcus*, and in these cases antibiotics may be the best method of treatment.

WHAT SHOULD I TAKE?

Bromelain • Quercetin • Vitamin A • Vitamin C

Quercetin may be helpful in preventing and treating allergic conjunctivitis. This flavonoid reduces the allergic response, perhaps by limiting the release of histamine and other inflammatory chemicals in the body. Histamine contributes to watery eyes and swelling. Using a combination supplement containing **bromelain** and quercetin may have a better effect than using quercetin alone. (For more information on bromelain and quercetin, see pages 54 and 236.)

Studies indicate that a deficiency of **vitamin A** may cause repeated bouts of conjunctivitis. Making sure that your levels of vitamin A are adequate may be one way to reduce the occurrence of chronic conjunctivitis. (For more information on vitamin A, see page 274.)

Vitamin C may prove helpful in treating several kinds of conjunctivitis by strengthening the immune system and reducing levels of

---

KITCHEN TIPS

SHAMPOO FOR YOUR EYES!

While getting shampoo in your eyes is something most people try to avoid, a well kept secret of treating conjunctivitis is to use baby shampoo and a clean washcloth. Simply wet a washcloth with warm water, apply a small amount of baby shampoo, and work into a lather. With the infected eye closed, gently glide the washcloth over the eye and rinse thoroughly with clean, warm water. Repeat one or two times daily.

histamine in the body, which can cause inflammation. (For more information on vitamin C, see page 284.)

MY SUPPLEMENT LIST—CONJUNCTIVITIS

SUPPLEMENT	RECOMMENDED DOSAGE
Bromelain	*Capsule:* Take 250 to 500 mg daily between meals. Look for a product containing 2,400 gelatin-dissolving units (GDU) or 3,600 milk-clotting units (MCU) per gram. *Note:* You may also purchase a combination supplement containing bromelain and quercetin (see below). Try to find a product that contains equal amounts of both supplements for the best effect.
Quercetin	*Capsule or Tablet:* Take 250 to 500 mg up to two to three times daily.
Vitamin A	*Capsule or Tablet: (Male 14 years and over):* Take 3,000 IU daily. *(Female 14 years and over):* Take 2,330 IU daily.
Vitamin C	*Capsule or Tablet:* Take 250 to 500 buffered mg twice daily with meals.

CONSTIPATION

CONSTIPATION IS ALMOST as uncomfortable to talk about as it is to experience firsthand. Although people may not want to freely discuss constipation, they are certainly spending money on ways to stop it. The American Gastroenterological Association reported that Americans spend an estimated $725 million on laxatives annually. However, laxatives are not the only answer for people suffering with constipation.

WHAT IS IT?

Constipation is defined as the infrequent and difficult passage of stool. While the normal frequency of bowel movements may differ greatly from one person to the next, it usually ranges from three movements a day to three a week. Generally, after 3 days without having a bowel movement, the intestinal contents harden, making it painful to move the bowels. Some common causes of constipation are poor diet (especially a diet without enough roughage such as raw vegetables or bran cereal), certain drugs, poor bowel habits, and pregnancy. Symptoms of constipation include bloating, stomach pains or cramps, excessive gas, lethargy, headache, and irritability.

Although constipation is often more bothersome than it is dangerous in the short term, it may signal a more serious health problem if it becomes chronic. (Be sure to consult with your doctor if you develop chronic constipation.) Constipation may contribute to hemorrhoids (see page 478), which can result from excessive straining or bearing down when trying to pass stool. If you suffer from alternating constipation and diarrhea, you may have irritable bowel syndrome (see page 520.)

WHAT SHOULD I TAKE?

Chamomile • Dandelion • Fiber • Flaxseed
Fenugreek • Magnesium • Vitamin C

Chamomile is a pleasant-tasting herb that may help gently stimulate the flow of digestive juices and intestinal movement. It may decrease spasms and inflammation in the digestive tract, and be useful for mild constipation. (For more information on chamomile, see page 67.)

While the leaves of **dandelion** are now appearing in farmers' markets and in delicious salad and vegetable dishes at fine restaurants, the roots of the dandelion plant are commonly used for the treatment of constipation. (For more information on dandelion, see page 96.)

It is well known that **fiber** aids in the prevention of constipation. Together with fluid and exercise, soluble fiber (fiber that dissolves in water) helps feces stay moist because it attracts water, making bowel movements easier. Because of its laxative effect, insoluble fiber (fiber that does not dissolve in water) also helps promote bowel movement, since it can pass through the digestive system relatively unchanged. (For more information on fiber, see page 120.)

Is the fiber found in oats and beans the same as the fiber found in whole grains and vegetables?

Fiber comes in two forms: soluble and insoluble. Many foods are particularly good sources of fiber, although knowing the difference between soluble and insoluble fibers—which together are good for adding bulk and softness to stool—can be tricky. Soluble fiber slows the digestion process and feeds beneficial bacteria in the intestines, helping the body to best absorb nutrients. Insoluble fiber helps food pass through the gastrointestinal tract and inactivates many toxins in the intestines. It is important to have a proper balance of both types of fiber in your diet. Putting an end to constipation does not have to be a complicated and confusing ordeal. Read on for ways you can eat good foods that also provide a healthy dose of fiber. (For more information on fiber, see above).

Soluble Fiber: Apples, barley, beans, citrus fruits, oat bran, strawberries, and squash.

Insoluble Fiber: Peppers, potatoes, vegetables, wheat bran, whole grains, and unrefined whole-grain bread.

Flaxseed has been used as a mild laxative because of its high content of fiber and mucilage—two substances that expand upon contact with water—which help to move stool through the intestinal tract. **Fenugreek** is also recommended to treat constipation because of its high-fiber content. (For more information on flaxseed and fenugreek, see pages 126 and 116.)

Magnesium acts as a mild to moderate laxative, depending on the type of magnesium you take. Magnesium oxide and citrate are more effective laxatives than magnesium glycinate. Magnesium works by drawing water into the intestines and stretching them, making stool soft and loose, and thus stimulating bowel movement. (For more information on magnesium, see page 203.)

Vitamin C acts as a gentle laxative when taken in a sufficiently high dose. (For more information on vitamin C, see page 284.)

FDA Says Prunes Are Not an Effective Laxative

Still in Debate

You may be surprised to hear that the U.S. Food and Drug Administration (FDA) has banned the use of prune concentrate or prune powders in laxatives. Despite the long traditional use of prunes and prune juice as natural laxatives, the FDA stated in 1990 that there is no proof of prunes' efficacy as a laxative. Furthermore, the FDA prohibits any statement on the labels of prunes or prune juice to claim that these foods serve as laxatives. These statements have upset many supporters of natural medicine. Ron McCaleb, president of the Herb Research Foundation—a private organization that strives to educate the world on the benefits of herbal medicine—insists that a lack of proof of effectiveness does not necessarily equate with proof of ineffectiveness.

News reporter Dan Rather, in an effort to get to the bottom of the prune-laxative confusion, conducted an interview about this with two knowledgeable guests, one whom was a member of the FDA and another who was not. When asked if prunes were a safe and effective laxative, botanist James Duke, who once served as a member of the U.S. Department of Agriculture

(USDA), and is a supporter of herbal medicine, suggested that Mr. Rather direct his question to the then director of the FDA member, Dr. David Kessler, who was the other guest on the program. If he answered no, Dr. Duke suggested that Mr. Rather ask Dr. Kessler to drink some prune juice and experience the results for himself. If he answered yes, he suggested that Mr. Rather ask why the FDA labeling regulations prohibit marketers of prune juice from stating that the juice is a safe, effective, and gentle laxative. Dr. Duke points out that people use prunes as a natural laxative all the time, no matter what the labels do or do not say. He and many others insist that despite the FDA ruling, prunes are not only safe and effective laxatives, but also inexpensive and a much more pleasant alternative to many other laxatives.

Interestingly enough, it seems that Americans are so set on the idea that prunes are indeed a natural laxative that in 2000, the California Prune Board applied to have "dried plum" serve as an official alternative name for prunes. The reason for another name? To broaden people's current image of prunes, since many eat them only when they need an effective laxative!

MY SUPPLEMENT LIST—CONSTIPATION

SUPPLEMENT	RECOMMENDED DOSAGE
Chamomile	*Tea:* Make chamomile tea by steeping 1 teabag or tbsp of dried chamomile in a cup of boiling water for 10 to 15 minutes. Drink up to four times daily between meals to relieve gas. *Capsule:* Take up to 2,400 mg daily, divided into several doses.
Dandelion	*Tea:* Steep 1–2 tsp of the cut root in 1 cup boiling water for 30 minutes, divide into two doses, morning and evening, on an empty stomach.
Fiber	*Capsule—Psyllium supplements:* Take 7 g in 8 ounces of liquid, as often as up to three times per day. *Methylcellulos (sold as Citrucel):* Take 10.2 g in 8 ounces of liquid, as often as three times per day. *Polycarbophil (sold as Fibercon):* Take 1 g (or 2 caplets) per day. Do not exceed 4 g per day.
Fiber	*Capsule:* Be sure to take the daily recommended dosage of fiber to prevent constipation: 20 to 40 mg once a day (or 4 tsp). Always drink 6 to 8 glasses of water when taking fiber. Start with a low dose and increase gradually.
Flaxseed	*Fresh:* Take 1 to 2 tsp of seeds freshly ground in a coffee grinder and sprinkled on salad or cereal, followed by 1 to 2 glasses of water as needed.
Magnesium	*Tablet:* Take 200 to 400 mg of magnesium oxide or citrate daily as needed.
Vitamin C	*Capsule or Tablet:* Take 1,000 mg twice a day. The dose may be increased by 1,000 mg a day (up to 5,000 mg a day) until bowel movements become regular.

COUGH

CHRONIC COUGH IS A COMMON condition for many people, especially smokers. Coughs may come in a variety of forms, from dry and fiery to hacking and phlegm-filled; they can be painful and exhausting, causing headaches, sore throats, and even sore muscles because of the jerking motions involved in coughing. However, a cough is not necessarily a bad thing; just as blinking your eye helps to keep dirt away, coughing is the body's way of keeping unwanted particles away from the throat and lungs.

WHAT IS IT?

A cough is a forceful release of air from the lungs that produces a sound. Coughing is the body's way of clearing the throat and airways. While some coughs are dry, other coughs, often called productive coughs, contain phlegm. There are two main categories of coughs: acute and chronic.

Acute coughs occur as the result of a cold, flu, or sinus infection. For this reason, making sure to keep your immune system strong (see page 507) and avoiding illness is one way to prevent a cough from developing. Acute coughs may last for up to 3 weeks before subsiding. Chronic coughs, on the other hand, last for longer than 3 weeks. The main causes of chronic cough are smoking, postnasal drip, asthma, gastroesophageal reflux, and chronic bronchitis.

If you have a chronic cough, see your doctor, since it may be symptomatic of a serious health condition.

WHAT SHOULD I TAKE?

Astragalus • Bromelain • Cordyceps • Elderberry • Eucalyptus Licorice • N-Acetylcysteine (NAC) • Peppermint • Slippery Elm

Astragalus has been used for centuries in Chinese medicine for strengthening the lungs. Astragalus is now being recognized in the U.S. for its immune-boosting powers, making it especially useful in people whose cough is a symptom of an overall cold, flu, or respiratory infection. (For more information on astragalus, see page 35.)

Aside from the immune-stimulating effects of **bromelain**, this pineapple-derived enzyme may be helpful when taken in conjunction with antibiotics. Studies indicate that taking bromelain with antibiotics may be more effective than taking antibiotics alone. Bromelain works especially well for people taking antibiotics for cough-causing conditions such as pneumonia, bronchitis, and sinusitis. (For more information on bromelain, see page 54.)

Preliminary studies indicate that **cordyceps** may be especially helpful for treating chronic cough that occurs after bronchitis. Studies suggest that this supplement may support the immune system and have antibiotic effects against various cough-causing bacteria. (For more information on cordyceps, see page 88).

Several studies have indicated that **elderberry** is useful in the treatment of influenza. Since cough is often one of the symptoms associated with the flu, elderberry may be an herb that you want to take when you are laid up with a nasty flu. (For more information on elderberry, see page 109.)

Eucalyptus oil is useful for treating coughs because it loosens phlegm in the respiratory tract, allowing better clearance of this phlegm from the body. Used in many over-the-counter cough suppressants, eucalyptus may be taken orally or inhaled as a decongestant and expectorant (an agent that loosens phlegm in the respiratory tract). (For more information on eucalyptus, see page 111.)

Licorice root is soothing to tissues and is commonly recommended by herbalists for a variety of respiratory ailments—including allergies, bronchitis, colds, and sore throats—because of its ability to soothe and coat the throat. (For more information on licorice, see page 192.)

N-Acetylcysteine (NAC)—a modified form of the dietary amino acid cysteine—may be especially helpful for people with a cough caused by chronic bronchitis. Studies show that NAC may reduce the frequency of bronchitis flare-ups caused by the chronic production of thick mucus in the respiratory tract. (For more information on NAC, see page 213.)

The menthol in **peppermint** may provide soothing relief from people suffering with a dry cough, as well as helping to loosen and break up phlegm when there is respiratory congestion. (For more information on peppermint, see page 226.)

The inner bark of the **slippery elm** tree has a gummy quality that is soothing to inflamed mucous membranes. This makes it a good treatment for sore throats, coughs, and respiratory dryness. (For more information on slippery elm, see page 256.)

MY SUPPLEMENT LIST—COUGH

SUPPLEMENT	RECOMMENDED DOSAGE
Astragalus	*Capsule:* Take 2,400 to 4,000 mg daily, divided into three or four doses, between meals.
Bromelain	*Capsule:* Take 250 to 500 mg daily between meals. Look for a supplement containing 2,400 gelatin-dissolving units (GDU) or 3,600 milk-clotting units (MCU) per gram.
Cordyceps	*Capsule:* Take 5 to 10 g daily divided into three or four doses, on an empty stomach. This amount may be taken in decoction, pill, or powder form.
Elderberry	*Tea:* Steep 3–5 g (½ to 1 tsp) of dried flowers in 1 cup of boiling water for 10 to 15 minutes. Drink three times daily. *Syrup:* Take from 2 tsp to 2 tbsp twice daily. *Note:* Elderberry syrup dosages may vary for different products. Be sure to read the individual product label for dosage information.
Eucalyptus	*Inhalant:* Bring 2 cups of water to a boil and add 10 drops of eucalyptus oil. Remove the pot of water from the heating source, lean over the water, and make a "tent" by draping a towel over your head and the water. Inhale the steam deeply. *Oral:* Eucalyptus can be found in a variety of over-the-counter products such as lozenges, cough syrups, and teas. Make sure to read individual product labels for dosage information.

(continued)

MY SUPPLEMENT LIST—COUGH (continued)	
SUPPLEMENT	**RECOMMENDED DOSAGE**
	Note: Pure eucalyptus oil should not be taken orally unless recommended by a doctor, since even small doses have caused toxic side effects and severe or even fatal reactions.
Licorice	*Tea:* Prepare tea by combining 1 cup of water with 1 tsp or teabag of licorice root. Steep for 5 minutes. Drink 1 cup daily before meals. *Capsule:* Take one to three capsules standardized to contain 200 mg of licorice root extract and 50 mg of glycyrrhizinic acid daily. *Lozenges:* Licorice can be found in many over-the-counter lozenges. Be sure to check the product label to make sure the lozenges contain real licorice, and for dosage information. Licorice supplements with glycyrrhizinic acid should not be used for more than 4 weeks at a time. *Note:* Licorice candy is made with artificial flavorings or anise and has no medicinal properties.
NAC	*Capsule:* Take 900 mg twice daily with meals.
Peppermint	*Tea:* Prepare tea by combining 1 cup of water with 1 tsp or teabag of peppermint. Steep for 5 minutes. Drink three or four times a day between meals. *Lozenges:* Peppermint can be found in many over-the-counter lozenges. Be sure to check the product label to make sure the product contains real peppermint, not artificial flavoring, and for dosage information.
Slippery Elm	*Tea:* Combine 1 cup of water with 1 tsp or teabag of loose bark. Steep for 5 minutes. Drink 1 cup three or four times daily. *Lozenges:* Slippery elm can be found in many over-the-counter lozenges. Be sure to check individual product labels for dosage information. *Capsule:* Take up to 4,800 mg daily.

DANDRUFF

WHITE FLAKES ARE GREAT during February when you're skiing. However, if it's June and you're wearing your favorite black shirt, you're probably cursing the flurry of "snow" coming from your head. Even though dandruff isn't contagious, it can be embarrassing, aggravating, and make a closet full of black clothes seem like a very fashionable nightmare. Fortunately, although dandruff can be annoying and unsightly, it is not typically a serious health threat.

WHAT IS IT?

Dandruff is marked by flaking of the scalp, as well as other oily areas of the skin, such as the eyebrows and nose. One frequent cause of dandruff is seborrheic dermatitis, a condition that may be caused by an overgrowth of a normally occurring yeast-like fungus called *malassezia.* This fungus feeds on oil secreted by the hair follicles, prompting skin cells to move through their life cycle and fall off more rapidly than normal, causing flaking.

Dandruff is usually characterized by flaky white bits of dead skin that appear in the hair and fall on the shoulders. Many conditions can cause dandruff, including psoriasis, cradle cap (in infants), and oily hair and skin. Men are more susceptible to dandruff than women, and certain factors can increase the risk for developing dandruff, such as age (dandruff usually occurs from puberty to age 40), oily skin, and certain diseases (particularly neurological conditions).

However, you don't have to retire your black clothes just yet! Many over-the-counter shampoos may help control dandruff and some supplements may also curb the flurry of flakes falling from your scalp.

WHAT SHOULD I TAKE?
Lavender • Omega-3 Fatty Acids • Selenium
Tea Tree Oil • Vitamin B Complex • Zinc

Delightful-smelling **lavender** contains essential oils that have antifungal properties and may therefore be useful in the treatment of dandruff. (For more information on lavender, see page 184.)

Omega-3 fatty acids, such as those found in fish oil, flaxseed oil, and evening primrose oil, are crucial for maintaining healthy skin and may also reduce the itching and inflammation associated with dandruff. (For more information on omega-3 fatty acids, see page 221.)

Selenium is a mineral that acts as an antioxidant and is useful in treating dandruff as well as other skin conditions, such as psoriasis (see page 569) and eczema (see page 427). (For more information on selenium, see page 253.)

In studies of people with mild to moderate dandruff, a 5 percent **tea tree oil** shampoo was effective, well tolerated, and particularly successful in reducing the greasiness and itchiness associated with dandruff. (For more information on tea tree oil, see page 265.)

Your skin and hair require plenty of **vitamin B complex** for proper health. Add this to your supplement plan to give your hair an additional amount of insurance. (For more information on vitamin B complex, see pages 277, 279, and 282.)

One component of some over-the-counter dandruff shampoos is **zinc**. This mineral regulates oil production by the glands in the skin and promotes healing by keeping the immune system healthy. (For more information on zinc, see page 304.)

KITCHEN TIPS

HONEY FOR YOUR HAIR
Not only does honey have nutritional value, it has antibacterial, antifungal, and antioxidant powers too! One study of people with dandruff showed that diluted (90 percent honey with 10 percent warm water), crude (raw) honey, when rubbed into the hair every other day for 2 to 3 minutes and left in the hair for three hours before rinsing with warm water, relieved the itching, skin irritation, and flaking associated with dandruff. When applied weekly, it also managed to prevent relapses.

MY SUPPLEMENT LIST—DANDRUFF

SUPPLEMENT	RECOMMENDED DOSAGE
Lavender Oil	*Shampoo:* Choose a shampoo and conditioner that contain pure lavender oil. Or, rub a few drops of the pure essential oil into your scalp at night, and rinse out in the morning.
Omega-3 Fatty Acids	*Capsule:* Take a product that includes 3 to 6 g of linoleic acid, 0.5 to 1 g docosahexaenoic acid (DHA), and 0.5 to 1 g of eicosapentaenoic acid (EPA) daily.
Selenium	*Tablet:* Take 100 to 200 mcg daily.
Tea Tree Oil	*Shampoo:* Tea tree oil shampoos and conditioners may be purchased in many health food stores. Be sure to buy a product containing 5% tea tree oil. Follow the directions on the product label for application instruction. *Note:* Some people are sensitive to some or all of tea tree oil's components, especially when used in too strong a dosage. Tea tree oil products should be tested on a small patch of skin in an unobtrusive area to make sure no allergic reaction occurs.
Vitamin B Complex	*Tablet:* Take a B-100 complex vitamin twice a day with meals.
Zinc	*Tablet:* Taking 15 mg daily will ensure that you do not have a deficiency of this nutrient. Discuss taking higher dosages of zinc with your doctor.

DEPRESSION

IN ANY GIVEN YEAR, ROUGHLY 10 percent of the American population will be caught in the grips of depression. For some people the depressive episode may be mild and last for a few weeks. For other people the depression may be debilitating and last for years. No age group is immune from depression—it can occur in children, adults, and the elderly. Women, however, experience depression twice as often as men, perhaps because of hormonal changes caused by childbirth, premenstrual syndrome, and menopause.

WHAT IS IT?

Typical symptoms of depression include sadness and a feeling of emptiness and hopelessness; lack of self-worth; decreased interest in normal hobbies or other pastimes; lack of energy; insomnia; anxiety; trouble with concentrating; changes in eating habits; and chronic physical pains and digestive upset. Symptoms of depression may be severe enough to interfere with one's ability to work or perform daily activities. Thoughts of suicide are common among people with depression and strongly indicate the urgent need for professional help.

One form of depression, called bipolar disorder, is marked by a cycle of depressive and manic episodes. During a manic episode, a person may be overly talkative, exhibit frantic behavior, be impulsive, and may experience delusions. An antidepressant agent, even an herbal one, can cause depression to swing into mania or hypomania, even if the person has no prior history of this type of illness. It's best to talk to your doctor before taking any supplements to treat depression. *Never* treat severe depression by self-medicating with supplements.

WHAT SHOULD I TAKE?

Dehydroepiandrosterone (DHEA) • Folic Acid • L-Carnitine
Multivitamin • Omega-3 Fatty Acids • SAMe
Selenium • St. John's Wort

Preliminary studies indicate that **DHEA** may be successful in treating mild to moderate depression. Double-blind trials have found that people with depression who took DHEA reported an increased feeling of physical and psychological well being, as well as a reduction in depression. Note, however, that while DHEA is available over-the-counter, it should be taken for depression only under the supervision of a doctor, who has documented low levels of DHEA-S with a blood test. (For more information on DHEA, see page 100.)

More than one-third of people with depression may have low levels of **folic acid** (vitamin B_9) in their bodies, and research has shown that people with a folic acid deficiency may not respond as well to a prescription antidepressant medicine. Thus, supplementation with this B vitamin may be a helpful alternative or addition to prescription drugs for this condition. (For more information on folic acid, see page 130.)

Regular Exercise Helps Stave Off Depression

Did You Know?

When you're feeling depressed, your instinct may be to curl up in a ball and wait for the terrible mood to pass; however, that couldn't be further from what your body needs! It is pretty clear that exercise improves mood: Over 1,000 studies have examined this phenomenon, and the consensus is that exercise may be just as effective in treating depression as psychotherapy.

Although the exact reason why exercise staves off depression remains unclear, one theory is that people who exercise experience an increase in self-esteem and confidence because of the active role they are taking to improve their health. The best news about exercise as a prescription for depression is that it doesn't seem to matter what type of exercise you choose. Whether you jog, swim, lift weights, hike, or play tennis, you can reap the mental-health rewards of exercise.

Studies indicate that **L-carnitine** may be successful in treating depression in the elderly, particularly in those with serious clinical symptoms of depression. (For more information on L-carnitine, see page 186.)

Taking a **multivitamin** may help to temper symptoms of depression. Other studies indicate that nutritional supplementation, when taken over a 1-year period, may help to improve mood. This makes good sense, since studies suggest that many cases of depression may be linked to vitamin deficiency. (For more information on multivitamins, see page 9.)

Much attention has recently been paid to **omega-3 fatty acids** for treating depression and bipolar disorder. Studies indicate that people with depression often have abnormally low levels of omega-3 fatty acids. In one study, people who ate fatty fish several times a week were found to have fewer symptoms of depression; in another study, people with manic depression who were given essential fatty acids along with their usual antidepressant medications had fewer episodes of depression and mania than those who were not. Preliminary studies have also found that supplementation with omega-3s may have positive short-term effect in people with bipolar disorder. (For more information on omega-3 fatty acids, see page 221.)

Rhodiola (*Rhodiola rosea*) is a multipurpose herb that is found in high altitudes in the arctic areas of Europe and Asia. While it has time-honored use in herbal medicine as an antidepressant, little research has been published recently in medical literature. (For more information about rhodiola, see page 243.)

Some research indicates that S-adenosylmethione, or **SAMe**, may be helpful in treating depression. Studies suggest that SAMe is effective in elevating mood in part by increasing levels of certain neurotransmitters, as do prescription medications, with far fewer side effects than prescription antidepressants. (For more information on SAMe, see page 247.)

A double-blind, crossover trial indicated that **selenium** may substantially improve mood after a period of 2 to 5 weeks. Other research indicates that people with diets high in selenium experience less anxiety, depression, confusion, and uncertainty than people whose diets are low in selenium. (For more information on selenium, see page 253.)

In the herbal world, **St. John's wort** is something of a celebrity. It has earned its status as a household name from its role in treating depression. The extensive studies conducted on St. John's wort have been almost as thorough as those necessary for prescription medications before their approval by the FDA. An overwhelming number of studies have found that St. John's wort works as well as several kinds of prescription antidepressants in treating mild to moderate depression. (For more information on St. John's wort, see page 262.)

Valerian is an herb with a reputation for alleviating anxiety. Depression and anxiety often occur together, and preliminary studies suggest that valerian and St John's wort may be useful in this setting, when used as a combination. (For more information on valerian, see page 272.)

MY SUPPLEMENT LIST—DEPRESSION

SUPPLEMENT	RECOMMENDED DOSAGE
DHEA	*Capsule or Tablet:* DHEA should be taken only under the supervision of a doctor. The ideal dose and long-term effects of this supplement are unknown. Ask your doctor to check your DHEA-S level to see if you are deficient in this hormone.
Folic Acid	*Tablet:* Take 400 to 800 mcg daily. In cases of extreme deficiency, a doctor may recommend taking a high dosage (such as 10 mg daily) for a short period of time, until levels of folic acid in the body are stabilized.
L-Carnitine	*Capsule or Tablet:* In studies, dosages of 500 mg taken three times daily were effective in decreasing symptoms of severe depression.
Multivitamin	*Tablet:* Take 1 chelated multivitamin/mineral supplement daily. See individual product labels for dosage information.
Omega-3 Fatty Acids	*Fish Oil—Capsule:* Studies suggested a benefit from dosages of 1.5 to 6 g daily of a fish oil supplement from marine sources. However, dosages often vary on an individual basis. Consult your doctor in order to determine a dosage that's suitable for you.
SAMe	*Tablet:* Take 800 mg twice daily on an empty stomach. *Note:* Take SAMe with vitamin B complex in order to prevent homocysteine levels from becoming too high.
Selenium	*Tablet:* Take 100 to 200 mcg daily. *Note:* Do not exceed dosages above 400 mcg daily unless recommended by your doctor.
St. John's Wort	*Capsule:* Take 300 mg of St. John's wort three times a day. It may take 4 to 6 weeks before you begin to see results. *Caution:* St. John's wort should not be used for cases of severe depression. Plus, St. John's wort may interact with prescription antidepressants. Consult your doctor before taking St. John's wort if you are taking a prescription antidepressant.

DETOXIFICATION

WHILE MOST PEOPLE ASSOCIATE the term "detoxification" with enemas, fasting, and colon cleanses, detoxification is actually an ongoing, naturally occurring process in the body. There is limited evidence that various self-induced methods of detoxification—including colon hydrotherapy, dieting, fasting, and the use of laxatives—are helpful in keeping the body free of toxins; however, there are ways in which you may be able to aid the body in its natural process of detoxification.

WHAT IS IT?

Detoxification is the body's way of neutralizing or "detoxifying" foreign substances that do not occur naturally in the body. These foreign substances, which may enter the body through the nose, eyes, mouth, and skin, include carcinogens (cancer-causing substances), insecticides, alcohol, drugs, and other substances, which are typically processed by the liver. Research suggests that when the body cannot properly carry out the detoxification process, it may be at an increased risk for certain diseases including cancer, Parkinson's disease, fibromyalgia, and chronic fatigue syndrome.

The process of detoxification is extremely complex but may be broken down into two phases: Phase 1 involves the breakdown of foreign substances into molecules that are extremely potent and potentially

Sauna Therapy May Have Detox Benefits

Did You Know?

Many alternative medicine specialists recommend sauna therapy for removing "stored" toxins from fat deposits and the liver. The belief behind this is that when the body reaches high temperatures, perspiration will promote the release of toxins through the skin. Studies show that sauna therapy has various health benefits, including restoring lost appetite, promoting weight loss in obese patients, and improving symptoms of lifestyle-related diseases such as high blood pressure, diabetes, and smoking-related sicknesses.

Sauna therapy has also been shown to alleviate complications from environmental toxins. In one study, a woman with multiple ailments caused by 20 years of exposure to toxic chemicals in the workplace had a significant overall improvement in her health after a regimen of sauna therapy combined with medicinal therapy. The evidence for the detoxification benefits of sauna is abundant, suggesting a bright future for sauna therapy in health care. However, it is important to note that no standardized recommendations exist for the temperature, humidity, and duration of sauna therapy, and that extreme heat can increase water loss and electrolyte (mineral) loss from the body, as well as increase the heart rate. While drinking plenty of water can help keep you from becoming dehydrated, you should consult your doctor before experimenting with sauna treatments.

more toxic than the original chemical substance that entered the body. If the detoxification process were to stop at this first phase (for example, in people with impaired detoxification), the body could experience severe damage to both RNA and DNA, leading to various diseases. The second phase of detoxification picks up where phase 1 left off, and further transforms the molecules produced in phase 1 into water-soluble compounds that can be excreted in the urine or feces.

Certain factors preferentially stimulate one or the other of the two phases of detoxification. For example, cigarette smoke, char-broiled meats, and certain medications (including steroids and certain anti-seizure drugs) induce phase 1 detoxification. Other beneficial factors may preferentially induce phase 2 detoxification, including garlic oil, rosemary, soy, cabbage, and brussels sprouts. Both phases of detoxification require "cofactors" to seamlessly complete the full detoxification process; These cofactors may be acquired by eating vegetables, fruits, whole grains, and dietary fats and taking various vitamins, minerals, and herbs.

WHAT SHOULD I TAKE?
Coenzyme Q10 (CoQ10) • Fiber • Ginger
Green Tea • Magnesium • Milk Thistle
N-Acetylcysteine (NAC) • Schisandra • Selenium
Vitamin C • Vitamin E

CoQ10 may help reduce levels of oxidative stress on the body, thus reducing the damage to cells and tissues caused by the "maverick" molecules known as free radicals. Studies indicate that CoQ10 increases levels of antioxidants in the blood and may reduce the risk of developing certain diseases. (For more information on CoQ10, see page 80.)

The fluid known as bile carries toxins from the liver to the small intestine, where these substances are flushed from the body in the stool. However, if adequate amounts of **fiber** are not consumed, the intestines can reabsorb toxins. Psyllium and flaxseed make excellent sources of supplemental fiber. (For more information on fiber, see page 120.)

The well-known ability of **ginger** to keep the digestive system working properly makes it an important player in helping to detoxify the body. Components in this knotty root encourage good peristalsis, which is the name for the wave-like muscle contractions that propel material through the digestive tract. (For more information on ginger, see page 136.)

FRIENDS AND FOES

Be sure to take **selenium** and **vitamin C** a few hours apart from each other, since vitamin C inhibits the body's ability to absorb selenium.

Studies suggest that **green tea** extract may have anticancer and antibacterial properties. Since research suggests that cancer may be one of the numerous diseases that may result from impaired detoxification, drinking a few cups of green tea daily may provide your body with additional health-promoting insurance. (For more information on green tea, see page 157.)

Magnesium may be helpful in supporting the phase 1 of detoxification, which is a necessary part of the overall detoxification process in the body. Since the benefits of magnesium in the body are widespread, taking supplements of this important mineral makes good sense in any event. (For more information on magnesium, see page 203.)

Milk thistle has acquired a reputation for its ability to promote and support healthy liver function. An active ingredient in milk thistle, called silymarin, protects the liver by reducing inflammation and promoting the regeneration of liver cells, allowing them to cleanse the blood more effectively. (For more information on milk thistle, see page 210.)

NAC plays a role in detoxification by increasing levels of glutathione in the body. In phase 2 detoxification, glutathione binds to various toxins and converts them to a form that can be excreted in the urine. Aside from its role as an antioxidant, glutathione is also used by the liver to convert toxins into forms that can be more easily excreted by the kidneys in the urine, in addition to being used to detoxify heavy metals such as mercury and lead. People with high levels of toxins in their bodies often have low levels of glutathione, which can allow damage to the liver. (For more information on NAC and glutathione, see pages 213 and 148.)

The active components in **schisandra**, called lignans, help protect the liver from damage as well as increasing the liver's ability to detoxify blood. Schisandra may also help to increase the body's ability to process waste and to deliver more oxygen to the body. (For more information on schisandra, see page 251.)

A deficiency of **selenium** compromises the liver's ability to use glutathione (see page 148) to reduce the harmful effects of toxins. Furthermore, selenium is a powerful antioxidant and may have cancer-fighting properties as well. Selenium is more effective when taken with vitamin E, which promotes the absorption of this mineral. (For more information on selenium, see page 253.)

Vitamin C aids in detoxification by helping the liver in its detoxifying processes and protecting it from damage. Vitamin C may also help the body to maintain glutathione levels. In one study, the glutathione content in the red blood cells of people taking a daily dose of 500 milligrams of vitamin C rose by almost 50 percent. (For more information on vitamin C, see page 284.)

Vitamin E is an antioxidant, meaning that it helps protect the liver from damage caused by the cell- and tissue-damaging molecules known as free radicals. (For more information on vitamin E, see page 292.)

MY SUPPLEMENT LIST—DETOXIFICATION

SUPPLEMENT	RECOMMENDED DOSAGE
CoQ10	*Softgel:* Take 30 to 90 mg daily.
Fiber	*Psyllium supplements:* Take 7 g in 8 ounces of liquid, as often as up to three times per day. *Methylcellulos (sold as Citrucel):* Take 10.2 g in 8 ounces of liquid, as often as three times per day. *Polycarbophil (sold as Fibercon):* Take 1 g (or 2 caplets) per day. Do not exceed 4 g per day. *Note:* Be sure to take the daily recommended dosage of fiber to prevent constipation: 20–40 mg once a day (or 4 tsp). Always drink 6 to 8 glasses of water when taking fiber. Start with a low dose and increase gradually.
Ginger	*Capsule:* Take 500 to 1,000 mg daily.
Green Tea	*Tea:* Steep 1 tsp of green tea leaves in 1 cup of boiling water for 3 minutes. Drink up to three times daily. *Capsule:* Take 100 mg of a decaffeinated extract three times daily.
Magnesium	*Capsule or Tablet:* Take 500 to 800 mg daily. This dosage may be higher than that found in most multivitamin/mineral supplements.
Milk Thistle	*Capsule:* Take 140 to 210 mg, three times daily, of an extract standardized to contain at least 70% silymarin.
NAC	*Capsule:* Take 250 to 1,500 mg daily.
Schisandra	*Capsule:* Take 200 to 800 mg daily. Dosages as high as 1 g three times daily have been recommended for detoxification, but consult your doctor before taking high dosages of schisandra.
Selenium	*Tablet:* Take 200 mcg daily. Be sure to take selenium a few hours apart from vitamin C supplements.
Vitamin C	*Capsule or Tablet:* Take 500 mg twice daily. *Note:* Be sure to use a buffered form of vitamin C. If taking vitamin C causes loose stools, decrease the dosage and then gradually increase the dosage as tolerated.
Vitamin E	*Capsule:* Take 400 IU daily in the form of natural vitamin E with mixed tocopherols with food.

DIABETES

EATING MAY BE EASY, but the process of turning the food you eat into fuel for your body is a little more complicated, especially if you have diabetes. After you eat, the digestion process begins, and the body begins to break down food for fuel and energy. Much of the food we eat is converted into the sugar known as glucose, which travels through the bloodstream and supplies most of the fuel our bodies use. However, glucose can't travel into the cells that use it for fuel by itself—for that, it depends on a hormone called insulin to let it through. Insulin is produced in the pancreas, the gland that is responsible for providing the body with enough of this hormone to move glucose through the bloodstream and into the cells. For the millions of people with diabetes, this process goes haywire.

WHAT IS IT?

Unfortunately, as 17 million Americans know all too well, diabetes (also called diabetes mellitus) is a problem in which the process of glucose transport breaks down. Diabetes takes one of three main forms—type 1, type 2, and gestational diabetes.

From 5 to 10 percent of people with diabetes have *type 1 diabetes*. This form of diabetes, also known as "insulin-dependant diabetes," occurs when the pancreas produces little or no insulin because the body's immune system attacks the pancreas, destroying the cells that

---

Are popular diets, such as the Atkins Diet and the South Beach Diet, recommended for people with diabetes?

Q & A

Low-carbohydrate, high-protein diets are not recommended for weight control in people with diabetes; however, the American Diabetes Association (ADA) insists that for people with diabetes, carbs really do count! The ADA advises that people with diabetes should monitor their carbohydrate intake, including foods such as bread, rice, crackers, cereal, fruit, potatoes, corn, peas, and sweets. According to the ADA, most people with diabetes should limit their carbohydrates to three or four servings per meal and to one or two servings in snacks.

Many foods that have a high carbohydrate content are also considered to have a high glycemic index. These include potatoes, instant rice, and white bread. The South Beach Diet provides instruction about using foods with a low glycemic index. As with counting carbohydrates, measuring the glycemic index of certain foods is a tool for measuring the impact a particular food will have on the body's blood sugar level. Foods with a high glycemic index are converted into sugar more quickly than foods with a low glycemic index, meaning that in order to keep blood sugar levels low, you should consume foods with a low glycemic index. Preliminary studies have shown that maintaining a low glycemic index diet may be beneficial to controlling diabetes.

produce insulin. (For additional information on such autoimmune diseases, see page 333.) Type 1 diabetes was once called "juvenile diabetes," since it is often diagnosed in children and young adults, although adults may also be found to have type 1 diabetes.

Type 2 diabetes was once referred to as "adult-onset diabetes" because it usually occurs in adulthood, although increasing numbers of young people are diagnosed with this condition. Type 2 diabetes is much more common than type 1, and often strikes people who are overweight. It occurs when the body becomes unable to properly use the insulin that the pancreas provides, and is also known as "insulin-resistant diabetes." Eventually, the pancreas starts pumping out less insulin.

Gestational diabetes usually develops in the second or third trimester of pregnancy. This type of diabetes occurs when certain hormones that occur during pregnancy affect the mother's production of insulin. Gestational diabetes often disappears after pregnancy, although about half of women who experience gestational diabetes can develop type 2 diabetes later in life.

Symptoms of diabetes include dramatic weight loss, unusual thirst, frequent urination, fatigue, and nausea. Additional symptoms associated with type 2 diabetes are gum or bladder infections, blurred vision, tingling or numbness in the hands and feet, and itchy skin. Symptoms of type 2 diabetes can occur gradually over time and may be so mild that they go unnoticed.

If you are overweight and have diabetes, it is very important that you gradually lose weight with a sensible diet. Cutting the three "evil whites" from your diet—white flour, white sugar, and white rice—and staying away from soda and fruit juice is a move in the right direction. Although there is no cure for diabetes, various supplements may help regulate levels of blood sugar in the body. However, it is crucial that you consult your doctor before taking any nutritional supplements for diabetes.

WHAT SHOULD I TAKE?

Diabetes is a potentially life-threatening disease. Make sure to consult your doctor before taking any type of supplement, especially if you have been diagnosed with diabetes or think you may have diabetes.

Aloe • Alpha Lipoic Acid • Bilberry • Biotin • Cayenne Chromium • Coenzyme Q10 (CoQ10) • Evening Primrose Oil Fenugreek • Fiber • Garlic • Ginseng

KITCHEN TIPS

RAW ONION MAY LOWER BLOOD SUGAR

Studies have shown that onions may effectively lower blood sugar levels. Certain oils found in onions, called volatile oils, have been shown to decrease blood sugar levels in both animals and humans. Researchers suspect that the onion oil increases the quantity of free insulin in the bloodstream. To reap the blood sugar-lowering benefits of onions, they must be eaten raw. Add raw onion to your salads or sandwiches to help regulate your blood sugar levels.

*Gymnema • L-Carnitine • Magnesium • Omega-3 Fatty Acids
Vitamin B₆ • Vitamin C • Vitamin E • Zinc*

Aloe (also called aloe vera) has been used traditionally in the Arabian peninsula for treating diabetes. Studies show that aloe vera juice may be effective in reducing both blood sugar levels and triglyceride levels in people with type 2 diabetes. (For more information on aloe, see page 27.)

Alpha lipoic acid (ALA) is a powerful antioxidant that may help reduce one of the complications of diabetes that affects the nerves—known as diabetic neuropathy—by improving communication in the nervous system. ALA has also shown promise in enhancing insulin function, especially when taken in conjunction with vitamin E (see page 414). (For more information on alpha lipoic acid, see page 29.)

Long before insulin was available for the treatment of diabetes, **bilberry** leaf was used as a treatment for this disease. Animal studies suggest that bilberry may be effective in reducing blood sugar levels. Bilberry may also decrease complications of diabetes, specifically retinopathy, a complication in which vessels in the eye become damaged and blocked, sometimes leading to blindness as well as other blood vessel problems. (For more information on bilberry, see page 44.)

Preliminary studies indicate that **biotin** may help control blood sugar levels and prevent symptoms of neuropathy in people with diabetes. (For more information on biotin, see page 46.)

Capsaicin, also known as **cayenne**, when applied topically, may be helpful in reducing nerve pain associated with diabetic neuropathy. In one study in which cayenne cream was applied to the feet of 13 people with diabetic neuropathy, symptoms improved greatly after 8 weeks, without any side effects. (For more information on cayenne, see page 64.)

Fairly strong evidence supports the use of **chromium**, especially in the form of chromium picolinate, for type 2 diabetes. Chromium may work to reduce triglyceride levels, improve glucose tolerance, and regulate insulin levels in people with diabetes. It may work in part because of its ability to help insulin draw blood sugar into cells. (For more information on chromium, see page 77.)

The body requires **CoQ10** in order to properly process blood sugar. However, studies show that people with type 2 diabetes may have lower than normal levels of this important antioxidant. Preliminary research indicates that supplementation with CoQ10 may help in regulating blood sugar levels and lowering blood pressure in people with type 2 diabetes. (For more information on CoQ10, see page 80.)

Evening primrose oil is rich in a substance called gamma-linolenic acid (GLA), and studies have shown that taking evening primrose oil is useful in reducing symptoms of nerve damage caused by diabetes. Some studies suggest that this effect is enhanced when evening primrose oil is taken with vitamin C. (For more information on evening primrose oil, see page 115.)

Studies indicate that the defatted portion of **fenugreek** seeds may reduce levels of glucose, insulin, total cholesterol, and triglycerides, as well as increasing HDL ("good") cholesterol levels. In studies of people with type 2 diabetes, powdered fenugreek seeds that had been soaked in water were found to significantly lower glucose levels. (For more information on fenugreek, see page 116.)

Studies show that a diet high in **fiber** may be as helpful in controlling blood sugar levels as some prescription medications. Studies have shown that people with diabetes who consume a high-fiber diet have lower levels of total cholesterol, triglyceride, and LDL ("bad") cholestserol in their blood, as well as having an increased ability to utilize insulin. (For more information on fiber, see page 120.)

Studies indicate that the active ingredient in **garlic**—called allicin—may reduce blood sugar levels. Although the exact reason for this is unknown, researchers believe that the allicin in garlic affects the liver by stopping it from inactivating insulin. (For more information on garlic, see page 135.)

Several double-blind studies have found that **ginseng** may help to lower blood sugar concentrations in people with type 2 diabetes, both during fasting and after meals. (For more information on ginseng, see page 141.)

Gymnema, a plant native to India, has a long history of use in treating diabetes. One study of people with type 2 diabetes who were taking prescription medication found that supplementation with gymnema helped to control blood sugar. As a result, 21 of the 22 study participants were able to reduce the dosage of their prescription medication, and 5 of the 22 study participants were able to stop taking their anti-diabetes medication entirely and take gymnema alone. (For more information on gymnema, see page 164.)

Preliminary research indicates that a deficiency of **L-carnitine** in people with diabetes may lead to complications associated with this condition including retinopathy, hyperlipidemia, and neuropathy. (For more information on L-carnitine, see page 186.)

Studies indicate that a deficiency of **magnesium** is more common in people with type 2 diabetes than in people without this condition. Magnesium supplementation may prevent diabetes-related complications, in addition to helping the body metabolize glucose. (For more information on magnesium, see page 203.)

Omega-3 fatty acids may help to reduce insulin sensitivity and glucose metabolism in people with diabetes. Other research indicates that these fatty acids may be especially helpful for women with diabetes, as they may reduce the risk of coronary artery disease. (For more information on omega-3 fatty acids, see page 221.)

Studies indicate that people with diabetes may have a deficiency in **vitamin B$_6$**. Studies indicate that supplementation with vitamin B$_6$ may be especially helpful in women with gestational diabetes or women who have glucose intolerance caused by oral contraceptives. (For more information on vitamin B$_6$, see page 279.)

Some people taking insulin for diabetes have low levels of **vitamin C**, even though they report an adequate intake from their diet. Since vitamin C facilitates the transport of insulin, people taking insulin often require higher than usual levels of this important vitamin. Furthermore, vitamin C is essential to proper wound healing and immunity, issues that are especially important in people with diabetes because of the increased risk of atherosclerosis and other complications resulting from this disease. (For more information on vitamin C, see page 284.)

Vitamin E is an antioxidant that can counteract the damaging effects of free radicals, which may be found in higher levels in people with diabetes. This vitamin may also help reduce excessively high blood sugar levels, reduce cholesterol levels, and help prevent long-term complications from diabetes. When taken in conjunction with ALA (see page 412), vitamin E may be especially helpful in preventing diabetes-related complications such as heart disease, nerve damage, vision trouble, and kidney disease. (For more information on vitamin E, see page 292.)

People with diabetes may have a deficiency of **zinc**, which they often excrete in large amounts in their urine. Zinc is an important element in wound healing and has also been found to improve insulin levels in people with diabetes. A deficiency of zinc may cause insulin resistance, also a precursor to diabetes. (For more information on zinc, see page 304.)

MY SUPPLEMENT LIST—DIABETES

SUPPLEMENT	RECOMMENDED DOSAGE
Aloe	*Gel:* Take 1 tbsp twice daily.
Alpha Lipoic Acid	*Capsule:* Take 600 to 800 mg daily.
Bilberry	*Capsule:* Take 80 to 160 mg of a bilberry fruit extract standardized to contain 25% anthocyanosides. *Note:* The ideal dose of bilberry leaf for lowering blood sugar is unknown. Consult your doctor to determine an appropriate dosage for you.
Biotin	*Capsule or Tablet:* Take 7,000 to 15,000 mcg daily.
Cayenne	*Topical—Cream:* Apply a topical cream containing 0.025 to 0.075% cayenne three to four times daily for neuropathy symptoms. *Note:* You may experience a burning sensation when applying cayenne cream, but this will subside with each use. Be sure to thoroughly wash your hands after each application in order to prevent the cream from entering your eyes, nose, or mouth.
Chromium	*Tablet:* Take 50 to 200 mcg daily for type 2 diabetes, in the form of chromium picolinate. Consult your doctor about taking higher doses of chromium if you have diabetes.
CoQ10	*Capsule:* Take 100 mg twice daily.
Evening Primrose Oil	*Capsule:* Take 4 to 6 g daily, in divided doses, with food, to treat diabetic nerve damage.
Fenugreek	*Capsule:* Take 5 to 30 g daily with each meal, or 15 to 90 g together with one meal. *Seeds:* Studies have used 15 g of powdered fenugreek seed soaked in water, with positive results. *Note:* Oral diabetes medications should not be taken together with fenugreek. Fenugreek may cause urine to have a maple syrup odor.
Fiber	*Diet:* Studies conducted on people who consumed 54 g of fiber daily yielded positive results.
Garlic	*Fresh:* Eat 1 clove of fresh garlic daily. *Note:* One to 1^1/$_2$ cloves of fresh garlic is equivalent to 10 g of fresh garlic, 18 mg of garlic oil, or 600 to 900 mg of garlic powder.

(continued)

MY SUPPLEMENT LIST—DIABETES (continued)	
SUPPLEMENT	**RECOMMENDED DOSAGE**
Ginseng	*Capsule:* Take 200 mg of a standardized extract containing 4% to 7% ginsenosides, divided in two doses daily.
Gymnema	*Capsule:* Take 1,000 mg twice daily. *Note:* It may take 6 to 12 months to notice the therapeutic effects of gymnema.
L-Carnitine	*Capsule or Tablet:* Take 1 to 3 g daily.
Magnesium	*Tablet:* Take 300 to 700 mg daily, in divided doses, with food. *Note:* Take in the form of magnesium glycinate to avoid loose stools. Large amounts of magnesium can cause diarrhea; if this becomes a problem for you, reduce your dosage.
Omega-3 Fatty Acids	*Fish Oil—Capsule:* Take enough fish oil to provide you with 3 g of total eicosapentaenoic acid (EPA) and docosahexaenoic acid (DHA), in divided doses, twice daily, with meals.
Vitamin B$_6$	*Tablet:* Dosages range from 30 to 200 mg daily. If you have gestational diabetes, talk to your doctor about an appropriate dosage of this supplement. *Caution:* If you have liver disease, consult your doctor before taking more than 50 mg of vitamin B$_6$ daily.
Vitamin C	*Capsule or Tablet:* Dosages as high as 1 to 2 buffered g a day (or even higher) with meals may be recommended for people managing their diabetes with insulin. Consult your doctor to find a dosage that is appropriate for you. High doses of vitamin C may have a laxative effect.
Vitamin E	*Capsule:* Take 400 IU each day of a natural product containing mixed tocopherols.
Zinc	*Tablet:* Dosages as high as 15 to 40 mg daily of zinc have been used for diabetes. Since zinc can have a negative effect on the body's absorption of copper at this high dosage, also take 1 to 2 g of copper daily (usually the amount in a multivitamin). *Caution:* High dosages of zinc, such as described above, should be taken only on the advice of a physician.

DIARRHEA

WHILE YOU MAY NOT KNOW the exact cause of your discomfort, what you do know is that you need to find the nearest bathroom . . . and fast! The normal rules of time and space lose all meaning when you're in the grips of a diarrhea attack. A bout of diarrhea can ruffle the feathers of even the most composed individuals, leaving them scratching their heads and wondering whether the cause was something they ate, all the undue stress they're experiencing, or a side effect of a recently prescribed medication.

WHAT IS IT?

In a healthy digestive system, the body digests nutrients properly— food and fluids are passed through the colon and absorbed, and the result is a formed stool. When diarrhea occurs, food and liquid sweep through the body too quickly to be absorbed, causing stools to become watery and loose.

According to the U.S. National Institutes of Health, the average American adult experiences a bout of diarrhea four times a year. Various factors can cause diarrhea, such as food sensitivity or allergy, bacterial or viral infections, parasites, certain medications, intestinal diseases, and functional bowel disorders (as in irritable bowel syndrome, see page 520). While diarrhea is usually not cause for alarm, prolonged cases of diarrhea can lead to dehydration or indicate a more serious health issue.

In many cases, diarrhea goes hand-in-hand with stomach cramps, abdominal pain, nausea, bloating, and, depending on the cause, fever. Short-term or acute diarrhea often lasts for up to 3 days, whereas long-term or chronic diarrhea can last for 3 weeks or more. Children often experience diarrhea, and it can be especially dangerous in infants and small children because it poses a greater risk of dehydration than in adults.

Useful steps in treating diarrhea include getting plenty of replacement fluids and electrolytes (such as sodium), and eating a bland diet that excludes sugar and dairy products. Medications, including antibiotics, may also be necessary in some cases.

WHAT SHOULD I TAKE?
Bilberry • Garlic • Goldenseal
Lactobacillus Acidophilus • Psyllium • Slippery Elm

The German Commission E approves the use of **bilberry** supplements for people with acute diarrhea. Some experts recommend bilberry fruit to both children and adults with diarrhea. (For more information on bilberry, see page 44.)

Because of its powerful bateria-killing properties, **garlic** may be useful in treating intestinal bacteria that can cause diarrhea. Not only do studies indicate that garlic may be effective in killing bacteria that are resistant to antibiotics, but it may also enhance the effect

CALL YOUR DOCTOR WHEN...

In some cases, diarrhea can indicate a more serious health problem. Make sure to consult your doctor if:

- Diarrhea has lasted for more than 3 days
- Diarrhea is accompanied by abdominal or rectal pain or a fever of 102° F or higher
- You have blood in your stool or the stool is black and tarry
- You have signs of dehydration (decreased urination, fatigue, and light-headedness)
- Your diarrhea is accompanied by fever, chills, rash, vomiting, changes in mental status, severe headache, or fainting.

Caution: Dehydration in children and elderly persons is a serious problem that warrants prompt medical attention. Make sure to call your doctor immediately in these cases.

KITCHEN TIPS

REHYDRATION MADE SIMPLE

While weak tea, flat soda, and Jell-O are often used to help rehydrate people with diarrhea, the best remedy for dehydration may be in your vegetable garden. When dehydration strikes, cook any vegetables you have in your home—celery, carrots, and greens such as spinach or broccoli are all good choices— in a pot of water, and let them simmer for one hour. The vegetables will make a broth that is rich in sugar, sodium, and potassium. Drink the broth to help eliminate dehydration.

of antibiotics when taken together with them. (For more information on garlic, see page 135.)

Goldenseal, because of its bacteria-killing component called berberine, may help relieve some cases of diarrhea caused by bacterial infection. (For more information on goldenseal, see page 151.)

A number of studies have found that **Lactobacillus acidophilus** bacteria are useful in treating diarrhea both in adults and young children. The studies included cases of diarrhea caused by viral infections and antibiotic medications. Antibiotic use can lead to a potentially serious overgrowth of harmful microbes, in which case supplementation with "good" bacteria, such as *Lactobacillus acidophilus* can help "crowd out" the bad ones. (For more information on Lactobacillus acidophilus, see page 180.)

Psyllium may be better known as a supplement for preventing constipation, but it also works to treat diarrhea. Psyllium, made from the husks of a certain kind of plant seed, may absorb excess fluids from loose stools, thus helping to "bulk up" loose stools. The German Commission E (see page 16) recommends psyllium for treating various types of diarrhea. Keep in mind, however, that when psyllium is used to treat diarrhea, it should be taken with about one-fourth of the recommended amount of water or it may cause loose stools. (For more information on psyllium and fiber, see page 120.)

Slippery elm, taken from the inner bark of the slippery elm tree, has a gummy texture, and herbalists have commonly recommended treatments containing slippery elm powder for coating and soothing the intestines in people with diarrhea. (For more information on slippery elm, see page 256.)

MY SUPPLEMENT LIST—DIARRHEA

Be sure to consult your doctor before administering any type of supplement to children.

SUPPLEMENT	RECOMMENDED DOSAGE
Bilberry	*Fruit:* Difficult to find in the United States, you may be able to find a dried product on the market. *Tablet:* Take 80 to 160 mg of an extract, standardized to contain 25% anthocyanosides, three times daily.
Garlic	*Capsule:* Take 600 to 900 mg daily of a preparation standardized to contain 5,000 to 6,000 mcg of allicin potential. Or crush a clove of raw garlic and take two to three times per day. Taking it with a bit of applesauce or yogurt may improve the palatability.

MY SUPPLEMENT LIST—DIARRHEA	
SUPPLEMENT	**RECOMMENDED DOSAGE**
Goldenseal	*Capsule or Tablet:* Take 1,000 mg of a standardized extract from one to three times daily.
Lactobacillus Acidophilus	*Capsule:* Adults should take enough of a supplement to provide 1 to 10 billion viable organisms per day. Follow the label directions for dosage information, since products will vary in their content of this supplement.
Psyllium	*Capsule:* Studies have typically used 7.5 to 30 g of psyllium daily, either in one dose or divided into several doses. *Note:* When using psyllium to treat diarrhea, take it with one-fourth of the recommended amount of water or fluid specified on the product label.
Slippery Elm	*Capsule:* Take up to 12 capsules daily containing 400 mg of slippery elm, as needed. *Tea:* Make a tea by combining 1 or 2 tsp or teabags of loose bark with 1 cup of boiling water; drink up to four times a day.

DIVERTICULAR DISEASE

IT WAS ONCE BELIEVED THAT IN industrialized nations of the Western world, people tend to eat more processed, refined foods than their global neighbors in Asia and Africa and that this was partly responsible for the greater incidence of diverticular disease in the west. However, diverticular disease is no longer limited to the United States. New research suggests that this condition is becoming an emerging problem in many areas of the African tropics, owing in part to the increase in highly processed food products in

Lifestyle Changes

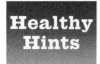

While certain common vices such as consuming alcoholic and caffeinated beverages may not have a direct effect on diverticular disease, some food and lifestyle choices can increase your chances of steering clear of symptoms of this condition. Read on for tips to avoid complications of diverticular disease:

- **Eat your vegetables.** A vegetarian diet may be beneficial for staving off diverticular disease. Although more research is needed, the Imperial Cancer Research Fund in England conducted a study and found that vegetarians may have a lower risk of developing certain diseases, including constipation and diverticular disease.

- **Quit smoking.** Although the results of studies remain inconclusive, there may be a correlation between smoking and diverticular disease. One study of 80 people with diverticular disease found that smokers seemed to have a predisposition to the disease.

- **Exercise!** Studies conducted at the Harvard School of Public Health found that people with a sedentary lifestyle have an increased risk of developing diverticular disease. Those who lead an active life, with more physical exercise, are less likely to develop diverticular disease.

supermarkets. Although such foods may be tasty and convenient, they also have a lower content of fiber, and consequently may come with a price—a higher incidence of diverticular disease.

WHAT IS IT?

Many people over the age of 60 have small, bulging pouches (or *diverticula*) in their digestive tracts, often caused by constipation from too little fiber in the diet. This condition is known as diverticulosis, and is often unnoticed and pain-free. In some cases, however, these pouches become inflamed, a more serious health condition known as diverticulitis.

Diverticulitis is often marked by abdominal pain, fever, nausea, or a change in bowel habits. Other symptoms of diverticulitis include painful urination, bloating, and rectal bleeding. Although many cases of diverticulitis can be treated through lifestyle changes and antibiotics, more serious cases may require surgery to remove diseased sections of the colon.

WHAT SHOULD I TAKE?

Fiber • Flaxseed • Glucomannan • Glutamine

A high-fiber diet is one of the most commonly recommended self-care methods for preventing and treating diverticular disease. In addition to eating plenty of fruits and vegetables, you may benefit from taking supplemental **fiber** in the form of psyllium, such as Metamucil. **Flaxseed** is another high-fiber supplement that may help treat diverticulosis. (For more information on fiber, see page 120.)

Glucomannan is a water-soluble dietary fiber derived from the root of the konjac plant *(Amorphophallus konjac)*. Preliminary studies indicate that glucomannan may be effective in reducing symptoms of diverticular disease. (For more information on glucomannan and fiber, see page 120.)

The amino acid **glutamine** may protect the lining of the digestive tract and may be useful in treating diverticular disease. (For more information on glutamine, see page 146.)

MY SUPPLEMENT LIST—DIVERTICULAR DISEASE

SUPPLEMENT	RECOMMENDED DOSAGE
Fiber	*Powder:* Take 7 g of psyllium in 8 oz of liquid from one to three times a day. Be sure to carefully follow the dosage instructions on your particular psyllium product.

MY SUPPLEMENT LIST—DIVERTICULAR DISEASE	
SUPPLEMENT	**RECOMMENDED DOSAGE**
Flaxseed	*Fresh:* Take 1 or 2 tbsp of seeds freshly ground in a coffee grinder and sprinkle on salad or cereal, followed by 1 to 2 glasses of water as needed.
Glucomannan	*Capsule:* Studies show that 3 or 4 g daily may be effective as a laxative.
Glutamine	*Capsule or Tablet:* Therapeutic dosages of glutamine range from 1.5 to 6 g daily. Consult your doctor to determine a dosage that is appropriate for you. *Note:* Avoid taking glutamine if you have liver or kidney disease.

EAR INFECTION

MANY PARENTS HAVE SPENT long nights trying to comfort a child with an ear infection. Among the most common childhood maladies, ear infections will affect almost all children at least once by the age of 7. Ear infections can range from being painful to excruciating and can be difficult to diagnose in children who do not yet have the language skills to communicate their symptoms. Ear infection can also occur in adults, especially those with allergies, although not as commonly as in children.

WHAT IS IT?

There are three main types of ear infection—outer, middle, and inner. An outer-ear infection, also called "swimmer's ear," occurs when the skin in the external part of the ear canal breaks and becomes irritated by too much water contact. This allows bacteria or fungi to more easily penetrate the skin and cause infection. An inner-ear infection is a very rare occurrence and is a complication of a middle-ear infection. Treatment methods for these infections require medical intervention.

Middle-ear infections—also called *otitis media*—are the most common type of ear infection. In order to understand this infection, it is important to understand the basic anatomy of the ear: The middle ear is located behind the eardrum, and is connected to the throat and nose via the eustachian tube. This tube allows the air pressure in the middle ear to remain the same as the atmospheric pressure in the immediate surroundings (as when flying in an airplane), and also allows fluid to drain away from the middle ear. When the draining action of the eustachian tube is hampered, often by a respiratory infection or allergy that causes the walls of the tube to become swollen, fluid can build up in the middle ear, providing a breeding ground for bacteria. The resulting infection—otitis media—is painful, interferes with hearing, and in some cases can even rupture the eardrum. Ear infections are more common in children because their eustachian tubes are shorter and positioned more horizontally than those of adults, making it more difficult for fluids to drain from the ear.

Treating the infection or allergy that blocks the eustachian tube is one way to prevent otitis media. Doctors commonly treat otitis media with antibiotics, although this approach is now controversial, since most children will get better without taking prescription medication. Placing drainage tubes in the eardrums is another common treatment for recurring ear infections, although this is usually done after numerous courses of antibiotics have failed.

WHAT SHOULD I TAKE?
Echinacea • Eucalyptus Oil • Herbal Eardrops (Garlic, Calendula, St. John's Wort, and Mullein Flower blend) Multivitamin with Selenium and Fish Oil • Xylitol

Immune-boosting **echinacea** may be helpful for warding off an ear infection and may also be beneficial if taken when symptoms of an ear infection first appear, to keep it from worsening. Echinacea is especially useful for ear infections that result from a respiratory infection. (For more information on echinacea, see page 107.)

While often used to treat the common cold, **eucalyptus** may also have a positive effect on otitis media, especially when used in the late stages of this condition. The oil is used in the form of a steam inhalation and may be effective in opening the passageways of the nose and throat. (For more information on eucalyptus, see page 111.)

Second-Hand Smoke Increases Risk of Children's Ear Infections

Did You Know?

According to a report published by the American Academy of Pediatrics, cigarette exposure is associated with 1.2 million or 7 percent of ear infections in the U.S. each year. Infants and children exposed to second-hand smoke are more likely to develop middle ear infections. Second-hand or "passive" smoke can come from two sources—the smoke exhaled by a smoker and the smoke emitted by a burning cigarette. Children exposed to smokers absorb the nicotine and other chemicals in cigarette smoke and are very vulnerable to these substances' potential hazards.

Children exposed to household smoke are also more likely to require surgery because of recurring ear infections, making up 14 percent of all ear tube insertions. Remember that if you smoke, your child is essentially also smoking and that you can add ear infections to the list of ways in which you may be harming your child.

Herbal eardrops consisting of garlic, calendula, St. John's wort, and mullein flower may help in treating the pain associated with an ear infection. An Israeli study of 103 children between the ages of 6 and 18 who had acute ear infections compared anesthetic eardrops with a proprietary blend of calendula, St. John's wort, mullein flower, and garlic. The study found the natural treatment to be as effective as the anesthetic eardrops and therefore an appropriate choice for reducing ear-infection pain. (For more information on garlic, calendula, and St. John's wort, see pages 135, 61, and 262.)

A preliminary study found that children with otitis media who were given daily supplements of cod-liver oil (for which **fish oil** may be substituted), **selenium**, and a **multivitamin** required less antibiotic than before receiving this supplementation. Additional research is needed to assess the effectiveness of these supplements in children with chronic ear infections. (For more information on fish oil, selenium, and multivitamins, see pages 221, 253, and 9.)

Xylitol, a sugar alcohol produced from birch sap, may be effective in preventing ear infections in children. In one study of 857 children, chewing gum containing xylitol was found to reduce the risk of ear infection by 40 percent. Xylitol syrup was less effective than the gum, and xylitol lozenges were the least effective form of xylitol. Although xylitol was effective in preventing ear infection, it does not appear to be effective in treating an ear infection once it has begun or in children who have drainage tubes. (For more information on xylitol, see page 300.)

MY SUPPLEMENT LIST—EAR INFECTION

Be sure to consult your doctor before administering any type of supplement to children.

SUPPLEMENT	RECOMMENDED DOSAGE
Echinacea Species	*Adults and children age 6 and over—Tea:* Make tea with one-half to 1 g of dried root, or 1 teabag, and drink three times daily. *Fluid Extract:* Take 1 to 2 ml of a fluid extract three times daily. *Capsule:* Take 150 to 300 mg of a powdered extract twice daily.
	Note: For children under age 6, use half these adult dosages.
Eucalyptus Oil	*Steam:* Use a tincture with 5% to 10% eucalyptus oil. Place in a vaporizer and use as a local inhalant. You may also place a few drops of oil in a pot of boiling water, drape a towel over your head and the pot, and breathe deeply to inhale the steam.

(continued)

MY SUPPLEMENT LIST—EAR INFECTION (continued)	
SUPPLEMENT	**RECOMMENDED DOSAGE**
	Note: Eucalyptus should not be used topically, especially on the nose or face of a young infant or child. Consult your doctor before applying eucalyptus oil topically.
Herbal Eardrops	*Eardrops:* A number of available products contain combinations of garlic, mullein, calendula, and St. John's wort. Follow the product label directions for dosage instruction. *Note:* Do not use this product if you think an infected eardrum has ruptured.
Multivitamin with Selenium and Fish oil	*Child age 1 to 4 years—Tablet:* Take 1 selenium-containing children's chewable multivitamin daily. *Liquid:* Take 1 tsp of cod-liver or fish oil daily.
Xylitol	*Chewing Gum:* For children with ear infections, chew 8.4 g of a xylitol-sweetened gum, four or five times daily. *Syrup:* Children should take 8.4 to 10 g daily, divided into five doses.

EATING DISORDERS

THE DIET INDUSTRY IS A 50-billion-dollar-a-year enterprise. This clearly shows that controlling weight and staying slender are great concerns for many people. *Why do last year's jeans suddenly feel too snug? Do we really need that last bite of food? If we eat that ice cream now, what will we have to avoid later?* For people with eating disorders, the problem goes far beyond this. In people with eating disorders, an acute concern about body image can combine with unhealthy eating patterns in a condition that can lead to malnutrition and menstrual irregularities, and may even cause organ damage or death. Eating disorders often strike people who also have depression and anxiety.

WHAT IS IT?

Eating disorders occur when a fixation on weight causes severe disturbances of healthy eating habits. The two most common eating disorders are *anorexia nervosa* and *bulimia nervosa*. Both of these conditions are most common in teenage girls and young women. Eating disorders can occur for a variety of reasons. Some studies show that certain personality types—those characterized by anxiety, perfectionism, and obsessive-compulsive behavior—are more likely to be accompanied by eating disorders. Research shows that heredity may also play a role in certain eating disorders. Psychological, social, and family problems, as well as the media, may create eating disorders.

According to government figures, roughly 4 percent of all women will experience anorexia during their lives. The condition is marked by an urge to stay excessively thin and a fear of becoming fat, as well as an inability to acknowledge being underweight because of a distorted body image. The person with anorexia may be obsessed about food, eat only tiny amounts, and exercise to an extreme, unhealthy degree.

People with bulimia—also known as the "diet binge-purge disorder"—often eat large amounts of food and feel that their eating is "out of control." They then take extreme measures to avoid gaining weight, such as vomiting, taking laxatives, fasting, or exercising furiously. When they are not binging, people with bulimia often diet, which makes them hungry and thus drives them to binge once again.

Eating disorders often need to be treated by a team of professionals, including a physician, a mental health professional, and a nutritionist, to deal with the physical and psychological triggers and consequences of the disorder. Overeaters Anonymous is a world-wide support group based on the Twelve Step concept (more information may be easily found online). People with severe eating disorders may even need to be hospitalized. The following supplements may be useful, in addition to professional care, for eating disorders.

WHAT SHOULD I TAKE?

Eating disorders are very serious conditions. Make sure to consult your doctor before taking any type of supplement. Be sure to speak with your doctor before administering any type of supplement to children or young adults.

Calcium • Dehydroepiandrosterone (DHEA) • Magnesium Multivitamin • Vitamin B Complex • Zinc

People with eating disorders tend to lack **calcium** in their diets, in addition to absorbing less of this mineral and excreting more of it from their bodies. This can contribute to decreased bone mineral density and an increased risk for osteoporosis. (For more information on calcium, see page 57.)

DHEA may reduce bone loss in people with eating disorders. In one study, 15 young women with anorexia showed significant improvements in bone health when given supplemental DHEA daily, including a reversal of bone loss. Women who had stopped menstruation also started to menstruate once again after taking DHEA. However, DHEA should be taken only under medical supervision. (For more information on DHEA, see page 100.)

FRIENDS AND FOES

Long-term **zinc** supplementation reduces levels of **copper** in the body. If you take zinc for more than 3 months, be sure to take 2 or 3 milligrams of a copper supplement daily.

People with eating disorders often have a deficiency of **magnesium**. When compared to a group of healthy patients, those with eating disorders and low magnesium levels often experienced greater muscle weakness and cramping, restlessness, difficulty concentrating, high blood pressure, heart problems, and short-term memory loss. These symptoms improved after supplementation with magnesium and returned when magnesium supplementation was discontinued. (For more information on magnesium, see page 203.)

People with eating disorders are at risk for a number of vitamin and mineral deficiencies that can cause serious health problems. A **multivitamin** can help to correct these vitamin deficiencies. (For more information on multivitamins, see page 9.)

Several studies have suggested that more than one-fifth of people with anorexia may be deficient in vitamins B_2 and B_6. People with anorexia and bulimia may also have a deficient intake of folic acid (vitamin B_9). Additionally, supplements of niacin (vitamin B_3) have been shown to be helpful in improving the appetite and mental state of people with anorexia. **B-complex** vitamins may also help reduce the stress and depression associated with eating disorders. (For more information on vitamin B complex, see pages 277, 279, and 282.)

A deficiency of **zinc** is commonly noted in people with eating disorders. Zinc deficiency can contribute to a loss of appetite, depression, and weight loss. Taking supplements to correct zinc deficiency has been shown in studies to improve appetite, emotional outlook, and the abil-

Communication May Prevent Eating Disorders

Did You Know?

With an estimated 11 percent of high school students having some type of eating disorder, and 40 percent of first- through third-grade girls admitting that they would like to be thinner, it is clear that eating disorders are a serious problem in adolescents and teenagers. However, there are many things you can do as a parent to prevent eating disorders in your children:

■ Maintain healthy attitudes and behaviors toward food and body image. Your children will follow your example.

■ Do not overemphasize the importance of beauty and

body shape. Do not reinforce the idea that fat is bad and thin is good.

■ Educate your children about the dangers of dieting and the benefits of nutritional health and exercise when practiced in moderation.

■ Help your children understand the ways in which television, magazines, and other media distort the reality and diversity of various body types. Explain that in order to be successful, powerful, popular, or beautiful, you do not need to be skinny.

■ Promote your children's self-esteem and self-respect. Teach them that there is no such thing as a "perfect" body type.

ity to taste foods. In one study, supplemental zinc may have been a factor in the improvement of women with bulimia who went on to develop a healthier body image. Other studies suggest that zinc may help to enhance weight gain and stabilize mood in people with anorexia. (For more information on zinc, see page 304.)

MY SUPPLEMENT LIST—EATING DISORDERS

SUPPLEMENT	RECOMMENDED DOSAGE
Calcium	*Capsule or Tablet: (Adults age 49 and under):* Take 1,000 mg of calcium citrate daily divided into two doses. *(Adults age 50 and over):* Take 1,200 mg of calcium citrate daily divided into two or three doses. Consult your doctor about determining a dosage that suits your particular needs.
DHEA	*Capsule or Tablet:* DHEA should be taken only under the supervision of a doctor. The ideal dose and long-term effects of this supplement are unknown. Ask your doctor to check your DHEA-S level to see if you need to take the hormone
Magnesium	*Tablet:* Take 500 to 800 mg daily, in divided doses. If it causes loose stools, try the magnesium glycinate form, which is often better tolerated.
Multivitamin	Take a multivitamin/mineral supplement daily. Follow the individual product label for specific dosage information.
Vitamin B Complex	*Tablet:* Take a B-complex vitamin daily. Be sure your formula includes all of the essential B vitamins, including vitamins B_1, B_2, niacin, B_6, folic acid, B_{12}, and biotin.
Zinc	*Tablet:* Take 15 mg daily.

ECZEMA

PLENTY OF RASHES CAN CAUSE you to itch, but eczema is known as "the itch that rashes." This maddeningly itchy skin condition can cause people to scratch so uncontrollably, particularly at night, that they damage their skin, leaving them prone to infection.

WHAT IS IT?

Eczema, also called "atopic dermatitis," usually affects the elbows, backs of the knees, and face, although it may affect other areas of the body as well. Eczema is usually triggered by allergies, and often affects people who have asthma and hay fever, although there is also a hereditary risk of this condition. The condition usually appears in infancy or childhood, but it can extend well into adulthood.

Eczema occurs when the immune system overreacts to certain allergens (such as soap, water, perfumes, certain fabrics, dust mites, and pet dander) and the skin releases chemicals that cause itching and inflammation. The inflamed skin may be red, cracked, and scaly, and it may also ooze fluid and become crusted. Long-term scratching may eventually cause the skin in an affected area to grow thick and leathery.

Although it may be unsightly, eczema is not contagious. Moreover, while there is no cure for the condition, there are ways to manage its symptoms. One key to preventing eczema is avoiding irritants and allergens. Treatments for the condition rest heavily on boosting the immune system and keeping the skin moisturized. Doctors also commonly recommend over-the-counter and prescription corticosteroid skin treatments for eczema. However, some physicians argue that steroid creams are absorbed into the circulation, causing suppression of the body's natural steroid-producing glands.

WHAT SHOULD I USE?

Calendula • Chamomile • Evening Primrose Oil
Lactobacillus Acidophilus • Licorice • Omega-3 Fatty Acids
Red Clover • St. John's Wort

Calendula cream is very popular in Europe for the topical treatment of eczema. The cream is often combined with chamomile (see below) for a variety of skin conditions, although further research on its effectiveness is needed. (For more information on calendula, see page 61.)

Food Allergies and Eczema

Did You Know?

Many experts believe that food allergy plays a role in eczema, particularly in children. The foods commonly implicated include dairy products (such as milk), eggs, wheat, sugar, peanuts, and soy. If you have eczema, an elimination diet (see page 449) may help you determine whether certain foods are triggering your symptoms. Eliminate each of these foods from your diet, one at a time, and record your body's reaction as you reintroduce them. Avoiding such "trigger" foods may help control the discomfort associated with eczema.

New mothers may be able to beat the odds of their children's developing eczema by choosing to breastfeed. Studies have shown that children who are exclusively breastfed early in life may be less likely to get eczema. However, mothers who are breastfeeding should take special care to avoid eating the common food allergens described above. Consult your doctor or a dietician to customize a food plan that will help beat eczema.

The German Commission E (see page 16) approves the use of topical **chamomile** for treating a variety of skin conditions. Topical chamomile treatments may reduce inflammation and allergic activity in affected areas of the skin, making them a popular choice for treating eczema in Europe. Chamomile is often combined with licorice (see below) or calendula (see above) in topical creams. (For more information on chamomile, see page 67.)

While studies examining the effects of **evening primrose oil** on eczema had mixed results, this supplement is widely used in Europe for treating eczema and may work in some people and not others. Your doctor may be able to advise whether it is worth giving this nutrient a try. (For more information on evening primrose oil, see page 115.)

When taken by pregnant and breastfeeding women, probiotic supplements of **Lactobacillus acidophilus** may help prevent eczema in babies at high risk for this condition. Two studies have found that babies of mothers who took probiotics while pregnant and breastfeeding were less likely to develop eczema before the age of 2. Also, acidophilus supplements may help reduce itching in people with low levels of these beneficial bacteria in their digestive systems. (For more information on acidophilus, see page 180.)

A component of **licorice**, called glycyrrhetinic acid, has an effect on eczema similar to that of hydrocortisone. In a study conducted in the 1950s, 9 of 12 patients with eczema had marked improvement after using an ointment containing this licorice ingredient. Finding a topical treatment containing glycyrrhetinic acid may, however, be difficult. Fortunately, taking licorice internally can also be effective for eczema because of the anti-inflammatory effect of licorice, and oral licorice supplements are easy to find in health-food stores. (For more information on licorice, see page 192.)

Research indicates that people with eczema have low levels of **omega-3 fatty acids**. Studies suggest that supplemental omega-3 fatty acids will reduce the severity and inflammation of eczema. (For more information on omega-3 fatty acids, see page 221.)

While there is little medical literature on the topical use of **red clover** for eczema, there is a long historic basis for this in herbal medicine. It is often found as an ingredient in topical herbal salves. (For more information about red clover, see page 238.)

St. John's wort has recently received study in the medical literature as a topical agent for the treatment of eczema. One of its chemical constituents, hyperforin, has antibacterial and anti-inflammatory effects. (For more information about red clover, see page 262.)

MY SUPPLEMENT LIST—ECZEMA

SUPPLEMENT	RECOMMENDED DOSAGE
Calendula	*Topical—Ointment:* Creams containing calendula are often applied topically two or three times daily. Follow the product label for application instruction.
Chamomile	*Topical—Ointment:* Look for a cream containing from 3% to 10% crude chamomile, and follow the individual product label for application instruction.
Evening Primrose Oil	*Oral—Capsule:* Take 3,000 mg daily.
Lactobacillus Acidophilus	*Capsule:* Take 1 to 2 billion colony-forming units (CFU) daily.
Licorice	*Oral—Capsule:* Take one to three capsules standardized to contain 20 mg of licorice root extract and 50 mg of glycyrrhizinc acid daily. Licorice supplements with glycyrrhizinic acid should not be used for more than 4 weeks at a time. *Topical—Gel:* Apply licorice root gel to affected areas of the skin. Read product label for application instruction. *Note:* Licorice candy is made with artificial flavorings and has no healing properties.
Omega-3 Fatty Acids	*Capsule:* In studies, dosages of 2 to 4 g daily were associated with reduced inflammation in people with eczema. Purchase a product containing both eicosapentaenoic acid (EPA) and docosahexaenoic acid (DHA). The amount of omega-3 fatty acid will vary by manufacturer, so be sure to check the product label carefully.
Red Clover	Look for herbal salves that contain this ingredient, and apply to affected areas several times per day.
St. John's Wort	*Oil:* Apply topically to the affected areas several times per day.

EMPHYSEMA

MANY PEOPLE ARE UNFAMILIAR with chronic obstructive pulmonary disease (COPD), an umbrella term that refers to the lung conditions known as emphysema and chronic bronchitis. COPD is the fourth leading cause of death in the United States, and 16 million Americans have it. Within this group are about 3 million Americans who have emphysema, a chronic lung disease marked by a constant shortness of breath and a chronic cough.

WHAT IS IT?

Emphysema occurs when there is an enlargement of the tiny air spaces in the lungs known as alveoli from which gasses pass to and from inhaled air and the blood, as well as damage to the tissues of the lung. It is often caused by smoking. In some cases a hereditary chemical damages the elastic fibers that allow the lungs to expand and contract. The substance that is defective in such cases is called alpha 1-antitrypsin (AAT).

Smoking accounts for 80 to 90 percent of all cases of COPD. With continued smoking, gradual damage is inflicted on the alveoli. Once the fragile walls of these tiny air sacs become permanently damaged, the alveoli can no longer effectively transfer oxygen to the bloodstream. The result is shortness of breath, one of the main symptoms of emphysema.

Aside from shortness of breath, symptoms of emphysema include chronic cough, fatigue, appetite and weight loss, and an increased risk of pneumonia, asthma, bronchitis, and other serious respiratory conditions.

Although there is no cure for emphysema, certain behaviors can help slow the progression of this disease. Quitting smoking before emphysema develops is the best way to prevent it. Breathing exercises may help promote lung strength and prevent additional damage to the lungs. Herbs and supplements may help to ease the symptoms and slow the progression of emphysema.

WHAT SHOULD I TAKE?

Emphysema is a very serious condition. Make sure to see your doctor before taking any type of supplement, especially if you have been diagnosed with emphysema or think you may have emphysema.

Bromelain • Coenzyme Q10 (CoQ10) • Cordyceps
Grape Seed Extract • L-Carnitine • Magnesium
N-Acetylcysteine (NAC)

Bromelain, an enzyme derived from pineapples, has a natural ability to break up mucus. This can be especially useful for treating the mucus-filled coughing and breathing that sometimes accompanies COPD. (For more information on bromelain, see page 54.)

Preliminary studies suggest that **CoQ10** may improve lung function in people with COPD. (For more information on CoQ10, see page 80.)

Cordyceps, a type of mushroom grown in China, has a long history of use in traditional Chinese medicine for treating coughing and wheezing. Although research on cordyceps in the United States is scant, studies indicate that it may strengthen the lungs and may thus be useful to people with emphysema. (For more information on cordyceps, see page 88.)

Preliminary studies indicate that **grape seed extract** may protect the lungs by scavenging cell- and tissue-damaging free radical molecules. Small, preliminary studies suggest that grape seed extract may also have promise as an anti-inflammatory agent that strengthens blood vessels. (For more information on grape seed extract, see page 155.)

Results from three studies suggest that **L-carnitine** may improve the ability to exercise in people with COPD, possibly by strengthening the lungs. L-carnitine is especially important for people with emphysema, who require exercise to strengthen damaged lungs. (For more information on L-carnitine, see page 186.)

Studies indicate that some people with COPD may have a deficiency of **magnesium**, and doctors sometimes give magnesium intravenously in severe COPD. While more research is needed to confirm the efficacy of supplemental or dietary magnesium in

Smoking Cessation

According to experts at the Harvard Medical School, smoking causes nearly all cases of COPD, including emphysema. If you quit smoking you can significantly decrease your chances of developing emphysema. Read on for some hints to help you kick the habit.

- **Set it up.** Set a date for quitting, and establish a nonsmoking environment by throwing away all cigarettes, cigars, or pipes and getting rid of all ashtrays in your home, car, and workplace.
- **Round up the troops.** When you're trying to break a habit, you need a good support system. Let everyone know that you are trying to quit smoking. Ask your friends and family for encouragement, and try to surround yourself with nonsmokers.

- **Trade in your habit.** People often smoke as a way to relieve stress or anxiety. Try to find a healthy way to reduce stress, such as walking or enrolling in a yoga class to stay calm and relaxed.
- **Call a professional.** Smoking is a serious addiction, and you may need professional assistance to ensure that you break the habit. Talk to your doctor about ways to quit, and consider seeking guidance from a counselor. Many hospitals and community centers offer programs that will help smokers become nonsmokers.
- **Be aware of obstacles.** If you have friends or co-workers who smoke, be aware that being with them while they smoke may make quitting more difficult. If you smoke in the evenings at your favorite hangout or while having a cocktail, you may want to seek out a new recreational routine.

COPD, making sure you get a healthy amount of this important mineral is always wise. (For more information on magnesium, see page 203.)

NAC is a variation of the amino acid cysteine. While researchers don't completely understand how NAC works, studies show that when people with COPD take NAC on a regular basis, they experience fewer attacks of severe bronchitis. (For more information on NAC, see page 213.)

MY SUPPLEMENT LIST—EMPHYSEMA

SUPPLEMENT	RECOMMENDED DOSAGE
Bromelain	*Tablet:* Take 250 to 500 mg daily between meals. Look for a supplement containing 2,400 gelatin-dissolving units (GDU) or 3,600 milk-clotting units (MCU) per gram.
CoQ10	*Softgel:* Take 30 to 300 mg daily, divided into several doses, with meals.
Cordyceps	*Capsule:* Take 5 to 10 g daily divided into three or four doses, on an empty stomach. This amount may be taken in decoction, pill, or powder form.
Grape Seed Extract	*Capsule:* Take 150–300 mg daily of an extract standardized to contain 92–95% oligomeric proanthocyanidins by weight.
L-Carnitine	*Capsule:* Take 500 to 1,000 mg three times a day, between meals.
Magnesium	*Tablet:* Take 500 to 800 mg daily, in divided doses, with meals. If this dose causes loose stools, try the glycinate form which is often more tolerable.
NAC	*Capsule:* Take 900 mg twice daily, between meals.

ENDOMETRIOSIS

THE BOTTOM LINE WITH endometriosis is that tissue is growing where it shouldn't. During healthy menstruation, women shed the lining of their uterus—the endometrium—each month, and the shed material is subsequently expelled from the body. Although many women would probably like to eliminate this monthly burden, the body has a fairly efficient system for eliminating the endometrium.

In endometriosis, however, cells from the uterine lining migrate from where they're supposed to be—inside the uterus—to other parts of the body. The cells may then multiply and grow at these sites, creating a buildup that can cause immense pain and lead to reproductive complications.

WHAT IS IT?

More than five million women in North America have endometriosis. Endometriosis occurs when endometrial cells from the uterine lining travel to areas outside the uterus, such as on the ovaries, the bladder, the bowel, and in rare cases even the lungs and other far-flung reaches of the body. This scattered tissue then swells and bleeds during every monthly menstrual period but cannot leave the body, as the endometrial tissue in the uterus does.

Symptoms of endometriosis include painful cramps or periods, heavy bleeding during periods, chronic pelvic pain, pain and cramping during sex, and painful bowel movements. Endometriosis is also one of the top three causes of infertility in women, rendering about one-third of women who have endometriosis unable to conceive. Fortunately, endometriosis-related infertility can often be corrected through the use of hormones and surgery.

The cause of endometriosis is unknown, and since there is no cure, treatment is aimed at relieving the symptoms that accompany this condition. The typical conventional medical treatment for endometriosis includes taking medications that act hormonally to stop menstruation. The following supplements may be used in addition to the steps recommended by your doctor.

WHAT SHOULD I TAKE?

Black Cohosh • Calcium • Chasteberry • Iron
Magnesium • Willow Bark

Women with Endometriosis May Be More Prone to Developing Other Health Conditions

Did You Know?

Researchers at the National Institute of Child Health and Human Development (NICHHD), at George Washington University, and at the Endometriosis Association have found that women with endometriosis are more likely than average to also have certain other diseases.

The researchers surveyed 3,680 women who had endometriosis and found that women with endometriosis are over a hundred times more likely than average to have chronic fatigue syndrome and are also at greater risk of having fibromyalgia, as well as eczema, asthma, or allergies. Sixty-one percent of participants reported allergies (compared to 18 percent in the general female population), and 12 percent had asthma (compared to 5 percent in the general female population). Twenty percent of the women in the survey had more than one other disease.

While these findings may seem alarming to women with endometriosis, researchers may be able to use this information to learn more about the causes of endometriosis and identify effective treatments for it.

Black cohosh is a common herbal treatment for menopausal complications and painful menstruation, and it may also be helpful for reducing the painful symptoms associated with endometriosis. (For more information on black cohosh, see page 48.)

Calcium and **magnesium** are minerals that aid the liver in properly metabolizing hormones, which play an important role in endometrial growth and menstruation. (For more information on calcium and magnesium, see pages 57 and 203.)

Chasteberry may decrease symptoms of endometriosis because of its ability to regulate hormones and balance hormonal fluctuations that may contribute to this condition. (For more information on chasteberry, see page 69.)

Excessive bleeding from endometriosis may contribute to **iron** deficiency. Taking an iron supplement can help boost iron levels in the body. (For more information on iron, see page 175.)

Willow bark may be helpful for reducing the pain associated with endometriosis. Although willow bark may take longer to work than conventional aspirin, studies show that its pain-relieving effects may actually last longer. (For more information on willow bark, see page 298.)

MY SUPPLEMENT LIST—ENDOMETRIOSIS

SUPPLEMENT	RECOMMENDED DOSAGE
Black Cohosh	*Capsule:* Take an extract standardized to provide 2.5% triterpene glycosides two to four capsules of 250 mg per day, in divided doses, between meals.
Calcium and Magnesium	*Capsule or Tablet:* Take 1,000 to 1,500 mg of calcium daily in 500 mg doses and 500 to 800 mg of magnesium daily. *Note:* Take magnesium in the form of magnesium glycinate to avoid loose stools. Large amounts of magnesium can cause diarrhea; if this becomes a problem for you, reduce your dosage.
Chasteberry	*Capsule:* Take 175 to 225 mg of an extract standardized to contain 0.5% agnuside each day before breakfast.
Iron	*Tablet:* A reasonable dosage for iron is 30 mg twice daily, but make sure to consult your doctor about your particular dosage needs.
Willow Bark	*Capsule:* Take a standardized extract containing 120 to 420 mg of salicin daily as needed. *Caution:* Do not take willow bark if you have an aspirin allergy, bleeding disorder, diabetes, or a peptic ulcer.

EXCESSIVE GAS

LET'S FACE IT. NO MATTER HOW old we get, gas still embarrasses us. A common misconception is that a normal, healthy digestive system shouldn't expel any gas until you eat a "trigger" food such as beans. In reality, most people produce about two pints of gas daily and release it about 14 times per day. So what you might consider "excessive" may be perfectly normal. Most gas is released from the body unnoticed; only when you do notice it does gas becomes a source of embarrassment or concern. The good news is that, although gas can be uncomfortable and unpleasant, it is—even in excess—not usually a serious health concern. In some cases, however, it can be a sign of digestion problems, food allergy, or bowel infection.

WHAT IS IT?

Gas can be expelled from the body in two forms: belching or flatulence. Belching expels air that has been swallowed into the stomach, which occurs when eating and drinking too quickly or when chewing gum. Carbonated beverages can also cause gas, which can be expelled by belching.

Swallowed air plays some role in flatulence, but the bigger culprits, are many of the foods we eat, which can cause gas to be produced in the large intestine. Certain foods contain components that don't digest well, and bacteria that live in the large intestine break down and ferment these foods, resulting in gas.

Foods known for gas-producing effects include those containing sulfur, such as beans, broccoli, and onions. People who have trouble digesting dairy products or who have lactose intolerance may also feel particularly gassy after eating products containing lactose. Drinking too much water with meals can also cause gas by diluting stomach acids and digestive enzymes.

Important steps for avoiding belching and flatulence include eating slowly, avoiding gas-producing foods (and dairy products if you're lactose-intolerant), and drinking fewer carbonated beverages.

Occasionally, gas can be a symptom of a more serious health problem, such as irritable bowel syndrome, food poisoning, or a stomach flu. The following supplements can help reduce uncomfortable gas as well as the embarrassment that often accompanies it.

WHAT SHOULD I TAKE?
*Betaine • Cayenne • Chamomile • Dandelion
Digestive Enzymes • Ginger • Lavender • Lemon Balm
Licorice • Peppermint • Valerian*

Betaine hydrochloride, a source of hydrochloric acid, is a naturally occurring chemical found in the stomach that aids in digestion. Betaine supplements may help the body to digest protein and other important nutrients, prevent the overgrowth of bacteria in the small intestine, and encourage the flow of various enzymes, all of which are important factors in healthy digestion. (For more information on betaine, see page 42.)

Although it may seem odd that the spicy **cayenne** pepper can aid in digestion, the German Commission E (see page 16) approves it for people with duodenal ulcers, which can often cause digestive upset. Additionally, studies suggest that cayenne may be useful in preventing gas caused by indigestion. (For more information on cayenne, see page 64.)

Among its many uses, **chamomile** is also used to treat digestive woes, including gas. Like ginger (see below), it is known as a *carminative,* meaning that it soothes the digestive tract. (For more information on chamomile, see page 64.)

Digestive enzymes may help alleviate gas by assisting your stomach and intestines in breaking down food so that gas does not form. (For more information about digestive enzymes, see page 102.)

If your gas is caused by food that has not been properly digested, **dandelion** may be helpful in promoting proper digestion and preventing unwanted gas. (For more information on dandelion, see page 96.)

Products made from **ginger** root are used to treat a range of digestive-upset symptoms, and ginger is also useful for easing gas. (For more information on ginger, see page 136.)

The German Commission E (see page 16) recommends **lavender** for "nervous stomach irritations" as well as for intestinal discomfort. A cup of lavender tea may be helpful in reducing the stomach upset that can produce gas. (For more information on lavender, see page 184.)

In addition to lavender (see above), the German Commission E (see page 16) recommends taking **lemon balm** for gastrointestinal discomfort. (For more information on lemon balm, see page 190.)

Because of its power as an anti-inflammatory agent, **licorice** root is often recommended as a treatment for gastric or duodenal ulcers. Licorice preparations may also be used to treat bloating, indigestion, and gas. (For more information on licorice, see page 192.)

Peppermint is another carminative herb (see Chamomile, above) and helps relieve gas by relaxing muscles in the digestive system. (For more information on peppermint, see page 226.)

Although more popular as a natural sleeping aid, **valerian** may also prove useful for treating gas, especially when the gas is accompanied by cramps. (For more information on valerian, see page 272.)

MY SUPPLEMENT LIST—EXCESSIVE GAS

SUPPLEMENT	RECOMMENDED DOSAGE
Betaine	*Capsule or Tablet:* Take betaine in the form of betaine hydrochloride. Dosages of betaine hydrochloride range widely, from 5 grains twice daily to 60 grains twice daily. Consult a doctor to determine the approrpiate dosage for you. *Note:* Betaine hydrochloride is measured in grains. One grain is equivalent to approximately 64.75 mg.
Cayenne	*Infusion:* Combine 1 cup of boiling water with ½–1 tsp of cayenne powder and let it sit for 10 minutes. Mix 1 tsp of this infusion with water and take three or four times a day. *Capsule:* Take 1,200 to 1,500 mg daily, divided into three doses.
Chamomile	*Tea:* Make chamomile tea by steeping 1 teabag or tbsp of dried chamomile in a cup of boiling water for 10 to 15 minutes. Drink up to four times daily between meals to relieve gas. *Capsule:* Take up to 2,400 mg daily, divided into several doses.
Dandelion	*Fresh:* Garnish your meal with fresh dandelion leaves to promote healthy digestion. *Capsule:* Take 1,500 mg of dried root three times daily.
Digestive Enzymes	*Capsule or Tablet:* Take 3 to 4 g in the form of 4x pancreatin daily with meals.
Ginger	*Fresh:* Take 3 to 10 g of fresh ginger daily. *Capsule:* Take 500 mg of an extract standardized to contain 5% gingerols up to four times daily, between meals. *Tea:* Steep 1 tsp or teabag of fresh ginger in 1 cup of boiling water for 10 minutes. Drink up to three times daily. *Fresh:* Take a piece of ginger and use a garlic press to squeeze out the juice. Mix 1–2 tbsp with some water and sip.
Lavender	*Tea:* Steep 1–2 tsp of lavender flowers in 1 cup of boiling water for 5–10 minutes. Drink up to three cups daily.

MY SUPPLEMENT LIST—EXCESSIVE GAS	
SUPPLEMENT	**RECOMMENDED DOSAGE**
Lemon Balm	*Tea:* Steep 1.5 to 4.5 g of fresh lemon balm in 1 cup of boiling water for 15 minutes. Drink several times daily. *Capsule:* Take up to 2,700 mg daily divided into three or four doses.
Licorice	*Chewable Tablet:* Take 200 to 300 mg of deglycyrrhizinated licorice (DGL) three times daily, with meals and before bedtime. *Note:* Licorice candy is made with artificial flavorings and has no healing properties.
Peppermint	*Tea:* Pour 1 cup of boiling water over 1 tsp, teabag, or 10 dried peppermint leaves, and steep for 5 minutes. Drink as needed.
Valerian	*Tea:* Pour 1 cup of boiling water over 1 tsp or teabag of dried valerian root. Steep for 5 to 10 minutes, and drink up to three times daily. *Capsule or Tablet:* Take 150 to 300 mg daily. *Note:* The strength of valerian products may vary greatly. Be sure to choose a standardized product and carefully follow the instructions on the label.

FEVER

CONTRARY TO POPULAR BELIEF, a fever isn't a disease or illness unto itself—it is a symptom. Nor is it necessarily a bad thing. Furthermore, there is no such thing as a "normal" temperature; most people's temperatures hover above the average 98.6°F. In infants and young children, however, even a low-grade fever can indicate serious illness. And in adults, a fever doesn't become a significant health concern until it's above 102°F or dangerous until it's above 103°F.

WHAT IS IT?

A fever is often a sign that the body is fighting off a viral or bacterial infection, such as the flu or an ear infection. Some experts believe that trying to reduce a fever of unknown origin may interfere with the body's immune response. Since some viruses, such as those that cause colds or respiratory infections, thrive at cool temperatures, running a fever may actually help the body fight off these viruses. Furthermore, many fevers subside naturally within a few days.

Certain other symptoms often accompany a fever, such as sweating, shivering, general weakness, and dehydration. Very high fever—in the range of 103°F to 106°F—may cause hallucinations, convulsions, and irritability. Although a fever can occur for a variety of reasons, identifying the symptoms that accompany it may help to determine the cause of the fever. (For additional information, see Q & A, below.) In some cases, fever may signal a serious health condition. Any fever that persists for more than a few days should be evaluated by a medical doctor.

WHAT SHOULD I TAKE?
Bilberry • Chamomile • Echinacea • Elderberry
Garlic • Goldenseal • Vitamin C • Willow Bark

Folk medicine suggests that **bilberry** may be useful for fevers caused by the common cold and by throat, skin, and urinary tract infections. (For more information on bilberry, see page 44.)

Fever is often accompanied by a host of other symptoms, such as a sore throat, wheezing, sleeplessness, and upset stomach. **Chamomile** may help temper these symptoms and reduce the discomfort that often goes hand in hand with fever. (For more information on chamomile, see page 67.)

Echinacea may be useful at treating the fever that often accompanies colds and flu. (For more information on echinacea, see page 107.)

Two studies have been published on the beneficial effects of **Elderberry**, such as alleviation of symtoms of influenza, including fever. (For more information on elderberry, see page 109.)

At what point should a person see a doctor for the treatment of a fever?

Knowing when to see a doctor for a fever varies according to age, the severity of the fever, and the accompanying symptoms. Read on for some quick tips that will help you determine when you or your child should see a doctor about a fever.

Infants under 1 month old:
■ Temperature above 100.4 °F rectally.

Infants 1 to 3 months old:
■ Temperature above 101.4°F (even if the child doesn't seem ill).
■ Temperature of 100.4°F for over 24 hours.
■ Fever accompanied by irritability.

Infants over 3 months:
■ Temperature is 101.4°F and rises or lasts for more than 3 days.

Children:
■ Fever accompanied by vomiting, headache, lethargy, or irritability
Note: Children often tolerate fever well. It is best to be guided by their other symptoms as well as by their particular temperature.

Pediatric Alert! Never give aspirin or medication containing aspirin to children with a fever. In rare cases, this may trigger a condition called Reye's syndrome, which can cause liver and brain damage and death.

Adults:
■ Temperature over 104°F.
■ Temperature of 101°F lasts for more than 3 days.
■ Fever accompanied by a major headache, stiff neck, confusion, skin rash, throat swelling, problems with breathing, or vomiting.

Garlic may give your immune system needed support while you're fighting an infection. Laboratory research indicates that garlic can kill many kinds of bacteria and may be especially useful when taken in conjunction with antibiotic drugs. (For more information on garlic, see page 135.)

Plants rich in a component called berberine have a long history of traditional use in treating fevers. Studies suggest that **goldenseal**—a plant with a high content of berberine—may have the ability to kill cold-causing viruses. (For more information on goldenseal, see page 151.)

Lemon balm is a mild herb that is historically considered useful for the relief of gas, causing a light sweat if one is sick, and the lowering of a fever. Modern studies in the test tube seem to confirm that this "balm" is good for what ails you, including a fever. (For more information on lemon balm, see page 190.)

Peppermint has been used by herbalists to "cool a fever." Studies now indicate that the essential oils have antibiotic activity against some of the bacteria that cause upper respiratory infections. (For more information on peppermint, see page 226.)

Antibiotic drugs often reduce the body's levels of **vitamin C**. Supplementing with vitamin C makes good sense if you're taking an antibiotic for an infection. Recent studies indicate that high doses of vitamin C may be effective in combating infection after surgery. Other studies show that vitamin C may be useful in restoring healthy numbers of blood cells in children with strep throat. (For more information on vitamin C, see page 284.)

Willow bark is often used as an alternative to aspirin for reducing fever, since it contains the compounds known as salicin and other salicylates, which are related to aspirin. (For more information on willow bark, see page 298.)

MY SUPPLEMENT LIST—FEVER

Be sure to consult your doctor before administering any type of supplement to children.

SUPPLEMENT	RECOMMENDED DOSAGE
Bilberry	*Capsule:* Take 240 mg three times daily of an extract standardized to contain 25% anthrocyanidins.
Chamomile	*Inhalant:* Bring 2 cups of water to a boil and add 10 drops of chamomile essential oil. Remove the pot of water from the heating source, lean over the water, and

(continued)

MY SUPPLEMENT LIST—FEVER (continued)	
SUPPLEMENT	**RECOMMENDED DOSAGE**
	make a "tent" by draping a towel over your head and the water. Inhale the steam deeply to treat respiratory inflammation, making sure not to burn yourself. *Tea:* Make tea by adding 2 to 3 tsp or teabags of chamomile flower to boiling water. Steep for 10 minutes and drink up to 3 times daily.
Echinacea	*Capsule:* Take up to 1,200 mg daily of an extract standardized to contain 125 mg of *E. augustfolia* root and at least 3.2% to 4.8% of echinacoside. Other echinacea species, such as *E. purpurea*, and *E. pallida* are also used.
Elderberry	*Tea:* Steep 3 to 5 g (1/2 to 1 tsp) of dried flowers in 1 cup of boiling water for 10 to 15 minutes. Drink three times daily. *Syrup:* Take from 2 tsp to 2 tbsp twice daily. *Note:* Elderberry syrup dosages may vary for different products. Be sure to read the individual product label for dosage information.
Garlic	*Fresh:* Eat 2 to 4 fresh, raw, chopped garlic cloves daily. *Capsule:* Take 900 mg daily of a garlic powder extract standardized to contain 1.3% allicin, providing about 12,000 mcg of allicin daily. Be sure the product you buy also has 4 to 5 mg of allicin potential.
Goldenseal	*Capsule or Tablet:* Take 250 to 500 mg three times daily of a preparation standardized to contain 5% berberine. *Note:* Do not use goldenseal for more than 3 weeks consecutively because it may lose its effectiveness. Goldenseal is not recommended for children under the age of 2 years. Do not give goldenseal to children without a doctor's supervision.
Lemon Balm	*Tea:* Steep 1.5–4.5 g of fresh lemon balm in 1 cup of boiling water for 15 minutes. Drink several times daily. *Capsule:* Take up to 2,700 mg daily divided into three or four doses.
Peppermint	*Tea:* Steep 1–2 tsp or teabags of dried peppermint leaf in 8 ounces of hot water for 5 minutes. Drink as needed. Add a few drops of the essential oil to some hot water, and inhale the vapors.
Vitamin C	*Capsule or Tablet:* Take 500 to 1,000 mg daily divided into two to four doses. *Note:* Be sure to use a buffered form of vitamin C. If taking vitamin C causes loose stools, decrease the dosage and then gradually increase the dosage as tolerated.
Willow Bark	*Capsule:* Take a standardized willow bark extract that provides 120 to 240 mg of salicin daily divided into three or four doses. Evidence suggests that taking standardized willow extracts (see previous page) at standard doses provides the equivalent of 50 mg of aspirin (a dose small enough for children). *Caution:* Avoid willow bark if you have an aspirin allergy, bleeding disorder, diabetes, or a peptic ulcer. Be sure to consult your doctor before giving willow bark to children.

FIBROCYSTIC BREASTS AND BREAST PAIN

FOR SOME WOMEN, premenstrual syndrome (PMS) can be accompanied by tenderness and lumps in the breasts, a painful condition clinically known as *cyclic mastalgia.* More than 50 percent of women have fibrocystic breast symptoms at some point in their lives, and this condition usually affects women between the ages of 30 and 50.

WHAT IS IT?

Fibrocystic breast disease is said to exist when swollen lumps in the breast become large enough to be classified as cysts. Symptoms of this condition include pain, tenderness, areas of thickening, and formation of scar-like connective tissue. Even though these cysts are difficult to distinguish from cancerous cysts in a mammogram, the two can be distinguished from one another, and fibrocystic breasts are not a risk factor for breast cancer.

Although it is not known exactly what causes fibrocystic breast disease, it has been suggested that high levels of the hormone prolactin or cyclical shifts in female hormone levels may be responsible,

A Low-Fat Diet May Suppress Symptoms of Fibrocystic Breast Disease

Did You Know? Decreasing dietary fat intake may reduce symptoms of fibrocystic breast disease including breast swelling and tenderness. In a double-blind, controlled study published in the medical journal *Lancet*, women who reduced their fat intake to 15 percent of their usual caloric intake found relief from breast pain.

Other research indicates that levels of certain growth hormones known as *lactogentic hormones* may be elevated in women who have cystic breast disease. A study of 16 women with cystic breast disease published in the *Journal of the National Cancer Institute* found that levels of these hormones were lowered when dietary fat intake was reduced to 20 percent of the total calorie content in the women's diets. When given a low-fat diet for 3 months, the women showed significant reductions in the levels of their lactogentic hormones. This is especially hopeful news because women with elevated lactogentic hormone levels appear to have an increased risk for developing breast cancer. If you have fibrocystic breast disease, consult your doctor about devising a diet plan that may not only decrease breast pain, but help stave off breast cancer as well.

And if a dietary change doesn't seem like the best treatment for you, simply opting for a more supportive, better-fitting bra may provide some relief from the pain and tenderness associated with fibrocystic breasts.

443

and some researchers claim that the cysts result from an imbalance of essential fatty acids in the body. Some studies suggest that a high intake of caffeine may contribute to the tenderness and pain associated with fibrocystic breasts. Nevertheless, if you detect one of these cysts during a self-examination, see your doctor. If it is noncancerous, the following natural herbs and supplements may help to banish the pain and discomfort, as well as the cysts themselves.

WHAT SHOULD I TAKE?

Chasteberry • Evening Primrose Oil • Flaxseed Oil
Ginkgo Biloba (Ginkgo) • Vitamin A • Vitamin B$_6$

Chasteberry naturally diminishes the release within the body of the hormone prolactin, which many researchers believe is what causes fibrocystic breast disease. As a result, a daily dose of chasteberry has demonstrated effectiveness in clinical studies for reducing breast tenderness and cysts. (For more information on chasteberry, see page 69.)

Evening primrose oil contains high levels of essential omega-6 fatty acids. Since researchers believe that imbalances in essential fatty acids can contribute to fibrocystic breasts, taking a daily dose of evening primrose oil may help prevent this. (For more information on evening primrose oil, see page 115.)

Some studies suggest that **flaxseed oil**, with evening primrose oil (see page 115) and chasteberry (see page 69) may reduce breast pain and tenderness. (For more information on flaxseed oil, see page 126.)

Although **ginkgo** is known to enhance memory and mental function, it also seems to relieve pain associated with fibrocystic breasts. In a study of 143 women with symptoms of PMS, ginkgo relieved all symptoms, but it seemed to be most effective in relieving breast pain. (For more information on ginkgo, see page 138.)

Supplementation with **vitamin A** before menstruation may be helpful in relieving the pain of fibrocystic breasts. In one study, women treated with 20 milligrams of beta carotene daily and 150 to 300,000 International Units of retinol every other day, beginning 7 days before menstruation, had relief from breast pain without any negative side effects. (For more information on vitamin A, see page 274.)

Some studies have shown a reduction of breast pain with **vitamin B$_6$** supplementation, although evidence suggests that this may only be slightly better than a placebo. More research is needed to explore the effects of vitamin B$_6$ supplementation on fibrocystic breast pain. (For more information on vitamin B$_6$, see page 279.)

MY SUPPLEMENT LIST—FIBROCYSTIC BREASTS AND BREAST PAIN

SUPPLEMENT	RECOMMENDED DOSAGE
Chasteberry	*Capsule:* Take 175–225 mg of an extract standardized to contain 0.5% agnuside each day before breakfast.
Evening Primrose Oil	*Capsule:* Take 4 to 6 g daily of a product containing 8% to 12% gamma linoleic acid (GLA).
Flaxseed Oil	*Fresh:* Take 1 to 4 tbsp daily divided into three or four doses.
Ginkgo	*Capsule:* Take 80 mg of a ginkgo extract twice daily. In the study mentioned in the What Should I Take section on page 437, women were given 80 mg of ginkgo twice daily, beginning on the 16th day of their menstrual cycle. This dosage was continued until day 5 of their next cycle and was then resumed on day 16 of that cycle.
Vitamin A	*Capsule or Tablet:* Take 20,000 IU daily. Use with caution if at risk for heart disease or osteoporosis.
Vitamin B$_6$	*Tablet:* Take up to 100 mg twice daily. *Note:* If you have liver disease, consult your doctor before taking more than 50 mg of vitamin B$_6$ daily. Do not take vitamin B$_6$ at this dosage for more than a 6-month period. If you experience numbness in the hands or feet, discontinue use of vitamin B$_6$ at this dosage and consult your doctor.

FIBROMYALGIA

FIBROMYALGIA IS A GOOD IMPERSONATOR—it can look like Lyme disease, chronic fatigue syndrome (see page 375), depression (see page 402), rheumatoid arthritis (see page 574), and many other conditions. Experts aren't sure what causes this condition, but it may be due to a dysfunction of the nervous and endocrine systems. It is also hard to pin down—doctors can't diagnose it by testing, and as a result, fibromyalgia often goes undiagnosed for 5 years or longer before being identified.

WHAT IS IT?

Despite its other elusive qualities, fibromyalgia does have some specific symptoms. Thus, people with this condition feel extreme tenderness in up to 18 "tender points" around their body. Other common symptoms include widespread musculoskeletal pain, extreme fatigue, depression, poor sleep, digestive upset, and in women, pelvic pain.

Helpful medical treatments for fibromyalgia include low doses of antidepressant and muscle relaxant medications. People with fibromyalgia can also help relieve its symptoms with massage and by making sure to get a good night's sleep and performing regular, gentle aerobic exercises, which helps keep muscles strong and more resistant to pain. In several recently published studies, acupuncture was found to be effective in alleviating some of the symptoms of fibromyalgia.

WHAT SHOULD I TAKE?
Calcium • Chamomile • Coenzyme Q10 (CoQ10)
5-Hydroxytryptophan (5-HTP) • Ginseng
Magnesium and Malic Acid • Melatonin
SAMe • Selenium • St. John's Wort • Valerian
Vitamin C • Vitamin D • Vitamin E

Studies indicate that people with fibromyalgia may have an increased risk for developing osteoporosis. Furthermore, many people with fibromyalgia are physically inactive, which increases their risk of having low bone density. Supplementation with **calcium**, **vitamin D**, and **magnesium** may help ensure adequate bone density and prevent osteoporosis. (For more information on calcium and vitamin D, see pages 57 and 289.)

Getting enough sleep is a problem for many people with fibromyalgia. However, some people may find the effects of the sleep-aiding supplement valerian (see page 272) too sedating. German **chamomile** may provide just the right amount of relaxation without causing excessive drowsiness. (For more information on chamomile, see page 67.)

CoQ10 is found naturally in cells, and its role is to help cells use their oxygen supply to generate fuel so that they can function properly. As a supplement, CoQ10 is also a powerful antioxidant, protecting cells from the damaging effects of free radical molecules. (For more information on CoQ10, see page 80.) For more information on a variety of herbs to help with sleep, see the section entitled "insomnia" on page 516.

A double-blind study of 50 people with fibromyalgia reported reduced sensitivity in their "tender points," as well as less pain, with **5-HTP**—a natural amino acid manufactured in the body—than with a placebo. Other improvements included less anxiety, stiffness, and fatigue, and improvements in sleep. Although more research on 5-HTP is needed, it may have a positive future in relieving fibromyalgia symptoms. Some research suggests that 5-HTP works by raising the concentration of serotonin in the blood, a substance important in nerve and muscle activity that many people with fibromyalgia have in short supply. (For more information on 5-HTP, see page 123.)

Ginseng is known as an *adaptogen*, which means that it can help you adapt to sleep deprivation and other stressful situations. It can also bolster your immune system and increase energy levels. These qualities make it a potentially useful treatment for fibromyalgia. (For more information on ginseng, see page 141.)

Magnesium and **malic acid** are commonly recommended supplements for treating fibromyalgia. Magnesium helps muscles to work properly (including helping them to relax), and malic acid—a component of apple juice—may help the body make better use of magnesium. A University of Texas study found that using a supplement containing both of these nutrients for more than 2 months significantly reduced pain and tenderness associated with fibromyalgia. (For more information on magnesium and malic acid, see page 203.)

Melatonin may be beneficial in people with fibromyalgia, although this is not firmly established. One small study indicated that people with fibromyalgia who took melatonin supplements experienced improvements in sleep as well as a reduction in tender points and overall disease symptoms. However, melatonin had only a modest effect in reducing pain and fatigue. (For more information on melatonin, see page 208.)

Preliminary studies suggest that **SAMe** may reduce pain, stiffness, and fatigue in people with fibromyalgia. It may also help with depression, which sometimes accompanies fibromyalgia. (For more information on SAMe, see page 247.)

The effect of the cell-and tissue-damaging molecules known as free radicals on fibromyalgia is controversial. Some research supports the theory that increased production of free radicals may contribute to the development of fibromyalgia. As a result, supplementation with **vitamins C**, **E**, and **selenium** may be useful for scavenging free radicals and possibly also for relieving muscle cramps in fibromyalgia. (For more information on vitamins C, E, and selenium, see pages 284, 292, and 253.)

Studies show that many tricyclic antidepressant medications—such as amitriptyline (Elavil)—can promote sleep and decrease pain. People who do not like taking prescription antidepressants may prefer **St. John's wort**, a natural supplement that may help people with fibromyalgia get a good night's sleep and help with depression as well. (For more information on St. John's wort, see page 262.)

A small study suggests that medicinal baths containing **valerian** oil may help improve the overall feeling of well-being and sleep in people with fibromyalgia. In addition to a valerian bath, taking whirlpool baths may help reduce the intensity of pain in cases of extreme tenderness from fibromyalgia. Valerian root may also be taken orally to help promote sleep. (For more information on valerian, see page 272.)

MY SUPPLEMENT LIST—FIBROMYALGIA

SUPPLEMENT	RECOMMENDED DOSAGE
Calcium	*Capsule or Tablet (Age 19 to 50):* Take 1,000 mg of calcium citrate daily divided into two doses. *(Age 51 years and over):* Take 1,200 mg of calcium citrate daily divided into two or three doses.
Chamomile	*Tea:* Add 3 g of dried flower heads to 1 cup of boiling water for 5 to 10 minutes. Drink up to three times daily.
CoQ10	*Capsule:* Take 50 to 100 mg once or twice a day.
5-HTP	*Capsule:* Take up to 100 mg three times daily.
Ginseng	*Capsule:* Take 200 mg of a standardized extract containing 4% to 7% ginsenosides, divided into two doses a day.
Magnesium and Malic Acid	*Tablet:* Take 200 mg of magnesium two or three times daily along with 1,200 mg of malic acid one or two times daily. *Note:* Take magnesium in the form of magnesium glycinate to avoid loose stools. Large amounts of magnesium can cause diarrhea; if this becomes a problem for you, reduce your dosage.
Melatonin	*Tablet:* Take 1 to 3 mg 2 hours before bedtime. Ask your doctor if a larger dose may be right for you.
SAMe	*Tablet:* Take 800 mg twice daily, one-half hour before meals.
Selenium	*Tablet:* Take 100 to 200 mcg daily.
St. John's Wort	*Capsule:* Take 300 mg up to three times daily of an extract standardized to contain 0.3% hypericin. *Tea:* Steep 2 to 4 g of dried herb in 1 cup of boiling water for 5 to 10 minutes. Drink up to three times daily.
Valerian	*Bath:* Add a few drops of a valerian oil to the water before taking a bath. *Capsule:* Take 400 to 900 mg daily, 2 hours before bedtime. *Tea:* Steep 2 to 3 g of valerian root in 1 cup of boiling water for 5 to 10 minutes. Drink up to three times daily. *Note:* The strength of valerian products may vary greatly. Be sure to choose a standardized product and carefully follow the instructions on the label.

MY SUPPLEMENT LIST—FIBROMYALGIA	
SUPPLEMENT	**RECOMMENDED DOSAGE**
Vitamin C	*Capsule or Tablet:* Take 500 mg twice daily. *Note:* Be sure to use a buffered form of vitamin C. If taking vitamin C causes loose stools, decrease the dosage and then gradually increase the dosage as tolerated.
Vitamin D	*Tablet:* Take 400–800 IU daily. *Note:* Elderly people may require a dosage of 800 to 1,000 IU of vitamin D daily for maximum effectiveness. Consult your doctor to perform a blood test to see if you are deficient in vitamin D.
Vitamin E	*Capsule:* Take 400 IU daily.

FOOD ALLERGY

WHAT EXACTLY IS A FOOD ALLERGY? It depends on who you ask. Some people who think they have a food allergy simply dislike a particular food or have an intolerance to it. For example, many people are intolerant to the flavor enhancer monosodium glutamate (MSG) or to the lactose in dairy products, but these intolerances aren't defined medically as allergies.

The foods that commonly cause allergic reactions in adults are shellfish and fish, peanuts, eggs, and tree nuts. In children, the most troublesome foods are eggs, milk, and peanuts. For an allergic individual, eating these foods may quickly trigger digestive upset, hives, asthma, or even anaphylactic shock (a life-threatening allergic reaction), which can lead to death.

WHAT IS IT?

An acute allergic reaction involves an antibody called IgE. If you're allergic to a particular food, your body produces a specific type of IgE that reacts with a component of that food. When you eat that food and the IgE encounters it, the IgE combines with the component of the food, known as antigen, and the combination results in what is known as immune complex. The complex then binds to the surfaces of cells known as mast cells, causing them to release the substance known as histamine. Depending on where in your body the histamine is released, it may cause you to develop hives, diarrhea, or other and sometimes potentially fatal symptoms, including difficulty in breathing from constriction of the windpipe (or trachea) and shock from a sudden reduction in blood pressure. Some doctors and health practitioners find that another type of antibody called IgG also plays a significant role in allergies by causing more delayed reactions.

A medical doctor is likely to consider a food allergy as a relatively rare occurrence, since it affects less than 2 percent of adults and 8 percent of children. Naturopathic doctors look for the IgG variety of food-allergy reactions, which can occur up to 72 hours after ingestion of a causative as well as the IgE variety.

Food allergies are thought to cause a wide variety of conditions, including ear infections, headaches, depression, gastrointestinal problems, and eczema.

The main way to control food allergies is to avoid the foods that trigger them. Avoiding even trace amounts of these foods may be a life-or-death matter for some people with acute allergies, such as those with peanut allergies. Your doctor may also suggest that you carry a syringe filled with epinephrine—which can relax a constricted windpipe and prevent severe shock—to halt an anaphylactic event. An elimination diet (see below) is often recommended for people attempting to discover the types of foods that cause them to have an allergic reaction.

The Elimination Diet May Help Control Allergies

Did You Know?

One very common tool that doctors use to identify the specific foods that cause a delayed IgG allergic reaction is an elimination diet. The goal of this diet is to isolate problem foods and avoid them, so as to prevent food-allergic reactions.

1. *Follow Your Gut.* Make a list of the foods you think are potential triggers for your allergy or intolerance.

2. *Eliminate.* Avoid these suspect foods completely. This includes whole foods as well as ingredients in foods. As you do this, record how you are feeling in a diary, and keep in mind that you may not feel better immediately. Sometimes you may even feel worse for a day or two.

3. *Challenge Yourself.* Slowly begin to reintroduce suspect foods into your diet, in small quantities, while making sure to record how you feel. Be sure to eat the suspect food twice a day. For the next 2 days, do not eat the suspect food, but continue to follow the elimination diet. You can have a reaction to a trigger food for up to 3 days after consuming it. Be sure to add back a suspect food to your diet every 3 days. If the food does not cause a reaction, it is safe to eat but should not be reincorporated into your diet until you have finished testing all suspect foods.

4. *Communicate.* Discuss your findings with your doctor so that he or she may have a better picture of your particular food-allergy profile.

WHAT SHOULD I TAKE?
Betaine • Bromelain • Digestive Enzymes
Lactobacillus Acidophilus • Omega-3 Fatty Acids
Quercetin • Vitamin C

Betaine (or betaine hydrochloride) may increase stomach acid production. Since people with food allergies may produce insufficient amounts of stomach acid, betaine can sometimes quell food allergy symptoms. (For more information on betaine, see page 42.)

According to some experts, food allergies may be caused by partially undigested proteins. **Bromelain** may digest these proteins and render them harmless, helping to reduce or prevent symptoms of food allergies. (For more information on bromelain, see page 54.)

Some alternative medicine practitioners theorize that **digestive enzymes** may reduce food allergy symptoms by eliminating undigested protein that leaks into the bloodstream, thus causing an allergic reaction. However, more scientific research is needed to confirm this theory. (For more information on digestive enzymes, see page 102.)

Taking supplements containing bacteria such as **Lactobacillus acidophilus**, which are known as probiotics and are friendly to the human digestive system, may help reduce the risk of food allergies. A medical philosophy known as "functional medicine" (which focuses on a patient-centered approach to medicine) proposes that a problem called increased intestinal permeability, or "leaky gut syndrome," plays a role in food allergies by allowing greater amounts of allergy-triggering food particles to pass from the intestine and get into the bloodstream, where they interact with IgE and other factors in the immune system. Probiotics help maintain intestinal health and may therefore prevent allergy and other factors in triggering food particles from entering the bloodstream. (For more information on Lactobacillus acidophilus, see page 180.)

Omega-3 fatty acids, like those found in fish oil, reduce inflammation in the digestive tract, which may be beneficial in treating food allergies. (For more information on omega-3 fatty acids, see page 221.)

Quercetin is a bioflavonoid found naturally in apples and onions. It minimizes the release of histamine from mast cells, and research has shown that it can lessen intestinal damage when a food allergen is eaten. (For more information on quercetin, see page 236.)

Vitamin C may also be helpful in treating food allergies, perhaps by helping the immune system to work better. (For more information on vitamin C, see page 284.)

MY SUPPLEMENT LIST—FOOD ALLERGY

SUPPLEMENT	RECOMMENDED DOSAGE
Betaine HCL	*Capsule or Tablet:* Take 125–525 mg with each meal.
Bromelain	*Capsule:* Take a supplement containing 250 to 500 milk-clotting units (MCU) or 333 gelatin-dissolving units (GDU) once daily.
	Note: Bromelain is measured in MCU or GDU. One GDU is the equivalent of 1.5 MCU. Follow individual product labels carefully since optimal dosages of bromelain vary widely from one product to another.
Digestive Enzymes	*Capsule or Tablet:* Take 3 to 4 g in the form of 4x pancreatin daily with meals.
Lactobacillus Acidophilus	*Capsule:* Adults generally take 1 to 10 billion viable cells daily.
Omega-3 Fatty Acids	Take 2–3 g of omega-3 fatty acids per day, in divided doses, with meals. The amount of omega-3 fatty acid will vary by manufacturer, so be sure to check the product label carefully.
Quercetin	*Capsule or Tablet:* Take 250 to 500 mg up to two to three times daily.
Vitamin C	*Capsule or Tablet:* Take 250 to 500 mg twice daily.
	Note: Be sure to use a buffered form of vitamin C. If taking vitamin C causes loose stools, decrease the dosage and then gradually increase the dosage as tolerated.

FUNGAL INFECTIONS OF THE SKIN

THEY'RE COMMON—affecting most people at one time or another—and they're sneaky, hiding in dark, damp places on the body. Fungal infections have many misleading names including ringworm, athlete's foot, and jock itch. Clearly, ringworm is not really a worm, and athlete's foot and jock itch are not limited to those who play sports. Fungal infections are contagious and come in many forms, affecting several parts of the body, but one thing is for sure—all of them are unpleasant!

WHAT IS IT?

Ringworm can be spread through contact with any human, animal, object, or soil that is infected with the parasitic fungal organism that causes it. Ringworm on the body takes the form of a red, scaly circle that spreads out along its edges, leaving the center clear (hence, the "ring"). When it strikes the scalp, ringworm creates an itchy red patch that may cause hair loss.

Athlete's foot is a very common condition that typically affects the areas between the toes but can also strike other parts of the feet, the groin, and other body parts. You can pick up an athlete's foot infection in warm, damp areas like a shower room at a gym. Wearing tight shoes or damp socks will increase the risk of developing athlete's foot, since the fungus that causes this infection thrives in moist climates.

Jock itch is a red, itchy fungal rash affecting the genital and buttock areas. Much like athlete's foot, this condition is acquired in warm, moist conditions. Jock itch is contagious and may spread through sexual intercourse and by sharing of towels or clothing with an infected individual.

WHAT SHOULD I USE?
Garlic • Lavender • Lemon Balm • Tea Tree Oil

Garlic has powerful fungus-killing abilities and is a useful and easy way to treat fungal infections. Some studies show that garlic-derived creams may have benefits in reducing fungal infections as well as preventing them from occurring in the first place. However, studies have not yet confirmed the ability of garlic taken internally to treat fungal infections. (For more information on garlic, see page 135.)

Plant Oils May Be the Key to Beating a Fungal Infection

Did You Know?

Many plant oils and extracts have been used traditionally to help eliminate fungal disorders. Recently, researchers have begun to investigate the medicinal effects of certain plant oils and extracts and their anti-fungal affects. One Australian study found that essential oils and extracts may have medicinal roles as anti-fungal agents. Of the 52 plant oils and extracts examined in the study, lemongrass and oregano oil had the strongest anti-fungal effects.

Oil of oregano has faired well in a number of studies. In a study conducted at the University of Tennessee, oregano showed the most promise in defense against infectious fungi of extracts from many different types of plants that are typically used as seasoning agents in foods and beverages.

Another effective anti-fungal oil appears to be sunflower oil. In a controlled study of patients with athlete's foot, a medicinal cream made from sunflower oil had a remarkable fungus-fighting effect. The cream was administered twice a day for 6 weeks to 100 patients. At the end of the study, 75 percent of the patients were completely cured of athlete's foot, and at a 6-month follow-up, they had experienced no recurrences of infection.

Lavender appears to have antifungal properties when tested in the lab. (For more information abour lavender, see page 184.)

Lemon balm is a time-honored remedy, recognized for its calming effects. Recent in vitro studies indicate that topical lemon balm oil is active as an antifungal agent. (For more information on lemon balm, see page 190.)

Tea tree oil is an effective treatment for fungal infections because of its antiseptic properties. A randomized, double-blind, controlled study of 158 patients with athlete's foot found that tea tree oil, as compared with a placebo, was effective in reducing the symptoms associated with this fungal infection. (For more information on tea tree oil, see page 265.)

MY SUPPLEMENT LIST—FUNGAL INFECTIONS OF THE SKIN

SUPPLEMENT	RECOMMENDED DOSAGE
Garlic	*Oral—Fresh:* Eat 1 or 2 cloves of raw garlic daily. *Topical—Paste:* Grind fresh garlic into a paste in a food processor and apply it to the area of fungal outbreak a few times each day; for athlete's foot, purchase a cream containing 0.4% ajoene (an antifungal compound in garlic) and apply it to affected areas once daily.
Lavender	*Essential oil—topically:* Apply sparingly directly to affected area. Or, use a cream that contains pure lavender essential oil.
Lemon Balm	*Essential oil—topically:* Apply sparingly directly to affected area. Or, use a cream that contains pure lemon balm essential oil.
Tea Tree Oil	*Topical—Oil:* Moderately apply an oil of 70% to 100% strength to affected areas two times a day for athlete's foot. *Note:* Tea tree oil products should be tested first on a small patch of skin in an unobtrusive area to make sure that no allergic reaction occurs.

GALLSTONES

WHEN YOU STRETCH, PAT YOUR BELLY, and order your after-dinner coffee at the end of a big meal, you may be relaxed, but your gallbladder is just beginning to get busy. This pear-shaped organ, which lies under your liver, is attached to your small intestine via a tube it shares with your liver and pancreas. The gallbladder doesn't get much attention, but it plays a very important role in digestion; it stores the fluid known as bile, made by the liver (about three cups' worth daily!), until you need it to digest fat in food.

WHAT IS IT?

Sometimes the components in bile—which contains enzymes and other ingredients that break up fat—crystallize and form lumps that can range in size from a grain of rice to a golf ball. These lumps in the gallbladder are called gallstones. About 80 percent of all gallstones are composed primarily of cholesterol, but some gallstones, called "pigment stones," are made mostly of bilirubin, a major component of bile.

About 1 million new cases of gallstone disease are diagnosed in the U.S. each year. Obesity, diabetes, or rapid weight loss can increase the risk of developing this condition. A gallstone can cause serious complications if it becomes lodged in the duct between the gallbladder and the intestine or if it blocks ducts coming out of the liver or pancreas. A gallstone "attack" typically occurs after eating a fatty meal and can cause abdominal pain, pain between the shoulder blades, nausea, and vomiting. Doctors often treat gallstones with surgery to remove the gallbladder, although they can sometimes use medications to dissolve the stones. Do not attempt to self-treat an attack unless under the direct supervision of a doctor. It is considered a medical emergency and can be fatal if not treated properly.

WHAT SHOULD I TAKE?

Calcium · Dandelion · Fiber · Peppermint
Vitamin C · Vitamin E

Both **calcium** and **fiber** may decrease the risk of developing gallstones. Calcium may work by lowering cholesterol levels in bile, thus reducing the risk of developing cholesterol gallstones. In one

Debunked Internet Claims for Gallstone Remedies

Many claims on the Internet support so-called "liver flush" products to rid the body of gallstones. Although the recipes for these products vary, they typically involve drinking a sizeable amount of olive oil, as well as apple juice, grapefruit juice, lemon juice, and/or Epsom salts. After drinking the liver flush, it is claimed to cause large numbers of green gallstones to pass out of the body in the stool. Some Web sites even post actual photos of these "globs"!

According to several alternative-health experts, the material that is passed is not actually gallstones—it is merely the olive oil mixed with the other ingredients of the flush that your gut has processed. And if you do have gallstones, such remedies can be dangerous, since drinking a large quantity of oil will cause your gallbladder to contract, thus releasing a stone and blocking the bile duct. However, a morning drink made with a tablespoon of olive oil and a crushed clove of garlic mixed with 4 ounces of fresh citrus juice can be a helpful liver tonic.

25-year study of 860 middle-aged men, the risk of developing gall-stones decreased with a higher intake of calcium. Additional studies show that people with high-fiber diets have lower rates of gallstone disease. Fiber reduces acids that contribute to gallstone formation and also prevents constipation, a condition linked to an increased risk of gallstone formation. Increasing your fiber intake with psylli-um may help prevent gallstones. (For more information on calcium and fiber, see pages 61 and 120.)

The German Commission E (see page 16) recommends **dande-lion** root for "disturbances in bile flow," and it may be helpful for preventing gallstones from forming. However, the use of dandelion for this purpose should be done only under the supervision of a doc-tor. (For more information on dandelion, see page 96.)

Peppermint leaf may be a useful addition to the treatment of gallstones. The German Commission E has approved its use for treat-ment of spastic discomfort of the upper gastrointestinal tract and bile ducts. (For more information of peppermint leaf, see page 226.)

Vitamins C and **E** may encourage increased bile production. Some studies suggest that vitamin C may help prevent gallstones from forming, specifically in women. (For more information on vitamins C and E, see pages 284 and 292.)

MY SUPPLEMENT LIST—GALLSTONES

SUPPLEMENT	RECOMMENDED DOSAGE
Calcium	*Capsule or Tablet:* Take 1,000 mg of calcium daily divided into two doses. Adults over age 51 should take 1,200 mg daily divided into two or three doses.
Dandelion	Dandelion should only be used under a doctor's supervision for treating gallstones. Consult your doctor in to determine an appropriate dosage of dandelion for you.
Fiber	*Capsule:* Take at least 5 g of a psyllium fiber supplement daily. *Seeds:* Take 2 tsp (5 g) of whole seeds daily.
Peppermint	*Tea:* Take 1 tbsp infused with 1 cup of boiling water for 10 minutes, take two to three times per day. *Leaf:* Take 3–6 g per day taken in capsules, divided doses, with meals.
Vitamin C	*Capsule or Tablet:* Take 1,000 mg twice daily. *Note:* Be sure to use a buffered form of vitamin C. If taking vitamin C causes loose stools, decrease your dosage and then gradually increase the dosage as tolerated.
Vitamin E	*Capsule:* Take 400 IU of a natural product containing mixed tocopherols daily.

GLAUCOMA

THEY MAY SEEM LIKE THE SAME, unchanging orbs day after day, with only a little redness or occasional tears to break up the routine, but your eyes are anything but static. A flow of fluid called *aqueous humor* is constantly running through your eyes, providing them with nourishment. This fluid comes from behind the iris (the colored ring in the eye) and flows through the pupil (the dark circle). It then moves around the *anterior chamber*, which is the clear space in the front of your eye that you see through. The fluid exits through a tiny mesh-like drain, which is located in a corner where the iris and cornea meet. While this often goes on daily without a hitch, trouble with the eyes' fluid and drainage system can result in glaucoma.

WHAT IS IT?

Glaucoma is a general term given to a group of diseases that damage the eye's optic nerve. For many people, glaucoma occurs when there is too much pressure inside the eye as the result of improper drainage of fluids from it. These fluids begin to accumulate, thereby increasing pressure in the eye. The increased pressure damages delicate cells in the optic nerve, which exits from the back of the eye and carries visual signals to the brain. This damage can cause the death of these cells, resulting in a loss of peripheral vision and eventually in total loss of vision.

Glaucoma comes in several varieties. In the most common form—*open-angle glaucoma*—the first symptom may be vision loss, which can take years to develop. Another form, called *angle-closure glaucoma,* can appear quickly, causing pain, vomiting, and vision loss within hours. People over the age of 60 or African-Americans over age 40 are at a particularly high risk for glaucoma. Traditional medical treatment for glaucoma consists of pressure-reducing eye drops and surgery.

WHAT SHOULD I TAKE?

Glaucoma is a serious condition. Make sure to consult your doctor before taking any type of supplement if you have been diagnosed with glaucoma or think you may have glaucoma.

Alpha Lipoic Acid • Ginkgo Biloba (Ginkgo)
Magnesium • Omega-3 Fatty Acids
Thiamine • Vitamin C • Vitamin E

Preliminary studies indicate that **alpha lipoic acid** (ALA) may benefit people with open-angle glaucoma. One study of 40 patients

CALL YOUR DOCTOR WHEN...

People over the age of 40 should get an eye checkup every year to allow detection and early treatment of the more gradual types of glaucoma. However, it is very important to also be aware of signs of acute angle-closure glaucoma, a serious condition that requires emergency medical attention. Be sure to call your doctor if:

■ You have blurry vision

■ You have acute pain in your eye or eyebrow

■ You see colored auras around lights

■ You experience persistent nausea

with open-angle glaucoma found that daily supplementation with ALA for 1 to 2 months improved visual function as well as the eyes' ability to properly drain fluid. (For more information on alpha lipoic acid, see page 29.)

Ginkgo may help treat glaucoma, by improving blood flow to the optic nerve. Researchers have theorized that ginkgo may work to not only reduce the constriction of blood vessels and improve blood flow in the eye but also to improve the flow of liquid in the eye, reduce cell death and damage, and improve vision in people with glaucoma. (For more information on ginkgo, see page 138.)

While more research is needed, studies show that **magnesium** may improve vision as well as blood circulation in the eye, especially those who have a constriction of blood vessels in the eye. In a Swiss study of 10 patients with glaucoma, vision was improved after taking 121 milligrams of magnesium twice daily for 1 month. (For more information on magnesium, see page 203.)

Some studies suggest that supplementation with **omega-3 fatty acids** and **vitamin E** may be beneficial in glaucoma by improving vision. Other preliminary research indicates that people who consume large amounts of omega-3 fatty acids are less likely to develop certain types of glaucoma. (For more information on omega-3 fatty acids and vitamin E, see pages 221 and 292.)

Research suggests that people with glaucoma may not effectively absorb **thiamine** (vitamin B_1). Supplementation with this vitamin

Promising Research Supports Acupuncture as Effective Treatment for Glaucoma

Did You Know?

Glaucoma is one of the chief causes of blindness, and as a result, many studies have been conducted to find effective, reliable treatments for this condition. Researchers have been exploring acupuncture—a technique in which very thin needles of varying lengths are inserted through the skin—as a possible treatment for glaucoma. In a study conducted in Germany, the effect of acupuncture therapy on glaucoma symptoms was evaluated in 18 glaucoma patients. The patients were given one session of a standardized acupuncture treatment. Researchers measured the intraocular pressure (pressure in the eye) in each patient before and after the acupuncture treatment. Fifteen minutes after treatment with acupuncture, the treated patients showed a significant decrease in intraocular pressure, and the improvement was still evident 24 hours later. Although more research is underway, acupuncture may show promise in the future of glaucoma treatment. To find a medical acupuncturist near you, contact the American Academy of Medical Acupuncture (http://www.medicalacupuncture.org/).

may help to maintain it at healthy levels in the body. (For more information on thiamine, see page 267.)

A number of studies have demonstrated that taking **vitamin C** reduces pressure in the eye, but the dosages needed for this were in some cases were very high (35 grams daily) and are not recommended without approval by your doctor. In one study, a group of people who took an average of 75 milligrams of vitamin C daily had significantly higher pressure in their eyes than a group that consumed an average of 1,200 milligrams of the vitamin. (For more information on vitamin C, see page 284.)

MY SUPPLEMENT LIST—GLAUCOMA

SUPPLEMENT	RECOMMENDED DOSAGE
Alpha Lipoic Acid	*Capsule:* Take 150 mg daily for 1 month.
Ginkgo	*Capsule or Tablet:* Take 120 to 240 mg daily, divided into three doses, of an extract standardized to contain 6% terpene lactones and 24% flavone glycosides.
Magnesium	*Tablet:* Take 240 mg twice daily. *Note:* Take magnesium in the form of magnesium glycinate to avoid loose stools. Large amounts of magnesium can cause diarrhea; if this becomes a problem for you, reduce your dosage.
Omega-3 Fatty Acids	Take 2–3 grams of omega-3 fatty acids per day, in divided doses, with meals. The amount of omega-3 fatty acid will vary by manufacturer, so be sure to check the product label carefully.
Thiamine	*Tablet:* Take 20 to 25 mg daily, a dosage that can be found in many multivitamins.
Vitamin C	*Capsule or Tablet:* Take 500 mg twice daily. *Note:* Be sure to use a buffered form of vitamin C. If taking vitamin C causes loose stools, decrease your dosage and then gradually increase the dosage as tolerated.
Vitamin E	*Capsule:* Take 400 IU of a natural product containing mixed tocopherols daily.

GOUT

BEING STUBBED INTO A COFFEE-TABLE leg is a bad thing for a big toe. So is having a dumbbell dropped on it. But these little miseries may pale in comparison to a disorder that is particularly excruciating for big toes: gout. One of the most painful forms of arthritis, gout is also one of the oldest recognized ailments and was once called the "disease of kings" because it was believed to be contracted by men who overindulged in rich foods and beverages.

WHAT IS IT?

Although gout often affects the big toes, it can also strike the knees, elbows, and other joints. Ordinarily, the kidneys eliminate uric acid—a waste product of metabolism—via the urine, but sometimes they don't remove it in adequate amounts, or there is too much uric acid circulating in the blood for the kidneys to remove it effectively. Gout results from such an overload of uric acid, which then accumulates in the form of shard-like needles in the joints between the bones.

Gout typically strikes adult men (although it can occur at any age) and people who are overweight; women are at a higher risk for gout after menopause. Acute attacks of gout cause severe pain as well as warmth and redness in the affected joints and typically last from 3 to 10 days. These attacks can progressively grow longer and more frequent, and long-term gout can cause permanent damage to the joints and kidneys.

To treat gout, your doctor may prescribe anti-inflammatory drugs or a drug to reduce uric acid levels in the body, such as allopurinol (Zyloprim). Good steps to take on your own to minimize problems from gout include drinking lots of water daily to dilute the uric acid in your system and minimizing your intake of foods high in purines, which break down into uric acid (see Diet and Gout, below).

Diet and Gout

Healthy Hints

The foods you eat (and those you don't eat) play an important role in controlling gout. Although some foods can help to ease gout, others may make it worse. Read on for hints that help prevent gout flare-ups.

■ **Hydrate.** Drink 2 1/2 liters of water every day. This will help prevent formation of painful urate crystals in the joints and kidneys and will also increase the body's excretion of uric acid.

■ **Make life a bowl of cherries.** Eating a half-pound of cherries daily—which are rich in the antioxidant substances called flavonoids—may help protect collagen in the body's connective tissue against oxidative damage, reducing inflammation. If that's too many cherries for you, try drinking 8 to 16 ounces of cherry juice daily.

■ **Stalk up.** Don't like cherries? Drinking celery juice is another traditional remedy for gout and is used widely in Australia. Celery seed have a high content of anti-inflammatory substances and might be worth a try. You can take them as a condiment in food or as an herbal extract.

■ **Stay away from…** Foods high in purine may contribute to the development of gout, especially in people who have an increased risk for developing this condition. Avoid high-purine foods including organ meats such as sweetbreads, liver, and kidney; young or small animals and fish, such as anchovies and scallops; veal and most game meats; legumes such as lentils, peas, beans, peanuts, and soybeans; and beer, coffee, tea, and caffeinated soda. Also avoid supplements that contain vitamin C or niacin.

WHAT SHOULD I TAKE?
Boswellia • Bromelain • Folic Acid • Licorice
Omega-3 Fatty Acids • Vitamin E • Willow Bark

Boswellia and **licorice** have anti-inflammatory effects. Boswellia has effects similar to that of nonsteroidal anti-inflammatory drugs (NSAIDs), while licorice has steroid-like effects. Both boswellia and licorice are useful in treating attacks of gout, and studies show that they may have fewer side effects than prescription medications. However, people taking licorice for prolonged periods of time should be closely monitored by a doctor for side effects. (For more information on boswellia and licorice, see pages 52 and 192.)

Bromelain—an anti-inflammatory enzyme found in pineapples—provides an effective way to reduce inflammation caused by gout. (For more information on bromelain, see page 54.)

Folic acid (vitamin B_9) works in a way similar to the drug allopurinol (Zyloprim) by inhibiting an enzyme in the body called xanthine oxidase, which plays a crucial role in the production of uric acid. (For more information on folic acid, see page 130.)

Omega-3 fatty acids are especially effective for controlling the pain and inflammation associated with gout. These fatty acids work by reducing the body's production of leukotrienes, which are inflammatory substances that cause much of the damage in gout. (For more information on omega-3 fatty acids, see page 221.)

Vitamin E also reduces leukotriene production, making it a useful addition to an anti-gout supplement regimen. (For more information on vitamin E, see page 292.)

The pain-relieving and anti-inflammatory properties of **willow bark** may reduce mild to moderate discomfort associated with gout. However, be sure to consult your doctor before using willow bark to treat gout symptoms. (For more information on willow bark, see page 298.)

MY SUPPLEMENT LIST—GOUT

SUPPLEMENT	RECOMMENDED DOSAGE
Boswellia	*Tablet:* Take 300 to 400 mg three times daily of an extract standardized to contain 70% boswellic acids between meals.
Bromelain	*Tablet:* Take 250 to 500 mg daily between meals. Look for a supplement containing 2,400 gelatin-dissolving units (GDU) or 3,600 milk-clotting units (MCU) per gram.

(continued)

MY SUPPLEMENT LIST—GOUT (continued)	
SUPPLEMENT	**RECOMMENDED DOSAGE**
Folic Acid	*Tablet:* Take 10–75 mg daily.
Licorice	*Capsule:* Take 200 mg of a licorice-root extract standardized to contain 50 mg of glycyrrhizinic acid daily. *Note:* Licorice candy is made with artificial flavorings and has no healing properties.
Omega-3 Fatty Acids	*Capsule:* Take 3–6 g of omega-3 fatty acids per day, in divided doses, with meals. The amount of omega-3 fatty acid will vary by manufacturer, so be sure to check the product label carefully.
Vitamin E	*Capsule:* Take 400 to 800 IU daily of a natural product containing mixed tocopherols.
Willow Bark	*Capsule:* Take a standardized extract containing 120 to 240 mg of salicin daily as needed. *Caution:* Consult your doctor before using willow bark to treat gout. Do not take willow bark if you have an aspirin allergy, bleeding disorder, diabetes, or a peptic ulcer.

HANGOVERS

PERHAPS A HANGOVER is Mother Nature's way of reprimanding us when we drink too much alcohol. Hangovers can incapacitate us, causing the passing minutes to feel like endless days. The feeling is often accompanied by a pounding headache rivaled only by an upset stomach and a serious hatred of all things noisy. While we vow never to drink again, the only thing that matters when we're in the throes of a hangover is how to end it so that we can make it through the day and go to sleep.

WHAT IS IT?

A hangover is a common malady; more than 75 percent of adults who have ever drunk alcohol have had one. Some research estimates that hangover-related work absenteeism and poor productivity cost the United States $148 billion annually.

A hangover does not necessarily occur after heavy drinking but can occur after even a few drinks, especially if you consume them quickly. Dehydration is one of the main reasons for a hangover; since alcohol is a diuretic and thus increases the flow of urine, it speeds the loss of water from the body, causing headaches and dizziness. Nausea, vomiting, and indigestion occur from alcohol irritating the lining of the stomach. Some studies show that forms of alcohol high in congeners—impurities which are found in greater quantities in dark liquors such as tequila and whiskey than in clear ones such as vodka and gin—tend to make hangovers worse.

Keep in mind that supplements will not protect you from the consistent and irresponsible consumption of alcohol. Some supplements may, however, help reduce the nasty symptoms of a hangover from more moderate drinking.

WHAT SHOULD I TAKE?
Fenugreek • Ginger • Green Tea
Milk Thistle • N-Acetylcysteine (NAC)
Vitamin B_6 • Vitamin C

Preliminary studies conducted on rats show that **fenugreek** may protect against alcohol poisoning by working as a powerful antioxidant that combats the free radical molecules that damage cells and tissues in the body and which are generated as the body breaks down alcohol. Although further research is needed to determine this, taking supplemental fenugreek for a hangover, in the form of a tea, may be beneficial. (For more information on fenugreek, see page 116.)

Ginger is an herb famous for its ability to temper the symptoms of nausea. When a hangover is accompanied by a sour stomach, taking

Avoiding Hangovers

Healthy Hints

Hangovers are really a matter of prevention rather than treatment. Although avoiding alcohol is the best defense against a hangover, you can take some measures to decrease the chances of experiencing a hangover if you do drink. Keep the following steps in mind before you lift that first glass:

■ **Hydrate with H_2O.** Drinking plenty of water will help you avoid the dehydrating effects of alcohol. Be sure to drink one glass of water between each alcoholic drink.

■ **Fill up on food.** Although a full stomach from eating won't actually absorb alcohol, as commonly thought, it may help protect the stomach from becoming irritated by alcohol.

■ **Go light.** Dark-colored drinks such as rum, tequila,

and whiskey are notorious for causing bad hangovers. Lighter liquors, such as vodka, decrease the chances of a hangover.

■ **Avoid cheap alcohol.** If you choose to drink cheap alcohol, you may suffer the consequences. More expensive brands of alcohol are usually better distilled, which means they contain fewer toxic byproducts and contaminants.

■ **Don't mix drinks.** Pick your favorite drink and stick to it! Drinking a variety of types of alcoholic beverages makes it harder for the body to metabolize the alcohol and other substances they contain.

■ **Avoid bubbly drinks.** Drinks such as champagne and sparkling wines tend to speed the body's absorption of alcohol.

ginger may help to reduce nausea. (For more information on ginger, see page 136.)

Similar in effect to fenugreek, **green tea** may work as a powerful antioxidant, thereby reducing the damage caused by free radicals generated during alcohol intoxication. Furthermore, green tea may be more beneficial to your health than a cup of coffee if you're looking for a beverage to help perk you up while you're trying to recover from a hangover. (For more information on green tea, see page 157.)

Milk thistle, a liver-protecting herb, may help reduce the misery of a hangover by helping the liver to rid the body of toxins. Additionally, alcohol damages the liver by depleting levels of glutathione, a protein that protects the liver from damage; the active ingredients in milk thistle—silymarin and silybin—have been shown to increase glutathione levels in rats. (For more information on milk thistle, see page 210.)

NAC is an amino acid that the body transforms into glutathione, which helps to detoxify harmful chemicals and protects the liver. NAC may be useful for relieving symptoms of a hangover as well as protecting the liver from alcohol-related damage. (For more information on NAC, see page 213.)

In a study that involved 17 party-goers, those who took **vitamin B_6** while they drank scored lower on a scale measuring 20 hangover symptoms than those who took a placebo. Further research is necessary to determine the effects of vitamin B_6 on hangovers. (For more information on vitamin B_6, see page 279.)

Another commonly recommended supplement for easing the effects of a hangover is **vitamin C**, which may speed the removal of alcohol from the body. (For more information on vitamin C, see page 284.)

MY SUPPLEMENT LIST—HANGOVERS

SUPPLEMENT	RECOMMENDED DOSAGE
Fenugreek	*Tea:* Take 1–2 tsp powdered seed in 1 cup boiling water, steep for 1 hour. Take 2–3 cups per day, as needed.
Ginger	*Capsule:* Take 1 to 4 g of powdered dry root to quell nausea on an as-needed basis. *Tea:* Steep 1 tsp or teabag of freshly shredded ginger root in boiled water. Drink two or three times daily. Make fresh ginger juice by squeezing a piece of ginger through a garlic press. Take 1–2 tbsp in water or juice, as needed.

MY SUPPLEMENT LIST—HANGOVERS	
SUPPLEMENT	**RECOMMENDED DOSAGE**
	Note: Most forms of ginger ale contain synthetic ginger and will not reduce nausea.
Green Tea	*Tea:* Combine 1 tsp or teabag of green tea leaves with 1 cup of boiling water and steep for 3 minutes. Drink up to 3 cups daily.
Milk Thistle	*Capsule:* Take 175 mg of a milk thistle extract, standardized to contain 80% silymarin, from one to three times daily.
NAC	*Capsule:* Take 900 mg one to two times per day with food.
Vitamin B$_6$	*Tablet:* In the study described in the "What Should I Take?" section on page 463, participants took 1,200 mg of vitamin B$_6$ divided into three doses while drinking. Do not take this high a dose for longer than 1 or 2 days.
	Note: If you have liver disease, consult your doctor before taking more than 50 mg of vitamin B$_6$ daily.
Vitamin C	*Capsule or Tablet:* Take 1,000 mg before bedtime after a bout of drinking.
	Note: Be sure to use a buffered form of vitamin C. If taking vitamin C causes loose stools, decrease your dosage and then gradually increase the dosage as tolerated.

HAY FEVER

ONCE UPON A TIME, someone must have thought "hay fever" sounded like a good name for the sneezing, stuffy-nosed, itchy-eyed malady that coincides with the harvest season. In reality, hay is only one of the variety of factors that can trigger this miserable state. Today, doctors refer to hay fever as "seasonal allergic rhinitis," because while it may occur at any time of the year, it most commonly occurs in the spring and fall.

WHAT IS IT?

More than 26 million Americans experience hay fever each year. Those who do are sensitive to various substances known as *allergens* that trigger the symptoms of this allergic condition. When they inhale these allergens, their bodies overreact by releasing an internal cascade of chemicals that cause inflammation in the eyes, nose, and throat. The results are congestion, sneezing, and itchy eyes, nose, and throat that typify hay fever. The leading allergens found outdoors are plant pollen and mold spores. Some people have particular problems with hay fever when certain kinds of plants release pollen or when large amounts of mold spores are floating in the air. People sensitive to allergens commonly found indoors—such as cockroach debris, dust mites, indoor mold, and pet dander—may have these symptoms year-round, a condition called *perennial allergic rhinitis*. Hay fever often goes hand-in-hand with asthma (see page 333), and it increases the risk of sinusitis (see page 580).

WHAT SHOULD I TAKE?

Acidophilus • Bromelain • Echinacea
Omega-3 Fatty Acids • Quercetin • Spirulina • Vitamin C

Acidophilus does more than just aid digestion. Two recent studies demonstrated that acidophilus (probiotics) were able to decrease the symptoms of allergic rhinitis (hayfever). (For more information on acidophilus, see page 180.)

Bromelain may be useful in treating hay fever because it can reduce swelling and inflammation, both of which are symptoms of hay fever. (For more information on bromelain, see page 54.)

Echinacea is often used to relieve the symptoms of colds and the flu, such as sore throat, runny nose, and coughing (see Colds and Flu, page 374). It may also be used to ease these symptoms in hay fever. (For more information on echinacea, see page 107.)

Omega-3 fatty acids may quiet allergy symptoms by making the body less prone to inflammation. The omega-3 fatty acids found in fish oil may be particularly helpful in this regard. (For more information on omega-3 fatty acids, see page 221.)

Tips for Escaping Hay Fever

For people who have it, hay fever may seem like inescapable misery, but there are some tips that can ease its symptoms:

■ **Spend mornings at home.** Pollen levels are often highest in the morning. To avoid the itching, sniffling, and sneezing pollen triggers, try to remain indoors in the morning when pollen counts are high.

■ **Shut up.** Although it's probably tempting to keep windows open in the spring and summer, open windows are an invitation for pollen to come indoors. Keep windows closed, and use an air conditioner or indoor fan to keep cool.

■ **Enlist yard help.** Mowing the grass or doing other yard work will exacerbate hay-fever symptoms. Ask a family member or friend to do these chores for you. (Of course, you may have to offer to do another chore in return!)

■ **Use the dryer.** Don't hang sheets or clothing outside on an outdoor clothesline when offending pollens are in the air. Pollen may get trapped in them and can remain in the fabric even after you bring the laundry inside.

■ **Stomp out cigarettes.** If your friends or family members smoke, ask them not to smoke around you, since cigarette smoke can aggravate hay fever. Also, ask your friends to refrain from wearing too much heavy perfume or using bug spray in your presence.

Quercetin, a substance found in plants and known as a flavonoid, limits the effects of histamine, an inflammation-inducing substance that the body releases in response to allergens. The antihistamine activity of quercetin can help reduce inflammation, which may in turn reduce the runny nose and swelling in the eyes, nose, and throat that occurs in hay fever. (For more information on quercetin, see page 236.)

Spirulina is a multipurpose food plant that appears to stimulate the immune system, and in preliminary studies shows promise for the treatment of allergies. (For more information about spirulina, see page 260.)

Vitamin C reduces inflammation by reducing the amount of histamine released in the body during an episode of hay fever. (For more information on vitamin C, see page 284.)

MY SUPPLEMENT LIST—HAY FEVER

SUPPLEMENT	RECOMMENDED DOSAGE
Lactobacillus Acidophilus	Capsule: Take 1- to 2-billion colony forming units (CFU) per day.
Bromelain	*Tablet:* Take 250 to 500 mg daily between meals. Look for a supplement containing 2,400 gelatin-dissolving units (GDU) or 3,600 milk-clotting units (MCU) per gram.
Echinacea	*Capsule:* Take up to 1,200 mg daily of an extract standardized to contain 125 mg of *E. augustfolia* root and at least 3.2% echinacoside. Other echinacea species, such as *E. purpurea* and *E. pallida* are also used.
Omega-3 Fatty Acids	Take 3–5 g of omega-3 fatty acids per day, in divided doses, with meals. The amount of omega-3 fatty acid will vary by manufacturer, so be sure to check the product label carefully.
Quercetin	*Capsule:* Take 250 to 500 mg two or three times a day.
Spirulina	*Capsule:* Take 3–5 g daily, divided into three doses.
Vitamin C	*Capsule or Tablet:* Take 250 to 500 mg twice daily.
	Note: Be sure to use a buffered form of vitamin C. If taking vitamin C causes loose stools, decrease your dosage and then gradually increase the dosage as tolerated.

HEADACHE

PROBLEM THAT JUST won't go away is sometimes referred to as a "headache." But anyone who suffers from recurring headaches will tell you that the pain is much more than

HOT PEPPER FOR YOUR HEAD

Although cayenne may not be the first ingredient that comes to mind when you think of treating a headache, a double-blind study has shown that cayenne—when administered under a doctor's supervision—may be helpful in treating cluster headaches, which often occur in groups over a long period of time. Other studies show that creams containing cayenne may also help in treating cluster headaches.

To make a topical cayenne-containing solution, combine a small amount of cayenne powder with water. Stir the solution and apply it to the nostril that is located on the same side of the head as the headache. Keep in mind, however, that the solution will burn—in some cases severely—when applied to the skin. Consult a doctor before using this treatment to be sure you are applying it correctly. Then, brace yourself: although cayenne may be painful, some headache sufferers have found relief with this natural treatment.

simply a problem! Headaches are all too common, last all too long, and can often be debilitating. Migraine headaches, commonly regarded as the epitome of bad headaches, are covered in a separate section (see page 529). Here we will discuss other common types of headaches that cause plenty of misery on their own.

WHAT IS IT?

The International Headache Society changed the name of tension headaches to "tension-type headaches." While physical tension was once believed to be the primary cause of these headaches, researchers now believe that factors beyond muscle tension—and including stress, depression, poor posture, and changes in brain chemistry—can trigger these headaches. Tension-type headaches are the most common form of headaches, affecting 9 of 10 adults at least once in their lifetime.

Although they are sometimes confused with tension headaches, sinus headaches occur when the sinuses become blocked, trapping air, mucus, and sometimes pus from an infection. The pain of sinus headaches often extends to the eyes, upper teeth, cheeks, and forehead. The way to relieving a sinus headache is to reduce swelling and inflammation of the sinuses and allow them to drain, thereby relieving the pressure that causes these headaches. Be sure to see Sinusitis on page 573 for ways to manage sinus infections as well as accompanying headaches.

Yet another type of headache, called a rebound headache, occurs as a response to the chronic use of prescription or over-the-counter headache medications. That is one good reason to consider the use of supplements as alternatives to medications for treating headaches. See below for a list of supplements that may help reduce tension headaches.

WHAT SHOULD I TAKE?
Calcium • Eucalyptus Oil • Magnesium
Peppermint Oil • Valerian • Willow Bark

Calcium and **magnesium** supplements are helpful for relaxing muscles, making these supplements useful for treating tension-type headaches. (For more information on calcium and magnesium, see pages 57 and 203.)

Preliminary research shows that **eucalyptus** oil, when combined with peppermint oil (see page 226), may be effective in reducing the muscle tension associated with tension-type headaches. (For more information on eucalyptus, see page 111.)

Peppermint oil, when applied topically, is a fresh-smelling way to ease a tension headache after a day of stress. Preliminary studies have shown that the topical application of peppermint oil, when applied to the temples 3 times over a 30-minute period, was better than a placebo and as good as acetaminophen in reducing tension-type headache pain. (For more information on peppermint, see page 226.)

Valerian helps relieve tension and anxiety and may also reduce spasms in the muscles, which may make this herb effective in treating tension-type headaches. (For more information on valerian, see page 272.)

Willow bark contains an ingredient similar to the key ingredient of aspirin, and this herb has been used for centuries as a pain relieving agent. Instead of taking aspirin for your next headache, consider trying this natural alternative. Keep in mind, however, that the regular use of willow bark may cause the same type of rebound headache that occurs with the chronic use of other pain relievers. (For more information on willow bark, see page 298.)

Acupuncture May Help Heal Headaches

Did You Know?

One of the oldest, most commonly used medical practices in the world, acupuncture is a form of traditional Chinese medicine that uses needles to unblock the flow of energy in the body, balancing the passive and active principles of *yin* and *yang,* respectively, to achieve spiritual, emotional, mental, and physical health. Acupuncture is very effective at releasing the muscle tension and postural dysfunction that can contribute to headaches. Widely practiced in the United States for the past 20 years, acupuncture is an effective treatment for chronic or recurring headaches and migraine headaches.

In this technique, an acupuncturist will place needles at various locations on the body. The needles are very thin, and the process does not hurt; indeed, many people find it very relaxing. The U.S. Food and Drug Administration (FDA) approved acupuncture by licensed practitioners as a health care technique in 1996, and many health insurance companies now cover much of the cost for this procedure. To find a medical acupuncturist near you, contact the American Academy of Medical Acupuncture (http://www.medicalacupuncture.org/).

MY SUPPLEMENT LIST—HEADACHE

SUPPLEMENT	RECOMMENDED DOSAGE
Calcium and Magnesium	*Capsule or Tablet:* Take 1,000 mg of calcium citrate and 1,000 mg of magnesium daily, dividing both into four 250-mg doses.

(continued)

MY SUPPLEMENT LIST—HEADACHE (continued)	
SUPPLEMENT	**RECOMMENDED DOSAGE**
	Note: Take magnesium in the form of magnesium glycinate to avoid loose stools. Large amounts of magnesium can cause diarrhea; if this becomes a problem for you, reduce your dosage.
Eucalyptus Oil	*Topical—Oil:* Combine 2 drops of peppermint oil with 1 drop of eucalyptus oil. Apply topically to the forehead and temples for 3 minutes. Avoid contact with the eyes.
Peppermint Oil	*Topical:* Put 2 drops of peppermint essential oil in a cup of water. Submerge a clean cloth in the water and press it to the back of your neck. You may also rub a solution containing 10% peppermint oil across your temples three times within a 30-minute period.
Valerian	*Capsule or Tablet:* Take 300 to 500 mg of a concentrated extract once or twice daily. Tea: Steep 1 tsp or teabag of valerian root in a cup of hot water for 20 minutes. Drink 2 to 4 cups daily as needed. *Note:* The strength of valerian products may vary greatly. Be sure to choose a standardized product and carefully follow the instructions on the label.
Willow Bark	*Capsule:* Take a standardized willow bark extract that provides 240 mg of salicin daily. Tea: Steep one-fourth to one-half tsp or teabag of willow bark in a cup of hot water for 10 minutes. Drink 2 to 4 cups daily as needed. *Caution:* Avoid willow bark if you have an aspirin allergy, bleeding disorder, diabetes, or a peptic ulcer.

HEART DISEASE

HEART DISEASE IS THE leading cause of death in the United States. In the year 2000, heart disease killed more than 700,000 people. While this number is staggering, you can make many lifestyle choices that can increase your chances of avoiding heart disease. Although certain risk factors for heart disease are beyond individual control (such as age and heredity), many common risk factors can be reduced. Eating a low-fat, low-cholesterol diet, quitting smoking, and getting plenty of physical activity are all steps that can help prevent and combat heart disease. Make sure to also read Weight Loss (page 614), High Cholesterol (page 489), and Hypertension (page 498) to help put you on the path to a healthy heart.

WHAT IS IT?

The term "heart disease" encompasses a number of conditions. The most common form is *coronary artery disease* (CAD), also known as coronary heart disease. This condition is caused by the build-up of deposits containing cholesterol and fat within the arteries that supply blood to the heart. CAD often develops slowly over time and is caused by lifestyle factors such as a diet with a high cholesterol content, smoking, and obesity.

Once the coronary arteries become clogged, less blood gets pumped to the heart, which can lead to the chest pain called angina. Angina often occurs after periods of severe stress and often causes a feeling of pressure in the chest, although angina may also occur during rest.

A *heart attack* occurs when a blockage within the arteries to the heart prevents blood from flowing through them. Warning signs of a heart attack include pressure or pain in the center of the chest that lasts for more than a few minutes; pain that extends to the left shoulder, arm, back, teeth, or jaw; shortness of breath; sweating; nausea and vomiting; and lightheadedness. Recurrent angina may be a warning sign of an impending heart attack.

CAD and heart attacks can both contribute to another condition, called *congestive heart failure*. This occurs when the heart becomes too weak or damaged to properly pump enough blood throughout the body. Symptoms of congestive heart failure include weakness, shortness of breath, waking at night, having to sit up in order to breathe, and swelling in the lower legs.

Heart disease is a serious condition. It must be treated under the supervision of a medical doctor. However, the supplements named in this section may be useful adjunctive treatments for heart disease. If you have a heart condition, steer clear of supplements containing ephedra and licorice root.

WHAT SHOULD I TAKE?

Heart disease can be life threatening. Make sure to consult your doctor before taking any type of supplement, especially if you have been diagnosed with a heart disease or think you may have a heart disease.

> *Alpha Lipoic Acid • Arginine • Astragalus • Betaine*
> *Coenzyme Q10 (CoQ10) • Folic Acid • Garlic*
> *Ginger • Hawthorn • L-Carnitine • Magnesium*
> *Omega-3 Fatty Acids • Vitamin B_6*
> *Vitamin B_{12} • Vitamin C • Vitamin E*

Although different studies have given conflicting information about their efficacy, antioxidants are often recommended as part of a plan for preventing heart disease, in part because they neutralize the cell- and tissue-damaging free-radical molecules that can contribute to

FRIENDS AND FOES

Resveratrol—a substance found in red wine, purple grape juice, and mulberries—may have heart-protecting effects. Not only is resveratrol an antioxidant, but it is also an anti-inflammatory agent and blood vessel dilator, and it prevents blood from clotting so it can flow freely to the heart. One glass of red wine contains 640 micrograms of resveratrol. Or try taking from 200 to 600 micrograms of a resveratrol supplement daily, divided into two doses.

the development and progression of many types of heart disease. Some studies suggest that taking antioxidants such as **alpha lipoic acid** (ALA), **vitamin C**, and **vitamin E** may help to protect the heart; however, strong evidence of such benefit is lacking. Other large studies show that antioxidants have no significant benefit for heart health. (For more information on alpha lipoic acid, vitamin C, and vitamin E, see pages 29, 284, and 292.)

The amino acid **arginine** may decrease symptoms associated with CAD as well as slow the development of atherosclerosis. The amount of arginine most people receive from food is often sufficient, although certain infections may deplete the amount of arginine in the body. A study published in the *Journal of the American College of Cardiology* in January 2002 found that a medical food bar with a high content of arginine and other vitamins increased the quality of life and exercise capacity of people with angina. Of the 36 participants in the double-blind study, all of whom had angina, those who received the arginine bar showed improvements in their electrocardiograms, a stronger capacity for exercise, and an overall improvement in their quality of life. Other studies indicate that supplemental arginine may improve heart function in elderly people with damaged endothelial cells (cells lining the heart). (For more information on arginine, see page 31.)

Astragalus may improve heart function, especially when it is taken after a heart attack. Studies suggest that astragalus improves heart function, specifically in the left side of the heart, and may also temper chest pain and discomfort and shortness of breath in people with a heart condition. (For more information on astragalus, see page 35.)

Studies suggest that **betaine** trimethylglycine may lower levels of homocysteine (a harmful byproduct of amino acid metabolism) in the blood. As a result, betaine may reduce the risk for developing atherosclerosis, a condition in which deposits of various harmful substances (including fat, cholesterol, and cellular byproducts such as homocysteine) build up in the arteries and reduce blood flow to the heart, increasing the risk of heart attack. (For more information on betaine, see page 42.)

CoQ10 may have some benefits in preventing and treating coronary artery disease and heart failure. Some medications prescribed to people with heart disease or related conditions—such as gemfibrozil (Lopid), and certain beta-adrenergic blocking drugs—may lower levels of CoQ10 in the body; thus, CoQ10 may be a wise adjunctive treatment with conventional medication. Studies also show that

CoQ10 may ease symptoms of angina including less chest pain and an increase in exercise ability. And preliminary research indicates that CoQ10 may improve recovery time in people who have recently undergone coronary artery bypass surgery. (For more information on CoQ10, see page 80.)

Vitamins B$_6$, B$_{12}$, and **folic acid** (vitamin B$_9$) are needed to keep the body's levels of homocysteine—an amino acid that contributes to the formation of cholesterol- and fat-containing plaque in arteries—from becoming too high, thus possibly preventing stroke and CAD. (For more information on vitamins B$_6$, B$_{12}$, and folic acid, see pages 279, 282, and 130.)

In some studies, **garlic** supplements have been shown to decrease blood clotting and the build-up of plaque. Because of its potential role as an antioxidant, garlic may be especially helpful in reducing the risk of atherosclerosis, specifically by stopping the oxidation of LDL ("bad") cholesterol, a key factor in the development of atherosclerosis. An analysis of 10 double-blind trials also found that garlic has a mild blood-pressure-lowering effect. (For more information on garlic, see page 135.)

Preliminary animal research indicates that **ginger** may keep blood from becoming abnormally likely to clot. Further research is needed to establish the role of ginger in preventing and treating heart disease and blood clots. (For more information on ginger, see page 136.)

The herb **hawthorn** is best known for its use in treating heart problems. It strengthens blood vessels, and evidence from laboratory

Women and Heart Disease

Did You Know?

While many women fear breast cancer as their primary health threat, heart disease is the number-one killer of women. One of every 2 women will die of heart disease, as opposed to 1 of 27 who will die of breast cancer. In the United States, 41.3 percent of all female deaths occur from some form of heart disease. Furthermore, the survival rate following a heart attack is significantly lower in women than in men.

Despite these frightening statistics, the common perception persists that heart disease is a man's disease. Many women are unaware of the dangers of heart disease and stroke. Surveys reveal that only 8 percent of women in the United States know that heart disease and stroke are their greatest health threats. And few women are aware of the increased risk of heart attack after menopause. Furthermore, women constitute only 25 percent of all participants in heart-related research studies.

Although the situation may sound grim for women, the good news is that women can take many steps to reduce their chances of cardiovascular disease. The first step, however, is awareness.

and animal studies indicates that it may help cut down plaque formation in the arteries. In human studies, patients with congestive heart failure who took hawthorn supplements showed better heart function and greater exercise capacity than those who did not. (For more information on hawthorn, see page 167.)

L-carnitine plays an important role in fueling muscles, including the heart. In several studies, taking carnitine supplements helped people with congestive heart failure to have better heart function, as evidenced by a greater ability to exercise. (For more information on L-carnitine, see page 186.)

Magnesium deficiency is often found in people with congestive heart failure, and research has shown that people with congestive heart failure who have lower levels of magnesium do not survive for as long as those with normal levels of this mineral. Magnesium also helps dilate blood vessels and is an extremely useful treatment after a heart attack when given intravenously. Unfortunately, the typical American diet, by itself, does not provide enough magnesium to meet the body's requirements for this mineral. (For more information on magnesium, see page 203.)

Studies indicate that people whose diets contain fish that provide high quantities of **omega-3 fatty acids**—such as salmon and mackerel—have a lower risk of death caused by cardiovascular disease. Omega-3 fatty acids may work against a variety of conditions that can compromise cardiovascular health. Research indicates that these fatty acids may decrease triglyceride levels, lower the risk of irregular heartbeat, improve the function of blood vessels, and reduce the chances of abnormal blood clot formation. Studies indicate that supplementation with omega-3 fatty acids may improve the elasticity of the arteries, increasing systemic arterial compliance—a measure that doctors use to predict an individuals' risk of heart disease. (For more information on omega-3 fatty acids, see page 221.)

MY SUPPLEMENT LIST—HEART DISEASE

SUPPLEMENT	RECOMMENDED DOSAGE
Alpha Lipoic Acid	*Capsule:* Take 50 to 100 mg once a day.
L-Arginine	*Tablet or Food:* Make sure that your intake of arginine is 6–9 g a day either in food or supplement form (as l-arginine). Foods that are high in arginine include nuts, grains, fish, and happily, chocolate! Large doses of l-arginine supplements may cause diarrhea.

MY SUPPLEMENT LIST—HEART DISEASE	
SUPPLEMENT	**RECOMMENDED DOSAGE**
Astragalus	*Capsule:* Take 300 to 600 mg of a standardized extract two or three times daily. *Tea:* Take 9–15 g sliced root, slowly boiled in 2–3 cups of water for 1 hour. Divide into two doses each day.
Betaine	*Capsule or Tablet:* Take 500 to 1,000 mg daily in the form of betaine trimethylglycine.
	Note: Some people may require dosages of up to 6g daily to lower levels of homocysteine in the blood. Consult your doctor to determine an appropriate dosage of betaine for you.
CoQ10	*Softgel:* Take 50 to 150 mg twice daily.
	Note: If you're taking the blood-thinning medication warfarin (Coumadin), consult your doctor before taking CoQ10.
Folic Acid	*Tablet:* Take 400 mcg daily.
Garlic	*Fresh:* Eat 4,000 mg (1 clove) of fresh, raw garlic daily. *Capsule or Tablet:* Take 600 to 900 mg daily of dried garlic powder, standardized to contain 1.3% allicin.
Ginger	*Fresh:* Cook thinly sliced pieces of fresh ginger root into food. *Capsule:* Take 500 to 1,000 mg of ginger daily. Higher dosages of ginger may be recommended. Consult your doctor to determine an appropriate dose of ginger for you.
Omega-3 Fatty Acids	*Fish oil:* Take 3–5 g of omega-3 fatty acids per day, in divided doses, with meals. The amount of omega-3 fatty acid will vary by manufacturer, so be sure to check the product label carefully.
Vitamin B$_6$	*Tablet:* Take 50–100 mg daily divided into two doses.
	Note: If you have liver disease, consult your doctor before taking more than 50 mg of vitamin B$_6$ daily.
Vitamin B$_{12}$	*Tablet:* Take 1,000–2,000 mcg daily.
Vitamin C	*Capsule or Tablet:* Take 500 mg three times daily. Use a buffered form of vitamin C. If taking vitamin C causes loose stools, decrease your dosage and then gradually increase the dosage as tolerated.
Vitamin E	*Capsule:* Take 400 IU daily of a natural product containing mixed tocopherols.

HEARTBURN

EVEN THOUGH IT MAY FEEL like a heart attack, the burning sensation that begins to creep its way toward your mouth from your stomach after you eat a bowl of chili is likely to be heartburn rather than a heart condition. Heartburn is the bane of spicy food lovers everywhere, a cruel companion to stress, and another good reason to quit smoking. If you experience heartburn, you are certainly not alone. A survey conducted in 2003 by the National Heartburn Alliance revealed that an estimated 54 million Americans experience frequent heartburn.

WHAT IS IT?

Heartburn is a common problem that almost everyone experiences at some point in their life. What causes the burning, tingling sensation of heartburn is the stomach acid backing up into the esophagus and toward the throat. This regurgitation is known as reflux, and it typically occurs after heavy meals, upon lying down before food is digested, or with smoking, stress, or alcohol intake.

Although occasional heartburn is very common, recurrent bouts of heartburn are known as gastroesophageal reflux disease (GERD). GERD usually denotes a greater problem within the digestive tract, and its symptoms are sometimes more severe than heartburn, including nausea and vomiting, hoarseness, and chest pain. GERD typically results from lifestyle choices, medication, or stress. Making changes in your diet and overall lifestyle can make a considerable difference in minimizing the symptoms of GERD. Avoiding heavy meals and acidic foods and alcohol, avoiding fatty foods, quitting smoking, and losing weight can all make a substantial difference in reducing persistent heartburn. Some nutritional and herbal supplements can also play a role in diminishing as well as preventing heartburn.

Extinguishing Heartburn

Healthy Hints

Although it may seem as though your heartburn comes and goes with no rhyme or reason, a number of behavioral and dietary factors can trigger heartburn. Try introducing some of these healthy habits to help eliminate indigestion and heartburn.

■ **Watch the clock.** Eating food immediately before going to bed may cause heartburn. Be sure to eat at least 2 to 3 hours before bedtime to avoid this problem.

■ **Get moving.** Excess weight contributes to heartburn—just one more reason to get exercise and shed those extra pounds.

■ **Stay away from...** Citrus fruits and other acidic foods, such as oranges and tomatoes, carbonated beverages, coffee, fatty foods, spearmint and peppermint, whole-fat milk, and other dairy products, are considered trigger foods, and people who experience frequent bouts of heartburn should avoid them.

■ **Cut back.** Eating several small meals as opposed to two or three large meals a day allows your digestive system to better break down food.

■ **Cook right.** The way food is prepared can make all the difference to a person prone to heartburn. Try steaming vegetables or poultry in wine or broth instead of sautéeing them or frying them with oils.

WHAT SHOULD I TAKE?
Bromelain • Calcium • Chamomile • Devil's Claw
Digestive Enzymes • Licorice • Slippery Elm

Bromelain is a natural enzyme found in pineapples, and it has enzymatic properties that make it useful in treating heartburn. Specifically, bromelain digests protein, which promotes good digestion, relieves upset stomach, and prevents heartburn. It is a natural alternative to over-the-counter medicines for heartburn relief. (For more information on bromelain, see page 54.)

Calcium, when taken in the form of calcium citrate powder, along with digestive enzymes (see below), may help to digest food when taken after meals. These two supplements may also work together to reduce the acidity of a meal. Although more research is needed to determine the benefits of calcium citrate on heartburn, doctors frequently recommend it in combination with digestive enzymes for relief from heartburn. (For more information on calcium, see page 57.)

Chamomile can be effective in reducing inflammation in the digestive tract and calming the stomach. (For more information on chamomile, see page 67.)

Devil's claw is a multipurpose herb approved by the German Commission E for the treatment of heartburn. (For more information on Devil's claw, see page 98.)

Digestive enzymes are often recommended for people experiencing frequent indigestion of unknown cause. Be sure to buy a product containing the enzymes lipase, amylase, protease, cellulase, and lactase for best effect. Many doctors recommend taking digestive enzymes along with calcium citrate (see above). (For more information on digestive enzymes, see page 102.)

Licorice root is a soothing herb, making it a natural choice for keeping heartburn at bay. It may serve as a natural alternative to prescription heartburn-relief medications. But the licorice must be deglycyrrhizinated when used for heartburn to prevent it from causing such side effects as fluid retention, increased blood pressure, and potassium loss. (For more information on licorice root, see page 192.)

Slippery elm, like licorice root, has a long history of use for digestive inflammation and ulcers. Its soothing, coating properties make it a nice complement to licorice for relief from heartburn. (For more information on slippery elm, see page 256.)

MY SUPPLEMENT LIST—HEARTBURN

SUPPLEMENT	RECOMMENDED DOSAGE
Bromelain	*Tablet:* Take 300 to 600 mg three times daily after meals. Look for a product containing 2,400 gelatin-dissolving units (GDU) or 3,600 milk-clotting units (MCU) per gram. *Note:* Follow individual product labels carefully because optimal dosages of bromelain vary widely from one product to another.
Calcium	*Powder:* Some doctors recommend taking one-half tsp of powdered calcium in the form of calcium citrate along with digestive enzymes after each meal. *Note:* Powder is the recommended form of calcium citrate for heartburn, since studies show that it works more effectively than tablets.
Chamomile	*Capsule:* Take 300 to 800 mg three times daily of a standardized extract between meals. *Tea:* Combine 1 tbsp of fresh flower with 1 cup of boiling water. Steep for 10 minutes and drink three times daily. You may also drink up to 4 cups of chamomile tea made from teabags only.
Devils' Claw	*Extract (root):* Take 500 mg (standardized to contain a minimum of 5% harpagosides), 1 capsule three times per day with meals. Some doctors recommend avoiding this herb if gastric or duodenal ulcer is present.
Digestive Enzymes	*Powder:* Many doctors recommend taking one-half tsp of digestive enzyme powder along with calcium citrate after each meal. *Tablet:* Take a product that 3 to 4 g of "4X pancreatin," which contains 100 mg of amilase, lipase, and protease, with meals.
Licorice	*Capsule:* Take 300 to 800 mg of deglycyrrhizinated licorice 20 minutes before each meal. *Alternate dose:* Take 200 mg of a licorice-root extract standardized to contain 50 mg of glycyrrhizinic acid daily. Do not take the glycyrrhiznic acid product for longer than 1 month. *Note:* Licorice candy is made with artificial flavoring and has no healing properties.
Slippery Elm	*Capsule:* Take up to 4,800 mg daily divided into three or four doses.

HEMORRHOIDS

I N AN OLD ADVERTISEMENT for hemorrhoid treatment, a burning match is used to illustrate the pain of a hemorrhoid. If you've ever suffered from this uncomfortable condition, you probably understand the metaphor all too well. Hemorrhoids have plagued humans since the beginning of time.

WHAT IS IT?

Hemorrhoids occur when a cluster of veins that are normally present in the rectum and anus become swollen. Constipation and hard stools, as well as prolonged and repeated sitting and inactivity, contribute to the development of hemorrhoids by causing the veins in the rectal area to become swollen. In some cases, a blood clot forms at the site, making a hemorrhoid even more uncomfortable. Internal hemorrhoids occur inside the rectum, and while not usually painful, they may bleed.

People in undeveloped countries rarely suffer from hemorrhoids. This is probably because of a high fiber content in their diet, which makes passing stools quite easy, as well as an active lifestyle. Modern Americans, however, rarely get enough fiber in their diets, and the result is hard stools that can lead to hemorrhoids. Pregnant women often develop hemorrhoids because of the excess pressure on the rectum from carrying a baby and giving birth.

Once a hemorrhoid has developed, typical symptoms include constipation, straining, discomfort, swelling in the rectum, itching, and in some cases rectal bleeding. Several over-the-counter remedies can provide immediate relief of hemorrhoid pain and laxatives can aid the passing of stools, but these treatments rarely get to the heart of the problem. Fortunately, nutritional supplements can play a role in healing hemorrhoids and preventing their recurrence.

WHAT SHOULD I TAKE?
Bilberry • Calendula • Fiber • Flaxseed
Horse Chestnut • Psyllium • Quercetin

As noted in the previous section, many women develop hemorrhoids during pregnancy and after childbirth. **Bilberry** may be a useful remedy for reducing the discomfort associated with these and other types of hemorrhoids and is a safe supplement to take during pregnancy and breastfeeding. (For more information on bilberry, see page 44.)

Witch Hazel May Offer Relief from Hemorrhoids

Did You Know?

Although there is little scientific evidence of its efficacy, witch hazel may offer soothing relief for hemorrhoids. The medicinal property of the witch hazel plant *(Hamamelis virginiana)* comes from water that is distilled from the bark and dried leaves of the plant. Witch hazel has been used traditionally to soothe the itching and burning associated with hemorrhoids, and Native Americans used liquid derived from leaves of the plant to treat hemorrhoids.

Witch hazel is available over the counter at most drug stores. Also available are disposable, medicated pads that contain witch hazel, such as Tucks hemorrhoidal pads. However, it may be more cost efficient to buy witch hazel in the bottle. When choosing bottled witch hazel, be sure to buy a product that has a low alcohol level. A solution with a high alcohol level could burn the delicate skin around a hemorrhoid.

Calendula, in the form of a topically-applied ointment, may help ease the burning and pain sometimes associated with hemorrhoids. (For more information on calendula, see page 61.)

Flaxseed is rich in fiber, making it a great supplement to add to your daily diet to relieve constipation and assist in more regular and softer stools. (For more information on flaxseed, see page 126.)

Fiber is a global term used to describe herbs such as flaxseed and psyllium seed. (For more information about other types of fiber and how to use them, see page 120.)

Horse chestnut extract is known historically for improving the strength of blood vessels, making it a vital part of a hemorrhoid treatment program. Studies show that horse chestnut extract reduces the symptoms of hemorrhoids. (For more information on horse chestnut, see page 171.)

Psyllium, much like flaxseed, is useful for bulking up stools, thereby preventing the constipation that can cause hemorrhoids. A double-blind study showed that 7 grams of psyllium taken twice daily reduced the pain and bleeding associated with hemorrhoids. (For more information on psyllium, see page 120.)

Quercetin is bursting with flavonoids, making it crucial in strengthening blood vessels. Studies indicate that bioflavanoids, when taken in dosages of 600 to 4,000 milligrams daily, help reduce the itching, bleeding, and discomfort associated with hemorrhoids. (For more information on quercetin, see page 236.)

MY SUPPLEMENT LIST—HEMORRHOIDS

SUPPLEMENT	RECOMMENDED DOSAGE
Bilberry	*Tablet:* Take 150 to 600 mg daily between meals of an extract standardized to contain 25% anthocyanosides, divided into two or three doses.
Calendula	*Topical—Lotion/Cream:* Apply a lotion or cream product containing calendula two or three times each day to the affected area. Follow the individual product label for application instructions.
Fiber	*Psyllium supplements:* Take 7 g in 8 ounces of liquid, as often as up to three times per day. *Methylcellulos (sold as Citrucel):* Take 10.2 g in 8 ounces of liquid, as often as three times per day. *Polycarbophil (sold as Fibercon):* Take 1 g (or 2 caplets) per day. Do not exceed 4 g per day. *Note:* To increase the fiber in your diet increase servings of well cooked beans, fresh fruits and vegetables, and whole grains.

MY SUPPLEMENT LIST—HEMORRHOIDS	
SUPPLEMENT	**RECOMMENDED DOSAGE**
Flaxseed	*Fresh:* Eat 1 heaping tbsp of ground flaxseed with cereal, apple juice, or another food product every day.
	Note: Be sure to drink plenty of water when taking fiber supplements.
Horse Chestnut	*Oral—Tablet:* Take 300 mg of an extract standardized to contain 16% to 21% aescin two to three times daily between meals. *Topical—Gel:* Apply a gel or cream containing 2% aescin to hemorrhoids two or three times daily.
Psyllium	*Seeds:* Take 2 tbsp of psyllium seeds or 1 tsp of psyllium husks, mixed with water or juice, two or three times daily.
	Note: Be sure to drink plenty of water when taking fiber supplements.
Quercetin	*Capsule:* Take 250 to 500 mg up to two to three times daily.

HEPATITIS

GETTING YOUR ABCS is a good thing when it comes to vitamins but not when it comes to your liver. Hepatitis A, B, and C are all caused by viruses. Although many people are familiar with the term "hepatitis" or have even received a vaccination against this condition, few people know the difference between them.

WHAT IS IT?

Hepatitis A can affect anyone, although it commonly affects children and young adults. The virus that causes it is often transmitted through contaminated food and water, or by contact with an infected person. Symptoms do not usually appear until 15 to 30 days after contracting the illness and include fatigue, poor appetite, fever, vomiting, and jaundice (yellowing of the skin and whites of the eyes). A vaccine for hepatitis A is an available form of protection against this disease.

Hepatitis B is a serious and potentially fatal condition that can result in lifelong infection by the virus that causes this disease, as well as cirrhosis of the liver, liver cancer, and liver failure. While anyone can contract hepatitis B, certain groups of people—such as drug abusers who share needles, men who have sex with multiple male partners, hemodialysis patients, and infants born to mothers who are carriers of the hepatitis B virus—are at an increased risk for getting this disease. Symptoms include those of hepatitis A as well as joint pain, hives, and rash. Hepatitis B is often transmitted through bodily fluids exchanged during sexual, not casual, contact. A currently available hepatitis B vaccine is the best form of protection against this disease.

Hepatitis C infects about 25,000 people each year and is transmitted via the blood of an infected person. This disease is most common in drug abusers who share needles and in people who had blood transfusions before July 1992. Most people with hepatitis C develop a chronic liver infection and have an increased risk of developing other liver diseases. There is no preventive vaccination for hepatitis C.

Alcoholic hepatitis is a syndrome of a progressive disease that occurs from chronic ingestion of alcohol. Symptoms of this condition include fever, jaundice (yellowing of the skin and whites of the eyes), fatigue, abdominal discomfort, weight loss, and nausea. Mild forms of alcoholic hepatitis may occur without these symptoms.

Although the prospects for people with hepatitis may seem troubling, nutrition can do quite a bit to minimize and reduce the severity of its symptoms.

WHAT SHOULD I TAKE?
Carnitine • Choline • Cordyceps • Licorice
Milk thistle • Schisandra • Selenium

Carnitine may be useful for alleviating the fatigue associated with hepatitis C. (For more information about carnitine, see page 186.)

Choline, when taken in the form of phosphatidylcholine (PC), may improve liver function in people with hepatitis B and C. A double-blind trial consisting of 176 people with hepatitis B and C found that when PC was taken along with interferon (Roferon-A; a drug commonly prescribed for treating hepatitis), not only did symptoms improve, but the improvement lasted for 24 weeks after supplementation was discontinued, suggesting that PC may enhance the effects of interferon. (For more information on choline, see page 71.)

Eat Your Brussels Sprouts!

Did You Know?

Plants in the cabbage family, including, brussels sprouts, broccoli, cauliflower, kale, mustard greens, and radishes, are sometimes called "cruciferous vegetables." These vegetables get this name from the word cruc, which means "to cross." They have flowers with four petals or leaves that form the shape of a cross.

You may already know that the vegetables named above have health benefits. Each is loaded with antioxidants and has a high content of fiber, vitamins, and minerals. Cruciferous vegetables are known for their cancer-preventing effects, but they also appear to help protect against hepatitis. These vegetables contain a compound, called indol-3-carbinol, that activates enzymes in the intestines and the liver that have detoxifying effects, helping to protect the liver and stave off hepatitis.

Studies indicate that **cordyceps**, a Chinese medicinal mushroom, may have liver-protecting effects in people with hepatitis B. (For more information on cordyceps, see page 88.)

Preliminary studies suggest that the combination of **milk thistle** and **selenium** may help protect the liver from damage, perhaps from the powerful antioxidant properties of this combination. Selenium help protect people with hepatitis from developing liver cancer, while milk thistle has been used historically to protect the liver, and studies have now given evidence that it protects the liver from damage caused by viruses and other toxins. (For more information on milk thistle and selenium, see pages 210 and 253.)

Licorice root is more than just a flavoring for candy. Glycyrrhizin, one of the active components in licorice, has been used intravenously for the treatment of hepatitis B and hepatitis C in Japan. Test-tube studies show that licorice may have the ability to prevent the hepatitis A virus from replicating. Licorice has been found to improve liver function and sometimes lead to a complete recovery from hepatitis. Trials have also found that when taken orally, licorice may be more effective than inosine polyIC, a drug often prescribed for people with hepatitis. (For more information on licorice, see page 192.)

Schisandra has been used in traditional Chinese medicine for a wide variety of health conditions and is currently being studied for use in treating hepatitis. In China, this herb is used to improve liver function in people with hepatitis. Some experts attribute schisandra's liver-protective effect to components called lignans, which may promote the regeneration of damaged liver tissue. (For more information on schisandra, see page 251.)

MY SUPPLEMENT LIST—HEPATITIS

SUPPLEMENT	RECOMMENDED DOSAGE
L-Carnitine	Take 1–3 grams per day in divided doses, with food. May cause a fishy body odor.
Choline	*Capsule or Tablet:* Studies using 1.8 g daily of phosphatidylcholine (PC) for 24 weeks have yielded positive results. Consult your doctor to determine an appropriate dosage for you.
Cordyceps	*Capsule:* Take 3 to 4.5 g twice daily on an empty stomach.
Licorice	*Capsule:* Studies have shown that taking 1,000 mg twice daily of licorice standardized to contain 750 mg of glycyrrhizin may work better than prescription drugs to treat hepatitis.

(continued)

MY SUPPLEMENT LIST—HEPATITIS (continued)	
SUPPLEMENT	**RECOMMENDED DOSAGE**
	Note: High doses of licorice can cause high blood pressure and other health problems. This dosage should only be taken under the supervision of a doctor. Licorice candy is made with artificial flavorings and has no healing properties.
Milk Thistle	*Capsule:* Take 300 mg of an extract standardized to contain 80% silymarin three times daily, along with selenium (see below).
Schisandra	*Capsule:* Take up to 3,000 mg daily divided into three doses.
Selenium	*Tablet:* Take 200 mcg twice daily, along with milk thistle (see previous page).

DIETARY DO'S AND DON'TS

Do. The amino acid lysine is especially beneficial for suppressing herpes outbreaks. To boost your lysine intake, try increasing your intake of beef, brewer's yeast, cheese, chicken, dairy products, eggs, fish, meat, milk, potatoes, soybeans, and yogurt. (For more information on lysine, see page 200.)

Don't. Just as lysine seems to inhibit the herpes virus, arginine—the *yin* to lysine's *yang*—can cause an outbreak when levels of this amino acid become too high. The best way to prevent elevated arginine levels is to avoid arginine-rich foods, such as chocolate, peanuts, nuts, seeds, oatmeal, raisins, coconut, caffeine, and whole wheat bread.

HERPES

HERPES IS THE MOST common sexually transmitted disease in America. Over 20 million Americans have herpes, with an average of 500,000 new cases breaking out each year. As many as 90 percent of people with genital herpes are unaware of their infection and unknowingly spread the virus that causes it—known as the Herpes Simplex virus—to other people, which is why new cases occur at such a rapid rate. Despite the scourge surrounding the condition, having herpes does not sentence you to a life of solitude and loneliness. Although there is no cure for herpes, you can manage the condition and live a healthy, productive, and sexually fulfilling life.

WHAT IS IT?

The Herpes Simplex virus is a relative of the Epstein-Barr virus, which causes mononucleosis, and of the varicella zoster virus, which causes chicken pox and shingles (see page 487). Infection with the herpes simplex virus takes two general forms: Type 1, often referred to as "fever blisters," and type 2, known as genital herpes.

The Herpes Simplex virus can be transmitted by sharing utensils or towels, and by kissing. Type 1 herpes appears in the form of cold sores, usually on the mouth, lips, nose, chin, or cheeks, although in rare cases type 1 herpes can develop in the genital area. The sores may spread if you touch them and then touch an unaffected part of your skin. Some people experience recurrent herpes infections, sometimes triggered by a fever, sun exposure, stress, or menstruation.

The symptoms of type 2 herpes include pain and itching in the skin around the genital area, pain in the buttocks or legs, and small red bumps, blisters, and open sores. This usually begins from 2 to 10 days after exposure to the virus, and the symptoms pass within a few days. On average, an individual with herpes will experience four or five outbreaks per year, although the frequency of recurrent outbreaks of genital herpes varies from one person to another. Sexual intercourse with someone who has herpes is the main cause of genital herpes.

Symptoms of herpes can be managed through antiviral medication and by keeping the area of an eruption clean and dry. To avoid spreading herpes, sex (including oral-genital contact) should be avoided during an episode of the disease, and condoms should always be used, even in the absence of an eruption. In addition, the nutritional remedies discussed below may hasten the healing of herpes and prevent outbreaks from occurring.

WHAT SHOULD I USE

Herpes Simplex is a serious condition. Make sure to consult your doctor before taking any type of supplement if you have been diagnosed with Herpes Simplex or think you may have Herpes Simplex.

Aloe • Cat's Claw • Echinacea
Lemon Balm • Licorice • Lysine • Propolis
Vitamin C • Vitamin E • Zinc

Applying a topical cream made with **aloe** (also called aloe vera) extract to affected areas may speed the recovery from outbreaks of genital herpes. Early studies also suggest that aloe may help reduce the number of recurring outbreaks. (For more information on aloe, see page 27.)

Research indicates that the herb known as **cat's claw**, when applied topically, may reduce the pain associated with herpes outbreaks in addition to speeding recovery and without reported side effects. (For more information on cat's claw, see page 63.)

Echinacea, when applied topically, may combat the Herpes Simplex virus. Studies have indicated that echinacea may be effective against numerous strains of this herpes virus even in cases in which the prescription antiviral medication acyclovir (Zovirax), often prescribed for herpes, is not. (For more information on echinacea, see page 107.)

Lemon balm is one of the most popular herbal remedies used for herpes. It has been found helpful in treating outbreaks of herpes, and in a large study in Germany in which lemon balm was used to treat primary herpes infection, no cases of recurrence were noted. This may indicate that lemon balm reduces the recurrence of outbreaks if it is used during the first occurrence of herpes infection. Lemon balm cream helps reduce the healing time for both genital and oral herpes. (For more information on lemon balm, see page 190.)

FRIENDS AND FOES

ZINC AND COPPER

Taking **zinc** on a long-term or high-dose basis may reduce the body's absorption of **copper**. If you plan to supplement with zinc for an extended period, take a copper supplement as well.

Licorice, a well-known anti-inflammatory agent, may also be useful in stopping the herpes simplex virus from growing. Topical applications of licorice may reduce the duration of eruptions in addition to decreasing the severity of oral herpes lesions. (For more information on licorice, see page 192.)

Studies have shown that **lysine** can inhibit the activity of the herpes virus itself. Not only is this amino acid valuable in a daily maintenance dose for preventing herpes outbreaks, but it can also be used during outbreaks to reduce their severity and duration. (For more information on lysine, see page 200.)

Propolis—a natural product derived from bees—may prevent the herpes virus from entering cells, thus keeping the virus from replicating. Studies hint even small amounts of propolis may achieve this. (For more information on propolis, see Q&A in Bee Pollen, page 37.)

Vitamin C may work orally and topically to reduce the healing time of herpes blisters during outbreaks, especially when used just before symptoms develop, when the skin is tender, painful, or tingling. (For more information on vitamin C, see page 284.)

Vitamin E oil, when applied directly to herpes lesions, may help reduce the pain associated with herpes outbreaks and speed the healing process. (For more information on vitamin E, see page 292.)

Zinc slows the reproduction of the herpes virus, helping to prevent and reduce the severity of outbreaks. When applied topically, creams containing zinc may be useful in treating both facial and genital herpes. (For more information on zinc, see page 304.)

MY SUPPLEMENT LIST—HERPES

SUPPLEMENT	RECOMMENDED DOSAGE
Aloe	*Topical—Cream:* Apply a cream containing 0.5% aloe to affected areas three times daily until sores disappear.
Cat's Claw	*Topical—Cream or Gel:* Apply a cream or gel containing cat's claw topically to affected areas once daily.
Echinacea	*Topical—Tincture:* Speak to an herbalist, who may recommend a tincture of echinacea for topical application to treat herpes eruptions.
Lemon Balm	*Topical—Cream:* Apply a cream containing lemon-balm extract to lesions from two to four times a day.
Licorice	*Topical—Tincture:* Use a cotton swab to apply a tincture containing licorice to affected areas three times daily until they have healed.

SUPPLEMENT	RECOMMENDED DOSAGE
	MY SUPPLEMENT LIST—HERPES
Lysine	*Oral—Tablet:* Take 500 mg of lysine daily and increase your intake to 1,000 mg three times daily with meals at the first sign of an outbreak until symptoms ease. *Topical—Cream:* Use lysine cream topically twice a day to treat herpes outbreaks.
Propolis	*Topical—Cream:* Apply a cream containing 0.5% propolis extract to affected areas at the first sign of herpes infection. Propolis cream may also be applied for up to 2 hours after an outbreak has occurred.
Vitamin C	*Oral—Capsule or Tablet:* Take 250 to 500 mg twice a day. *Topical—Solution:* Apply a topical solution containing vitamin C three times for 2 minutes each at 30-minute intervals on the first day of an outbreak to speed healing. *Note:* When taking vitamin C orally, be sure to use a buffered form of vitamin C. If taking vitamin C causes loose stools, decrease the dosage and then gradually increase it as tolerated.
Vitamin E	*Topical—Oil:* Squeeze the liquid from a vitamin E capsule onto a cotton swab and apply it directly to affected areas every 8 hours as needed.
Zinc	*Oral—Tablet:* Take 25 mg once a day. *Topical—Cream:* Apply a cream containing zinc oxide/glycine or zinc sulfate to affected areas. Follow individual product labels for application instructions.

HERPES ZOSTER (SHINGLES)

SHINGLES MAY WELL BE CALLED "chickenpox redux." Remember the itchy, painful chickenpox you experienced as a child? If you had chickenpox as a child, the varicella virus lies dormant in cells around the spinal cord, waiting to make a comeback. When certain factors including age, illness, medication, or stress reawaken the virus, you are forced to relive the nightmare all over again.

WHAT IS IT?

Herpes zoster, also known as shingles, is characterized by a red rash and blisters that last for 2 to 3 weeks before they give way to scabs. The rash and blisters typically occur around the trunk, spreading around the abdomen and chest and down the arms and legs, following the course of a nerve. Shingles may be accompanied by pain and intense itching as well as fever and headaches. In some cases, however, the pain of shingles can occur without a rash, a condition known as *zoster sine herpete*. This usually occurs in elderly people and produces symptoms that include burning or shooting pain, numbness, tingling, itching, headache, fever, chills, and nausea.

If you seek medical attention immediately at the onset of an outbreak of shingles, your doctor may be able to ease the outbreak with a dose of antiviral medication. But if you have had the rash for 3 days or more, you will probably have to live with the outbreak until it passes. One area to watch carefully in a case of shingles is the region around the eyes, since the virus can cause an eye infection. If an eruption of shingles occurs in this area, seek immediate medical attention. Once the rash of shingles clears up, you may still experience pain, known as *postherpetic neuralgia.* This complication can be difficult to treat; however, when a rash first develops, the doctor may prescribe medication to help prevent persistent pain after the rash leaves, such as opiates.

Always see your doctor if you have a painful rash, even if you have had it for several days. Not all painful rashes are shingles, and it's best to play it safe and have your doctor make a correct diagnosis of any rash. Furthermore, if you do have shingles, it may be highly contagious to someone who has never had chickenpox, and this can be extremely dangerous to adults and seniors. Herbs and supplements may be a helpful addition to the treatment prescribed by your doctor.

WHAT SHOULD I TAKE?
Cayenne • Licorice • Vitamin E

Capsaicin, the active component in **cayenne** peppers, is available over the counter in a cream. It may be helpful in relieving pain and itching,

Hypnosis May Help Alleviate the Pain of Shingles

Did You Know?

The pain of shingles is often exacerbated by the postherpetic neuralgia that follows this disorder. This neuralgia is characterized by pain over the entire body, and although it is not fatal, this pain can be debilitating.

Hope for relief from the pain of postherpetic neuralgia can be found in hypnosis. Studies have shown that hypnosis benefits patients with shingles and postherpetic neuralgia. Hypnosis was approved in 1985 by the American Medical Association for treating pain, and its popularity in pain management is growing. The way in which hypnosis works in easing pain is not fully understood, but researchers have observed that it helps patients to control their responses to pain, making the pain more bearable.

Clinicians who use hypnosis have been able to control dermatologic pain, including the pain associated with shingles and neuralgia, with hypnotherapy. Consult your health care provider to see if hypnotherapy can help you to manage the pain of shingles.

including the pain associated with postherpetic neuralgia. However, cayenne cream should not be used to treat a rash that has not yet healed. (For more information on cayenne, see page 64.)

Licorice-containing gels have been used traditionally to treat shingles. Preliminary research suggests that the component of licorice known as glycyrrhizin may keep the varicella zoster virus from spreading. However, licorice gels are not easily available and may need to be obtained from a doctor who uses or specializes in herbal medicine. (For more information on licorice, see page 171.)

Some studies suggest that when applied topically or taken orally, **vitamin E** may help people with shingles. Long-term application of vitamin E oil to affected areas may hasten healing of the blisters that occur in shingles. Oral supplementation with vitamin E may also help to ease postherpetic neuralgia, even if it has been a source of pain for several years. (For more information on vitamin E, see page 292.)

MY SUPPLEMENT LIST—HERPES ZOSTER

SUPPLEMENT	RECOMMENDED DOSAGE
Cayenne	*Topical—Cream:* Studies using creams containing 0.025% to 0.075% capsaician have yielded positive results. Apply such a cream three or four times daily. *Note:* It may take at least 2 weeks of treatment to reach the full benefit of capsaicin-containing creams.
Licorice	*Topical—Gel:* Licorice gel may be applied to affected areas three times daily. Follow the individual product label information for specific application instructions.
Vitamin E	*Oral—Capsule:* (Note: Only use this large of a dose under the direct supervision of your physician.) Take 1,200 to 1,600 IU of vitamin E daily. *Topical—Oil:* Apply vitamin E oil directly to affected areas of skin as needed. *Note:* It may take several months of continuous topical application of vitamin E to achieve benefits.

HIGH CHOLESTEROL

DESPITE COMMON MISCONCEPTIONS, cholesterol is not necessarily the root of all evil. Actually, this soft, waxy substance is a normal component of the fatty substances that circulate in the bloodstream and constitute important "building blocks" for hormones, cells, and tissues. Cholesterol is important in maintaining overall health, helping to form cell membranes, the coating of nerve cells, and certain hormones, and in other necessary functions. Problems with cholesterol arise when our dietary and lifestyle choices cause it to increase to dangerous levels in the blood and to clog blood vessels, blocking the flow of blood and causing heart attacks, strokes, and other serious health problems.

WHAT IS IT?

Cholesterol in the bloodstream exists in two major forms. One of these, known as low-density lipoprotein (LDL) or "bad" cholesterol, is the type of cholesterol that tends to form deposits in the walls of arteries, leading to their obstruction and to serious diseases such as heart attack and stroke. The other, known as the "good" type of cholesterol or high-density lipoprotein (HDL) cholesterol, tends to keep away from blocking your arteries and causing disease. Having a high level of HDL cholesterol and low level of LDL cholesterol in the blood is therefore considered quite healthy.

New Research on Fat Intake, Cholesterol, and Heart Disease

It is widely believed that a direct link exists between dietary fat, cholesterol levels, and heart disease. However, new research suggests that this link may be more myth than truth, and several studies have contradicted its existence. Thus, for example, a study of Japanese immigrants in the United States found that Japanese food—which is lean, low in dietary fat, and often believed to be heart-friendly—did not appear to decrease their risk of having heart attacks. In fact, those immigrants who were brought up in a more Americanized fashion but continued to eat lean Japanese food suffered from heart attacks twice as often as those who were brought up in typical Japanese fashion but consumed a fatty and more "American" diet.

In East Africa, the Masai people have the highest intake of animal fat in the world. Yet they exhibit fewer heart-related abnormalities in the electrical measurements of heart function known as electrocardiography than do Americans. "Hardening" of the arteries, from the formation on cholesterol depostis and blood clots in the artery walls, is also rare in the Masai people. In southern India, where people tend to eat 19 times more fat than those in northern India, the number of deaths from coronary artery disease is seven times lower than the number in northern India. Furthermore, the average age of death from coronary disease in the south of India is 44 years, compared to 52 in the north.

Beyond these findings, not one of twenty-one studies of more than 150,000 people with and without coronary artery disease found that a heart-friendly diet of low-fat, low-cholesterol foods played a role in the prevalence of heart disease. If the surprising results of these studies are confirmed by future studies, current dietary approaches to preventing high cholesterol may have to be reevaluated.

Cholesterol can become a health concern when LDL cholesterol levels become too high (160 mg/dL and above) and HDL levels become too low (less than 40 mg/dL). If you are obese or inactive, levels of LDL cholesterol may gradually increase in your bloodstream, leading to clogged arteries and heart disease, stroke, or other disease.

Smoking, high blood pressure, diabetes, and heredity can all increase the chance of high LDL levels leading to heart disease. A high level of such cholesterol causes no symptoms until damage to the blood vessels is quite advanced, by which time heart disease may have already developed. The best way to keep your blood cholesterol levels in check is to get tested frequently. Doctors recommend that you take your first cholesterol test in your 20s, and follow up with additional tests every 3 to 5 years. Diet, exercise, and overall health and well-being are important cholesterol-lowering elements. Herbs and supplements, along with an overall healthy diet and lifestyle, can play a key role in reducing dangerous levels of cholesterol in your body.

WHAT SHOULD I TAKE?

Beta-Sitosterol • Chromium • Fenugreek • Fiber
Green Tea • Guggul • Magnesium • Niacin • Policosanol
Red Yeast Rice • Vitamin C • Vitamin E

Studies indicate that **beta-sitosterol**, a plant sterol found in soy, may reduce levels of cholesterol in the body by blocking the absorption of cholesterol. (For more information on beta-sitosterol, see page 40.)

Although study results are conflicting, some research suggests that **chromium** may increase HDL ("good") cholesterol while lowering total cholesterol levels. In a double-blind trial, when chromium was taken in conjunction with daily exercise, it decreased total cholesterol levels by almost 20 percent in 13 weeks. Chromium may be especially helpful in reducing cholesterol levels in people taking beta-adrenergic blocking medication. (For more information on chromium, see page 77.)

Preliminary evidence suggests that **fenugreek** may be beneficial to people with high cholesterol, perhaps due to its content of saponins—compounds that appear to increase cholesterol secretion in the gastrointestinal tract, consequently lowering serum cholesterol levels. (For more information on fenugreek, see page 116.)

Substantial research indicates that soluble **fiber**, which is fiber that dissolves in water, is an effective cholesterol-lowering agent. Insoluble

FRIENDS AND FOES

Cholesterol-lowering medicines of the statin type belong to the family of drugs known as HMG-CoA reductase inhibitors. Studies indicate that HMG-CoA reductase inhibitors interfere with the body's production of **coenzyme Q10** (CoQ10), and use of these drugs should be therefore accompanied by supplementation with CoQ10. Consult your doctor about taking supplemental CoQ10 if you are taking red yeast rice (which contains the monacolins also found in some prescription cholesterol-lowering drugs) or a statin drug. Consult your doctor immediately if you are taking red yeast rice or a statin drug and experience muscle weakness or pain.

fiber, or fiber that does not dissolve in water, may also play a role in lowering cholesterol. One study found that 20 grams of either soluble or insoluble fiber significantly reduced cholesterol levels for an extended period of time. (For more information on fiber, see page 120.)

Green tea is a relative newcomer to the cholesterol-cutting supplement scene, but recent studies seem to suggest its effectiveness. Catechins—the active ingredients in green tea—block the absorption of cholesterol in the intestines, preventing it from making its way into the bloodstream and promoting its excretion from the body. (For more information on green tea, see page 157.)

Research shows that some of the compounds found in **guggul**, known as guggulsterones, may significantly lower triglyceride and LDL ("bad") cholesterol levels in the blood. Guggul also raises HDL ("good") cholesterol and because of its power as an antioxidant may prevent cholesterol from oxidizing, which is a major cause of the condition known as atherosclerosis, in which there is a buildup of plaque in the arteries. One study found that guggul was equal in effect to the prescription medication clofibrate (Atromid-S), often used to treat high cholesterol. (For more information on guggul, see page 162.)

Preliminary research indicates that **magnesium** may help to lower cholesterol levels, especially in people with diabetes. One study of 40 people with type 2 diabetes found that after 12 weeks of supplementation with magnesium, the levels of total cholesterol in their blood had fallen, as had their LDL and triglycerides, whereas the levels of HDL cholesterol in their blood had risen, with no negative effect on their blood sugar levels. (For more information on magnesium, see page 203.)

Niacin has been well studied in major clinical trials and has become an accepted treatment for lowering LDL cholesterol while raising HDL cholesterol levels; it has also been shown to reduce the risk for cardiovascular disease when taken on a long-term basis. There is one caveat: The dosage of niacin needed to lower LDL cholesterol levels can cause liver damage as well as "niacin intolerance"—a side effect with symptoms including flushing of the face. It is important to consult your doctor if you are thinking about taking niacin as a supplement. (For more information on niacin, see page 219.)

Policosanol, a substance derived from sugar cane, shows promise in reducing cholesterol levels by slowing the synthesis of cholesterol in the liver. The results of various studies suggest that policosanol both reduces LDL cholesterol levels and increases HDL cholesterol levels. (For more information on policosanol, see page 232.)

Monacolins, compounds found in **red yeast rice**, slow the production of cholesterol-generating enzymes in the liver. A synthetic form of one such monacolin—monacolin K (which is one of the many monacolins found naturally in red yeast rice)—is also known as lovastatin (Mevacor), and is an important prescription medication for lowering cholesterol levels. Red yeast rice also contains a number of sterols, isoflavones, and unsaturated fatty acids that add to the cholesterol-lowering effects of the monacolins. (For more information on red yeast rice, see page 241.)

Vitamin C has properties that enable it to reduce high cholesterol levels. Studies suggest that taking vitamin C every day can decrease LDL cholesterol levels as well as increase HDL cholesterol levels. (For more information on vitamin C, see page 284.)

Although the evidence is conflicting, **vitamin E** may keep LDL cholesterol from forming plaque and clogging arteries. Vitamin C helps to reactivate vitamin E when the latter has become "spent," which is why these two vitamins are effective when taken together. (For more information on vitamin E, see page 292.)

MY SUPPLEMENT LIST—HIGH CHOLESTEROL

SUPPLEMENT	RECOMMENDED DOSAGE
Beta-Sitosterol	*Capsule or Tablet:* Dosages range from 50 mg to 10 g daily. Consult a doctor to determine an appropriate dosage for you.
Chromium	*Capsule:* Take 200 mcg daily. *Note:* Dosages as high as 1,000 mcg may be taken to lower cholesterol but only under the supervision of a doctor.
Fenugreek	*Capsule:* Take 5 to 30 g of defatted fenugreek with meals three times daily.
Fiber	*Diet:* A diet high in oats, legumes, barley, apples, citrus fruits, and oats will provide a generous source of fiber. *Powder:* Take 7 grams of psyllium powder in 8 ounces of liquid, up to three times daily.
Green Tea	*Capsule:* Take 125 to 500 mg per day of a standardized extract. *Tea:* Make a tea by combining 1 tsp or teabag of green tea with 2 cups of boiling water. Steep for 5 minutes and drink 3 cups daily. *Note:* Decaffeinated green tea products are available for those who do not wish to consume caffeine.

(continued)

MY SUPPLEMENT LIST—HIGH CHOLESTEROL (continued)	
SUPPLEMENT	**RECOMMENDED DOSAGE**
Guggul	*Capsule:* Be sure to take a supplement that provides 25 mg of guggulsterones three times daily.
Magnesium	*Tablet:* Take 500 to 600 mg daily in the form of magnesium glycinate.
Niacin	*Tablet:* Begin taking 250 mg daily. Dosages may be raised to 2,000 mg a day, but only under a doctor's supervision.
Policosanol	*Capsule or Tablet:* Take 20 mg one or two times daily with meals.
Red Yeast Rice	*Capsule:* Take 1,200 mg twice daily.
	Caution: Do not take red yeast rice if you are allergic to yeast or have liver disease. Red yeast rice can cause muscle problems similar to those of statin cholesterol-lowering medications. This supplement should be taken for long term only under the supervision of a medical doctor.
Vitamin C	*Capsule or Tablet:* Take up to 3,000 mg divided into several doses each day.
	Note: Be sure to use a buffered form of vitamin C. If taking vitamin C causes loose stools, decrease your dosage and then gradually increase the dosage as tolerated.
Vitamin E	*Capsule:* Take 400 IU daily.

HIV AND AIDS

AIDS—ACQUIRED IMMUNE deficiency syndrome—is a globally epidemic disease, affecting more than 40 million people worldwide, with 5.3 million people infected in 2001 alone. The problem of AIDS is most devastating in Africa, where it is estimated that in highly infected regions, 20 million children will lose one or both parents to AIDS within the next 8 years. For the first time in history, as many women as men are infected with the human immunodeficiency virus (HIV) that causes AIDS. Although the AIDS epidemic is most severe in Africa, there are 800,000 to 900,000 Americans living with this disease.

WHAT IS IT?

HIV attacks the body's immune system, damaging and destroying cells until the body can no longer effectively fight off infection. AIDS occurs in the later stages of HIV infection. As a result, infections that a healthy immune system would normally prevent become life-threatening in people with AIDS. HIV can remain in the body for up to 11 years before developing into AIDS. HIV infection is most commonly spread through sexual contact with an infected individual, but it can also be spread through shared needles and syringes, infected blood, and from mother to child during pregnancy or through breast milk.

In its early stages, HIV infection is symptom-free. After 2 to 6 weeks of infection, a flu-like illness commonly develops. Since there is no distinction between the symptoms of this illness and the symptoms of other common illnesses, such as influenza, it is hard to identify early HIV infection. Nevertheless, at this stage of the illness, it is possible to infect others, even though no symptoms exist. As HIV progresses, symptoms include swollen lymph nodes, diarrhea, weight loss, fever, and shortness of breath. During the last phase of HIV infection—AIDS—more serious symptoms begin to appear, such as vision problems, white spots or lesions on the tongue and mouth, persistent headaches, shaking chills, long-term fever, and fatigue.

Although there is no cure for HIV infection or AIDS, in the past 8 years the available number of medications for treating AIDS has more than tripled, and new treatments can now extend and improve the quality of life for those infected with HIV. Along with conventional medical treatment, nutritional and herbal supplements can help reduce symptoms of HIV infection, decrease the adverse side effects of medications for treating AIDS, and improve the overall sense of well-being of people with HIV and AIDS.

WHAT SHOULD I TAKE?

HIV and AIDS are life-threatening illnesses. Make sure to consult your doctor before taking any type of supplement, especially if you have been diagnosed with HIV or AIDS or think you may have HIV or AIDS.

Alpha Lipoic Acid • Echinacea • Ginseng • Glutamine L-Carnitine • Multivitamin • N-Acetylcysteine (NAC) Selenium • Vitamin B Complex • Vitamin C • Vitamin E

Preliminary studies suggest that **alpha lipoic acid** (ALA) may be helpful in managing HIV. Not only is ALA a powerful antioxidant that helps to scavenge the cell- and tissue-damaging molecules known as free radicals, but it helps to raise levels of glutathione in the body, an amino acid that is crucial to maintaining healthy immune-system function. ALA may also curb the replication of HIV by slowing the replication process. (For more information on alpha lipoic acid, see page 29.)

Echinacea and **ginseng** may be useful herbs for helping to strengthen and support the immune system in people with HIV. Test-tube studies suggest that these herbs may help people who have compromised immune systems, such as those with HIV, to fight off infection. (For more information on echinacea and ginseng, see pages 107 and 141.)

Glutamine may help people with HIV to maintain a healthy body weight by preventing the loss of protein from the body's own tissues. Additionally, anecdotal evidence suggests that many patients taking the anti-HIV drugs known as protease inhibitors find glutamine helpful, particularly with diarrhea, a side effect associated with this type of medication. (For more information on glutamine, see page 146.)

L-Carnitine may be useful in tempering some of the side effects of commonly prescribed anti-HIV medications. Research indicates that people taking zidovudine (Retrovir) or didanosine (Videx) who experience side effects have lower levels of carnitine than those not taking these drugs. Further research is needed to study the effects of L-carnitine on HIV. (For more information on L-carnitine, see page 186.)

Many people with AIDS have deficiencies of several nutrients. One study found that HIV-infected people who took a **multivitamin**

Home Tests for HIV

The only way to know if you are infected with HIV is to have an HIV test. Until recently, only a healthcare professional could administer an HIV test, but the U.S Food and Drug Administration (FDA) has since approved a test for HIV infection that individuals can use in the privacy of their own homes. The test is called the "Home Access Express HIV-1 Test System," and is manufactured by the Home Access Health Corporation. The kit for performing the test is available from doctors and health clinics.

The test uses a simple process in which you prick your skin, collect a blood sample, and mail it to a laboratory along with a confidential and anonymous personal identification number (PIN). Professional clinicians in a certified medical laboratory analyze the blood sample in the same way a blood sample taken at a hospital or clinic would be analyzed. There is a toll-free number to call to receive test results, and post-test counseling is available at this number as well.

Be aware that the Home Access Express HIV-1 Test System is the only test approved by the FDA for HIV infection, and it can only be obtained at a clinic or through your doctor. A number of other HIV home test systems and kits that are marketed on the Internet and in magazines are not approved and should not be used. Such tests promise rapid results and may even falsely claim to be FDA approved. Be sure to use only the FDA-approved test system to get valid HIV results.

experienced a slower onset of AIDS than those who did not take a multivitamin. (For more information on multivitamins, see page 9.)

NAC may be helpful in improving immune function in people with HIV, as well as slowing the progression of the infection caused by the virus. In one study, supplementation with 800 milligrams of NAC daily improved immune function in people with HIV. (For more information on NAC, see page 213.)

Selenium works along with vitamin B complex (see below) to help the body fight the physical stress of HIV infection. (For more information on selenium, see page 253.)

Vitamin B complex may help the body fight the extreme physical stress it undergoes as the result of HIV infection. A 9-year study showed that not only did low levels of vitamin B_{12} serve as an early marker of HIV disease progression, but that the development of AIDS occurred an average of 4 years sooner in people with low levels of vitamin B_{12}. (For more information on vitamin B complex, see pages 277, 279, and 282.)

According to a 1998 study, **vitamin C** has the antioxidant potential to minimize cell damage and reduce the overall amount of HIV in the body. Injections of vitamin C in extremely high doses seemed to hinder the growth of the HIV virus. (For more information on vitamin C, see page 284.)

Vitamin E has had effects similar to those of vitamin C (see above) in inhibiting HIV and its damage to the body, as well as helping people infected with the virus to maintain a healthy body weight. If you have HIV, ask your doctor about adding vitamins C and E to your supplement regimen. (For more information on vitamin E, see page 292.)

FRIENDS AND FOES

ST. JOHN'S WORT AND GARLIC

St. John's wort and **garlic** may decrease levels of certain AIDS medications in the blood, inhibiting these drugs' effectiveness. It is important to speak with your doctor if you have AIDS and are taking supplements. Since many people with AIDS take large amounts of herbs, vitamins, and prescription medications, the possibility of interactions between these agents is high.

MY SUPPLEMENT LIST—HIV AND AIDS

SUPPLEMENT	RECOMMENDED DOSAGE
Alpha Lipoic Acid	*Capsule:* Take 450 mg daily.
Echinacea	*Capsule:* Take up to 1,200 mg daily of an extract standardized to contain 125 mg of *E. augustfolia* root and at least 3.2% to 4.8% echinacoside. Other echinacea species, such as *E. purpurea* and *E. pallida* are also used. To be used as an adjunctive treatment of infections in people living with AIDS, not as a stand alone treatment.
Ginseng	*Capsule:* Take 100 to 200 mg daily of an Asian ginseng extract standardized to contain 5% to 7% ginsenosides. Nonstandardized extracts should be taken in higher doses of 1 to 4 g daily.

(continued)

MY SUPPLEMENT LIST—HIV AND AIDS (continued)	
SUPPLEMENT	**RECOMMENDED DOSAGE**
	Note: Discontinue ginseng use after 2 to 3 weeks and resume after 1-week.
Glutamine	*Capsule or Tablet:* Take 10 g three times daily for weight gain. Ask your doctor about taking a supplement with beta-hydroxy-beta-methylbutyrate (HMB), L-glutamine, and L-arginine.
L-Carnitine	*Capsule:* Take 1 g three times daily. May cause fishy body odor.
Multivitamin	Take a multivitamin/mineral supplement every day. Follow the individual product label for dosage information.
NAC	*Capsule:* Take up to 600 mg four times a day.
Selenium	*Tablet:* Take 200 mcg daily.
Vitamin B Complex	*Tablet:* Take vitamin B complex in a dose of 75 to 100 mg daily. Read the individual product label for dosage information.
Vitamin C	*Capsule or Tablet:* Take 1,000 mg daily.
	Note: Be sure to use a buffered form of vitamin C. If taking vitamin C causes loose stools, decrease your dosage and then gradually increase the dosage as tolerated.
Vitamin E	*Capsule:* Take 400 IU every day.

HYPERTENSION

YOU SHOULD LOOK AT your blood pressure in the same way that Tiger Woods looks at his golf score—the lower the better! One of the greatest health problems in America is high blood pressure, or hypertension. Hypertension is often referred to as "the silent killer" because about one-third of the 50 million Americans who have it are completely unaware that they do.

WHAT IS IT?

The ideal blood pressure reading is around 120/80 mmHg for adults. The first number, 120, refers to the systolic pressure, which is the pressure the heart generates when pumping out blood. The second number, 80, is the diastolic pressure, or the pressure in the arteries when the heart rests between beats. Both readings are measured—like the barometric pressure of the earth's atmosphere—in millimeters of mercury (mm/Hg). A blood pressure reading of 130 to 139 mmHg systolic over 80 to 89 mmHg diastolic is considered a high risk for subsequent hypertension and should be cause for close monitoring. A blood pressure reading of 140/90 mmHg or higher is considered high and is typically treated with medication.

Hypertension often shows no signs or symptoms. There are, however, a few warning signs that affect a small number of people, such as a dull ache in the back of the head in the morning, frequent nosebleeds, and dizziness; However, these symptoms usually occur in late-stage hypertension, when the condition may already be life-threatening. The best way to keep tabs on your blood pressure is to have it checked at least every 2 years by your physician. If your blood pressure is above the healthy range, you should have it checked more often.

You can do quite a bit to keep hypertension under control: Eating a healthy diet that includes whole grains, fresh fruits, and vegetables and that limits sugar, salt, and processed foods is a good place to start. In addition to diet, exercising frequently, reducing stress, and curbing excess alcohol and all tobacco use can all help to prevent or reduce high blood pressure. And lowering your weight is the most important factor in controlling hypertension.

WHAT SHOULD I TAKE?
Arginine · Calcium · Coenzyme Q10 (CoQ10)
Garlic · Hawthorn · Magnesium
Omega-3 Fatty Acids · Potassium · Vitamin C · Vitamin E

Studies suggest that even modest increases in the intake of **arginine** may have the ability to lower blood pressure. Arginine is a precursor to nitric oxide, a substance that dilates blood vessels and lowers blood pressure. Maintaining healthy levels of arginine may therefore prevent blood pressure from rising. (For more information on arginine, see page 31.)

While studies have given conflicting results, **calcium** may be beneficial in reducing high blood pressure. One study of the famous Dietary Approaches to Stop Hypertension (DASH) diet for lowering blood pressure found that a diet with low-fat dairy products, fruits, and vegetables did more to reduce blood pressure than fruits and vegetables alone. Other studies show that calcium may reduce blood pressure, particularly in African Americans, pregnant women, and people whose blood pressure is sensitive to their salt intake. (For more information on calcium, see page 57.)

CoQ10 has tested well in several studies in reducing both systolic and diastolic blood pressure in patients with hypertension. Furthermore, 39 percent of people with hypertension have been shown to have a deficiency of CoQ10. (For more information on CoQ10, see page 80.)

Small studies show that **garlic** may lower blood pressure. An analysis of 12 clinical trials that included 415 participants showed that garlic was beneficial in achieving this. (For more information on garlic, see page 135.)

Hawthorn may help in reducing both systolic and diastolic blood pressure. In one study, 36 women with mild hypertension showed improvement in their blood pressure after taking hawthorn supplements for 10 weeks. Not only did hawthorn lower blood pressure in this study, it reduced anxiety levels as well, which in turn can lower blood pressure levels even further. (For more information on hawthorn, see page 167.)

Diet May Be as Effective as Medication in Easing Hypertension

The U.S. National Heart, Lung, and Blood Institute (NHLBI) developed the DASH diet as an eating plan to stop hypertension, and researchers have since found that this diet plan significantly reduces and prevents high blood pressure.

The DASH diet is rich in vegetables and fruits that are high in fiber, and low in saturated fats (fats from meat and dairy products). The DASH diet forbids foods high in cholesterol and allows only low-fat dairy products.

The DASH diet includes the following daily servings:
■ Seven or eight servings of grains, including whole grain bread, rice, pasta, or cereal
■ Four or five servings of vegetables; raw leafy vegetables are especially helpful
■ Four or five servings of fruits, including sugar-free dried fruit, fresh fruit, or canned fruit
■ Two or three servings of low-fat or fat-free dairy products, including an 8 ounce glass of milk or 1 cup of yogurt
■ Two or fewer servings of lean meats, poultry, and fish

The NHLBI conducted a study of 459 participants who followed the DASH diet. They found that the DASH diet significantly lowered blood pressure (as well as cholesterol and heart disease risk). Further studies revealed that the DASH diet produced results similar to those with anti-hypertensive medications.

To get started on the DASH diet, follow some of these tips:
■ If you normally eat only one or two vegetables a day, try adding one more serving of vegetables at lunch and another serving at dinner.
■ Cut your intake of butter or margarine by half.
■ Gradually increase your intake of low-fat dairy products to three servings per day. For example, drink low-fat (1 percent) or fat-free (skim) milk with lunch or dinner, instead of soda, juice, or alcohol.
■ When you go to the grocery store, buy less meat than you usually would. If you don't have meat in your home, you'll eat less of it.
■ If you eat large portions of meat, cut them back gradually, by a half or a third at each meal.
■ Introduce one or two vegetarian meals to your weekly dinner schedule.
■ Replace snacks with a few of these snack ideas: nuts mixed with raisins; low-fat and fat-free yogurt and frozen yogurt (without sugar) ; plain popcorn with no salt or butter added; and raw vegetables.

Magnesium may be an up-and-coming supplement in the world of hypertension. Researchers believe that magnesium may work to lower blood pressure because of its ability to relax smooth muscles in the walls of blood vessels. While additional studies are being conducted to test the effectiveness of magnesium in high blood pressure, supplementation with magnesium makes good sense because of its widespread use for a variety of other ailments. (For more information on magnesium, see page 203.)

Omega-3 fatty acids, the essential fatty acids found in cold-water fish such as salmon, mackerel, and tuna, have tested well in studies for significantly lowering blood pressure. The active ingredients in fish oil supplements—eicosapentaenoic acid (EPA) and docosahexaenoic acid (DHA)—may be taken to reduce blood pressure levels. One study found that DHA, when taken alone, may be especially useful for lowering blood pressure. (For more information on omega-3 fatty acids, see page 221.)

Well-documented studies show that **potassium**—which is found in high amounts in bananas and oranges—may be very effective in lowering blood pressure. However, over-the-counter potassium supplements, when taken in high doses, may irritate the stomach. If you have high blood pressure, speak to your doctor about taking potassium supplements. (For more information on potassium, see page 233.)

Some evidence indicates that blood pressure decreases with an increased intake of **vitamin C**. In one recent study, vitamin C reduced blood pressure by an additional 10 percent in people already taking prescription blood pressure medication. (For more information on vitamin C, see page 284.)

One triple-blind, placebo-controlled trial observed that **vitamin E** may lower blood pressure in people with mild hypertension. The study found that not only did vitamin E substantially decrease systolic blood pressure, but that it also decreased diastolic blood pressure, although not as dramatically. (For more information on vitamin E, see page 292.)

MY SUPPLEMENT LIST—HYPERTENSION

SUPPLEMENT	RECOMMENDED DOSAGE
L-Arginine	*Capsule:* Therapeutic dosages range from 6 to 20 g daily and are usually based on individual cases. Consult your doctor to determine an appropriate dosage for you.

(continued)

MY SUPPLEMENT LIST—HYPERTENSION (continued)	
SUPPLEMENT	**RECOMMENDED DOSAGE**
Calcium	*Capsule or Tablet:* Take 800 to 1,200 mg of calcium at bedtime for 2 months. Discontinue it if it is not effective in lowering blood pressure levels.
CoQ10	*Capsule:* Take 120 mg one to two times daily.
Garlic	*Capsule:* Take 600 to 900 mg daily of an extract standardized to contain 5,000 to 6,000 mcg of allicn potential.
Hawthorn	*Capsule:* Up to 5 g per day of nonstandardized capsules. If standardized, dose range is 160–900 mg per day.
Magnesium	*Tablet:* Take 500 mg twice daily. *Note:* Take in the form of magnesium glycinate to avoid loose stools. Large amounts of magnesium can cause diarrhea; if this becomes a problem for you, reduce your dosage.
Omega –3 Fatty Acids	Take 1–2 grams of omega-3 fatty acids per day, in divided doses, with meals. The amount of omega-3 fatty acid will vary by manufacturer, so be sure to check the product label carefully.
Potassium	*Tablet:* Dosages of 2,400 mg daily are often required to lower blood pressure; however, dosages this high are not available without a doctor's prescription. Speak with your doctor about taking potassium supplements if you have high blood pressure. *Note:* People taking potassium-sparing diuretics should not take potassium supplements.
Vitamin C	*Capsule or Tablet:* Take 500 mg two times daily. *Note:* Be sure to use a buffered form of vitamin C. If taking vitamin C causes loose stools, decrease the dosage and then gradually increase the dosage as tolerated.
Vitamin E	*Capsule:* Take 400 IU daily of a natural product containing mixed tocopherols.

HYPERTHYROIDISM AND HYPOTHYROIDISM

FOR SUCH A TINY ORGAN, the thyroid certainly has a big impact on human health. This small gland that rests at the base of the neck produces hormones that regulate the body's entire metabolism, from how quickly we burn calories to how quickly or slowly our heart beats. Keeping in mind the important role of the thyroid, it makes perfect sense that thyroid problems can have a serious health impact if left untreated. Two of the most common thyroid problems are hyperthyroidism and hypothyroidism.

WHAT IS IT?

Hyperthyroidism occurs when the thyroid produces too much of the hormone thyroxine; hypothyroidism occurs when the thyroid does not produce enough of this hormone. Hyperthyroidism typically occurs in people between the ages of 20 and 40 and can strike after extreme stress or during pregnancy. Symptoms of hyperthyroidism can vary widely, making it a difficult condition to diagnose. Sudden weight loss while eating the same or increased amounts of food is one indication of hyperthyroidism. Other symptoms include protruding eyeballs, irregular heartbeat, nervousness and irritability, sweating, sensitivity to heat, fatigue and muscle weakness, and difficulty sleeping. These symptoms result from an increased rate of metabolism caused by the thyroid's overproduction of hormones, putting the body into "overdrive."

By contrast with hyperthyroidism, hypothyroidism slows down metabolism, making you feel sluggish and lethargic. Unexpected and uncontrollable weight gain, elevated cholesterol levels, and depression are common effects of an underactive thyroid. An estimated 11 million people have hypothyroidism, and middle-aged women seem to be the most vulnerable to this condition. It is also likely to occur in people who have undergone radiation therapy, thyroid surgery, or treatment with radioactive iodine, or who have an autoimmune disease.

Although there is still much that doctors don't know about hyperthyroidism and hypothyroidism, early diagnosis of both conditions has been made fairly easy with the latest tests of thyroid function. Medication for hypothyroidism and surgery for hyperthyroidism can usually put an end to these conditions.

In addition, natural herbs and supplements can do quite a bit to prevent and regulate the symptoms of hypothyroidism and hyperthyroidism.

WHAT SHOULD I TAKE?

Both hypothyroidism and hyperthyroidism are serious conditions. Make sure to consult your doctor before taking any type of supplement if you have been diagnosed with either one of these conditions.

Iodine • Selenium • Vitamin A • Vitamin B Complex
Vitamin C • Vitamin E • Zinc

CALL YOUR DOCTOR WHEN...

Thyroid conditions are best treated when detected early. However, the symptoms of hyperthyroidism may not be obvious, making it important to know how to identify them. *Be sure to call your doctor if:*

- You experience unexplained weight loss
- You feel like your heart is beating rapidly
- You notice unusual sweating
- Your neck swells at the base

The symptoms of hypothyroidism are very different from those of hyperthyroidism and are just as important to recognize. *Be sure to call your doctor if:*

- You feel tired for no reason
- Your skin is unusually dry
- Your face is puffy and pale
- You experience prolonged constipation
- Your voice is hoarse

Adequate **iodine** intake is key to a properly functioning thyroid. While iodine deficiencies rarely occur in the United States, an inadequate intake of iodine can result in hypothyroidism. Although iodine supplements are unnecessary for most people, especially if they put iodized salt on their food even occasionally, such supplements are useful for people with deficiencies. Speak to your doctor to see whether you need iodine supplements, since taking supplemental iodine when it is unnecessary can actually cause hyperthyroidism.

Since **selenium** has a role in maintaining thyroid hormone metabolism, a deficiency of this mineral may further impair thyroid function, especially in the elderly. Be sure that your intake of selenium is adequate to avoid a deficiency in this important nutrient. (For more information on selenium, see page 253.)

Vitamin B complex may help in the fight against hypothyroidism or inadequate thyroid function. The entire cast of B vitamins support and regulate healthy thyroid hormone production. Taking a vitamin B complex is the best way to get all of the B-vitamin benefits at once. (For more information on vitamin B complex, see pages 277, 279, and 282.)

Oxidative stress is increased in people with hypo- and hyperthyroidism. Nutritional support with the antioxidants **vitamins A**, **C**, and **E** may help in neutralizing cell- and tissue-damaging free radical molecules from the body and reducing oxidative stress. (For more information in vitamins A, C, and E, see pages 274, 284, and 292.)

Some research shows that people with hypothyroidism have trouble metabolizing **zinc**. Taking a zinc supplement may be helpful for people who have an underactive thyroid. (For more information on zinc, see page 304.)

MY SUPPLEMENT LIST—HYPERTHYROIDISM AND HYPOTHYROIDISM

SUPPLEMENT	RECOMMENDED DOSAGE
Iodine	*Tablet:* Iodine is considered safe when taken in dosages of up to 1 or 2 mg daily, although this is 10 times the amount needed to keep levels of this nutrient within a normal range (150 mcg per day). It is not necessary to take iodine supplements unless you have an iodine deficiency. Consult your doctor before taking iodine supplements.
Selenium	*Tablet:* Take 200 to 300 mcg daily.

MY SUPPLEMENT LIST—HYPERTHYROIDISM AND HYPOTHYROIDISM	
SUPPLEMENT	**RECOMMENDED DOSAGE**
Vitamin A	*Tablet:* For hypo- or hyperthyroidism, take 20,000 IU daily.
Vitamin B Complex	*Tablet:* For hypothyroidism, take 50 to 100 mg daily.
Vitamin C	*Capsule or Tablet:* For hypo- or hyperthyroidism, take 500 mg from two to four times daily.
	Note: Be sure to use a buffered form of vitamin C. If taking vitamin C causes loose stools, decrease the dosage and then gradually increase the dosage as tolerated.
Vitamin E	*Capsule:* Take 400 to 800 IU daily of a natural product containing mixed tocopherols.
Zinc	*Tablet:* Take 30 mg of zinc daily.

HYPOGLYCEMIA

WE ARE CONSTANTLY BEING told by doctors that we consume entirely too much sugar. How, then, can anyone have low blood sugar? One of the greatest ironies of modern medicine is that a condition characterized by low blood sugar is in fact caused by too much sugar intake in the first place. In the past few years, hypoglycemia has become a buzzword, and many people claim to have this condition if they feel lightheaded after skipping a meal or having a late lunch. Real hypoglycemia is, however, a recognized medical condition and often symptomatic of other, more serious illnesses.

WHAT IS IT?

Hypoglycemia occurs when the body experiences abnormally low levels of sugar in the blood. Symptoms of this condition include headaches, depression, nervousness, hunger, perspiration, shakiness, dizziness, fatigue, and anxiety. Hypoglycemia can have a host of causes, including certain medications, alcohol, insulin treatments, and hormonal deficiencies, as well as diseases of the liver, kidneys, and heart that cause the body to overproduce insulin. People with diabetes often experience hypoglycemia, caused by an overadministration of insulin.

Serious problems can occur if hypoglycemia is not treated immediately. Vision can become blurred and the heart can begin to palpitate, which not only increases the heart rate but also raises blood pressure. In extreme cases, hypoglycemia can result in seizures, unconsciousness, and even death.

Fortunately, hypoglycemia can usually be controlled by eating regular meals, avoiding refined sugars and simple carbohydrates, and working with your doctor or nutritionist to develop an appropriate diet. However, because hypoglycemia is often a symptom of another more serious health condition, it is important to speak with your doctor if you have unexplained symptoms. Mother Nature can also lend a hand in maintaining sugar levels.

WHAT SHOULD I TAKE?

Chromium • L-Carnitine • Magnesium
Vitamin B₃ • Vitamin C (for people with diabetes)
Vitamin E (for people with diabetes)

Chromium seems to be a superstar when it comes to reducing sugar cravings by regulating glucose levels in the blood. (For more information on chromium, see page 77.)

Hypoglycemia may be a sign of an **L-carnitine** deficiency, so it's not surprising that supplementation with L-carnitine may be beneficial in this condition. Additionally, carnitine may help decrease fatigue, a common symptom of hypoglycemia. (For more information on L-carnitine, see page 186.)

Magnesium is a mineral that helps regulate glucose levels in the blood and may be beneficial for people with hypoglycemia. (For more information on magnesium, see page 203.)

Foods to Avoid

Healthy Hints

Because hypoglycemia is directly related to diet, it is very important for someone with hypoglycemia to make informed food choices. Read on for tips to help temper hypoglycemic symptoms.

■ **Say no to sugar.** Avoid cakes, cookies, candies, ice cream, and soft drinks, among other foods containing sugar. Instead, look for sugar-free goodies, such as candy and desserts that are made for people with diabetes.

■ **Steer clear of carbs.** Eliminate simple carbohydrates or processed foods (such as white bread) from your diet, as well as instant rice and potatoes. Replace them with multigrain breads, brown rice, and unprocessed foods.

■ **Don't drink.** Drinking alcoholic beverages, especially on an empty stomach, may cause hypoglycemia, even a day or two later. If you drink an alcoholic beverage, make sure you eat a snack or meal at the same time.

■ **Choose decaf.** Caffeine may increase the body's susceptibility to hypoglycemia. If you tend to experience hypoglycemia, eliminate caffeine, such as in coffee, tea, soda, and chocolate, from your diet.

■ **Keep a schedule.** Remember to eat at regular intervals every day, without skipping meals. Make sure to eat small meals on a frequent, steady basis rather than a few very large meals each day.

Preliminary research shows that supplemental **vitamin B$_3$** (niacinamide) may be helpful for people with hypoglycemia. (For more information on vitamin B$_3$, see page 219.)

Vitamins C and **E** may help regulate blood-sugar levels in people with diabetes. (For more information on vitamins C and E, see pages 284 and 292.)

MY SUPPLEMENT LIST—HYPOGLYCEMIA

SUPPLEMENT	RECOMMENDED DOSAGE
Chromium	*Tablet:* Take 50 to 200 mcg of chromium picolinate three times a day with meals.
L-Carnitine	*Capsule:* Take 1 to 3 g daily divided into two or three doses.
Magnesium	*Tablet:* Take 200 mg two or three times each day.
	Note: Take in the form of magnesium glycinate to avoid loose stools. Large amounts of magnesium can cause diarrhea; if this becomes a problem for you, reduce your dosage.
Vitamin B$_3$	*Tablet:* Take 500 to 1,000 mg two or three times daily.
Vitamin C	*Capsule or Tablet:* Take 250 to 500 mg twice a day.
	Note: Be sure to use a buffered form of vitamin C. If taking vitamin C causes loose stools, decrease your dosage and gradually increase as tolerated.
Vitamin E	*Capsule:* Take 400 IU daily of a natural product containing mixed tocopherols.

IMMUNE-SYSTEM SUPPORT

D O YOU FEEL THAT whenever a new strain of the flu comes around, you're the first to get it? The most effective way to avoid illness is to make sure you have a healthy immune system. After all, the only thing better than knowing how to treat illness is to prevent it from occurring in the first place!

WHAT IS IT?

Think of the immune system as the body's natural defense department, working tirelessly to fight off illness and protect your health. The immune system is composed of the white blood cells called neutrophils, granulocytes, monocytes, and lymphocytes, which spring into action whenever infection and illness threaten your health. When your immune system isn't "up to snuff," you just don't feel right, even though your symptoms may seem a bit vague. It's a feeling many people refer to as the "blahs." Signs that your immune system is not quite up to snuff include lethargy, a slow recovery time from illness, and frequent illness. Not only is it important to support your immune system on a regular basis, but when you do contract a cold, flu, or other illness, you can bolster your immune system in order to battle it.

Whether you want to protect your immune system because you are sick or you are trying to support your immune system in order to stay healthy, supplements and herbs can help arm this vital component of your body's natural defenses.

WHAT SHOULD I TAKE?

Astragalus • Cordyceps • Echinacea • Garlic
Ginseng • Glutamine • Goldenseal
Lactobacillus Acidophilus • Quercetin • Selenium
Spirulina • Vitamin C • Vitamin E • Zinc

Astragalus is a well-known herb derived from traditional Chinese medicine with modern potential in boosting the immune system. Studies have shown its specific ability to boost the function of the white blood cells known as T cells, which are important members of the immune system and destroy invading germs. (For more information on astragalus, see page 35.)

Tips for Boosting Immunity

Healthy Hints

People lead very full lives today, balancing work, family, and hobbies. Sometimes it may seem like there is hardly time to breathe! And with such hectic lifestyles, the immune system is often the first element of your health to suffer. Read on for some useful tips to help keep your immune system healthy:

■ **Say no to soda.** One 12-ounce bottle of soda contains 100 grams (about 24 teaspoons) of sugar! Consuming this much sugar can inhibit white blood cells' ability to kill germs, making the immune system up to 40 percent less effective in staving off viral infections and other diseases.

■ **Opt for water.** Hydration is a crucial element for healthy immunity. Drinking water will help the body to flush out toxins through sweat and urine.

■ **Cut out refined carbs.** Studies show that reducing the amount of refined carbohydrates in the diet —such as white rice, white bread, sugar cereal, and pasta or noodles made from white flower—can help improve the immune system.

■ **Walk it out.** Research shows that moderate daily exercise, such as walking for 20 to 30 minutes each day, will not only help you to lose weight, but may directly boost immune function by flushing carcinogens (cancer-causing cells) and bacteria from the body.

■ **Get your sleep.** Studies show that lack of adequate sleep (less than 8 hours a night) decreases immune responsiveness. Be sure to get a good night's rest each night to ward off infection.

Cordyceps—a Chinese medicinal mushroom—may strengthen the immune system by boosting levels of cells that help protect the body against infection and disease. (For more information on cordyceps, see page 88.)

Clinical studies indicate that **echinacea** may be successful in reducing the severity of flu-like symptoms. Studies also suggest that echinacea may fight fungal, viral, and bacterial infections—the three major types of infectious illness that your body can face. (For more information on echinacea, see page 107.)

Along with echinacea, add **garlic** to your supplement regimen. It's a natural antibiotic that may have the ability to get the immune system up and running. While a clove of good old-fashioned raw garlic is the best way to take garlic, capsules of deodorized garlic can be effective as well. (For more information on garlic, see page 135.)

In traditional Chinese medicine, **ginseng** has been used to prevent respiratory infections as well as colds and flu. Ginseng may work by helping the body to better adapt to stress, in addition to helping the liver remove toxins from the body. (For more information on ginseng, see page 141.)

Supplemenation with **glutamine**, the most abundant amino acid in the body, may benefit the immune system. Glutamine may feed immune cells, specifically in the stomach, which is the greatest user of glutamine in the body. In endurance athletes, a depletion of glutamine makes it harder for the body to recuperate between workouts, leaving the body susceptible to infection. (For more information on glutamine, see page 146.)

In traditional herbal medicine, **goldenseal** is often recommended along with echinacea. Preliminary animal studies show that supplementation with goldenseal may help boost the immune system, but the benefits disappeared after about 2 weeks of treatment. More research is needed to test goldenseal's effectiveness as an immune stimulator. (For more information on goldenseal, see page 151.)

Lactobacillus acidophilus may be helpful, especially for people experiencing an age-related decline in their immune system function. While research is preliminary, one study found that supplementation with acidophilus helped to improve immune function in elderly people. Acidophilus may also help prevent a number of ailments, including infectious diarrhea, urinary tract infection, and yeast infection. (For more information on Lactobacillus acidophilus, see page 180.)

Polyphenols such as **quercetin** are effective in strengthening the immune system and protecting body tissue from damage. Quercitin may have additional benefits by also working as an antihistamine. (For more information on quercetin, see page 236.)

While many studies show that **selenium** may effectively support immunity and reduce the risk of certain types of cancers, it may also play a role in boosting general immunity, especially when taken in conjunction with zinc (see page 304). Since many people have an inadequate intake of selenium, a selenium supplement may help support the immune system, especially during the cold and flu season. However, keep in mind that excessive amounts of selenium may actually impair the immune system. (For more information on selenium, see page 253.)

Spirulina contains many important nutrients, including all of the essential amino acids, vitamins, minerals, and essential fatty acids. Research conducted on human immune cells shows that spirulina may inhibit the growth of certain viruses, suggesting that this botanical supplement may have the potential for strengthening the immune system. (For more information on spirulina, see page 260.)

Vitamin C is an extremely popular and well-known immune booster. Vitamin C also protects against illness by preventing viruses from penetrating into cells. Clinical studies show that taking 1 gram of vitamin C daily during the cold and flu season can reduce the risk of catching a cold by almost 20 percent and can reduce the duration of illness by almost 40 percent. (For more information on vitamin C, see page 284.)

Some research suggests that **vitamin E** supplementation may help elderly people to maintain a healthy immune system. Studies indicate that intakes of 200 International Units per day of vitamin E are the ideal dosage, with lower or higher dosages lacking the same positive effect on the immune system. (For more information on vitamin E, see page 292.)

Zinc, found in many over-the-counter cold lozenges, is helpful in reducing the severity and duration of colds, especially when taken at the onset of symptoms. While its distinct taste may be hard for some people to tolerate, zinc, when taken with selenium (see page 246), may help bolster the immune system. Conversely, and much like selenium, high dosages of zinc can impair the immune system. (For more information on zinc, see page 304.)

MY SUPPLEMENT LIST—IMMUNE-SYSTEM SUPPORT

SUPPLEMENT	RECOMMENDED DOSAGE
Astragalus	*Capsule:* Take 400 mg of a standardized extract one to three times daily.
Cordyceps	*Capsule:* Take 4 to 15 g daily divided into three doses between meals.
Echinacea	*Capsule or Tablet:* Take 300 mg every 2 hours on the first day that you are sick, followed by 300 mg three times daily for 7 to 10 days. *Note:* Because of the various forms of echinacea readily available in the market, it is important to select a standardized product to ensure that you receive the proper dosage.
Garlic	*Fresh:* Eat 1 to 2 cloves of raw garlic daily. *Capsule:* Take 600 to 900 mg daily, divided into two or three doses, of a standardized extract that delivers about 5,000 to 6,000 mcg of allicin potential.
Ginseng	*Capsule:* Take 100–200 mg, three times per day—in the form of Asian ginseng—of a supplement standardized to contain approximately 4% to 7% ginsenosides.
Glutamine	*Capsule or Tablet:* Take 1.5 to 6 g daily divided into several doses (to be taken only if you have low muscle mass and difficulty fighting off infections).
Goldenseal	*Capsule:* Take 250 to 500 mg three times daily of an extract standardized to contain approximately 5% berberine or total alkaloids. *Note:* Do not use goldenseal for more than 3 consecutive weeks, and take a break of 2 weeks between each use, since its effectiveness may otherwise diminish.
Lactobacillus Acidophilus	*Capsule:* Take a supplement containing 1- to 2-billion colony-forming units (CFU) daily.
Quercetin	*Capsule:* Take 400 to 500 mg three times daily.
Selenium	*Tablet:* Take 100 to 200 mcg of selenium daily.
Spirulina	*Capsule:* Take 3 to 5 g daily, divided into three doses.
Vitamin C	*Capsule or Tablet:* Take 500 mg three times daily. *Note:* Be sure to use a buffered form of vitamin C. If taking vitamin C causes loose stools, decrease the dosage and then gradually increase the dosage as tolerated.
Vitamin E	*Capsule (Seniors):* Take 400 IU daily of a natural product containing mixed tocopherols.
Zinc	*Lozenge:* Take 13 to 23 mg of zinc in lozenge form every 2 to 3 hours, for up to 2 weeks, to reduce cold symptoms. Try choosing a sugar-free form of zinc, since sugar binds to zinc, reducing its effectiveness. *Note:* Dosages of zinc above 300 mg daily may impair the immune system.

INFERTILITY

ATTEMPTING TO CONCEIVE a baby can be an exciting venture in a couple's life. But having trouble conceiving can be frustrating, trying, and emotionally exhausting. Conception is a complex process, with many coincidences needed in order for it to be successful. There is a 24-hour period every month when a woman's egg is in just the right place for fertilization in the fallopian tube that leads sperm from the ovary to the uterus. Sperm are only viable for about 72 hours, and they must be present in the fallopian tube at the exact same time as the egg. Moreover, a single sperm must breach the surface of the egg within this period for fertilization to occur!

WHAT IS IT?

Infertility can occur in both men and women and is usually reflected by a failure to conceive during a year of unprotected sexual intercourse. The causes of infertility can be difficult to assess, and it can be equally difficult to discern whether male or female infertility is the problem in a couple's inability to conceive.

In men, inadequate quantity and quality of sperm is the chief cause of infertility. When men produce little or no sperm (conditions known as *oligospermia* and *azoosperimia*, respectively), infertility occurs. In other instances, infertility in men is caused when sperm become misshapen or do not successfully reach the egg before dying.

Acupuncture for Infertility

Did You Know?

Acupuncture—the ancient Chinese practice that uses very thin needles inserted into various points on the body to treat disorders—may offer help for both male and female infertility. By inserting needles at specific points, acupuncturists seek to unblock blocked energy and help the body's energy flow in a more healthy and balanced manner.

Several studies have been conducted to evaluate the efficacy of acupuncture in treating infertility in both men and women. One controlled study of 16 infertile men found that acupuncture increased their sperm counts. The men in the study received acupuncture twice a week for 5 weeks, and all experienced positive results.

Some promising research also supports a benefit from acupuncture for infertility in women, including three studies suggesting such a benefit. Studies dating back to 1976 suggest that acupuncture has an effect on female reproductive hormones. Other, more recent studies have found that acupuncture may induce ovulation as well as improve pregnancy outcomes after in vitro fertilization.

Consult your doctor to determine whether acupuncture may be an appropriate therapy for you to explore in case of infertility. To find a medical acupuncturist near you, contact the American Academy of Medical Acupuncture (http://www.medicalacupuncture.org/).

In rare cases, infertility is caused by a genetic disorder such as Parkinson's disease (see page 548) or a chromosomal abnormality. In women, a disorder of ovulation is the most common cause of infertility. Infertility in women may also occur when the fallopian tubes become blocked because of a condition such as endometriosis (see page 433) or a previous pelvic inflammatory disease.

Everything from stress and psychological issues to environmental issues and diet can play a role in both male and female infertility. Some specific inhibitors of fertility include alcohol and tobacco, a high caffeine intake, vitamin deficiencies, stress, and sexually transmitted diseases. It is important to keep in mind that conceiving a child takes time. However, if conception has not occurred after 1 year of unprotected intercourse, it may be time to talk to your family doctor. He or she can help you get to the heart of the problem and refer you to a specialist if necessary. In conjunction with the doctor's advice, supplements may help boost fertility in both men and women.

WHAT SHOULD I TAKE?

Women of child-bearing years should not use supplements, herbs, and greater than the RDA for any vitamin if they are not using birth control, unless they are not sexually active. The suggestions that follow are to be used prior to attempts at conception, not during. For more specific advice, consult with your doctor before taking any herbs or supplements as fertility aids.

Arginine • Chasteberry • Coenzyme Q10 (CoQ10)
Folic Acid • Ginseng • L-Carnitine
Red Clover • Selenium • Vitamin B$_{12}$
Vitamin C • Vitamin E • Zinc

Studies show that supplementation with the amino acid **arginine** may be helpful in promoting fertility in women who have had a history of failed attempts at conception via test-tube fertilization. It may also help with infertility. Some studies indicate that several months of arginine supplementation may increase sperm count and quality and fertility in men whose sperm count is 10 million per milliliter. (For more information on arginine, see page 31.)

Chasteberry could be the herbal answer to infertility in women. It balances levels of progesterone and estrogen, both of which are needed to facilitate conception. For this reason, chasteberry is often helpful to women who have recently stopped taking birth control pills, since female hormones are typically unbalanced at this time. (For more information on chasteberry, see page 69.)

Although the way in which **CoQ10** works in forming sperm is unknown, studies have shown increased sperm counts and sperm motility in men taking small dosages of CoQ10. Another study suggested a significant improvement in test-tube fertilization after CoQ10 supplementation. More research is needed to determine the effect of CoQ10 on infertility in men. (For more information on CoQ10, see page 80.)

Folic acid (vitamin B_9) prevents birth defects during pregnancy, but it is also a key player in helping men with infertility. Studies have shown that folic acid, when taken in combination with zinc (see page 304), can improve the sperm count as well as increase the overall percentage of healthy sperm. (For more information on folic acid, see page 130.)

Ginseng has a history of use in Chinese medicine to revive the male Qi (pronounced "chi"), a term used to describe the body's vital energy. A double-blind study of infertile men found that supplementation with 4 grams of ginseng daily for 3 months increased sperm counts and improved sperm motility. Animal studies have shown that ginseng helps improve sperm development and increases testosterone levels, which are a key factor in sperm production. (For more information on ginseng, see page 141.)

L-carnitine is necessary for the healthy function of sperm cells. Supplementation with L-carnitine may help promote the movement of sperm in men with low sperm quality. (For more information on L-carnitine, see page 186.)

Red clover may help balance estrogen levels in women, which makes it a good supplement to take in conjunction with chasteberry (see page 508). Using red clover with chasteberry can help to resolve seesawing variation between estrogen and progesterone levels in a woman's body. (For more information on red clover, see page 238.)

Selenium may increase sperm motility, although studies do not indicate that it has the ability to increase sperm count. In one double-blind, placebo controlled study, supplementation with selenium significantly improved sperm motility. (For more information on selenium, see page 253.)

Preliminary research indicates that injection or oral supplementation with **vitamin B_{12}** may help increase sperm count and sperm activity in men. (For more information on vitamin B_{12}, see page 282.)

Vitamin C seems to play a major role in improving sperm count and motility, and it reduces sperm clustering in men. Vitamin C may be especially helpful in improving the quality of sperm in men who smoke. (For more information on vitamin C, see page 284.)

Animal studies show that a deficiency in **vitamin E** may lead to infertility. One preliminary human study showed that infertile couples who were receiving vitamin E supplements had an increase in fertility. However, additional research is needed to determine the effectiveness of vitamin E for treating infertility. (For more information on vitamin E, see page 292.)

Zinc is another key mineral linked to sperm count and sperm motility in men. Studies have shown that zinc is most effective in fighting infertility when taken along with folic acid (see page 130). Other studies indicate that a deficiency in zinc may lead to a low sperm count and impotence, whereas still other research shows that a high concentration of zinc in sperm is related to decreased sperm movement and infertility in men. Consult your doctor in order to determine whether zinc supplementation is appropriate for you and what the proper dosage for your condition would be. (For more information on zinc, see page 304.)

MY SUPPLEMENT LIST—INFERTILITY

SUPPLEMENT	RECOMMENDED DOSAGE
L-Arginine	*Tablet (Female):* Studies have used 16 g of arginine daily to achieve positive results. *(Male):* Take up to 4 g daily for several months.
Chasteberry	*Capsule:* Take 175 to 225 mg daily of an extract standardized to contain 0.5% agnuside.
CoQ10	*Tablet:* Dosages range from 10 to 60 mg daily. Consult your doctor to determine an appropriate dosage for you.
Folic Acid	*Tablet:* Men should take 5 mg of folic acid daily, along with zinc (see next page).
Ginseng	*Capsule:* Studies using 4 g of Asian ginseng daily for 3 months have yielded positive results.
L-Carnitine	*Capsule:* In studies, dosages of 3 to 4 g daily for 4 months were effective in improving sperm motility in men.
Red Clover	*Capsule:* Take an extract standardized to provide 40 mg of isoflavones twice daily. Take red clover in conjunction with chasteberry (see above).

(continued)

MY SUPPLEMENT LIST—INFERTILITY (continued)	
SUPPLEMENT	**RECOMMENDED DOSAGE**
Selenium	*Tablet:* Studies have shown positive results with 100 mcg taken three times daily for 3 months.
Vitamin B$_{12}$	*Tablet:* Take 300–1,000 mcg daily. *Injection:* Discuss vitamin B$_{12}$ injections with your doctor to determine if this is the appropriate form of supplementation for you.
Vitamin C	*Capsule or Tablet:* Take 1,000 mg daily. *Note:* Be sure to use a buffered form of vitamin C. If taking vitamin C causes loose stools, decrease the dosage and then gradually increase the dosage as tolerated.
Vitamin E	*Capsule:* Both men and women should take 200–400 IU daily of a natural product containing mixed tocopherols.
Zinc	*Tablet:* Take 30 mg of zinc twice daily. *Note:* People taking zinc over the long term should also take 1–2 g of copper daily to prevent a copper deficiency.

INSOMNIA

EVERYONE EXPERIENCES AN occasional sleepless night, often caused by stress, too much caffeine, schedule changes, or illness. When it happens, you spend hours tossing and turning, thinking about how tired you'll be the next day and trying to will your body to sleep. And when trouble with sleeping occurs on a frequent basis, it can have a detrimental effect on your health and well-being and may be classified as a sleep disorder.

WHAT IS IT?

Insomnia is the inability to sleep at night. While a "good night's sleep" may last anywhere from 7^{1}/$_{2}$ to 10 hours a night, the constant inability to sleep can be a serious problem. Symptoms of insomnia include difficulty falling asleep, waking up in the middle of the night or too early in the morning, feeling tired even after a full night's sleep, and daytime irritability and fatigue. It is not surprising that insomnia is such a common problem in America. Although 8 hours of sleep every night are recommended, only about 35 percent of Americans meet that quota.

There are two main forms of insomnia: *primary* and *secondary*. Primary insomnia occurs when trouble with sleeping is not directly related to any other health condition or problem. Secondary insomnia is the result of a specific health condition, such as depression, heartburn, menopause, or arthritis; pain; medication; or consumption of a substance such as alcohol or caffeine. Insomnia can be a short-term problem, lasting from one night to a few weeks, and may come and go, or it may be a long-term or chronic problem. Chronic insomnia is categorized by the inability to sleep for 3 nights a week for a period of 1 month or longer. Smokers experience insomnia more frequently than do non-smokers.

There are many ways to fight back against insomnia. Getting healthy amounts of physical activity, managing stress, reducing caffeine intake, and creating a less hectic schedule can all help to prevent insomnia. Doctors may prescribe medication or recommend various behavioral therapies such as relaxation exercises, sleep restriction therapy, and reconditioning for chronic insomnia. In severe cases your doctor may refer you to a sleep clinic for more thorough evaluation. For additional support, herbs and supplements have a long history in helping people get the sleep they so urgently require.

Sleep-Promoting Tips

Healthy Hints Although insomnia is the most common sleep complaint, you can develop many habits that will help put an end to sleeplessness. Sometimes just altering your bedtime routine can help you get the rest you need. Try some of these hints and you may soon be dreaming!

■ **Take a bath.** Naturopathic doctors often recommend taking hot Epsom-salt baths for insomnia because they help relax muscles, thus promoting sleep. If you're having trouble sleeping, try soaking for 15 to 20 minutes in a hot bath containing one quart of Epsom salts to relax tense muscles. You can also add a few drops of lavender and lemon balm essential oils to the bath water.

■ **Curb your late-night appetite.** Eating late at night or eating heavy meals late in the day is a bad idea if you're having trouble sleeping. Having a light snack before bedtime, however, may help to promote sleep.

■ **Put worries to rest.** If you find yourself lying awake and worrying about things when you should be asleep, try writing a to-do list before bedtime. This will help you let go of your cares overnight, so that you may deal with them the next day after you have had a solid nights' sleep.

■ **Lay off…** Caffeine, nicotine, and alcohol can interfere with a good night's sleep. While caffeine and nicotine are stimulants that make it hard to fall asleep, alcohol can cause midnight waking and interfere with your sleep quality.

■ **Develop a routine.** Try to go to sleep at the same time every night and wake up at the same time each morning. Avoid naps during the day, since they will only make you less sleepy at night.

WHAT SHOULD I TAKE?

Chamomile • 5-Hydroxytryptophan (5-HTP)
Kava • Lavender • Lemon Balm
Magnesium • Melatonin • Schisandra • Valerian

Chamomile has been used traditionally as a sleep aid both in tea form and, when inhaled, as aromatherapy. Small studies suggest that chamomile has sleep-inducing properties, although larger studies are needed to confirm these findings. (For more information on chamomile, see page 67.)

Preliminary studies suggest that **5-HTP**, a substance that is converted in the body to serotonin—which is essential for transmitting signals within the nervous system—may help people with insomnia. One study indicated that people who were given supplements of 5-HTP had improved rapid eye movement (REM) during sleep, suggesting improved sleep quality. (For more information on 5-HTP, see page 123.)

Kava (also known as kava kava) is an herb well-known for its relaxing effects on the body and mind, and in clinical studies it has been shown quite effective for helping to produce a good night's sleep. Kava also works to reduce stress and anxiety, which makes it particularly good for stress-related insomnia. However, keep in mind that kava should not be taken in conjunction with anti-anxiety drugs (such as diazepam [Valium]), since this can severely depress the nervous system. (For more information on kava, see page 178.)

Lavender is recognized by the German Commission E (see page 16) for treating insomnia. Whether taken internally in the form of tea or inhaled as aromatherapy, lavender can be soothing and very helpful for treating sleeplessness. A trial involving elderly people suggested that lavender oil, when inhaled, was as effective as tranquilizers in promoting sleep. (For more information on lavender, see page 177.)

Among its other uses, **lemon balm** has been used traditionally for treating difficulty in sleeping. A small study found that a combination of lemon balm and valerian (see page 272) had similar effects to those of Halcion (triazolam), a popular prescription sleep-promoting medication. The German Commission E (see page 16) recommends lemon balm for treating sleeping disorders related to nervous states. (For more information on lemon balm, see page 190.)

Research indicates that **magnesium** may be a helpful sleep aid, especially in the elderly, who often experience changes in their sleeping patterns. Other studies indicate that stress of any sort, particularly the type that causes insomnia, may be a sign of magnesium deficiency. (For more information on magnesium, see page 203.)

Recent studies have shown **melatonin** to be effective in promoting sleep, increasing the number of sleeping hours, and boosting daytime alertness. Melatonin may be a welcome alternative to over-the-counter and prescription sleep medications, since it is inexpensive and non-habit forming. (For more information on melatonin, see page 208.)

Schisandra, an herb commonly used in Chinese medicine, has been prescribed traditionally for sleeping disorders including insomnia, dream-disturbed sleep, and night sweats. Recent studies have confirmed the effectiveness of schisandra's traditional uses, suggesting that this herb may help people with insomnia. (For more information on schisandra, see page 251.)

Valerian is the herbal superstar of sleep aids. Numerous studies have shown that its mildly sedative effects help people sleep longer, fall asleep earlier, and improve overall sleep quality. (For more information on valerian, see page 272.)

MY SUPPLEMENT LIST—INSOMNIA

SUPPLEMENT	RECOMMENDED DOSAGE
Chamomile	*Tea:* Combine 2 or 3 (heaping) tsp or teabags of fresh chamomile flower heads. Steep for 5 minutes and drink three times daily. *Inhalant:* Put 4 drops of chamomile essential oil in a bowl of steaming hot water. Cover your head with a towel and inhale the vapors deeply.
5-HTP	Consult your doctor to determine an appropriate dose of 5-HTP for you.
Kava	Consult your doctor before taking kava. Kava may cause liver damage when taken in high dosages. Kava may also enhance the effects of alcohol, antidepressant medications, and sedative medications.
Lavender	*Tea:* Steep 1 or 2 tsp or teabags of flowers in a cup of boiling water for 5–10 minutes. Drink as often as three times daily. *Inhalant:* Put 4 drops of lavender oil in a bowl of steaming hot water. Cover you head with a towel and inhale the vapors deeply. *Caution:* Do not ingest lavender oil.
Lemon Balm	*Tea:* Steep 1.5 to 4.5 g of lemon balm in 1 cup of boiling water for 10 to 15 minutes. Drink as needed. Valerian may be added to the mixture, although it is very bitter and often preferably consumed in capsule or tablet form.

(continued)

MY SUPPLEMENT LIST—INSOMNIA (CONTINUED)	
SUPPLEMENT	**RECOMMENDED DOSAGE**
Magnesium	*Tablet:* Take 400 mg twice daily. Or, try taking 800 mg before bed. *Note:* Take in the form of magnesium glycinate to avoid loose stools. Large amounts of magnesium can cause diarrhea; if this becomes a problem for you, reduce your dosage.
Melatonin	*Tablet:* Take one 1 to 10 mg before bedtime to promote sleep. Discontinue use after 2 weeks if there is no marked improvement in sleep patterns.
Schisandra	*Capsule:* Take 400 to 450 mg three times daily.
Valerian	*Capsule or Tablet:* Take 300 to 500 mg of an extract standardized to contain at least 0.5% volatile oils, 1 hour before bedtime. You can also try valerian tincture, 1–2 tsp before bed. Beware that it may aggravate gastroesophageal reflux disease (GERD). *Note:* The strength of valerian products may vary greatly. Be sure to choose a standardized product and carefully follow the instructions on the label.

IRRITABLE BOWEL SYNDROME

BLOATING, CONSTIPATION, cramps, diarrhea, and gas. Many people with irritable bowel syndrome (IBS) are all-too-familiar with these symptoms. IBS occurs so frequently that it is surpassed only by the common cold as a cause for lost work time. IBS is also responsible for 3 million physician visits in the United States every year. That's 12 percent of all visits to primary-care physicians, surpassing the percentages of visits for high blood pressure, asthma, and coronary artery disease.

WHAT IS IT?

IBS was once thought to be psychological condition rather than a physical problem. Although experts still don't know exactly what causes IBS, they do know that it occurs when the muscles in the intestines do not function properly. In the case of IBS, muscles can contract too quickly, causing food to pass through the intestines at an accelerated rate, which leads to cramping, bloating, gas, and diarrhea. At other times, food is passed through the intestines too slowly, and the stool becomes hard and dry from loss of water, resulting in constipation. As a result, IBS is often marked by alternating periods of diarrhea and constipation. People with IBS have an increased sensitivity to certain "trigger" factors such as stress, certain types of foods and medications, or emotional turmoil. However, while stress may aggravate symptoms of IBS, it does not cause them. On a positive note, IBS is not a life-threatening condition, and it does not increase your risk of intestinal cancer or other serious gastrointestinal conditions.

Symptoms of IBS can be managed through appropriate relief of stress, adding fiber to the diet, eating regular meals, and drinking plenty of fluids. Some people find that eliminating sugar, wheat, and dairy products is all it takes to relieve their symptoms of IBS. In addition, supplements may help to cut out cramps and constipation, ditch diarrhea, and beat bloating.

WHAT SHOULD I TAKE?
Chamomile • Digestive Enzymes • Fiber • Flaxseed
Lactobacillus Acidophilus • Peppermint

Chamomile is an herb traditionally used to provide soothing relief to irritated digestive tracts. Furthermore, chamomile may relieve cramping and irritation in the intestines, a common malady in IBS. This herb may be especially useful for people with IBS accompanied by alternating bouts of constipation and diarrhea. (For more information on chamomile, see page 67.)

Digestive enzymes may reduce the bloating, gas, and feeling of fullness that can follow a high-fat meal. Taking digestive enzymes helps to support healthy digestion, potentially reducing symptoms of IBS. (For more information on digestive enzymes, see page 102.)

Ground **flaxseed** is a good source of **fiber**, helping to regulate the digestive tract and aid in healthy digestion. In a small study involving 55 people with constipation caused by chronic IBS, those who took flaxseed every day for 3 months had reduced abdominal pain, bloating, and constipation. (For more information on flaxseed and fiber, see pages 126 and 120.)

Lactobacillus acidophilus, a beneficial species of bacteria naturally found in the intestines, has shown positive effects in IBS. In multiple studies, acidophilus' greatest attributes were in reducing gas and relieving pain. (For more information on Lactobacillus acidophilus, see page 180.)

While more study is necessary, **peppermint**, when taken in capsule form, may be quite beneficial in relieving symptoms of IBS if taken immediately after meals. Peppermint oil may relieve symptoms including abdominal pain, distention, frequency of bathroom visits, and flatulence. (For more information on peppermint, see page 226.)

DIETARY DO'S AND DON'TS

Do. Eat foods high in fiber such as bran, whole-grain bread, cereal, fruits, and vegetables. Remember that it is important to add fiber-rich foods to your diet slowly: Begin with 20 to 30 grams per day, since eating too much fiber at once may cause gas and trigger other symptoms of IBS. If you have IBS, try eating four or five small meals a day because eating larger meals can often cause cramping and diarrhea. Drink a minimum of 8 glasses of water a day to keep fiber-rich foods from causing constipation.

Don't. Do not eat processed foods and beverages high in food additives, fats, or sugar such as snack chips and sodas. Avoid foods high in saturated fat such as fried food and milk products such as cheese, butter, and red meat. Also, steer clear of caffeine, alcohol, and chocolate, which may irritate the digestive organs.

MY SUPPLEMENT LIST—IRRITABLE BOWEL SYNDROME

SUPPLEMENT	RECOMMENDED DOSAGE
Chamomile	*Tea:* Make a tea by combining 2 or 3 g of fresh herb with 1 cup of water. Steep for 10 minutes. Drink up to three times daily. If preparing tea with a teabag, you may drink up to four cups daily.
Digestive Enzymes	*Tablet:* Take a product that 3 to 4 g of "4X pancreatin," which contains 100 mg of amilase, lipase, and protease, with meals.
Fiber	*Capsule:* Take 3.25 g of fiber in the form of psyllium seed husk three times daily. *Powder:* Mix one-half to 2 tsp of a psyllium supplement in 1 cup of water, stir, and drink. If you are just starting to take psyllium, consider using a low dosage at first and then gradually increasing it. Alternately, you can stir 1 to 3 tbsp of bulk ground flaxseed in 5 to 15 oz of water and drink this preparation daily as necessary. *Note:* Be sure to drink plenty of water when taking psyllium.
Flaxseed	*Ground:* Take 1 or 2 tbsp daily.
Lactobacillus Acidophilus	*Capsule:* Choose a well-regarded supplement that provides 3 to 5 billion live organisms daily.
Melatonin	Take 3 mg at night.
Peppermint	*Capsule:* Take 1 or 2 capsules that supply 0.2 to 0.4 ml of peppermint oil three times a day after meals. *Note:* Peppermint oil capsules should be enteric-coated to prevent them from causing stomach distress. Do not take undiluted peppermint oil, since it may be irritating to the esophagus.

KIDNEY STONES

IN MUMMIES MORE than 7,000 years old, researchers have found evidence of small, crystallized minerals on the inner surface of the kidneys—kidney stones. This bit of historical insight shows just how long this common and excruciatingly painful condition has been a part of the human state.

WHAT IS IT?

Passing a kidney stone is a painful experience that you are not likely to forget. Ten percent of people will have a kidney stone at some point in their lives, and the number is steadily increasing. Men tend to develop kidney stones more often than women.

The formation of a stone begins in the bean-shaped kidneys—which are located toward the back on either side of the body—when calcium, oxalate, uric acid, and cystine collect and from hard deposits in these organs. Normally, these substances remain in a dissolved state in the fluid that is filtered through the kidneys, but when the balance that keeps them in a dissolved state is disrupted—usually as a result of dietary factors—these elements begin to crystallize, forming the hard deposit or "stone." An excess of calcium is usually the culprit.

Once a kidney stone forms, it begins to move around in the kidneys. The result is pain in the back and side that persists for as long as the stone continues to move. The pain may extend toward the groin area as the stone heads for the ureter (the tube that transports urine from the kidney to the bladder), and if the stone "passes" out of the ureter and into the bladder, the pain can be tremendous. Symptoms include bloody or foul-smelling urine, nausea and vomiting, and a more persistent urge to urinate.

Diet and Kidney Stones

Healthy Hints
There are many ways to reduce your chances of developing kidney stones through changes in diet. However, when it comes to warding off kidney stones, fluids are the key. Make sure to drink plenty of water and stay well hydrated to keep stones from forming.

■ **Stay hydrated.** A high fluid intake has been shown to prevent kidney stones as well as keeping stones from recurring. Be sure to compensate for fluid loss in hot weather or after periods of heavy exercise or sweating. Use caution, however, when drinking mineral water—if it has a high calcium content it may actually cause kidney stones.

■ **Don't overeat meat.** Diets with a high meat and protein content are often associated with kidney stones. Eating protein increases the quantities of uric acid, calcium, and oxalates in the urine and reduces the content of citrate. Keep in mind that meat protein generates more acid in the body than vegetable protein.

■ **Be salt-free.** High levels of salt intake can increase the amount of calcium in urine, which may lead to the development of kidney stones. A high sodium intake also increases the uric acid content of urine. Whenever possible, avoid using too much salt.

■ **Say no to soda.** A 3-year study showed that men with one kidney stone who drank at least 1.1 liters per week of soda were less likely to develop another stone when they reduced their consumption of soda.

■ **Avoid oxalates.** People with calcium oxalate kidney stones should steer clear of certain foods that contain oxalates. Foods that are infamous for increasing the urinary oxalate content include spinach and other green, leafy vegetables, rhubarb, beets, chocolate, peanuts, tea, wheat bran, and almonds. Boiling the foods first will greatly decrease the soluable oxalates in food.

■ **Eat seeds.** Two trials from Thailand found that eating pumpkin seeds—in amounts less than a handful of seeds—may help reduce the urinary risk factors of forming kidney stones. Although more research is needed, eating a handful of pumpkin seeds daily can't hurt.

Most kidney stones can be prevented by drinking adequate amounts of water. A diet with low salt and a low content of animal protein may also help. Although it was once believed that high intakes of vitamin C caused kidney stones, recent research shows that there is no justification for this claim.

WHAT SHOULD I TAKE?
Magnesium • Potassium • Vitamin B$_6$

Magnesium may break down the components of a kidney stone, including calcium oxalate and calcium phosphate, which are the main components of 75 to 80 percent of all kidney stones. Population-based studies show that in areas where the drinking water has a high magnesium content there is a lower incidence of kidney stones. (For more information on magnesium, see page 203.)

Potassium may play a role in preventing stones formed from uric acid. However, using potassium to prevent calcium-based kidney stones rather than uric acid–based kidney stones should be done only under the supervision of a doctor. (For more information on potassium, see page 233.)

Vitamin B$_6$, when taken at levels that exceed the normal upper limit, may help break down oxalic acid, a component of many kidney stones. A study involving 85,000 women with no history of kidney stones showed that those with a higher intake of vitamin B$_6$ had a reduced risk of developing kidney stones. More research is needed to determine the effect of vitamin B$_6$ on kidney stones. (For more information on vitamin B$_6$, see page 279.)

MY SUPPLEMENT LIST—KIDNEY STONES

SUPPLEMENT	RECOMMENDED DOSAGE
Magnesium	*Tablet:* Take 200 to 400 mg daily in the form of magnesium citrate with meals. Take a lower dose if you experience diarrhea or loose stools.
Potassium	Consult your doctor about increasing your potassium intake through diet and/or with supplements in order to prevent kidney stones. Most research involving potassium supplementation and kidney stones use the mineral in the form of potassium citrate.
Vitamin B$_6$	*Tablet:* Studies have used high dosages of vitamin B$_6$ to prevent kidney stones. Consult your doctor about determining your own proper dosage of vitamin B$_6$ for preventing kidney stones. *Note:* If you have liver disease, consult your doctor before taking more than 50 mg of vitamin B$_6$ daily.

MACULAR DEGENERATION

MY EYES AREN'T WHAT they used to be" is a phrase you've probably heard a parent, grandparent, or older friend say many times. For most people, a decline in eyesight is a natural accompaniment to the aging process. In some other cases, however, a change in vision with aging may result from a condition known as macular degeneration.

WHAT IS IT?

As we age, our eyes tend to age with us and the result can be an eye disease that gradually robs us of our vision. Macular degeneration commonly affects older Americans and is the leading cause of blindness in millions of people age 55 and over. About one-fourth of Americans over age 65 show signs of macular degeneration, and for those over 80, the proportion rises to one of every three people.

This gradual loss of vision in macular degeneration is caused by the breakdown of the macula, the central portion of the retina, which is the part of the eye upon which images are formed. As the macula breaks down, the central field of vision is first blurred and then lost, with loss of all ability to see detail and color. Macular degeneration is a stealthy disease, since it evolves so slowly that there is never an abrupt loss of vision. It is also painless, making the victim oblivious to its onset. Environmental, nutritional, and medical factors all play a role in the progression of macular degeneration; cigarette smoke, sun exposure, high blood pressure, diabetes, and heart disease can all speed the progression of this condition.

The best way to prevent the onset of macular degeneration is to have regular eye examinations, adhere to healthy lifestyle choices, and use the following supplements.

WHAT SHOULD I TAKE?

Bilberry • Carnitine • Coenzyme Q10 • Ginkgo Biloba (Ginkgo)
Grape Seed Extract • Lutein • Lycopene • Selenium
Omega-3 fatty acids • Vitamin C • Vitamin E • Zinc

Research indicates that people with low antioxidant levels sustain more damage to their eyes from free radicals. Therefore, **bilberry** may be useful for macular degeneration. (For more information on bilberry, see page 44.)

Carnitine, in the form of acetyl-n-carnitine, when taken in combination with **coenzyme Q10** and **omega-3 fatty acids**,

CALL YOUR DOCTOR WHEN...

While our vision tends to become less sharp as we age, some visual symptoms are not a natural part of aging, but rather a sign that something more serious is occurring. Macular degeneration develops slowly and the symptoms may be subtle, but it is preceded by specific warning signs of which you should be aware as you age. Be sure to call your doctor if:

- You notice that you need brighter light when reading
- Printed words appear increasingly blurry when you read
- Colors appear washed out and dull
- A blind spot or blurry spot occurs in the center of your visual field
- You notice visual distortions, such as a straight line appearing crooked or blurry

was found to be useful in the treatment of macular degeneration in a recent medical study. (For more information on this, see page 186.)

Studies indicate that **ginkgo** may halt and lessen some retinal problems, even after they have begun to occur. Experts have attributed ginkgo's abilities to help vision problems to its high levels of flavonoids. (For more information on ginkgo, see page 138.)

Grape seed extract, like ginkgo, is also bursting with flavonoids, and clinical studies have indicated its ability to retard vision loss and improve visual sharpness. (For more information on grape seed extract, see page 155.)

Lutein and **lycopene** are both antioxidants that may have protective effects against macular degeneration. Lutein is found naturally in the part of the retina where macular degeneration occurs. Studies suggest that lutein-containing supplements may help protect eyes from damage caused by the sun, as well as prevent age-related macular degeneration. Lycopene—a red pigment found only in plant sources—may also have protective effects against age-related macular degeneration. Lutein may be found in high levels in spinach, kale, and collard greens; lycopene can be found in many red- or pink-colored foods, including tomatoes, guava, pink grapefruit, and watermelon. (For more information on lutein and lycopene, see pages 195 and 197.)

Selenium and **zinc** are both vital minerals that gradually decrease in the body with age. By maintaining the levels of these minerals through supplementation, you can strengthen your immune system and possibly prevent the progress of macular degeneration and other vision problems. (For more information on selenium and zinc, see pages 253 and 304.)

Vitamin C is another tried-and-true antioxidant to add to the list of supplements for preventing macular degeneration. Studies have shown that taking a single antioxidant by itself does little to reverse or prevent health problems, but by combining antioxidants you can do a lot to protect your vision. (For more information on vitamin C, see page 284.)

Vitamin E was the subject of a recent vision-related study in France. In a study of 2,584 adults age 60 and older, those with high levels of vitamin E were 82 percent less likely to experience the later stages of macular degeneration than those with low levels of vitamin E. This provides some evidence that vitamin E might help protect vision. (For more information on vitamin E, see page 292.)

MY SUPPLEMENT LIST—MACULAR DEGENERATION

SUPPLEMENT	RECOMMENDED DOSAGE
Bilberry	*Capsule or Tablet:* Take 240 to 1,800 mg once a day of an extract standardized to contain 25% anthocyanosides divided into one to three doses.
L-Carnitine	*Acetyl-n-carntine:* Take 500–1,000 mg twice daily, with meals. It may work best when taken together with coenzyme Q10 and omega-3 fatty acids.
Coenzyme Q10	Take 120 mg once daily, with food.
Ginkgo	*Capsule or Tablet:* Take 120 to 240 mg once daily of an extract standardized to contain 24% ginkgo flavone glycosides and 6% terpene lactones divided into two or three doses.
Grape Seed Extract	*Capsule:* Take 150 to 300 mg daily divided into two or three doses.
Lutein	*Capsule:* Take 20 mg one or two times daily with a fatty meal for optimal absorption.
Lycopene	*Diet:* Eat five or more servings of foods containing processed tomatoes, such as tomato sauce or juice, or cooked tomatoes each week. Cooked tomatoes appear to be more effective than raw ones for providing lycopene. *Capsule:* The ideal dose of lycopene is unknown. Studies have used dosages of 4 to 6.5 mg daily with positive results.
Omega-3 Fatty Acids	Take 1–2 g of omega-3 fatty acids per day, in divided doses, with meals. The amount of omega-3 fatty acid will vary by manufacturer, so be sure to check the product label carefully.
Selenium	*Tablet:* Take 200 to 500 mcg daily.
Vitamin C	*Capsule or Tablet:* Take 500 to 1,000 mg daily in 1 or 2 divided doses. *Note:* Be sure to use a buffered form of vitamin C. If taking vitamin C causes loose stools, decrease the dosage and then gradually increase the dosage as tolerated.
Vitamin E	*Capsule:* Take 400 IU daily.
Zinc	*Tablet:* Take 30 to 50 mg daily. *Note:* When taking zinc at high dosages for more than a 1-month period, add a 1- to 3-mg supplement of copper daily. A dosage higher than 30 mg may cause nausea.

MENOPAUSE

MENOPAUSE IS NOT A DISEASE. Although it was once believed to be an estrogen-deficiency disorder, menopause is now recognized as a natural process and not an abnormal occurrence. Yet, despite this, menopause has a stigma surrounding it. One reason for this is the unpleasant symptoms it brings, most notably irritability and the infamous "hot flashes." Another is that for some women, menopause is synonymous with old age, signifying a major passage in life. However, much like puberty, menopause simply marks the beginning of a new stage of life.

WHAT IS IT?

As women get older, estrogen and progesterone levels in their bodies diminish, causing various changes to occur, especially in the menstrual cycle. Because of these hormonal changes, the monthly cycle of ovulation becomes less regulated, and eggs have a decreased chance of being fertilized. Over the course of time, the menstrual cycle stops completely, and with it the possibility of becoming pregnant. Menopause is defined as a 12-month period of amenorrhea after the final menstrual period.

The most common side effects of menopause are hot flashes and night sweats (also known as vasomotor symptoms), which can begin from 1 to 1^1/$_2$ years before the onset of menopause. Hot flashes are uncomfortable waves of heat that can occur at any time and may be joined by other symptoms such as insomnia, nausea, and anxiety. In addition to hot flashes, menopausal women will often experience vaginal dryness and itching, as well as urinary changes and a decrease in libido. Mood changes, and even depression, are not uncommon symptoms of menopause. Weight gain may also be a problem, or the weight distribution of weight around the body can shift. Additionally, over time, low levels of estrogen bring other health problems such as osteoporosis (see page 551), heart disease (see page 470), and macular degeneration (see page 525).

Among the keys to a healthy menopause are a good attitude, plenty of exercise (shown to be beneficial in menopause in a number of studies), and a healthy diet. A number of herbs and supplements that may also help ease menopausal symptoms.

WHAT SHOULD I TAKE?
Black Cohosh • Calcium • Chasteberry
Dong Quai • Kava • Magnesium
Red Clover • St. John's Wort

Black cohosh is the most well-known, well-studied, and perhaps the most effective herb for treating the symptoms associated with menopause. Studies indicate that it may reduce symptoms including hot flashes, vaginal dryness, irritability, mood swings, and depression and may even prevent osteoporosis. However, black cohosh should not be confused with blue cohosh, another herb, that is potentially more toxic and dangerous than black cohosh. (For more information on black cohosh, see page 48.)

Calcium is vital in maintaining bone mass and strength as women age (see also Osteoporosis, page 551). During menopause, when estrogen levels decline, women have a greater risk for developing osteoporosis. Taking a daily calcium supplement can act as bone insurance against this condition. Be sure to take a magnesium supplement along with calcium to maximize the absorption of calcium. (For more information on calcium, see page 57.)

Preliminary studies indicate that **chasteberry** may reduce menopausal symptoms, although more research is needed to confirm this suggestion. (For more information on chasteberry, see page 69.)

Traditionally, **dong quai** is believed to have estrogen-like properties, and therefore may be useful in treating symptoms of menopause. However, more scientific research is needed to confirm this theory. (For more information on dong quai, see page 105.)

Kava (also called kava kava) may help to reduce the anxiety often associated with menopause. One study of 40 women with menopause found that kava reduced its psychological symptoms (including anxiety and depression) without diminishing the effect of hormone replacement therapy on diseases such as osteoporosis and heart disease. (For more information on kava, see page 178.)

The Scoop on Soy

Still in Debate

Years ago researchers thought that the plant estrogens (known as phytoestrogens) in soy-based foods could eliminate or ease symptoms associated with menopause. These phytoestrogens belong to a group of substances known as isoflavones, and supplementation with soy isoflavones in high doses became common practice among menopausal women.

Recently, however, studies—albeit incomplete—have shown a link between isoflavones and an increased risk of breast and uterine cancer. What is puzzling, however, is that some studies have shown an increased risk of such cancers with isoflavone supplementation while other studies have shown a decreased risk of such cancers with the same supplementation.

Because of this controversy, the current recommendation of the North American Menopause Society is to consume your isoflavones in soy rather than through supplementation. Tempeh and miso are two forms of soy most easily digested in the body.

Magnesium helps the body absorb calcium and should therefore be taken together with calcium (see previous page). Also, because magnesium levels appear to drop along with estrogen levels during menopause, supplemental magnesium may help alleviate menopausal symptoms such as hot flashes. (For more information on magnesium, see page 203.)

Although more research is needed to test the effectiveness of **red clover** in treating menopause, some research suggests that the herb may benefit the function of arteries, making it a useful supplement for women whose menopause is associated with high blood pressure. Other studies indicate that red clover may also reduce hot flashes, although the results for this are mixed. (For more information on red clover, see page 238.)

Short-term supplementation with **St. John's wort** may be helpful in treating mild or moderate depression as well as assisting sexual well-being during menopause. (For more information on St. John's wort, see page 262.)

MY SUPPLEMENT LIST—MENOPAUSE

SUPPLEMENT	RECOMMENDED DOSAGE
Black Cohosh	*Capsule:* Take 20 to 40 mg twice daily of an extract standardized to contain 1 mg of 27-deoxyactein for every 20 mg of product.
Calcium	*Capsule or Tablet:* Take 1,200 mg of a calcium citrate daily divided into two or three doses. Postmenopausal women should take 1,500 mg of calcium daily divided into three doses if they are not receiving estrogen therapy. Women who are receiving estrogen therapy should take 1,000 mg daily divided into two doses.
Chasteberry	*Capsule:* Take 175 to 225 mg daily of an extract standardized to contain 0.5% agnuside. *Note:* The dosages of chasteberry products may vary widely. Be sure to read individual product labels for dosage information.
Dong Quai	The optimal dosage of dong quai varies. Consult your doctor or herbalist to determine an appropriate dose for you. It is typically taken together with other herbs.
Kava	*Capsule:* Studies of 100 mg of kava extract, standardized to contain 70% kavalactones and taken three times daily, yielded positive results for easing menopausal symptoms. *Note:* Consult your doctor before taking kava. Kava may cause liver damage when taken in high dosages. Kava may also enhance the effects of alcohol, antidepressant medications, and sedative medications.

SUPPLEMENT	RECOMMENDED DOSAGE
MY SUPPLEMENT LIST—MENOPAUSE	
Magnesium	*Tablet:* Be sure to take magnesium in a 1:2 ratio with calcium. For example, if you are taking 600 mg of magnesium, take it with 1,200 mg of calcium. *Note:* Take magnesium in the form of magnesium glycinate to avoid loose stools. Large amounts of magnesium can cause diarrhea; if this becomes a problem for you, reduce your dosage.
Red Clover	*Tea:* Mix 10 to 15 g with 1 cup of boiling water. Steep for 10 to 15 minutes and drink up to three cups daily. *Capsule or Tablet:* Take an extract standardized to contain 40 mg of isoflavones twice daily.
St. John's Wort	*Capsule:* Take 300 mg of a product standardized to .03% hypericin three times a day.

MENSTRUAL PROBLEMS

WHILE MENSTRUATION MAY not be the highlight of the month for most women, regular menstruation is usually an important sign that a woman's body is in good health. Menstrual cycles vary from one woman to another in the degree of menstrual flow and whether or not menstruation is accompanied by symptoms such as cramps and bloating. However, heavy bleeding can sometimes be problematic, especially when it occurs on a frequent basis.

WHAT IS IT?

Two dysfunctions can occur in the menstrual cycle: *menorrhagia* and *dysmenorrhea.* Almost no woman is immune to either condition, and the chances are that sooner or later every woman will experience both. Some women, however, experience these conditions more often than others.

Menorrhagia is characterized by a heavy, steady menstrual blood flow that quickly soaks through sanitary pads and tampons. Menorrhagic periods may last longer than the typical 7 days and may include blood clotting as well. Often, these heavy periods can interfere with day-to-day activities and result in anemia from blood loss, which in turn can cause fatigue or shortness of breath. A number of factors—from hormonal imbalance to medication—can cause heavy bleeding, while in other cases the cause is unknown.

Heavy bleeding itself can lead to dysmenorrhea. *Primary dysmenorrhea* (dysmennorhea that occurs without another underlying health problem) is characterized by menstrual cramping and pain. This condition is typified by throbbing pain in the lower abdomen, which sometimes also affects the back or thighs. In some cases, vomiting, sweating, or dizziness can occur. Most women probably experience primary dysmenorrhea at one point or another. *Secondary dysmenorrhea* is defined as dysmenorrhea resulting from another disease such as endometriosis, pelvic inflammatory disease, or polyps. Alleviation of secondary dysmenorrhea may require treatment of the underlying disease.

The discomfort and bleeding associated with menorrhagia and dymenorrhea can be helped with the use of herbs and supplements. Dietary changes—such as avoiding red meat, poultry, and whole milk—along with the use of herbal and other supplements, may ease menstrual symptoms.

WHAT SHOULD I TAKE?

Women of child-bearing years should not use supplements, herbs, and greater than the RDA for any vitamin if they are not using birth control, unless they are not sexually active.

Black Cohosh • Bromelain • Calcium • Chamomile
Chasteberry • Iron • Magnesium • Niacin
Omega-3 Fatty Acids • Vitamin E • Willow Bark

Black cohosh has been used historically to provide relief from menstrual cramps. This herb is approved by the German Commission E (see page 16) for the treatment of premenstrual discomfort and dysmenorrhea. (For more information on black cohosh, see page 48.)

Bromelain may be helpful for decreasing spasms in the cervix in dysmenorrhea. Some experts believe bromelain exerts this effect by relaxing muscles in the uterus, thus decreasing cramping. (For more information on bromelain, see page 54.)

The benefit of **calcium** for menstrual cramps is theoretical. Calcium is known to maintain muscle tone. In people who are calcium deficient, muscles may have a tendency to cramp more easily. The use of calcium to prevent menstrual cramps is based on some studies indicating that using calcium may help reduce the pain associated with dysmenorrhea. (For more information on calcium, see page 57.)

Chamomile is a mild herb with analgesic properties. A recent study found that chamomile elevated glycine levels in the body. Since glycine is a chemical that relieves muscle spasms and can act as a nerve relaxant, this may serve to relax the uterus, which explains why the tea appears to relieve menstrual cramps. (For more information on chamomile, see page 67.)

Chasteberry may be useful in balancing a woman's hormonal system and easing painful menstruation. However, it is unlikely to provide immediate relief from menstrual symptoms and may take a few months to exert its effects. (For more information on chasteberry, see page 69.)

A frequent side effect of heavy menstrual bleeding is anemia, which is characterized by fatigue, dizziness, and weakness. Taking a daily **iron** supplement can help reduce these symptoms. However, iron should be taken only by women who are at risk for or who have a deficiency of iron. Consult your doctor to determine if iron supplements are appropriate for you. (For more information on iron, see page 175.)

Besides helping the body to absorb calcium, **magnesium** may help reduce menstrual pain associated with dysmenorrhea. Studies show that supplementation with magnesium helps to temper symptoms associated with magnesium deficiency, possibly by promoting muscle relaxation, which may in turn decrease menstrual cramps. (For more information on magnesium, see page 203.)

Niacin may be effective in tempering the pain of dysmenorrhea. A preliminary study of 200 women with painful menstruation found that supplementation with 200 milligrams of niacin daily was effective in alleviating pain in 87 percent of the group. More research is needed to study the effectiveness of niacin in alleviating dysmenorreah, but the results so far look promising. (For more information on niacin, see page 219.)

Irregular Periods May Be a Red Flag for Osteoporosis

Did You Know?

Skipped or erratic menstrual periods are common in young women. However, according to a preliminary study conducted by researchers at the National Institute of Child Health and Human Development (NICHHD), irregular menstrual periods may signal a shortage of hormones that can lead to osteoporosis later in life. The study involved women diagnosed with a condition known as premature ovarian failure, which occurs when the ovaries stop producing eggs and reproductive hormones well before natural menopause.

Most of the women with this condition reported that they had a history of amenorrhea—the absence of menstrual periods. Of the 89 study participants, 67 percent had developed osteopenia, a state of low-bone density that is a precursor to osteoporosis. Many of the women in the NICHHD study said that they didn't consider an absence of periods to be cause for concern.

Although further research is necessary, a skipped menstrual period should never be taken lightly. It is important to speak with your doctor to determine the cause of your missed periods and to ensure that your health is not at risk.

Women who do not have an adequate intake of **omega-3 fatty acids** may be more prone to menstrual pain. Studies indicate that supplementation with fish oil—a good source of omega-3 fatty acids—may help reduce painful menstruation. (For more information on omega-3 fatty acids, see page 221.)

Vitamin E has anti-inflammatory properties, and in one study was equal to ibuprofen in relieving the pain associated with menstruation. Because of its anti-clotting properties, however, vitamin E is not recommended if heavy bleeding is a problem. (For more information on vitamin E, see page 292.)

Studies show that **willow bark**, which is both an anti-inflammatory and a painkiller, may have effects comparable to those of aspirin in relieving pain and cramping. However, although the effects of willow bark last longer than those of aspirin, it may take longer to begin working. (For more information on willow bark, see page 298.)

MY SUPPLEMENT LIST—MENSTRUAL PROBLEMS

SUPPLEMENT	RECOMMENDED DOSAGE
Black Cohosh	*Capsule:* Take 20 to 40 mg twice daily of an extract standardized to contain 1 mg of 27-deoxyactein for every 20 mg of product.
Bromelain	*Tablet:* Take 300 to 600 mg three times daily between meals. Look for a product containing 2,400 gelatin-dissolving units (GDU) or 3,600 milk-clotting units (MCU) per gram.
Calcium	*Capsule or Tablet:* Some experts recommend taking 1,000 mg of calcium daily and 250 to 500 mg every 4 hours during painful cramping to a maximum of 2,000 mg a day. *Note:* Calcium is better absorbed when taken with a magnesium supplement. Be sure to take calcium with magnesium in a 2:1 ratio. For example, take 1,000 mg of calcium with 500 mg of magnesium.
Chamomile	*Tea:* Prepare a chamomile tea by adding from 3–10 g of fresh flowers to 1 cup of boiling water. Steep for 5–10 minutes and drink up to three times daily.
Chasteberry	*Capsule:* Take 175–225 mg per day of a extract standardized to 0.5% anguside, in divided doses. *Note:* Chasteberry should not be used by pregnant women or women who are using oral contraceptives. It may take 3 months in order to experience chasteberry's therapeutic effects.
Iron	*Tablet:* General dosage recommendations for iron range from 100 to 200 mg daily. *Note:* Consult your doctor before taking iron supplements.

MY SUPPLEMENT LIST—MENSTRUAL PROBLEMS	
SUPPLEMENT	**RECOMMENDED DOSAGE**
Magnesium	*Tablet:* Take 500 to 1,000 mg daily, beginning on day 15 of the menstrual cycle. Continue until menstruation begins.
	Note: Take magnesium in the form of magnesium glycinate to avoid loose stools. Large amounts of magnesium can cause diarrhea; if this becomes a problem for you, reduce your dosage.
Niacin	*Tablet:* Take 200 mg of niacin throughout the menstrual cyle. During menstruation, take niacin every 2 to 3 hours when you experience menstrual cramps.
	Note: Niacin may not be effective unless taken for about 1 week before menstruation.
Omega-3 Fatty Acids	Take 1–2 g of omega-3 fatty acids per day, in divided doses, with meals. The amount of omega-3 fatty acid will vary by manufacturer, so be sure to check the product label carefully.
Vitamin E	*Capsule:* Take 400 IU daily of a natural product containing mixed tocopherols.
Willow Bark	*Capsule:* Take an extract standardized to contain 60 to 240 mg of salicin daily.
	Caution: Avoid willow bark if you have an aspirin allergy, bleeding disorder, diabetes, or a peptic ulcer.

MIGRAINE HEADACHES

FOR 26 MILLION Americans, the terrible pain of a migraine headache is an all-too-familiar sensation. While all headaches are unpleasant, migraines are in a class of their own, with the ability to incapacitate someone for hours or even days.

WHAT IS IT?

Researchers believe migraines result from changes in the trigeminal nerve system, a network of nerves in the head that send messages to the brain. What researchers know is that a migraine headache often begins with intense pain on one side of the head that gradually spreads to other areas. Symptoms of migraine include blurred vision, acute sensitivity to sound, weakness, and numbness in the face, hands, or legs, and speech difficulties. For some people, migraines are preceded by visual auras, which consist of vision loss or seeing flashing lights or "squiggly" lines. Migraine headaches may begin during the aura, shortly after the aura ends, or up to an hour after the aura passes.

The patterns of migraine headaches are often difficult to follow. Some people experience them several times a month, others just once or twice a year. Women seem to bear the brunt of migraine headaches—70 percent of the people they affect are women. In

Do. Ask your doctor for a list of foods that may cause migraines, and work with him or her to create an elimination diet that will pinpoint exactly which foods trigger your migraines. Do eat meals at regular times; skipping meals may trigger a migraine.

Don't. Foods and beverages containing the substance called tyramine, including beer, ale, robust red wines, Chianti, vermouth, homemade breads, cheese, sour cream, bananas, red plums, figs, raisins, avocados, fava beans, Italian broad beans, green bean pods, eggplant, pickled herring, liver, canned meats, salami, yogurt, commercial gravies, chocolate, and soy sauce may trigger migraine headaches. Aspartame (NutraSweet), which is an artificial sweetener used in many diet foods and drinks, has also been linked to migraine headaches and should be avoided. Stay clear of foods containing monosodium glutamate (MSG), which is often used in Chinese food and can bring on migraine headaches.

women, migraines may occur during menstruation (sometimes beginning with the first period) and improve with the approach of menopause. Often, migraines occur suddenly and without cause, although factors such as stress, muscle tension, fatigue, irregular sleep habits, cigarette smoke, changes in weather, and certain medications can trigger migraines or exacerbate their symptoms. Dietary factors may also trigger migraines, including foods containing the amino acids aspartame and glutamate and the irregular intake of products high in caffeine (see Dietary Do's and Don'ts, alongside).

WHAT SHOULD I TAKE?

*Black Cohosh • Calcium • Chasteberry • Feverfew
5-Hydroxytryptophan (5-HTP) • Magnesium
Melatonin • Omega-3 Fatty Acids • Vitamin B₂ • Willow Bark*

Black cohosh and **chasteberry** may be helpful for relieving headaches associated with menstruation, which are often caused by hormonal fluctuations. (For more information on black cohosh and chasteberry, see pages 48 and 69.)

Calcium can help relieve migraine headaches caused by muscle cramping. This mineral should be taken in the evening, in conjunction with evening primrose oil (see page 115). (For more information on calcium, see page 57.)

Feverfew is the most well-known and well-studied herb used medicinally for migraine headaches. It has been shown in clinical studies to reduce both the frequency and the intensity of these headaches. (For more information on feverfew, see page 118.)

Some experts believe that migraine headaches are caused by abnormal serotonin function in the blood vessels. **5-HTP** may help to correct this abnormality because the body converts 5-HTP to serotonin. Studies have found that 5-HTP may reduce the occurrence of migraine headaches, and when taken in large doses (600 milligrams daily) this supplement may be as effective as prescription medications for reducing the occurrence of migraine headaches. (For more information on 5-HTP, see page 123.)

Many studies testing the effectiveness of **magnesium** on migraines have been conducted with the intravenous administration of magnesium and have shown positive results. Preliminary studies indicate that magnesium taken orally may be effective in easing symptoms of migraine headaches. Other studies have noted that women with a deficiency of magnesium may be more prone to migraine headaches during menstruation. (For more information on magnesium, see page 203.)

There is some research indicating that **melatonin** may be useful in the prevention of migraines, though it's probably best to use this under a doctor's supervision. (For more information on melatonin, see page 208.)

Omega-3 fatty acids seem to offer some help in reducing the frequency and severity of migraines. Taking a daily fish oil supplement is a good way to add omega-3 fatty acids to your nutritional intake. (For more information on omega-3 fatty acids, see page 221.)

Riboflavin, or **vitamin B$_2$**, tested very well when studied for its effects on migraine headaches. In one clinical study, vitamin B$_2$ was very effective in reducing the frequency and duration of migraine attacks. (For more information on vitamin B$_2$, see page 245.)

Willow bark has analgesic properties that may be useful in the treatment of migraines. (For more information about willow bark, see page 298.)

MY SUPPLEMENT LIST—MIGRAINE HEADACHES

SUPPLEMENT	RECOMMENDED DOSAGE
Black Cohosh	*Capsule:* Take 20 to 40 mg three times daily of an extract standardized to contain 1 mg of deoxyactein per 20 mg of extract.
Calcium	*Capsule or Tablet:* Take 1,200 mg of calcium citrate before bedtime, along with evening primrose oil.
Chasteberry	*Capsule:* Take 30 to 40 mg once in the morning for several months. Be sure to look for chasteberry products under the name Vitex, the plant's botanical name.
	Note: Chasteberry may be more effective if taken with black cohosh.
Feverfew	*Capsule:* Take 250 to 300 mg twice a day.
5-HTP	*Capsule:* Take 200 mg daily.
	Note: Consult your doctor about taking higher dosages to reduce the occurrence of migraine headaches if this dosage is not effective.
Magnesium	*Tablet:* Take 600 mg daily divided into two or three doses.
	Note: Take in the form of magnesium glycinate to avoid loose stools. Large amounts of magnesium can cause diarrhea; if this becomes a problem for you, reduce your dosage.

(continued)

MY SUPPLEMENT LIST—MIGRAINE HEADACHES (continued)	
SUPPLEMENT	**RECOMMENDED DOSAGE**
Melatonin	Ask your doctor if using melatonin as a preventative treatment for migraines may be right for you.
Omega-3 Fatty Acids	*Capsule:* Take 1,500 to 3,000 mg of omega-3 fatty acids in the form of fish oil supplements daily, in divided doeses, with meals.
Vitamin B$_2$	*Tablet:* Take 200 mg twice daily for 3 months.
Willow Bark	*Capsule:* Take an extract standardized to contain 60 to 240 mg of salicin daily.

MULTIPLE SCLEROSIS

AFTER DECADES OF RESEARCH, the exact origin of multiple sclerosis (MS) is unknown. Recent theories hypothesize that MS is an autoimmune disease, in which the immune system begins to attack the body as it would a foreign invader. In the case of MS, the result is a chronic and sometimes debilitating condition.

WHAT IS IT?

In multiple sclerosis, the immune system attacks the protective sheath that covers the nerves in the brain and spinal cord. As a result, the sheath and the nerves within it become damaged, impairing vision, muscle coordination, and other nerve-related activities.

The severity of MS symptoms can vary greatly from mild illness to permanent disability. At the onset of MS, its symptoms include lack of coordination and unsteady gait, impaired vision, fatigue, dizziness, numbness, and paralysis. As the disease progresses, it causes slurred speech, loss of vision, bladder problems, muscle spasms, paralysis, and occasionally forgetfulness and confusion.

Multiple sclerosis affects women twice as often as men, and the main cause of the disorder seems to be heredity, although doctors believe that environmental factors also seem to play a role. Although MS has no cure, most people with the disease can still lead active lives and manage symptoms. The keys include plenty of rest and aerobic exercise, avoiding long soaks in hot water (since a change in core body temperature may worsen the symptoms of MS), using air conditioning, and eating a healthy, well-balanced diet. Keeping your immune system strong through proper nutrition together with a reasonable array of nutritional supplements is also very important.

WHAT SHOULD I TAKE?

MS is a serious condition. Make sure to consult your doctor before taking any type of supplement if you have been diagnosed with MS.

Calcium • Carnitine • Magnesium •
Omega-3 Fatty Acids • Selenium • Vitamin B$_{12}$
Vitamin C • Vitamin D • Vitamin E • Zinc

Calcium keeps bones and joints strong, helping to prevent the debilitating effects of MS. **Carnitine** (in the form of L-carnitine) may help with the fatigue associated with medication used to treat multiple sclerosis. In one recent study, the majority of patients taking immunosuppressive or immunomodulatory therapies who also took L-carnitine had decreased fatigue intensity. (For more information on carnitine, see page 186.)

Magnesium is another crucial mineral that should be taken every day to support a healthy immune system and help the body to absorb calcium. (For more information on calcium and magnesium, see pages 57 and 203.)

Still in Debate: Mercury and MS

Still in Debate

An ongoing controversy has surrounded the possible link between mercury exposure and an increased predisposition to autoimmune diseases such as MS, lupus, and epilepsy. Many experts believe that exposure to mercury can increase the risk and worsen the severity and of autoimmune diseases. Because the greatest source of mercury exposure for many people comes from dental fillings, dental fillings made with mercury plus other metals—called dental amalgam—have come under heavy attack in recent years.

At present, there is no definitive evidence that mercury fillings cause or worsen MS. Some studies have claimed that the low level of mercury exposure from dental fillings is insufficient to cause systemic health problems such as MS. However, proponents of the mercury–MS connection claim that studies have shown an improvement in MS patients who have had mercury-containing dental fillings removed. Some studies have shown that patients with MS who have mercury amalgam fillings have poorer mental health than those who do not. A study conducted at the University of Maryland School of Medicine found that even low levels of mercury exposure hastened autoimmune disease in mice and in some cases worsened its symptoms.

Undoubtedly, further research will be performed to determine more definitive answers regarding the connection between mercury toxicity and MS. If you decide to have your mercury fillings removed before then, find a dentist who specializes in this, so that you do not inhale the mercury as it is being removed from your mouth. Recently, there has been growing awareness regarding the mercury content of certain fish, such as king mackerel, tuna, swordfish, tilefish, and shark. If you are concerned about your mercury intake, it's probably best to avoid eating these foods.

Various studies indicate that supplementation with **omega-3 fatty acids** may be beneficial to people with MS. One study found that supplementation with essential fatty acids, such as omega-3 fatty acids, reduced the severity and frequency of relapses and provided a slight overall benefit to people with MS. (For more information on omega-3 fatty acids, see page 221.)

Selenium may be an important element in reducing the severity of MS symptoms. People with MS should take it every day, along with vitamins C and E (see pages 284 and 292). (For more information on selenium, see page 253.)

Some studies have found a deficiency of **vitamin B$_{12}$** in people with MS, which may aggravate the symptoms of MS or make its treatment more difficult. Other studies indicate that a deficiency of vitamin B$_{12}$ may play a role in the early onset of MS (prior to age eighteen). Vitamin B$_{12}$ levels may also be low in people who are receiving treatment with intravenous steroids for MS. (For more information on vitamin B$_{12}$, see page 282.)

Vitamin C and **vitamin E** are just two of a handful of antioxidants that should be taken supplementally in high doses in MS. Indeed, studies have shown the full range of antioxidant supplements to be helpful in MS, and other studies have found that levels of antioxidant vitamins are low during periods of worsened MS symptoms. (For more information on vitamins C and E, see pages 284 and 292.)

Research indicates that people with a deficiency of **vitamin D** may be more prone to developing MS. Additionally, regular supplementation with vitamin D may help to reduce symptoms of MS as well as prevent MS in people with a genetic predisposition to the disease. (For more information on vitamin D, see page 289.)

Zinc is an important mineral for effective functioning of the immune system. Some studies indicate that zinc levels may be deficient in people with MS. (For more information on zinc, see page 304.)

MY SUPPLEMENT LIST—MULTIPLE SCLEROSIS

SUPPLEMENT	RECOMMENDED DOSAGE
Calcium	*Capsule or Tablet:* Take 1,000 mg daily divided into two doses.
L-Carnitine	Take 2 g daily of proprionyl-L-carnitine divided into two doses, between meals.
Magnesium	*Tablet:* Take 500 mg daily divided into two or three doses along with calcium (see previous page).

MY SUPPLEMENT LIST—MULTIPLE SCLEROSIS	
SUPPLEMENT	**RECOMMENDED DOSAGE**
	Note: Take in the form of magnesium glycinate to avoid loose stools. Large amounts of magnesium can cause diarrhea; if this becomes a problem for you, reduce your dosage.
Omega-3 Fatty Acids	*Fish Oil—Capsule:* Take 2–3 g of omega-3 fatty acids per day, in divided doses, with meals. The amount of omega-3 fatty acid will vary by manufacturer, so be sure to check the product label carefully.
Selenium	*Tablet:* Take 200 mcg daily.
Vitamin B$_{12}$	Consult your doctor to determine an appropriate dosage of vitamin B$_{12}$ for you. Some people may require injections or sublingual (under the tongue) forms of this vitamin for better absorption.
Vitamin C	*Capsule or Tablet:* Take 500 mg twice a day with meals.
	Note: Be sure to use a buffered form of vitamin C. If taking vitamin C causes loose stools, decrease your dosage and then gradually increase the dosage as tolerated.
Vitamin D	*Tablet:* Take 400 IU daily.
	Note: If you think you have a vitamin D deficiency, consult a doctor to check for this and determine an appropriate dosage of this vitamin for you. Some doctors may recommend dosages of vitamin D as high as 10,000 IU daily, but don't take this high dose on your own without supervision.
Vitamin E	*Capsule:* Take 400 IU daily of a natural supplement containing mixed tocopherols.
Zinc	*Tablet:* Take 30 mg daily.

MUSCLE PAINS AND CRAMPS

EVERYONE HAS EXPERIENCED the unpleasant sensation of a "Charley horse," particularly a few days after a great workout at the gym or a day spent gardening outdoors. You may wake up in the middle of the night and stretch your body, only to suddenly feel a fiery pain in your leg, back, abdominal, or arm muscles. For a few seconds you toss and turn, waiting for the feeling to pass, and then it finally subsides as quickly as it came.

WHAT IS IT?

With more than 600 muscles in the human body, quite a bit can go wrong with their tone and functioning. In athletes, the overuse, stress, and dehydration of muscles can lead to recurrent cramping and pain. Even gardening, painting, or pursuing other activities that involve repetitive movements can lead to muscle pain and cramping. And at age 30, we all enter a natural process of losing some of our muscle mass year after year, making muscle pain and cramping typically more frequent with age.

Occasional muscle aches and pains can often be managed with simple self-care techniques. However, muscle pain that becomes frequent and severe should prompt a talk with a doctor. Drinking lots of water, particularly during periods of high activity, and stretching before and after exercise may help prevent muscle pain. When muscle pain occurs, self-massage and the application of hot and cold compresses may make it more tolerable.

WHAT SHOULD I TAKE?
Bromelain • Ginger • L-Carnitine
Magnesium • Vitamin C

Bromelain, an enzyme naturally derived from pineapples, breaks down proteins in the muscle in a process that eases pain and cramping. The result may also be a more rapid recovery from pain, soreness, and bruising. (For more information on bromelain, see page 54.)

Ginger is an herb well known for its anti-inflammatory properties. It also has enzymes similar to those in bromelain, which help break down proteins in the muscle to ease pain and soreness. Preliminary studies of ginger for muscle pain have been very promising, suggesting it can be a safe and effective treatment for this. (For more information on ginger, see page 136.)

A controlled study found that **L-carnitine** may help prevent muscle injury and pain when taken before physical exercise. However, other studies have been less conclusive about L-carnitine, and more research is needed to determine its effect on exercise-related muscle soreness. Don't forget about Epsom salts, which are magnesium sulphate. A nice warm soak in an Epsom salt bath, with a little powdered ginger, is often effective at relieving cramped muscles. (For more information on L-carnitine, see page 186.)

Deficiencies of the mineral **magnesium** play a role in muscle tension and nighttime leg cramps. Consequently, supplemental magnesium may help alleviate muscle pain. Studies suggest that women who experience leg cramps during pregnancy may benefit from magnesium supplementation. Magnesium may also help relieve the twitches and tics that often accompany muscle pains and cramps. (For more information on magnesium, see page 203.)

Vitamin C may affect muscle pain and cramping through its strong antioxidant properties. Muscles produce many more cell- and tissue-damaging free radical molecules during strenuous activity than they normally do. Vitamin C may help alleviate muscle tenderness by scavenging the excess free radicals. It seems that vitamin C may be particularly helpful for muscle pain that follows strenuous exercise, especially in people who are not usually physically active, and some studies have found that vitamin C may be helpful in easing delayed muscle soreness. Plus, vitamin C helps build collagen, the tissue that holds muscles together. (For more information on vitamin C, see page 284.)

MY SUPPLEMENT LIST—MUSCLE PAINS AND CRAMPS

SUPPLEMENT	RECOMMENDED DOSAGE
Bromelain	*Tablet:* Take 250–500 mg daily between meals. Look for a product containing 2,400 gelatin-dissolving units (GDU) or 3,600 milk-clotting units (MCU) per gram.
Ginger	*Capsule:* For acute pain, take six 500-mg capsules of concentrated ginger extract daily.
L-Carnitine	*Capsule:* Take 1–3 g once daily.
Magnesium	*Tablet:* Take 500 to 800 mg daily. It's also helpful to use magnesium topically, in the form of Epsom salts (magnesium sulphate). Take a warm bath with about 1–2 quarts of Epsom salts. Add several tablespoons of freshly grated ginger to the water. Powdered ginger (use less, 1–2 tsp) may be used but should be mixed in 1 cup of water first, and then added to the bath, to avoid inhaling the powder. *Note:* Take in the form of magnesium glycinate to avoid loose stools. Large amounts of magnesium can cause diarrhea; if this becomes a problem for you, reduce your dosage.
Vitamin C	*Tablet:* Take up to 1,000 mg twice daily, with meals. *Note:* Be sure to use a buffered form of vitamin C. If taking vitamin C causes loose stools, decrease the dosage and then gradually increase the dosage as tolerated.

NAUSEA, VOMITING, AND MORNING SICKNESS

NO ONE IS IMMUNE FROM feeling nauseous. Whether you are prone to getting motion sickness, are in the early stages of pregnancy, or simply ate a meal that did not agree with you, nausea is one of the most unpleasant yet common conditions that people of all ages experience. Whether it leads to vomiting or not, suppressing the feeling of nausea is a high priority for anyone feeling queasy.

WHAT IS IT?

While they may be unpleasant, nausea and vomiting do occur for a reason. They are protective mechanisms, the body's way of cleansing itself of a toxic substance. Nausea typically precedes vomiting—it is often described as coming in waves. What is really occurring is that the brain is signaling the mouth to increase saliva production, telling the digestive tract to get ready to vomit, and informing the windpipe that it needs to close. Other symptoms include chills, sweating, weakness, dizziness, and loss of appetite. After nausea sets in, the next step is retching, in which the stomach and esophagus begin to spasm. Vomiting usually follows shortly afterward.

Since nausea and vomiting are protective measures that keep your body safe during a flu, infection, or after ingesting something that disagrees with us, in most cases it's best to just give in and let nature run its course. There are times, however, when waves of nausea can be frequent, persistent, and downright frustrating. It is important to stay

Practical Tips to Preventing Nausea

Healthy Hints

Nausea can occur for a variety of reasons. Below are custom-designed tips to help prevent and minimize queasy stomachs.

Morning Sickness

- **Snack in bed.** Try sipping some tea or nibbling on crackers before getting out of bed. Don't get up too quickly, and give your body adequate time to digest your snack before rising.
- **Rest.** Feeling sleepy can cause nausea, especially in pregnancy. Make sure to get adequate sleep each night.
- **Avoid bad odors.** Make sure to avoid odors that trigger your nausea.

Motion Sickness

- **Stay centered.** When traveling by boat, make sure to sit in the middle of the ship. When flying, make sure to sit near the front edge of the wing of the airplane.

When traveling by train, sit in a forward-facing window seat. When traveling by car, sit in the front passenger seat.

- **Focus.** Focus on the horizon line, or on a distant, nonmoving object.
- **Don't indulge.** Avoid drinking alcohol and eating large meals before traveling.

Food Poisoning

- **Rehydrate.** Since bouts of food poisoning often include vomiting and diarrhea, drink plenty of fluids, especially those containing electrolytes (such as chicken broth) in order to prevent dehydration.
- **Eat smart.** Avoid illness altogether by staying away from contaminated foods. Make sure to prepare and store foods wisely.
- **Seek help.** Make sure to call your doctor if your symptoms do not improve and if you are having an acute episode of diarrhea or vomiting.

hydrated when having episodes of vomiting, since it results in a loss of bodily fluids, especially if accompanied by diarrhea. During pregnancy, the first trimester is the most common period for nausea and is commonly referred to as "morning sickness." If you experience morning sickness or frequent waves of nausea for other reasons, you can take steps to prevent it or ease the feeling once it has begun.

WHAT SHOULD I TAKE?

The safety of many herbs for use during pregnancy is not clearly established. If you are pregnant, never take any supplement without first consulting your doctor.

Chamomile • Ginger • Peppermint • Vitamin B$_6$

Chamomile has traditionally been used to treat digestive upset. If your nausea is due to indigestion, a cup of chamomile tea may be a tasty solution to your discomfort. (For more information on chamomile, see page 67.)

Ginger is the herb of choice when it comes to preventing nausea and vomiting. The oils in ginger work to calm an upset stomach, aid digestion, and relax the muscles of the digestive tract. Although most sources agree that ginger is safe and probably effective for use during pregnancy, some controversy surrounds its use. If you are pregnant, consult your doctor before using this herb. (For more information on ginger, see page 136.)

That after-dinner mint may be more important than you think! **Peppermint** oil can help to soothe stomach cramps typically associated with nausea. (For more information on peppermint oil, see page 226.)

Vitamin B$_6$ is recommended to combat nausea and vomiting related to morning sickness during pregnancy. In studies, women who took a daily preventive dose of vitamin B$_6$ had significantly fewer episodes of nausea and vomiting than those who did not. (For more information on vitamin B$_6$, see page 279.)

MY SUPPLEMENT LIST—NAUSEA, VOMITING, AND MORNING SICKNESS

SUPPLEMENT	RECOMMENDED DOSAGE
Chamomile	*Tea:* Combine 2 or 3 (heaping) tsp of fresh flower with 1 cup of boiling water. Steep for 10 minutes and drink as needed.

(continued)

MY SUPPLEMENT LIST—NAUSEA, VOMITING, AND MORNING SICKNESS (continued)	
SUPPLEMENT	**RECOMMENDED DOSAGE**
Ginger	*Capsule:* Take 1 to 4 g daily, divided into two or four doses; to prevent motion sickness, begin taking ginger 1 to 2 days before traveling and continue taking ginger during travel. *Tea:* Add thinly sliced ginger root to a cup of boiling water. Boil for 5–10 minutes. Drink up to four times daily.
Peppermint	*Tea:* Pour 1 cup of water over 1 (heaping) tbsp or 5 g of dried peppermint leaves. Let steep for 5–10 minutes. Drink three or four cups daily between meals. *Capsule:* Take 1 or 2 peppermint oil capsules three times a day between meals.
Vitamin B$_6$	*Tablet:* Take 50 mg daily, to prevent morning sickness. *Note:* If you are pregnant, do not take vitamin B$_6$ without first consulting your doctor.

DIETARY DO'S AND DON'TS

Do. Certain foods may help strengthen the adrenal glands and perhaps help to ease neuralgic pain. If you have neuralgia, be sure to eat adrenal-supporting foods, including almonds, avocados, bananas, fish, garbanzo beans, and shrimp. **Don't.** Some foods may aggravate neuralgia symptoms. If you experience neuralgic pain, be sure to avoid salt and salty foods; foods with saturated fats, including meat and eggs, or foods made from them; sugar and sweets such as candy, cake, and cookies; and stimulants, including coffee, soda, and alcohol.

NEURALGIA

SEARING, BLINDING, out-of-the-blue pain. It's unexplained, unprovoked, and can at times be so painful that it brings those who have it to their knees. The condition is known as neuralgia, and the cause of the pain is often unknown.

WHAT IS IT?

Nerve pain and discomfort can occur with a variety of medical conditions. Pain that extends along the course of a nerve is called *neuralgia.* All types of neuralgia are characterized by jabbing, sharp, and deep pain.

In cases of *postherpetic neuralgia,* dormant chickenpox virus in the body becomes reactivated when the immune system is weakened by age, illness, stress, or certain medications. The virus passes from the cells that harbor it, and travels along nerve fibers, causing pain. Once it reaches the skin, it causes a rash and blisters known as shingles (see Herpes Zoster, page 487). Many people continue to feel severe pain even after the blisters have healed. Postherpetic neuralgia is characterized by pain that often occurs where the rash was present, but it may affect other parts of the body as well.

Trigeminal neuralgia, also called "tic douloureux," is caused by a disturbance in the trigeminal nerve—one of 12 cranial nerves in the skull—which carries sensation from the region of the face to the brain. As a result, the sharp pain of trigeminal neuralgia affects the face and can be triggered by everyday activities involving the face or head, such as shaving, brushing your teeth, chewing, or talking.

Doctors have been somewhat successful in treating neuralgia with medication, and occasionally surgery is done a last resort.

Studies are underway to investigate appropriate supplements for alleviating neuralgia. Currently, your best bet may be to obtain nutrients from foods that support the nervous system (see Dietary Do's and Don'ts on the previous page).

WHAT SHOULD I TAKE?

Devil's Claw • Peppermint Oil • St. John's Wort

Devil's claw, when taken internally, and **peppermint oil**, when applied topically, are approved by the German Commission E (see page 16) for treating the pain associated with neuralgia. (For more information on devil's claw and peppermint oil, see pages 98 and 226.) **St. John's wort** oil, when applied topically, may help alleviate the pain associated with neuralgia. (For more information on St John's wort, see page 262.)

MY SUPPLEMENT LIST—NEURALGIA	
SUPPLEMENT	**RECOMMENDED DOSAGE**
Devil's Claw	*Oral—Capsule:* Take 750 mg of an extract standardized to contain 3% iridoid glycosides 3 times daily.
Peppermint Oil	*Topical—Oil:* rub 2 to 3 drops of peppermint oil into affected areas as needed. If you find that peppermint oil is too strong, you may dilute the oil with a carrier oil such as avocado, olive, almond, or jojoba.
St. John's Wort	*Oil:* Apply full strength St. John's wort oil topically to the affected area several times per day.

OSTEOARTHRITIS

SEWING. WOODWORKING. Cooking. Gardening. There are so many hobbies and everyday tasks in which we are wholly dependent on our hands to enjoy. It seems tragic that the most common medical problem in the world is one that can rob these hobbies and tasks from us with crippling and debilitating pain. Osteoarthritis (OA) is a condition affecting one in three people, often turning the things that we love to do into challenging hurdles. OA typically affects the hands, knees, hips, feet, and back.

WHAT IS IT?

OA is the most common form of joint disease. It occurs when there is a breakdown of cartilage—the tough tissue in a joint that cushions the

FRIENDS AND FOES

Folic acid helps the action of **SAMe** in the body. People with OA who have a low intake of folic acid should consider increasing their intake of this vitamin through dark leafy green vegetables or supplementation.

bones of the joint—and allows them to glide over one another. When cartilage deteriorates, bones begin to rub against each other, causing friction, pain, and loss of movement. Although increasing age may put you at risk for OA, many factors can cause this condition. Obesity can cause OA, especially in the knees, since excess weight puts more strain on weight-bearing joints. People with sports injuries may be at increased risk for OA as well, especially if they have had repeated injuries to their joints. In some cases, people are born with defective cartilage, which may deteriorate, increasing the risk of OA.

There is no cure for OA, but there is some good news for those who have it. By taking steps such as weight loss, regular exercise, and a healthy diet, you can prevent OA or reduce its symptoms if they have begun. In conjunction with lifestyle changes, nutritional and herbal supplements can also do quite a bit to help.

WHAT SHOULD I TAKE?

Boron • Boswellia • Bromelain • Cat's Claw • Cayenne
Chondroitin • Devil's Claw • Ginger • Glucosamine
Niacinamide • S-Adenosylmethionine (SAMe)
Vitamin D • Willow Bark

Boron has been a popular supplement in Australia mainly because the soil is deficient in this trace element, making it hard to provide boron-containing foods in the diet. Boron supplements in Australia sold at a whopping 10,000 bottles per month and were particularly popular for treating OA. Preliminary studies are now showing that boron may help people with OA who do not get enough boron from the foods they eat, particularly in vegetables and nuts. (For more information on boron, see page 50.)

Studies indicate that **boswellia** may help to reduce inflammation and pain and to increase flexibility in OA of the knees. In one study in which people with OA of the knee were given supplemental boswellia, not only were pain and inflammation decreased, but walking distances became easier with increased flexibility of the knees. (For more information on boswellia, see page 52.)

Bromelain—an enzyme derived from pineapples—is well known for its anti-inflammatory properties. Bromelain may be useful for reducing the swelling and tenderness associated with OA. One study comparing bromelain to diclofenac (Voltaren)—a medication commonly prescribed for people with OA or rheumatoid arthritis—found that bromelain was as effective as diclofenac in reducing joint tenderness, swelling, and pain. (For more information on bromelain, see page 54.)

Preliminary research suggests that **cat's claw**, in the form of *Uncaria guianensis*, may be effective in treating osteoarthritis of the knee. A study of 45 people with osteoarthritis found that cat's claw effectively reduced osteoarthritis pain in the knee within 1 week of cat's claw treatment. (For more information on cat's claw, see page 63.)

When applied topically, creams containing capsaicin, which is derived from the **cayenne** plant, may help to reduce the pain and tenderness associated with OA. (For more information on cayenne, see page 64.)

Many people with OA experience a loss of **chondroitin** as their cartilage erodes. Chondroitin is a main component of cartilage and helps to keep water and nutrients in cartilage, thus making its preservation beneficial in OA. Some studies have found that chondroitin and glucosamine (see below) work best when taken together. (For more information on chondroitin, see page 74.)

Several studies have found that **devil's claw** may be effective in reducing OA pain, and in Europe devil's claw is an extremely popular treatment for various types of arthritis including OA. Studies suggest that devil's claw may relieve pain and improve mobility in people with OA. (for more information on devil's claw, see page 98.)

Several studies indicate that **ginger** offers moderate relief for the swelling and pain associated with osteoarthritis, particularly in the knee. (For more information on ginger, see page 136.)

Glucosamine works along with chondroitin (see above) in the prevention and treatment of OA pain. Like chondroitin, glucosamine works better than many over-the-counter treatments in

Avocado and Soybeans May Help Alleviate OA

Did You Know?

Special extracts of avocado and soybean, called "avocado/soybean unsaponifiables" (ASU), appear to reduce the pain and inflammation caused by OA. In a double-blind, controlled study in which 260 people with OA of the knee were given 300 to 600 milligrams daily of ASU, it was found that over the 3-month period, ASU was significantly more effective than placebo in easing the pain and inflammation of their OA.

A study published in 2003 concluded that evidence for ASU as an effective treatment for OA is convincing but recommended conducting further research. An article in the journal of the *American Academy of Family Physicians* recommended 300 milligrams of ASU daily to help reduce symptoms of OA. If you have OA, this supplement may be worth investigating.

decreasing pain and improving the range of motion of joints. Combination glucosamine–chondroitin supplements may be purchased, allowing both supplements to be taken together. (For more information on glucosamine, see page 144.)

Studies indicate that **niacinamide** (a form of niacin or vitamin B_3) may reduce the inflammation associated with OA. One study of niacinamide found that people taking non-steroidal anti-inflammatory drugs (NSAIDs), such as aspirin, to reduce inflammation were able to reduce their dosage of medicine when they also took niacinamide supplements. (For more information on niacinamide, see Niacin, page 219.)

Experts are unsure of exactly how **SAMe** works when it comes to treating OA, but the studies indicate that it works as well as some conventional medications in reducing the pain, swelling, and morning stiffness often associated with OA. (For more information on SAMe, see page 247.)

Vitamin D deficiency is quite common in people who have OA. Maintaining normal vitamin D levels through supplementation can prevent the breakdown of cartilage and preserve bone health. Ask your doctor to check your Vitamin D level, and try to get out in the sunshine each day. (For more information on vitamin D, see page 289.)

Willow bark contains a substance known as salicin, which has greatly reduced the pain of OA in clinical studies. (For more information on willow bark, see page 298.)

MY SUPPLEMENT LIST—OSTEOARTHRITIS

SUPPLEMENT	RECOMMENDED DOSAGE
Boron	*Tablet:* Take 1 to 9 mg daily.
Boswellia	*Tablet:* Take a supplement containing 150–300 mg of boswellic acid two or three times daily. Take with food if necessary.
Bromelain	*Tablet:* Take 250–500 mg daily between meals. Look for a product containing 3,600 milk-clotting units (MCU) per gram.
Cat's Claw	*Capsule:* Take 100 mg of a standard extract in the form of *Uncaria tomentosa* or *Uncaria guyanensis* one to three times daily according to the manufacturer's directions.
Cayenne	*Topical—Cream:* Apply a cream containing .025% to .075% capsaicin four times daily for 2 weeks; after 2 weeks, the dosage may be reduced to three times daily.
Chondroitin	*Tablet:* Take 600 mg twice daily with meals.

MY SUPPLEMENT LIST—OSTEOARTHRITIS	
SUPPLEMENT	**RECOMMENDED DOSAGE**
Devil's Claw	*Capsule or Tablet:* Take up to 100 mg three times daily, with meals, of an extract standardized to contain 3% iridoid glycosides or 50 mg of harpagoside.
Ginger	*Capsule:* Take 1 to 4 g daily of a concentrated ginger extract divided into two to four doses daily, with meals. Start at a low dose, to avoid digestive upsest. *Fresh:* May also use up to 50 g of fresh ginger per day (one ounce is equal to 28 g). Take a 1 ounce piece of the fresh root, and squeeze it through a garlic press. Add the juice to water or other beverage to dilute it. Take in divided doses throughout the day.
Glucosamine	*Capsule or Tablet:* Take 500 mg three times daily with meals, or 1,500 mg at night with dinner.
Niacinamide	*Tablet:* Take 500 mg daily.
SAMe	*Enteric-coated Tablet:* Take 800 to 1,200 mg twice daily, on an empty stomach. *Note:* Take SAMe with a vitamin B complex to prevent high levels of homocysteine from developing.
Vitamin D	*Tablet:* Take 400 to 600 IU daily. Ask your doctor to check your vitamin D level.
Willow Bark	*Capsule:* Take a standardized extract containing 120 to 240 mg of salicin daily as needed. *Caution:* Do not take willow bark if have an aspirin allergy, bleeding disorder, diabetes, or a peptic ulcer.

OSTEOPOROSIS

BRITTLE BONES ARE OFTEN thought of as going hand in hand with aging—the older you get, the more brittle your bones become, and there is little you can do to stop it. But osteoporosis, with its loss of bone mass and brittle, fragile bones that result, is not a necessary evil of aging. The first step in preventing osteoporosis is knowing how and why it occurs in the first place.

WHAT IS IT?

In osteoporosis, key minerals are leeched from the bones, causing them to deteriorate and become increasingly brittle. Until age 30—when bones are the strongest—the body works tirelessly to replenish new bone and remove old bone. However, after age 30, the body begins to remove old bone faster than it produces new bone. Osteoporosis can occur if the body does not have enough strong bone mass by the age of 30 or if bone loss after age 30 occurs too quickly. Late warning signs of osteoporosis include back pain, loss of height, stooped posture, and easy bone fracture.

In the United States, osteoporosis affects 8 million women and 2 million men. The reason for this unbalanced statistic is that in women, estrogen levels drop at the onset of menopause, causing bone loss to accelerate from 1 to 3 percent each year. Risk factors for developing osteoporosis may be genetic, environmental, or related to diet and lifestyle. Thin women of Asian or Caucasian descent are at particular risk for this condition. Certain medications can also increase the risk for developing osteoporosis. Ask your doctor if any medication you're taking increases your risk of developing osteoporosis, and see if you can be given a safer alternative.

Building up bone mass early in life through proper nutrition is crucial to preventing osteoporosis, but that doesn't mean there's nothing you can do to strengthen your bones as you grow older. Although your body becomes prone to losing bone mass as you age, you can take many steps to keep your bones strong even in your golden years. A strict regimen of bone-building nutritional supplements is definitely part of this initiative.

WHAT SHOULD I TAKE?

Boron • Calcium • Copper • DHEA • Ipriflavone • Magnesium
Omega-3 Fatty Acids • Vitamin D • Soy • Vitamin K

Preliminary research suggests that **boron** may benefit bone health. Boron may affect the body's absorption of calcium, magnesium, and vitamin D, all of which are key players in bone maintenance and in fighting osteoporosis. Other research suggests that boron may reduce the body's loss of calcium in the urine, which could also help prevent osteoporosis. (For more information on boron, see page 50.)

Soy for Bone Strength

Still in Debate Years ago, medical research seemed to indicate that plant hormones known as phytoestrogens that are found in soy could have beneficial effects on bones, particularly in postmenopausal women who had decreasing estrogen levels as part of the normal aging process. Since then, some research indicates that soy milk has bone-protective effects and is especially useful for women as an alternative to hormone replacement therapy.

However, recent reports have also suggested that soy products, such as soy milk and tofu, may contain substances (phytates) that prevent the absorption of key nutrients in soy. Fortunately, the fermentation of certain soy products, such as tempeh and miso, allows the nutrients in soy to be more readily absorbed.

While the scientists sort out this issue, there is no reason to stop enjoying your favorite soy recipes in moderation, although there is no guarantee that they will be beneficial to your bones.

Calcium deficiency is the number-one cause of osteoporosis, and ensuring a high intake of calcium is therefore the best thing you can do for preventing or delaying the onset of osteoporosis. An adequate intake of calcium can be derived from the right foods, including dark green, leafy vegetables, squash, legumes, nuts, whole grains, and broccoli. Choosing a good calcium supplement is also quite helpful. Calcium citrate may be the best bet for this, since studies show that it is the form of calcium best absorbed by the body. Also, be sure the product you choose is made by a company that checks for heavy metal contamination such as by lead, mercury, or aluminum. Steer clear of bone-derived calcium supplements, since studies indicate they may have a high content of lead. (For more information on calcium, see page 57.)

Increasing evidence suggests that **copper** may help in preventing osteoporosis. While copper is needed for healthy bone synthesis, most people do not have an adequate intake of this trace mineral. One study found that 2-year supplementation with copper was effective in reducing bone loss. Although many people increase their intake of milk products to help provide calcium for bone health, milk and milk products have a very low copper content, and researchers believe that lactose—the major sugar in milk—may even interfere with copper metabolism, further weakening the effects of inadequate intake of copper. Supplementation with copper may help in preventing a deficiency of this important mineral, thus protecting bones and staving off osteoporosis. (For more information on copper, see page 84.)

DHEA (dehydroepiandrosterone) is a supplement that may, for some people, be of benefit in the treatment of osteoporosis. But it's best not to take this without first having your doctor measure your blood levels of DHEA-S. If they are low, your doctor might suggest augmenting them with a DHEA supplement. (For more information on DHEA, see page 100.)

Ipriflavone may help treat osteoporosis, and then again, it may not. In other words, the research thus far has been somewhat contradictory as to the effect of this supplement on osteoporosis. (For more information on ipriflavone, see page 172.)

Magnesium is another crucial mineral for keeping bones healthy. Some studies suggest that a deficiency of magnesium, rather than calcium, may be the real culprit in osteoporosis. One study found that people with osteoporosis did not absorb magnesium as effectively as those without osteoporosis. In another 2-year study, supplementation with magnesium either stopped bone loss or increased bone mass in 87 percent of people with osteoporosis. (For more information on magnesium, see page 203.)

Preliminary studies suggest that **omega-3 fatty acids** may be helpful in preventing bone loss. However, these important fatty acids offer so many health benefits for the cardiovascular, nervous, and immune systems that it is a good idea to include this nutrient in your daily regimen in any case. (For more information on omega-3 fatty acids, see page 221.)

Soy and all its manifestations (soy milk, tofu, miso, tempe) may be useful in the overall prevention of osteoporosis. (For more information on soy, see page 257.)

Because **vitamin D** helps the body to absorb calcium, it is important to include vitamin D into your osteoporosis prevention plan. Without proper calcium absorption, the effectiveness of calcium supplementation is greatly diminished. When taken in conjunction with calcium, vitamin D may decrease the risk of bone fracture with aging. (For more information on vitamin D, see page 289.)

Preliminary research indicates that **vitamin K** may improve bone density in women. This vitamin may also play a role in decreasing the risk of fractures. Although study results are conflicting, some studies suggest that supplementation with vitamins D and K in postmenopausal women may increase bone mass. Other studies have found that a low dietary intake of vitamin K may lead to low bone density in women. While most people can get an adequate intake of vitamin K from food or a multivitamin, supplementation with this vitamin may be necessary if you have a deficiency of it. (For more information on vitamin K, see page 295.)

MY SUPPLEMENT LIST—OSTEOPOROSIS

SUPPLEMENT	RECOMMENDED DOSAGE
Boron	*Tablet:* Take 1 to 9 mg daily.
	Note: There is no evidence that boron supplementation is necessary for people who consume adequate amounts of boron in their diet.
Calcium	*Tablet or Capsule:* Take 1,200 mg of a calcium citrate supplement at bedtime. Postmenopausal women should take 1,500 mg of calcium a day divided into three doses if they are not receiving estrogen therapy. Women who are receiving estrogen therapy should take 1,000 mg of calcium daily divided into two doses.
	Note: Take calcium with magnesium (on the next page) and vitamin D (on the next page).

MY SUPPLEMENT LIST—OSTEOPOROSIS	
SUPPLEMENT	**RECOMMENDED DOSAGE**
Copper	*Tablet:* Some doctors recommend taking from 1 to 3 mg of copper daily. Zinc lowers levels of copper in the body. If you are taking zinc supplements, consider taking 2 to 3 g of copper daily. *Note:* Copper may be best absorbed by the body when it is taken in the form of copper sulfate, cupric acetate, and alkaline copper carbonate. Cupric oxide—a form of copper found in most multivitamin/mineral supplements—may be poorly absorbed by the body, according to animal studies.
DHEA	Ask your doctor to check your DHEA-S level to determine if you need to take this supplement.
Ipriflavone	Take 300 mg three times per day, with meals.
Magnesium	*Tablet:* Take 400 to 800 mg twice daily. *Note:* Take in the form of magnesium glycinate to avoid loose stools. Large amounts of magnesium can cause diarrhea; if this becomes a problem for you, reduce your dosage.
Omega-3 Fatty Acids	*Capsule:* 1–2 g of omega-3 fatty acids per day, in divided doses, with meals. The amount of omega-3 fatty acid will vary by manufacturer, so be sure to check the product label carefully
Soy	Have a serving of a soy product each day, such as soy milk, tofu, miso, or tempe. Since the overall effects of soy on osteoporosis are controversial, it's probably best not to over do it.
Vitamin D	*Tablet:* Take 400 to 600 IU daily. For people deprived of sunlight, a daily dosage of 600 to 1,000 IU may be necessary. Consult your doctor to determine an appropriate dosage for you. Ask your doctor to check your vitamin D level.
Vitamin K	*Tablet:* Take 75 to 100 mcg each day. *Note:* Vitamin K supplementation is not necessary unless you have a deficiency of this vitamin. Consult your doctor before taking supplemental vitamin K.

PARKINSON'S DISEASE

CAN YOU IMAGINE living with trembling, muscle stiffness, difficulty with walking, and problems in keeping your balance and coordination every day? For over 1 million Americans, this is the stark reality of Parkinson's disease. This progressive disease generally develops in people over the age of 50, although it can strike those younger. While Parkinson's disease is not curable, it is treatable, and researchers are working on finding new, better treatments and a cure for this disorder.

DIETARY DO'S AND DON'TS

Do. Eat fruits and vegetables—and drink wine! Fruits and vegetables contain antioxidants called polyphenols. Polyphenols appear to protect against many diseases, including Parkinson's. You can also get these antioxidants from nuts, whole grains, and soybeans. Grapes and red wine have high concentrations of polyphenols, which may make red wine may the drink of choice if you have Parkinson's disease.

Don't. Studies indicate that eating large amounts of protein may increase tremors associated with Parkinson's disease. To decrease amounts of protein in your diet, avoid foods high in protein such as poultry, meat, fish, and egg whites. It seems that diets high in calories and fat —particularly animal fat—contribute to the tremors of Parkinson's disease. Decrease red meat intakes and reduce your overall fat and calorie intake. You should also steer clear of aspartame, an artificial sweetener found in sugar-free yogurt and diet soda that, while controversial, is associated with neurological symptoms.

WHAT IS IT?

Parkinson's disease is the most common degenerative disease of the motor system, and after Alzheimer's disease, the second most common neurodegenerative disease. The disease affects the nerve cells in the brain that control muscle movement. The loss of dopamine cells in a specific region of the brain is part of the disease. The onset of Parkinson's disease is slow, but the symptoms gradually worsen over time. At first, the disease may produce a mild twitch in the fingers or lack of energy. Gradually, the symptoms progress to the point at which it's difficult to perform routine daily tasks.

Researchers are uncertain about exactly what causes Parkinson's disease, but they do know that genetics and exposure to environmental chemicals can play a role in the development of the disease. Parkinson's disease can improve somewhat with oral drug therapy. Levodopa (Larodopa)—a drug that provides dopamine to brain cells—along with other drugs, is the mainstay of Parkinson's treatment, although with time these drugs' effectiveness tends to diminish. Deep brain stimulation, a procedure that involves implanting an electrical stimulator in the brain resembling a pacemaker for the heart, has shown some promise in the treatment of Parkinson's disease, and research into stem cell implants to replace damaged dopamine-using neurons in the brain is ongoing. There are some supplements that also may be useful in reducing symptoms and slowing the onset of Parkinson's disease.

WHAT SHOULD I TAKE?

Parkinson's disease is a very serious condition. Make sure to consult your doctor before taking any type of supplement, especially if you have been diagnosed with Parkinson's disease or think you may have Parkinson's disease.

Alpha Lipoic Acid • Choline • Coenzyme Q10 (CoQ10) N-Acetylcysteine (NAC) • Nicotinamide Adenine Dinucleotide (NADH) • Phosphatidylserine • Riboflavin SAMe • Vitamin C • Vitamin E

The precursors of glutathione—**alpha lipoic acid** (ALA) and **NAC**—may reduce oxidative stress in the brain, which can help slow the progression of Parkinson's disease, and glutathione levels have been shown to be low in people with this disease. One study noted increased brain activity in people with Parkinson's disease who were given 500 milligrams a day of ALA. Giving glutathione itself, rather than in its precursors, would have to be done intraveneously. (For more information on alpha lipoic acid and NAC, see pages 29 and 213.)

CDP-**choline**, which is closely related to choline, may enhance the effectiveness of levodopa (Larodopa), a prescription medication commonly given to people with Parkinson's disease. CDP-choline seems to increase dopamine levels in the brain, reducing the overall symptoms of the disease. However, this supplement may need to be given by injection to be effective. (For more information on CDP-choline, see page 71.)

CoQ10 has been shown to slow the progression of Parkinson's disease in clinical studies. In a study of people with Parkinson's disease, CoQ10 seemed to halt the onset of the disease. Other studies suggest that CoQ10 may slow the functional decline in Parkinson's. (For more information on CoQ10, see page 80.)

Preliminary studies suggest that **NADH** may improve the effectiveness of the drug levodopa (Larodopa) in treating Parkinson's disease and increase the length of time during the day when this drug is most beneficial. (For more information on NADH, see page 216.)

Phosphatidylserine is a type of lipid important for normal brain function and the effective transmission of nerve impulses. Low levels of phosphatidylserine are associated with Parkinson's disease. (For more information on phosphatidylserine, see page 229.)

One study showed that taking **riboflavin** (vitamin B_2), in addition to a non-red-meat diet, led to the recovery of some motor function in people with Parkinson's disease. (For more information on riboflavin, see page 245.)

SAMe may be useful for people with Parkinson's disease and who also have depression. Studies indicate that people with Parkinson's disease have lower-than-normal levels of SAMe in their blood, and SAMe may be an effective alternative to antidepressants. (For more information on SAMe, see page 247.)

Antioxidants such as **vitamin C** and **E** reduce oxidative stress in the brain, slowing the progression of Parkinson's. Additionally, vitamin C may have a promising future in tempering some of the side effects of levodopa (Larodopa)—very often prescribed for Parkinson's disease—according to the results of a small study. In particular, many people taking levodopa experience an "on-off" effect, in which improved mobility occurs for a few hours and is followed by impaired mobility.

Vitamin C seemed to slightly reduce these side effects. (For more information on vitamins C and E, see pages 284 and 292.)

MY SUPPLEMENT LIST—PARKINSON'S DISEASE

SUPPLEMENT	RECOMMENDED DOSAGE
Alpha Lipoic Acid	*Capsule:* Take 250 mg, 2–4 capsules daily, in divided doses, with meals.
CDP-Choline	*Capsule or Tablet:* Take 400 mg of CDP-choline three times a day. *Note:* Some people may experience a fishy body odor when taking choline at this dosage.
CoQ10	*Softgel:* Take up to 1,200 mg daily in divided doses.
NAC	*Capsule:* Take 600 mg two to three times per day.
NADH	NADH was given intravenously in the few published studies on Parkinson's disease. Ask your neurologist if this might be useful for you.
Phosphatidyl-serine	*Capsule:* Take 100 mg three times per day, with meals.
Riboflavin	*Capsule or Tablet:* Studies using 30 mg three times a day found positive results. Consult your doctor to determine an appropriate dosage of riboflavin for you.
Vitamin C	*Capsule or Tablet:* Take 800 mg daily of buffered vitamin C divided into two or three doses, with meals. High doses of vitamin C may have a laxative effect.
Vitamin E	*Capsule:* Take 1,200 IU daily of a natural product containing mixed tocopherols. *Note:* This is a high dose of vitamin E and should only be taken under a doctor's supervision.

POISON IVY

AS THE SAYING GOES, "Leaves of three, let them be." For centuries, this simple utterance has inspired fear in the hearts of many. And when you consider the plant to which it refers, the fear is well justified—it is the scourge of family vacations, the bane of avid hikers and wanderers in the woods, and a financial goldmine for the calamine lotion industry. The plant is none other than the seemingly benign but persistently aggravating poison ivy.

WHAT IS IT?

Upon first glance, this stubby green weed with clusters of three irregularly shaped leaves doesn't look like it could do much harm.

However, contained within those leaves is an oily resin known as urushiol, the most potent allergen in the world. More than 50 percent of all people are allergic to urushiol, which is also the reactive substance in poison oak and poison sumac. Since an allergy to poison ivy can develop at any time in life, immunity in youth is no guarantee against future outbreaks. In addition, just 1 nanogram (1 billionth of a gram) of the stuff is all that's needed to cause a rash.

If you have ever been unlucky enough to brush against poison ivy, you are no doubt aware of the results. Typically within 24 to 48 hours, severe itching occurs, followed by a red inflammation and skin blisters. In severe cases, the blisters begin to ooze, an especially unpleasant side effect. Luckily, poison ivy is rarely life-threatening (see Did You Know? below), and the irritating symptoms it causes generally subside in 7 to 10 days. Despite the common misconception, poison ivy is not contagious and does not spread from an eruption site to other areas of the body; the only areas affected are those exposed to urushiol oil.

The first step in treating poison ivy is to wash it as soon as possible with soap and cold water. If you can wash the contact site within 3 minutes, you may actually have a chance of stopping the reaction before it starts. If you don't succeed, read the tips that follow for natural ways to soothe and even reduce an allergic reaction to poison ivy.

WHAT SHOULD I USE?
Aloe • Calendula • Chamomile • Vitamin C

Aloe (also called aloe vera) is well known for its soothing, itch-relieving properties, and this also applies to the itching and burning of poison ivy. Use fresh juice from the leaves of the aloe vera plant to relieve the itchy

When Ivy Turns Dangerous

Did You Know?

Although the symptoms of poison ivy are troubling, they are rarely life-threatening. Often, the rash and itching subside within 7 to 10 days. About 15 percent of the 120 million Americans allergic to poison ivy will break out in a rash within 4 to 12 hours after contact with the plant. Swelling will soon follow and may be so severe that if it affects the eyelids, it will swell them shut. In these rare instances, fluid-filled blisters are also known to break open on the skin. If you happen to be one of the unlucky few who have a severe reaction to poison ivy, seek medical attention immediately.

rash, since you can be more certain of its potency than with some commercial brands. (For more information on aloe, see page 27.)

While no specific research has been performed on the effect of **calendula** on the rash of poison ivy, calendula has some documented anti-inflammatory effects on the skin. (For more information on calendula, see page 61.)

Chamomile is perhaps the most aggressively tested herbal remedy for skin inflammation, or *dermatitis*, which includes poison ivy. Some human studies suggest that chamomile ointment may actually work better than hydrocortisone cream in easing dermatitis, and it has been shown to improve wound healing when applied topically. (For more information on chamomile, see page 67.)

Vitamin C is well-known for its anti-inflammatory and histamine-blocking properties—both big pluses when dealing with an allergic reaction such as poison ivy. Although the effectiveness of "mega-doses" of vitamin C is questionable, many people have experienced diminished itching and improved healing of the poison ivy rash when taking large oral daily doses of this vitamin. (For more information on vitamin C, see page 284.)

MY SUPPLEMENT LIST—POISON IVY

SUPPLEMENT	RECOMMENDED DOSAGE
Aloe	*Topical:* Use juice from an aloe vera plant to relieve itching. Simply break off part of the plant and squeeze the juice onto the skin as needed.
Calendula	*Topical:* May be used to decrease the inflammation of the rash. Apply as needed.
Chamomile	*Topical—Ointment:* Use chamomile ointment to relieve itching and speed healing. Simply spread the ointment over the affected area as needed.
Vitamin C	*Oral—Capsule or Tablet:* Take 1,000 mg from two to four times daily.

PREMENSTRUAL SYNDROME

SOME PEOPLE THINK THERE IS NO SUCH THING as premenstrual syndrome (PMS). But tell that to the scores of women who experience some kind of premenstrual symptoms every month and you may have your work cut out for you! Over the past several decades, few medical conditions have received as much attention and stirred up as much controversy as PMS. Although PMS is now recognized as a legitimate, cyclical set of physical and behavioral symptoms, part of the confusion surrounding it comes from the vast number of symptoms that can accompany the syndrome. Researchers have discovered more than 150 different maladies that can be classified as reflecting PMS.

WHAT IS IT?

Although the term PMS can cover a laundry list of symptoms, the most common include bloating, weight gain, mood swings, anxiety, depression, breast swelling and tenderness, headaches, lack of concentration, and changes in appetite and sexual desire. PMS affects about 75 percent of women in varying degrees, and the most popular current theory attributes its cause to changes in hormonal balance before the beginning of the menstrual cycle. Luckily, the onset of PMS is usually predictable. PMS can typically be expected from 7 to 14 days before the start of the menstrual cycle.

PMS does *not* have to be an inevitable and dreaded part of your monthly menstrual cycle. Studies indicate that herbs and supplements may reduce and prevent symptoms of PMS in some cases with great effectiveness.

WHAT SHOULD I TAKE?
Black Cohosh • Calcium • Chasteberry
Dong Quai • Evening Primrose Oil • Ginkgo Biloba (Ginkgo)
Magnesium • St. John's Wort • Vitamin B₆ • Vitamin E

Although **black cohosh** may be better known for tempering symptoms of menopause, the German Commission E (see page 16) approves it for PMS as well as dysmnenorrhea, or painful menstruation. (For more information on black cohosh, see page 48.)

PMS shares many of the same symptoms as **calcium** deficiency, and research indicates that supplemental calcium alleviates most of the mental and physical symptoms associated with PMS. One study of 497 women with PMS, found that those who took 1,200 milligrams of calcium a day had a 48 percent overall reduction in symptoms. (For more information on calcium, see page 57.)

Chasteberry is an herb that combats PMS by relieving irritability, depression, headache, and breast tenderness. Chasteberry does not, however, have an immediate effect. A minimum of 3 months of taking this supplement is recommended, and as long as 6 months may be needed to experience the therapeutic effects of chasteberry. (For more information on chasteberry, see page 69.)

Traditionally, **dong quai** has been used to treat menstrual cramps and general discomfort accompanying PMS, although more research is needed to determine its effectiveness. (For more information on dong quai, see page 105.)

Some studies suggest that **evening primrose oil**, which is rich in essential fatty acids, may reduce PMS-related discomfort such as breast pain, depression, and bloating. (For more information on evening primrose oil, see page 115.)

In a single trial, **ginkgo** showed great promise as an herbal treatment for symptoms of PMS. A standardized extract of ginkgo was shown to decrease the congestive symptoms of PMS caused by the accumulation of excess blood or fluid, and including water retention, weight gain, and breast tenderness. (For more information on ginkgo, see page 138.)

Magnesium was shown to be most effective for relieving PMS symptoms when taken together with vitamin B_6 (see page 279). Magnesium should also be taken with calcium (see above), since calcium can maximize the body's absorption of this important mineral. Conversely, a high intake of refined sugar will increase the amount of magnesium excreted in urine, and dairy products interfere with the body's absorption of magnesium. (For more information on magnesium, see page 203.)

St. John's wort may hold promise for relieving symptoms of PMS. A 3-month study of 19 women with PMS found that St. John's wort decreased overall symptoms of PMS by half in two-thirds of the women. (For more information on St. John's wort, see page 262.)

Tips for Tempering PMS

Healthy Hints

You can temper symptoms of PMS in a variety of ways. Read on for tips to keep the misery of PMS at bay.

■ **Exercise regularly.** Studies show that daily, regular exercise for 30 to 60 minutes helps to ease all symptoms of PMS.

■ **Skip salt.** Women who have PMS consume 78 percent more sodium than they should, accounting for a lot of unnecessary bloating! Despite common cravings for french fries and other salty foods, salt will only increase fluid retention and cause more bloating and discomfort.

■ **Stick to decaf.** A 1990 study showed that women who consumed caffeinated coffee were more likely to have PMS, and that the more they consumed the worse their symptoms became.

■ **Keep a record.** Although guidelines exist for universal triggers of PMS, every woman's body will react individually to different foods. Keep a journal of all the foods you eat and your symptoms to help determine which foods trigger your PMS.

Vitamin B₆ increases the speed at which the body absorbs magnesium. When taken in combination with magnesium, vitamin B_6 has shown some effectiveness in alleviating PMS. Vitamin B_6 also plays an important role in the breakdown and processing of important brain-regulating chemicals, which may further help to temper symptoms of PMS. (For more information on vitamin B_6, see page 279.)

Preliminary studies indicate that **vitamin E** may help relieve the breast swelling and tenderness associated with PMS. Try taking vitamin E supplements if breast discomfort is your most painful PMS symptom. (For more information on vitamin E, see page 292.)

MY SUPPLEMENT LIST—PREMENSTRUAL SYNDROME

SUPPLEMENT	RECOMMENDED DOSAGE
Black Cohosh	*Capsule:* Take an extract standardized to provide 2.5% triterpene glycosides 2–4 capsules of 250 mg per day, in divided doses, between meals.
Calcium	*Capsule or Tablet:* Take 1,200 mg daily divided into two or three doses. *Note:* Studies indicate that calcium carbonate is the most effective form of calcium for reducing PMS symptoms.
Chasteberry	*Capsule:* Take 175 to 225 mg of an extract standardized to contain 0.5% agnuside each day before breakfast. *Note:* Chasteberry should not be used by women who are pregnant or nursing. It may take 3 months to experience chasteberry's therapeutic effects.
Dong Quai	*Capsule:* Take 3,000 to 3,600 mg daily divided into three doses between meals. *Note:* In traditional Chinese medicine, dong quai is often prescribed with other herbs, including black cohosh. The optimal dosage of dong quai varies. Consult your doctor or herbalist to determine an appropriate dose for you. It is typically taken together with other herbs.
Evening Primrose Oil	*Capsule:* Take up to 2–4 g per day, in divided doses, with meals. The dosage is based on a gamma-linolenic acid (GLA) content of 9% to 12%.
Ginkgo	*Capsule:* Take 120 to 160 mg once daily of an extract standardized to contain 24% ginkgo flavone glycosides and 6% terpene lactones. May increase the dose to 240 mg daily as needed.
Magnesium	*Tablet:* Take 400 mg every day and twice daily 1 week before menstruation. *Note:* Take in the form of magnesium glycinate to avoid loose stools. Large amounts of magnesium can cause diarrhea; if this becomes a problem for you, reduce your dosage.

(continued)

MY SUPPLEMENT LIST—PREMENSTRUAL SYNDROME (continued)	
SUPPLEMENT	**RECOMMENDED DOSAGE**
St. John's Wort	*Capsule:* Take 300 mg daily of an extract standardized to contain 900 mcg of hypericin 0.3% three times daily, between meals.
Vitamin B$_6$	*Tablet:* Take 50 mg up to three times daily. *Note:* If you have liver disease, consult your doctor before taking more than 50 mg of vitamin B$_6$ daily.
Vitamin E	*Capsule:* Take 400 to 600 IU daily of a natural supplement containing mixed tocopherols.

PROSTATE HEALTH

HERE'S A QUICK RIDDLE: What begins with the size of a pea, ends with the size of a walnut, and is the source of most male urinary problems? Answer: The tiny organ called the prostate that rests just below the male bladder.

WHAT IS IT?

The most common prostate problems include prostate enlargement, prostate infection or inflammation, and prostate pain. Most benign prostate problems begin when men reach their forties, which is when the prostate undergoes its second "growth spurt." However, prostate problems can begin for some men in their twenties. At about age 40, cells in the prostate begin to reproduce rapidly, and the tissues of the prostate often become enlarged. By the time they reach their eighties, 80 percent of men will experience prostate enlargement.

Also called benign prostatic hyperplasia (BPH), prostate enlargement is a common problem and may be a natural part of aging. Some BPH symptoms are urinary urgency or frequency, awaking at night with the urge to urinate, a weak urine stream, a flow that stops and starts during urination, and urinary incontinence. BPH is associated with an inability to fully empty the bladder and, in extreme cases, can cause blood to enter the urine or lead to urinary tract infection.

Prostatitis (the suffix "*itis*" means inflammation) is an inflammation of the prostate gland. This inflammation can occur with or without a bacterial infection. In fact, only 5 percent of men with prostatitis have bacterial prostatitis. Acute prostatitis is the least common but most severe form of prostatitis. It occurs with an onset of symptoms including fever, chills, burning during urination, difficulty in urinating, and pain in the lower back, bladder region, or behind the scrotum. These symptoms warrant an immediate visit to your doctor.

Chronic bacterial prostatitis is a long-standing prostate condition. It may be caused by a recurring or incompletely cured infection. Although symptoms of this condition are milder than those of acute prostatitis, they often last longer and are harder to treat. Relatively long courses of broad-spectrum antibiotic therapy are often required to eradicate this disease.

Chronic nonbacterial prostatitis is a condition with symptoms similar to those of chronic bacterial prostatitis. However, no bacterial or other infection of any sort exists in chronic nonbacterial prostatitis; rather this condition is caused by muscle tension in the pelvis. Treatment for this condition involves biofeedback, therapeutic exercises, acupuncture, psychotherapy, and perhaps herbs and supplements to decrease pelvic muscle tension.

Sometimes, symptoms of prostate problems are minor enough that treatment is not necessary. At other times, they may be an indication of a more serious health concern. It is important to communicate any symptoms of prostate problems to your doctor. Despite the variety of problems that affect the prostate, it can be maintained and kept healthy by an effective regimen of nutritional supplements and herbs.

KITCHEN TIPS

OPT FOR PUMPKIN SEEDS

Studies have shown that pumpkin seeds, which have a high content of zinc, encourage improvement of BPH symptoms, especially at an early stage of this condition. If you have BPH or if you have a high risk of developing it, consider eating a handful of pumpkin seeds every day. You may also drizzle pumpkin seed oil over salads, meat, or chicken to get a healthy dose of pumpkin seeds.

Prostate Cancer Warning Signs

Did You Know?

Prostate cancer is the most common type of cancer in men, affecting 30 percent of American males. The average age at diagnosis is 72 years. Early detection of catching the cancer while it is still confined to the prostate is associated with greater cure rate. Treatment becomes increasingly challenging once the cancer has spread beyond the prostate. The American Urological Association (AUA) recommends screening for prostate cancer through annual prostate examinations and blood tests for all men over 50 years of age. For African American men and men with a family history of prostate cancer, the AUA recommends screening beginning at age 40 and over.

The problem with diagnosing prostate cancer is that its symptoms are difficult to detect in the early stages of this disease or mimic the symptoms of other prostate problems. It is important to be aware of the symptoms of prostate cancer in order to detect it at an early stage. Its symptoms include:

- Dull pain in the pelvic area
- Urgent and painful urination
- Difficulty in starting urination
- Weak urine flow
- A sensation that the bladder is full
- Frequent nighttime urination
- Blood in the urine
- Painful ejaculation
- Pain in the lower back, hips, or upper thighs
- Appetite and weight loss
- Persistent bone pain

If you are experiencing any of these above symptoms, see your doctor immediately. Remember, early detection is crucial to beating prostate cancer!

FRIENDS AND FOES

ZINC AND COPPER

Taking zinc at dosages above 30 mg a day may lead to **copper** deficiency. Be sure to take a copper supplement if you plan to take zinc in a high dosage. Most doctors recommend taking 2 to 3 mg of copper a day along with zinc.

WHAT SHOULD I TAKE?

The following supplements are intended to keep the prostate healthy. If you think you have a prostate problem make sure to consult your doctor before taking any supplements.

Bee Pollen • Beta-Sitosterol • Bromelain • Cranberry Flaxseed • Kava • Quercetin • Red Clover • Saw Palmetto Selenium • Uva Ursi • Vitamin C • Zinc

Because of its anti-inflammatory properties, Cernilton—a proprietary blend of **bee pollen** extract—may be helpful in improving symptoms of prostatitis. Preliminary studies indicate that Cernilton tablets were effective in treating chronic prostatitis, without the side effects often associated with prescription medication. Other research suggests that bee pollen may be effective in inhibiting the growth of prostate cancer cells. More research is needed to determine bee pollen's exact role in improving prostate health. (For more information on bee pollen, see page 37.)

Beta-sitosterol may have a positive effect on some of the symptoms associated with BPH. In a study of 200 men with BPH, supplementation with beta-sitosterol for 6 months, as compared to a placebo, improved urinary flow and produced an overall improvement in symptoms. The placebo group in the study reported no change in symptoms. (For more information on beta-sitosterol, see page 40.)

Cranberries contain proanthocyanidins—substances that may have bacteria-fighting properties. Cranberries are often recommended for the treatment of urinary tract infections (see page 605), and may help in preventing prostatitis resulting from recurrent urinary tract infection. (For more information on cranberry, see page 90.)

Research indicates that people with a high dietary intake of omega-3 fatty acids may have a decreased risk for developing prostate cancer. One study suggests that a low-fat diet supplemented with **flaxseed** may help thwart prostate cancer. Other studies have found that men who ate fish more than three times a week had a reduced risk of prostate cancer. One population-based study of 6,272 men found that after 30 years, those who ate no fish had two- to threefold greater incidence of prostate cancer than those who did. Although some of this may be due to the high content of omega-3 fatty acids in fish, other factors may also play a role. Besides their potential cancer-fighting effects, omega-3 fatty acids may show promise for people with BPH. A preliminary study found that supplementation with flaxseed oil reduced the amount of urine retained in the bladder in BPH. It also increased libido, reduced the size of the enlarged prostate, and in most cases stopped nighttime urination. More research is needed into the effects of flaxseed supplements on BPH. (For more information on omega-3 fatty acids and flaxseed, see pages 221 and 126.)

Kava (also called kava kava), may be useful for relaxing muscles in people with chronic nonbacterial prostatitis. Studies have found that kava compared favorably with benzodiazepine (Valium)—a prescription sedative medication. (For more information on kava, see page 178.)

Quercetin—a flavonoid derived from plants—may help to ease chronic nonbacterial prostatitis. Quercetin is has anti-inflammatory as well as antibacterial properties, and studies have found that supplementation with quercetin may decrease symptoms of chronic nonbacterial prostatitis. Other studies suggest that **bromelain** may help the body to absorb quercetin, in addition to its own anti-inflammatory effects. (For more information on bromelain and quercetin, see pages 54 and 236.)

Preliminary research indicates that **red clover** may help prevent prostate cancer and may even kill cancerous cells in men with prostate cancer. (For more information on red clover, see page 238.)

Saw palmetto is the herbal gold standard when it comes to BPH, and studies have shown it to be as effective as finasteride (Proscar)—a prescription drug commonly used to treat BPH—without the unwanted side effects. Choose a standardized extract of saw palmetto, since it seems to be more effective than a tea or a tincture of this herb. A 3-year study in Germany found that saw palmetto extract reduced nighttime urination and improved urinary flow in BPH. However, a study recently published in the *New England Journal of Medicine* did not confirm these results. Saw palmetto has also been used traditionally to treat the inflammation and swelling associated with prostatitis. (For more information on saw palmetto, see page 249.)

Research indicates that blood levels of **selenium** may be low in people with prostate cancer. One double-blind trial involving 1,312 people with a history of skin cancer found that after 3 years, supplementation with selenium had no effect on their skin but did reduce the incidence of prostate cancer by 63 percent. Many experts recommend supplementation with 200 micrograms of selenium to reduce the risk as well as slow the progression of prostate cancer. (For more information on selenium, see page 253.)

The leaves of the **uva ursi** plant contain compounds that are effective in fighting a number of bacteria that cause prostatitis. However, uva ursi should not be used for more than 1 week because of its high tannin content. (For more information on uva ursi, see page 270.)

Vitamin C, among its many other medicinal properties, has been shown in test-tube studies to slow the growth of the bacteria known as *Escherichia coli*, a common cause of both acute and chronic bacterial prostatitis. Although additional studies are needed to test the efficacy of vitamin C in prostatitis, many doctors recommend taking vitamin C for this condition when its cause is the *Escherichia coli* bacteria. (For more information on vitamin C, see page 284.)

Preliminary research suggests that when taken in high doses, **zinc** may reduce the size of the prostate in BPH. Other research suggests that zinc may help reduce the risk of prostatitis-induced infertility. Consult your doctor to determine whether zinc supplementation is appropriate for you. (For more information on zinc, see page 304.)

MY SUPPLEMENT LIST—PROSTATE HEALTH

SUPPLEMENT	RECOMMENDED DOSAGE
Bee Pollen	The ideal dosage of bee pollen is unknown. Follow individual product labels for specific dosage information.
Beta-Sitosterol	*Capsule or Tablet:* Take 60–120 mg of a standardized extract daily divided into two or three doses.
Cranberry	*Capsule:* Take 2,700–4,500 mg daily divided into three or four doses. *Juice:* Drink 16 oz of unsweetened cranberry juice every day (which may be diluted with water).
Flaxseed	*Flaxseed Oil:* Take 1 tbsp daily, with meals.
Kava	*Capsule:* Take 200 mg extract (standardized to contain 60 mg kavalactones), two capsules, two-three times per day, between meals. *Note:* Consult your doctor before taking kava. Kava may cause liver damage when taken in high dosages. Kava may also enhance the effects of alcohol, antidepressant medications, and sedative medications.

SUPPLEMENT	RECOMMENDED DOSAGE
MY SUPPLEMENT LIST—PROSTATE HEALTH	
Quercetin and Bromelain	*Capsule or Tablet:* Take 200–500 mg of quercetin two or three times daily between meals; take 250–500 mg of bromelain two to three times daily between meals; look for a bromelain product containing 2,400 gelatin-dissolving units (GDU) or 3,600 milk-clotting units (MCU) per gram.
Red Clover	*Tea:* Mix 1–2 tsp of red clover dried flower tops with 1 cup of boiling water. Steep for 10–15 minutes and drink up to three cups daily. *Capsule or Tablet:* Follow individual product labels for specific dosage information.
Saw Palmetto	*Capsule:* Take 320 mg twice a day of an extract standardized to contain 80% to 90% fatty acids.
Selenium	*Tablet:* Take 200 mcg daily.
Uva Ursi	*Tea:* Add 3 g of ground herb to 5 oz of boiling water. Drink up to four times daily. *Capsule:* Take 700 to 1,000 mg three times a day of an extract standardized to contain 20% arbutin. *Note:* Do not take uva ursi for more than 7 days or if you have kidney disease.
Vitamin C	*Capsule or Tablet:* Take 250–500 mg twice a day in the form of buffered ascorbic acid. May cause loose stools.
Zinc	*Tablet:* Take 50 mg daily. *Note:* Be sure to take 2–3 mg of copper every day along with zinc to avoid a copper deficiency.

PSORIASIS

PSORIASIS IS A CHRONIC condition affecting about 0.5 to 1.5 percent of people in North America. Although the severity of psoriasis may vary individually, most people with this disorder experience it in its mildest form. While not contagious, psoriasis can be uncomfortable, unsightly, and embarrassing—especially in the summer, when more skin is exposed.

WHAT IS IT?

Psoriasis is a chronic condition characterized by raised, pink areas of skin with silver scales. It most commonly affects the knees, elbows, groin, and scalp, and many people experience periodic flare-ups of the condition alternating with periods when it subsides. Psoriasis may be limited to a small area of the body or can cover large areas simultaneously. Its symptoms include sore, painful, and extremely itchy skin. At times, psoriasis breakouts can occur on the soles of the feet and palms of the hands, causing oozing blisters. Although people with psoriasis generally function normally, the condition often causes problems with self-esteem. The unsightly appearance of affected, psoriatic skin can make social interactions difficult and embarrassing, causing anxiety and depression. There are also times when psoriasis causes pain and can interfere with daily routines. It is important to see a doctor in these instances.

Some research indicates that alcohol consumption may increase the frequency of flare-ups of psoriasis, and curbing alcohol intake therefore makes good sense for people affected by this condition. Other studies show that smoking and environmental or emotional stress may be associated with an increased risk of psoriasis and psoriatic flare-ups. Common treatments for psoriasis include skin creams, ointments, oral medications, and ultraviolet-light therapy. In addition, numerous studies have shown that nutritional supplements can play a key role in relieving the pain and itching of psoriasis, and even in preventing breakouts of this condition.

Stress Plays a Role in Psoriasis Flare-Ups

Flare-ups of psoriasis appear to be triggered by stress. A study published in the *Archives of Dermatology* suggests that people who are anxious, worried, or experiencing high levels of stress are less likely to respond to treatment for psoriasis. Furthermore, high stress and anxiety levels can actually worsen psoriasis symptoms. One of the best things to do for people with psoriasis is therefore simply to relax. But because eliminating stress or anxiety is easier said than done, experts have begun to use certain psychological therapies for easing the symptoms of psoriasis.

A specific and fairly new therapy used primarily for treating people with post-traumatic stress disorder but which also seems promising for psoriasis is eye movement desensitization and reprocessing (EMDR). EMDR integrates various elements of psychotherapy with one another, including psychodynamic, cognitive behav-

ioral, interpersonal, experiential, and body-centered therapies. In one 12-month study of EMDR for stress-induced psoriasis, four patients received from three to six sessions of EMDR for 4 to 12 weeks, and all patients experienced improvement. When the researchers who conducted the study re-examined the patients 6 to 12 months later, all four had maintained a significant improvement in their symptoms.

Another seemingly promising psychological therapy for psoriasis is music therapy. A German study found that patients with psoriasis who had Medical Resonance Therapy Music (MRT-Music) three times a day for 30 minutes, in addition to their regular regimen of treatment for psoriasis, had a reduced heart rate and blood pressure and also a decrease in their dermatological symptoms.

Although more research is needed to secure psychological therapy as an effective component of treatment for psoriasis, research on this technique is promising.

WHAT SHOULD I TAKE?
Aloe • Folic Acid • Milk Thistle
Omega-3 Fatty Acids • Slippery Elm • Zinc

A study of **aloe** (also called aloe vera), when applied directly from an aloe plant, found that it produced significantly better results in relieving pain and itching and eliminating psoriatic patches of skin than did a placebo. (For more information on aloe, see page 27.)

Methotrexate (Trexall), a medication that is often prescribed to treat psoriasis, may impair the body's ability to absorb **folic acid** (vitamin B_9). Discuss taking folic acid supplements with your doctor if you are taking methotrexate, so that you can maintain healthy levels of this important nutrient. In conjunction with folic acid, you may add **milk thistle** to your supplement regimen if you are taking methotrexate for psoriasis. Methotrexate can be damaging to the liver, and milk thistle is known for its liver-protecting effects. (For more information on folic acid and milk thistle, see pages 130 and 210.)

Omega-3 fatty acids, in the form of fish oil, may help reduce the itching, redness, and scaling of psoriatic lesions. Preliminary research indicates that fish oil preparations may also be helpful when applied topically to psoriatic lesions. A further benefit of fish oil is that it may reduce triglyceride levels in the blood that commonly occurs with the vitamin-A derived medications known as retinoids that are commonly prescribed for psoriasis. (For more information on omega-3 fatty acids, see page 221.)

Slippery elm has not received scientific study for the treatment of psoriasis. However, it was part of the Edgar Cayce recommendation, in conjunction with a special diet. (For more information about slippery elm, see page 256.)

Although studies of **zinc** in preventing psoriasis have given mixed results, it has been found that people with persistent psoriasis are often zinc deficient. (For more information on zinc, see page 304.)

MY SUPPLEMENT LIST—PSORIASIS

SUPPLEMENT	RECOMMENDED DOSAGE
Aloe	*Topical—Gel:* Apply aloe gel directly from the plant to psoriatic lesions three times daily for 4 weeks. Aloe gel may also be purchased from your local health-food store or drugstore.
Folic Acid	Consult your doctor about folic acid supplementation if you are taking the prescription medication methotrexate to treat psoriasis.

(continued)

MY SUPPLEMENT LIST—PSORIASIS (continued)	
SUPPLEMENT	**RECOMMENDED DOSAGE**
Milk Thistle	Consult your doctor about milk thistle supplementation if you are taking the prescription medication methotrexate to treat psoriasis.
Omega-3 Fatty Acids	*Oral:* Take 1–2 g of omega-3 fatty acids per day, in divided doses, with meals. The amount of omega-3 fatty acid will vary by manufacturer, so be sure to check the product label carefully. *Topical—Cream:* Apply a preparation that contains 10% fish oil to lesions twice daily. Results may be seen after 7 weeks of treatment.
Slippery Elm:	*Capsule:* Take up to twelve 400 mg per day.
Zinc	*Tablet:* Take 30 mg once a day.

RESTLESS LEGS SYNDROME

WHETHER DURING A LONG business meeting, a weekend with in-laws, or a painfully boring seminar, everyone has experienced restlessness. For about 2 to 10 percent of Americans, however, restlessness, specifically in the legs, is such an uncomfortable sensation that it creates an uncontrollable urge to get up and move around. This malady is known as restless legs syndrome (RLS).

WHAT IS IT?

Doctors still don't know exactly what causes RLS, although many believe that iron deficiency and heredity may play a role. The problem may also be related to the body's inability to process iron, even when an individual does not have iron deficiency. Other recent studies suggest that RLS may occur when particular areas of the brain do not get the iron they need (see Did You Know, below). There are two main forms of RLS. The first of these is a mixed type of RLS, which may be characterized by a tingling, tickling, or jittery sensation in the legs during periods of inactivity. Most people who have this type of RLS experience their most severe symptoms at night when they are trying to sleep, although they can have these uncomfortable feelings in their legs while in a car, on an airplane, or at a movie theater. The second form of RLS produces the same tingling effects as the first form, but without the accompanying pain. Additionally, women with RLS may have more headaches than the general population.

One of the most detrimental effects of RLS is sleep deprivation, since the uncontrollable urge to move around usually awakens the people it affects (as well as their spouses!) in the middle of the night. Periodic limb movements during sleep, such as involuntary kicking (which can occur hundreds of times a night) is another problem that may occur in RLS. Although there is no known cure for RLS, medications and self-care may ease its symptoms. The use of muscle relaxants and sleep medications are common conventional methods for treating RLS. Other helpful approaches are baths and massages, applying warm and cool packs to the legs, meditation, yoga, and exercise. Going hand in hand with this approach is a solid regimen of supplements that relieve the pain and help allow sleep.

WHAT SHOULD I TAKE?
Folic Acid • Iron
Magnesium • Vitamin E

Certain people with RLS may respond to supplementation with **folic acid** (vitamin B$_9$). Some studies show that RLS may occur during pregnancy because of a folic acid deficiency. In these cases, increasing folic acid intake to healthy levels may ease the pain and discomfort associated with RLS. (For more information on folic acid, see page 130.)

Numerous studies have shown a link between **iron** deficiency and RLS, particularly in the elderly. Increasing your iron intake beyond what you may get from a multivitamin may help deter or ease the symptoms associated with RLS. However, this must be done only under the supervision of a doctor. (For more information on iron, see page 175.)

Along with folic acid and iron, **magnesium** deficiency may occur in people with RLS. Making sure your body has adequate amounts of magnesium may help to ease RLS. (For more information on magnesium, see page 203.)

In a small study, **vitamin E** produced positive results in easing the discomfort associated with RLS. Although the study involved only nine people, all of the participants experienced partial or full relief of symptoms with vitamin E supplementation. (For more information on vitamin E, see page 292.)

MY SUPPLEMENT LIST—RESTLESS LEGS SYNDROME

SUPPLEMENT	RECOMMENDED DOSAGE
Folic Acid	*Tablet:* Take 5–30 mg daily for up to 1 month.
	Note: Pregnant women should consult their doctor before taking any type of supplement. Consult your doctor before taking this dosage of folic acid, as it is extremely high.
Iron	*Tablet:* Take 100–200 mg daily for up to 1 month.
	Caution: Ask your doctor to check your iron level. Only take iron supplements if you are iron deficient.
Magnesium	*Tablet:* Take 400 mg two times daily, 800 mg at bedtime.
	Note: Take in the form of magnesium glycinate to avoid loose stools. Large amounts of magnesium can cause diarrhea; if this becomes a problem for you, reduce your dosage.
Vitamin E	*Capsule:* Take 400–800 IU daily of a natural product containing mixed tocopherols.

RHEUMATOID ARTHRITIS

RHEUMATOID ARTHRITIS (RA), one of the most debilitating forms of arthritis, affects 2.1 million Americans. Experts are still unsure of what causes RA. What they do know is that it affects women three times as often as men and that it generally strikes between the ages of 20 and 50.

WHAT IS IT?

RA is an inflammatory disease that typically occurs in the small joints of the hands and feet. It can flare up and subside at random and may cause generalized stiffness and soreness simultaneously in various joints throughout the body. As RA progresses, it can result in deformity and loss of movement of the afflicted joints. Although the precise cause of RA is unknown, it is believed to be an autoimmune disorder (see page 340) in which the body's immune system attacks healthy joint tissue, causing it to become inflamed.

While RA may not be curable, many steps are available to allow those who have it to live healthy, active lives. Medications are available to relieve symptoms and slow the progression of the disease. Other important steps include weight control, a healthy diet, avoiding allergy-causing foods, regular exercise, and relaxation techniques. A solid regimen of symptom-relieving and disease-slowing supplements may play a crucial role in a personal program for managing RA.

WHAT SHOULD I TAKE?
Boswellia • Cat's Claw • Evening Primrose Oil
Ginger • Omega-3 Fatty Acids • Vitamin E • Willow Bark

Preliminary research indicates that **boswellia** may reduce the pain and swelling associated with RA, although more research is needed to confirm its effectiveness. (For more information on boswellia, see page 52.)

Cat's claw may reduce pain in joints that are affected by RA. In preliminary studies, cat's claw faired better than placebo in alleviating tenderness in arthritic joints. (For more information on cat's claw, see page 63.)

Evening primrose oil is one of the richest herbal sources of omega-6 fatty acids. These essential fatty acids stop joint pain, swelling, and morning stiffness in their tracks. Evening primrose oil also has the benefit of enhancing the effectiveness of nonsteroidal anti-inflammatory drugs (NSAIDs) such as aspirin or ibuprofen. (For more information on evening primrose oil, see page 115.)

Ginger, when taken as a supplement or tea, has been traditionally used in Ayurvedic and Chinese medicine as a remedy for inflammation. Preliminary evidence indicates that ginger may be an effective anti-inflammatory agent in people with RA. (For more information on ginger, see page 136.)

KITCHEN TIPS

OLIVE OIL MAY PREVENT RHEUMATOID ARTHRITIS

When sautéing or otherwise cooking vegetables, use olive oil. Cooking with olive oil may help prevent RA. A study published in the *American Journal of Clinical Nutrition* found that people who had a diet rich in vegetables cooked in olive oil had a lower risk for developing RA than those who did not.

Alleviating Arthritis Aches

Healthy Hints

Lifestyle changes may help control the pain of RA. Read on for some helpful hints to alleviate arthritis-related aches and pains.

■ **Cut the caffeine.** Drinking 4 or more cups of coffee a day may increase your risk of RA. Limit coffee intake to less than 4 cups a day.

■ **Try a vegan diet.** Research has shown that a vegan diet (a diet with absolutely no animal products), which is high in vegetables and fiber, may be beneficial for people with RA. *Note:* Be sure to consult your doctor before changing to a vegan diet.

■ **Go Mediterranean.** If a vegan diet seems too drastic for you, try a Mediterranean diet. Studies have shown that a Mediterranean diet, with its high content of olive oil, cooked vegetables, and fish, appears to ease symptoms of RA.

■ **Kick the habit.** Scientific study has shown a correlation between smoking and the risk of developing RA. Smoking puts stress on connective tissue, bringing unwelcome pain to people with RA.

Omega-3 fatty acids, in the form of fish oil supplements, have had moderate success in controlling RA. Regular supplementation with fish oil for up to 3 months has reportedly helped to reduce morning stiffness and joint tenderness associated with RA. Fish oil taken in conjunction with NSAIDs, such as aspirin and ibuprofen, has also shown benefits, although more study of this is needed. (For more information on omega-3 fatty acids, see page 221.)

Vitamin E may help alleviate pain associated with RA. Some reports suggest that low levels of vitamin E may increase the risk for developing RA. Additionally, vitamin E may increase the effectiveness of standard anti-inflammatory agents, as does evening primrose oil (see page 115). A German study found that vitamin E was as effective as diclofenac (Cataflam)—a commonly prescribed NSAID with potentially serious side effects—in treating RA. (For more information on vitamin E, see page 292.)

Salicin and other salicylates—compounds that are similar in structure to aspirin—give **willow bark** its pain-reducing and anti-inflammatory properties. Willow bark may not relieve rheumatoid arthritis pain as quickly as aspirin, but its effect may last longer, and it is gentler on the stomach. (For more information on willow bark, see page 298.)

MY SUPPLEMENT LIST—RHEUMATOID ARTHRITIS

SUPPLEMENT	RECOMMENDED DOSAGE
Boswellia	*Tablet:* Take 300 to 400 mg three times daily of a standardized extract that contains 37.5% boswellic acids.
Cat's Claw	*Capsule:* Take a standard extract in the form of *Uncaria tomentosa* or *Uncaria guyanensis* one to three times daily according to the manufacturer's directions.
Evening Primrose Oil	*Capsule:* Take up to 2–4 g per day, in divided doses, with meals. The dosage is based on a gamma-linolenic acid (GLA) content of 9% to 12%.
Ginger	*Tea:* 1 tsp or teabag of dried root steeped in 1 cup of water for 5 to 10 minutes. Drink up to four times daily. *Fresh:* Take 500 to 1,000 mg three to four times daily divided into several doses. To prepare the root, it's possible to press out the juice with a garlic press. Alternately, use a grater and swallow the grated ginger by placing it on the back of your tongue. *Extract:* Take 500 mg (standardized to contain 5% gingerols), 1–4 capsules per day, in divided doses, with food.
Omega-3 Fatty Acids	*Oral:* Take 5 g of omega-3 fatty acids per day, in divided doses, with meals. The amount of omega-3 fatty acid will vary by manufacturer, so be sure to check the product label carefully.

MY SUPPLEMENT LIST—RHEUMATOID ARTHRITIS	
SUPPLEMENT	**RECOMMENDED DOSAGE**
Vitamin E	*Capsule:* Take 1,200 IU daily divided into three doses of a natural product containing mixed tocopherols.
	Note: Only take this high a dose of vitamin E under a doctor's supervision.
Willow Bark	*Capsule:* Take 120 to 240 mg of a standardized extract daily.
	Caution: Do not take willow bark if you have an aspirin allergy, bleeding disorder, diabetes, or a peptic ulcer.

SEXUAL DYSFUNCTION

WHETHER YOU'RE A MAN OR a woman, problems in the bedroom, physical or emotional, are never easy to face. Just getting past the embarrassment of admitting there is a problem may be a daunting ordeal. However, almost everybody faces sexual dysfunction of one kind or another at some time in his or her life. For 20 to 30 million men, sexual dysfunction is a persistent and frustrating disorder. And although it's less publicized, a nearly equal number of women—an estimated 43 percent—face the problem as well.

WHAT IS IT?

Sexual dysfunction is a general term for complications of a sexual relationship, such as male impotence, vaginal spasms, painful intercourse, and decreased libido. Although sexual dysfunction typically occurs later in life, it is not a necessary part of the aging process.

Sexual dysfunction can have physical or psychological roots. Psychologically, diminished sexual desire may accompany depression. In such cases, antidepressant medications can be helpful for both

Changing Habits to Improve Male Sexual Dysfunction

Healthy Hints

Certain lifestyle habits may be particularly important for maintaining sexual function in men. Read on for tips on improving male sexual health.

■ **Exercise.** A study of men over age 50 found a correlation between erectile dysfunction and lack of exercise.

■ **Lose weight.** Obesity appears to play a role in the risk of sexual dysfunction in men. If you are overweight, this is just one more good reason to discuss a weight-loss plan with your doctor.

■ **Stay away from TV.** Believe it or not, a study of sexual dysfunction in men found that sitting in front of the tube for extensive periods of time seemed to increase the risk of erectile dysfunction.

■ **Don't drink.** Alcohol consumption may contribute to erectile dysfunction in men over age 50. Consider decreasing your alcohol intake if you experience difficulties with sexual function.

men and women. (However, some antidepressants may also cause sexual dysfunction.) Physically, sexual dysfunction both in men and in women may come from reduced blood flow to the sexual organs, usually as a consequence of poor overall circulation (great reason to stop smoking now). Other important causes of sexual dysfunction may be a dysfunction of the nervous system, such as from diabetes or spinal cord injury.

Since sexual dysfunction may be the first sign of a more serious medical condition, it is important to communicate it openly to your doctor to ensure that your health is sound. Along with your doctor's advice, natural herbs and supplements may help put a spark back in your sex life.

WHAT SHOULD I TAKE?
Arginine • Ginkgo Biloba (Ginkgo) • Ginseng
Pycnogenol • Vitamin C • Yohimbe

I was told that I would need a prescription from my doctor in order to take yohimbe, but I have seen yohimbe supplements sold over-the-counter in health-food stores. Is this supplement approved by the FDA?

Every once in a while, the evidence of an herbal product's medicinal value is so irrefutable that it breaks through into the realm of conventional medicine. Such is the case with the herb yohimbe, undoubtedly one of the most effective and popular remedies for erectile dysfunction. Yohimbe has received its fair share of attention in the medical community, and it has been the focus of many clinical trials.

Yohimbe was approved by the U.S. Food and Drug Administration (FDA) as a prescription medication for sexual dysfunction. As a result, several prescription drugs containing yohimbe have been developed for erectile dysfunction. Over-the-counter products containing yohimbe are available in most health-food stores, although this does not mean that they are necessarily safe. Yohimbe has a list of side effects ranging from headaches and anxiety to more serious conditions such as high blood pressure and heart palpitations. Many experts believe that the risks of taking yohimbe outweigh the benefits. If you decide to take yohimbe, it is very important to speak with your doctor first.

Your doctor may feel more comfortable about writing a prescription for a yohimbe-containing medication, which comes in a standardized dose, than about recommending an over-the-counter product containing yohimbe, in which the active ingredients often vary greatly. Nevertheless, with their doctors' approval, many men have found yohimbe to be an effective alternative to prescription medication.

Studies have found that supplementation with **arginine** and **pycnogenol** may yield substantial improvements in men with erectile dysfunction. One study found that after supplementation with the combination of arginine and pycnogenol, 92 percent of 40 men who had erectile dysfunction experienced a normal erection without any side effects. (For more information on arginine, see page 31.)

Ginkgo improves circulation throughout the body and therefore may play a role in reinvigorating blood flow to the sexual organs and improving sexual function. Studies show that men with erectile dysfunction may benefit from taking supplemental ginkgo. Additionally, preliminary research shows that ginkgo may be used to treat sexual dysfunction caused by antidepressant drugs. (For more information on ginkgo, see page 138.)

Ginseng—in both its Panax and Siberian forms—has been shown to play a positive role in increasing energy and libido. Preliminary data show that creams containing ginseng may be useful for men who have a decreased libido or difficulty with erections. One double-blind study found that men with erectile dysfunction had an increase in libido and the ability to maintain erections after daily supplementation with Panax ginseng. (For more information on ginseng, see page 141.)

Vitamin C stands out for its value in preserving healthy arteries. Taking a dose of vitamin C daily supports the integrity of the veins and minimizes the risk of sexual dysfunction due to poor circulation. A study of 42 healthy young adults found that supplementation with vitamin C resulted in an increase in frequency of their sexual activity. This effect was most noted in couples who had not been having intercourse before the study. (For more information on vitamin C, see page 284.)

Yohimbe has a long history of use as an aphrodisiac and has been used for centuries to treat erectile dysfunction, primarily because of its ability to dilate blood vessels and therby promote erection. However, because of its potentially negative side effects, which can include high blood pressure and heart palpitations, yohimbe should be taken only under a doctor's supervision. (For more information on yohimbe, see page 302.)

MY SUPPLEMENT LIST—SEXUAL DYSFUNCTION

SUPPLEMENT	RECOMMENDED DOSAGE
Arginine	*Tablet:* Take 2 g of L-arginine daily.

(continued)

MY SUPPLEMENT LIST—SEXUAL DYSFUNCTION (continued)	
SUPPLEMENT	**RECOMMENDED DOSAGE**
Ginkgo	*Capsule:* Take 120 to 240 mg in divided doses, daily between meals, of an extract standardized to contain 24% ginkgo glycosides and 6% terpene lactones.
Ginseng	*Capsule—Siberian Ginseng:* Take 1,000 mg two to three times a day, between meals, of an extract standardized to contain at least 1% eleutherosides. *Asian Ginseng:* Take 100 to 200 mg once a day of an extract standardized to contain 4% to 7% ginsenosides.
Pycnogenol	*Capsule:* Take 100 mg (standardized to contain 65% to 75% proanthocyanins) one to two times per day, between meals.
Vitamin C	*Capsule or Tablet:* The study described in the What Should I Take section on previous page used 3,000 mg daily of vitamin C. *Note:* Be sure to use a buffered form of vitamin C. If taking vitamin C causes loose stools, decrease your dosage and then gradually increase the dosage as tolerated.
Vitamin E	*Capsule:* Take 400 IU daily of a natural product containing mixed tocopherols.
Yohimbe	Yohimbe should only be used under medical supervision, by prescription. Consult your doctor to determine if prescription yohimbe is appropriate for you.

SINUSITIS

CHANCES ARE THAT YOU MAKE it through most days without devoting a single thought to your sinuses. All the while, the sinuses—located above, behind, and below your eyes—work tirelessly for you, clearing away dust, pollen, and other particles that enter your nose and mouth to prevent you from their potentially harmful effects. In most cases, your sinuses are very *good* things to have.

WHAT IS IT?

Good as your sinuses are, you probably weren't exactly singing their praises if you've ever experienced a sinus infection. Instead, you were likely cursing their very existence as your head filled up with mucus, your breathing became difficult and congested, and your nose began running like a leaky faucet. With these symptoms you may also have had pain, fever, a reduced sense of smell and taste, and fatigue.

If any three of the symptoms mentioned above linger for more than a week, then you have sinusitis—a sinus inflammation. Sinusitis most frequently develops as a nasty side effect of a lingering cold or infection, but allergies and nasal polyps (tissue growths in the nose) can also be culprits in this condition. Luckily, most bouts of sinusitis pass after just a few days without the use of medications. If symptoms linger for more than a few days, it is essential to consult a doctor. In the meantime, herbs and supplements may speed healing and reduce symptoms of sinusitis.

WHAT SHOULD I TAKE?

*Astragalus • Bilberry • Bromelain • Chamomile
Echinacea • Elderberry • Eucalyptus • Garlic • Ginger
Ginseng • Goldenseal • Lavender • N-Acetyl Cysteine (NAC)
Peppermint • Quercetin • Selenium • Vitamin A
Vitamin C • Vitamin E*

Preliminary studies suggest that **astragalus** may have antiviral and antibacterial effects. Astragalus may also boost blood cells' ability to absorb waste and fight harmful microorganisms in the bloodstream. (For more information on astragalus, see page 35.)

Bilberry has been used traditionally to ease minor mucous membrane inflammation and may therefore soothe irritated mucous membranes in the throat that become inflamed due to sinusitis. (For more information on bilberry, see page 44.)

Bromelain and **quercetin** are excellent anti-inflammatory supplements that can ease pain, and bromelain offers the additional benefit of helping to break up mucus. (For more information on bromelain and quercetin, see pages 54 and 236.)

The German Commission E (see page 16) has approved **chamomile** for the treatment of mucous membrane inflammation. Inhaling the vapor from boiling water containing a few drops of chamomile oil may help soothe swollen sinuses. (For more information on chamomile, see page 67.)

Echinacea is an herb that is also well known for its immune-boosting potential, particularly during cold and sinus infections. Echinacea as both a solid and liquid extract and as a tea may be quite helpful for sinusitis. (For more information on echinacea, see page 107.)

Preliminary studies suggest that **elderberry**—when used in combination with antibiotic medications or other herbs—may relieve symptoms of sinusitis including headache, nasal congestion, and swollen mucus membranes. Herbal products containing elderberry have been shown to speed the recovery of acute sinusitis when taken together with antibiotic drugs. Further research is needed to determine elderberry's effect when used alone. (For more information on elderberry, see page 109.)

CALL YOUR DOCTOR WHEN...

If you exhibit only mild symptoms of sinusitis, you can probably weather the storm. However, some symptoms of sinusitis may necessitate a visit to the doctor's office. Be sure to call your doctor if:

- You have pain and swelling on your face or around your eyes
- You experience unusual confusion
- Your neck is stiff
- You have a prolonged, severe headache
- You have a temperature above 101° F

Often compared to menthol, **eucalyptus** may be effective in clearing sinus congestion. The leaves and oil of eucalyptus have a long history of traditional medicinal use. Preliminary studies suggest that when applied topically, eucalyptus may even fight infection and bacteria as well as clearing nasal passages. In combination with **lavender**, eucalyptus may be helpful when inhaled in a steam vapor for clearing clogged sinuses. (For more information on eucalyptus and lavender, see pages 111 and 184.)

When brewed together in a tea, **garlic** and **ginger** promote mucus drainage and stimulate the immune system. (For more information on garlic and ginger, see pages 135 and 136.)

Ginseng stimulates the immune system, making it a useful addition to the herbal prescription for sinusitis. (For more information about ginseng, see page 141.)

Goldenseal is one of the most effective antiviral and antibacterial herbs, making it quite useful for speeding the healing process in cases of infection caused by viruses and bacteria. Goldenseal is helpful in both supplement and tea form. (For more information on goldenseal, see page 151.)

NAC is an amino acid that has antioxidant properties and may also break up mucus, making it a useful supplement in treating sinusitis. (For more information on NAC, see page 213.)

Several recent studies indicate that **peppermint** oil has anti-inflammatory effects and may also be beneficial for fighting fungal and bacterial infections. (For more information on peppermint, see page 226.)

To fend off sinus infections, it is important to have a healthy, stable immune system. **Vitamins A** and **E** and **selenium** are just a few supplements that help keep the immune system strong. For more information on other ways to bolster the immune system, see Immune-System Support on page 507. In addition, **vitamin C** with flavonoids is a well-known immune-boosting supplement duet that can speed healing. (For more information on vitamins A, C, and E, and selenium, see pages 274, 284, 292, and 253.)

MY SUPPLEMENT LIST—SINUSITIS

SUPPLEMENT	RECOMMENDED DOSAGE
Astragalus	*Tea:* Simmer 9–15 g of dried astragalus root in 3 cups of boiling water for 20–30 minutes. Drink 1 cup twice daily. *Capsule:* Take 500 mg daily, divided into 2 doses.

MY SUPPLEMENT LIST—SINUSITIS	
SUPPLEMENT	**RECOMMENDED DOSAGE**
Bilberry	*Mouthwash:* Gargle with a mouthwash containing 10% bilberry as needed.
Bromelain	*Tablet:* Take 200 to 500 mg two or three times a day between meals. Look for a product containing 2,400 gelatin-dissolving units (GDU) or 3,600 milk-clotting units (MCU) per gram.
Chamomile	*Inhalant:* Add 2 or 3 drops of chamomile oil to a steam vaporizer or pot of boiling water. Deeply inhale the steam to clear sinus congestion.
Echinacea	*Tea:* Mix 1 tsp or 1 teabag of dried herb with 1 cup of hot water and steep for 5 to 10 minutes. Drink up to three times daily. *Capsule:* Take 300 mg three times daily.
Elderberry	*Oral—Tea:* Steep one-half to 1 tsp of dried flowers in 1 cup of boiling water for 10 to 15 minutes and drink three times a day. *Syrup:* Take from 2 tsp to 2 tbsp twice daily. *Note:* Elderberry syrup dosages may vary for different products. Be sure to read the individual product label for specific dosage information.
Eucalyptus	*Inhalant:* Add 2 or 3 drops of eucalyptus oil to a steam vaporizer or pot of boiling water. Inhale the steam to clear sinus congestion. *Note:* Do not take eucalyptus oil internally without a doctor's supervision.
Garlic and Ginger	*Tea:* Mix 2 or 3 cloves of garlic with 2 or 3 slices of fresh ginger and boil in 2 cups of water. Strain and drink as needed.
Ginseng	*Asian Ginseng:* Take 100–200 mg once a day of an extract standardized to contain 4% to 7% ginsenosides.
Goldenseal	*Tea:* Brew goldenseal in a tea by mixing 1 tsp or 1 teabag of dried herb with 1 cup of hot water and steeping for 5 to 10 minutes. You can mix goldenseal with echinacea (see above) and licorice. *Capsule:* Take 200–500 mg of an extract standardized to contain 8% to 12% of goldenseal alkaloids three times a day. *Note:* After taking goldenseal for 3 weeks, it may be useful to discontinue use for 2 weeks before taking goldenseal again.
Lavender	*Inhalant:* Add 2 or 3 drops of lavender oil to a steam vaporizer or pot of boiling water. Deeply inhale the steam to clear sinus congestion. Lavender may be combined with eucalyptus (see above) and peppermint oil (see below) when inhaled.
NAC	*Capsule:* Dosages may range from 250 to 1,500 mg daily. Consult your doctor to determine appropriate dosage information for you.
Peppermint	*Tea:* Steep 5 g of dried peppermint leaves in 1 cup of boiling water for 5 to 10 minutes. Drink up to four times daily. *Inhalant:* Add 2 or 3 drops of peppermint oil to a steam vaporizer or pot of boiling water. Deeply inhale the steam to clear sinus congestion. You may also add 1 drop each of eucalyptus and lavender to the steam.

(continued)

SUPPLEMENT	RECOMMENDED DOSAGE
	MY SUPPLEMENT LIST—SINUSITIS (continued)
Quercetin	*Capsule or Tablet:* Take 500 mg three times a day between meals, as needed.
Selenium	*Tablet:* Take 100 to 200 mcg once daily.
Vitamin A	*Capsule or Tablet:* Take 5,000 to 10,000 IU once daily. *Note:* Women who are pregnant or who are expecting to become pregnant should take vitamin A only under the supervision of a doctor.
Vitamin C	*Capsule or Tablet:* Take 1,000 mg of vitamin C with 500 mg of flavonoids three times a day. *Note:* Be sure to use a buffered form of vitamin C. If taking vitamin C causes loose stools, decrease the dosage and then gradually increase the dosage as tolerated.
Vitamin E	*Capsule:* Take 200 to 400 IU once daily of a natural product containing mixed tocopherols.

SKIN HEALTH

BEAUTY MAY BE ONLY SKIN deep, but most people can agree that wrinkles and age spots are an unwelcome part of the aging process. Since skin is the largest, most visible organ of the body, maintaining skin health is an important element for many people who want to look good and feel good about themselves.

WHAT IS IT?

Over the course of youth and middle age, the increased wear and tear on the skin leads to an accumulation of skin-cell damage. Some of the more harmless markers of aging skin include wrinkles, dryness, spots, growths, and a slower rate of healing. Other, more serious occurrences, such as skin cancer, require medical attention. Some of the symptoms of aging skin can be prevented and addressed with a variety of vitamins and supplements.

You probably already know the basic elements of good skin care: avoid too much sunlight, eat a healthy diet, don't smoke, drink alcohol in moderation, drink lots of water, and stay active. Mother Nature may help out with the battle with the supplements named below.

WHAT SHOULD I USE?
Alpha Lipoic Acid · Green Tea
Omega-3 Fatty Acids · Vitamin C · Vitamin E

Preliminary research suggests that **alpha lipoic acid** (ALA), when applied topically, may help slow the aging process of the skin caused by sun damage. A study of 33 women with an average age of 54 years noted significant improvements in skin appearance after treatment with ALA. Through its power as an antioxidant, ALA may also help to protect the skin from oxidative damage. (For more information on alpha lipoic acid, see page 29.)

Green tea extract, in a topical concentrated form, has shown noteworthy results in protecting the skin from sun damage, reversing sun damage, delaying the aging of collagen, and preventing skin cancer. This may be due to the high level of antioxidant polyphenols in green tea. A specific polyphenol in green tea—called epigallocatechin gallate (EGCG)—may have the ability to reactivate dying skin cells. Additional human studies are needed to confirm the effects of green tea on skin. (For more information on green tea, see page 157.)

Some studies suggest that **omega-3 fatty acids**, in the form of fish oil supplements, may be able to reduce skin sensitivity to ultraviolet (UV) rays, especially in people who are sensitive to the sun. Other preliminary studies indicate that omega-3 fatty acids may have a protective role against skin cancer, although further research is needed to confirm these findings. (For more information on omega-3 fatty acids, see page 221.)

Vitamin C is a good standby when it comes to antioxidants, protecting the face and skin from the damage caused by free radical molecules when taken orally or applied topically. Topical vitamin C may minimize sunburn damage when applied directly after exposure to the sun. One study found that topical vitamin C, when applied from 30 to 60 minutes after exposure to UV rays, decreased the amount of sunburned cells and began to repair damaged skin. Animal studies have found that oral supplementation with vitamin C may help reduce the rate of tumors caused by UV exposure. (For more information on vitamin C, see page 284.)

Recent studies suggest that as a powerful antioxidant, **vitamin E** may help to neutralize free radicals, preventing the damage they often cause with aging. Other studies have found that vitamin E may reduce the damage caused by sunburn as well as curb the production of potentially cancerous cells. Topical vitamin E can also help to moisturize dry or rough skin. When taken orally, vitamin E may reduce the occurrence of wrinkles and sun damage and improve the overall texture of skin. (For more information on vitamin E, see page 292.)

KITCHEN TIPS

EATING ORANGE PEELS MAY LOWER RISK OF SKIN CANCER

A recent study found that consuming the peel of oranges and other citrus fruits, such as grapefruits and lemons, may decrease the risk of a specific type of skin cancer called *squamous cell carcinoma* (SCC). It appears that simply drinking citrus juices or eating citrus fruits does not have the same anti-cancer effect and that to reap the protective benefits of these fruits, you will have to bite into the peel. If you find this prospect slightly unappealing, try adding a twist of grapefruit or lemon to your favorite drinks or scraping a lemon peel to add zest as a topping for your foods. Studies show that the more peel you consume, the better your chance of beating SCC.

Note: Choose organic peels to avoid ingesting pesticides.

MY SUPPLEMENT LIST—SKIN HEALTH

SUPPLEMENT	RECOMMENDED DOSAGE
Alpha Lipoic Acid	*Topical—Cream:* Use a topical cream containing 5% ALA twice daily for 12 weeks to reduce the effects of sun damage.
Green Tea Extract	*Topical:* Look for skin creams, moisturizers, and other products with high levels of green tea extract. Read individual product labels for application instruction.
Omega-3 Fatty Acids	*Oral:* Take 1–2 g of omega-3 fatty acids per day, in divided doses, with meals. The amount of omega-3 fatty acid will vary by manufacturer, so be sure to check the product label carefully.
Vitamin C	*Oral—Capsule or Tablet:* Take 500 to 1,000 mg once a day. *Topical—Cream:* Apply up to 30 minutes after sun exposure as needed. *Note:* Be sure to use a buffered form of vitamin C. If taking vitamin C causes loose stools, decrease the dosage and then gradually increase the dosage as tolerated.
Vitamin E	*Oral—Capsule:* Take 400 to 800 IU daily. *Topical—Cream:* Apply vitamin E in the form of d-alpha-tocopherol before and after exposure to the sun as needed.

SPRAINS AND STRAINS

WE LIKE TO THINK OF our bodies as temples, but unbeknownst to us, those temples can have loose foundations and creaky walls that, if pushed too far, just might break apart. When this happens, the result is often a sprain or strain.

WHAT IS IT?

Sprains and strains are generally grouped together into one medical category, owing to the similarity of their symptoms and treatment. In reality, however, they are two very different conditions. Sprains occur when ligaments (tissues that connect bone or cartilage) are either stressed or torn. Because blood vessels often burst in sprains, they are often accompanied by swelling, inflammation, or skin discoloration in the affected area, which is usually at or near a joint. Strains occur when there is damage to a muscle and particularly when a muscle is torn and may cause bleeding within the affected muscle.

Both sprains and strains can result from overexertion, falls, impacts, and accidents. Strains and sprains can vary greatly in their severity. Symptoms can range from mild pain, stiffness, and swelling to the inability to move the affected joint or muscle or put weight on it. In the case of a severe strain, internal bleeding may occur, and surgery may be necessary.

For either strains or sprains, you should seek medical attention immediately if you experience intense pain, swelling, or a popping sound when the injury occurs. You should also see a doctor if a strain or sprain occurs and the stiffness doesn't improve in 2 to 3 days. The following herbs and supplements can help to heal faster. Read on for tips to speed up the rebuilding of your temple.

WHAT SHOULD I TAKE?
Boswellia • Bromelain • Chondroitin
Devil's Claw • Eucalyptus • Glucosamine
Quercetin • Vitamin E • Willow Bark

Its effectiveness as an anti-inflammatory agent may make **boswellia** helpful for reducing the pain and inflammation associated with sprains and strains. Not only do some studies suggest that boswellia works as well as many nonsteroidal anti-inflammatory drugs (NSAIDs), but when taken for long periods, boswellia does not cause stomach irritation, a common side effect of many NSAIDs. (For more information on boswellia, see page 52.)

Bromelain is one of the best supplements for strains and sprains because it is known to ease pain by reducing swelling and inflammation. (For more information on bromelain, see page 54.)

Chondroitin and **glucosamine** may be useful for treating strains and sprains because they help the body to produce glycosaminoglycans, which are important in the growth and repair of tendons, ligaments, and joints. Preliminary trials have suggested that these two supplements may promote tissue recovery and the healing of injuries to tendons and joints, especially in cases of sports-related injuries. (For more information on chondroitin and glucosamine, see pages 74 and 144.)

Devil's claw, a plant native to southern Africa, may be helpful for reducing the inflammation and pain associated with sprains and strains. However, unlike boswellia, devil's claw promotes the secretion of stomach acid and should be avoided by people with duodenal or gastric ulcers. (For more information on devil's claw, see page 98.)

Eucalyptus oil, when applied topically, may provide injured muscles with heat that helps promote blood flow to and from them, as well as soothing sore muscles. Try rubbing eucalyptus oil on sprains and strains to ease muscle discomfort. (For more information on eucalyptus, see page 111.)

CALL YOUR DOCTOR WHEN...

Sprains and strains will often heal with just a little extra TLC. However, certain symptoms of these injuries may require immediate medical care. Be sure to call your doctor if:

- You hear a popping sound in the joint at the time of injury
- You have considerable swelling and are unable to use the injured area
- You are unable to bear weight on the injured body part or feel unstable
- You have a fever
- The area is inflamed, red, and hot
- You experience swelling and stiffness that do not improve within 2 or 3 days

Quercetin, a flavonoid antioxidant derived from the skins of apples and oranges, may help to reduce inflammation in people with sprains or strains. (For more information on quercetin, see page 236.)

Vitamin E has strong antioxidant properties that help the healing of muscles and connective tissue. A recent study found that vitamin E was useful in reliving pain and decreasing inflammation. Since vitamin E has many health benefits besides this, you may want to consider adding it to your supplement list, especially if you are trying to recover from a recent injury, and then continuing to use it once the injury has healed. (For more information on vitamin E, see page 292.)

Studies indicate that **willow bark** may be as effective as aspirin in easing pain, without the unpleasant side effects often associated with aspirin and other over-the-counter pain relievers. Many people refer to willow as herbal aspirin, and its ability to reduce pain and inflammation make it useful for easing the pain associated with sprains and strains. (For more information on willow bark, see page 298.)

MY SUPPLEMENT LIST—SPRAINS AND STRAINS

SUPPLEMENT	RECOMMENDED DOSAGE
Boswellia	*Tablet:* Take 300 to 400 mg three times daily of a standardized extract containing 70% boswellic acids between meals.
Bromelain	*Tablet:* Take 250 to 500 mg daily between meals. Look for a product containing 2,400 gelatin-dissolving units (GDU) or 3,600 milk-clotting units (MCU) per gram.
Chondroitin	*Capsule or Tablet:* Take 400 mg three times daily with meals, or 1,200 mg with dinner.
Devil's Claw	*Capsule:* Take 800 to 1,000 mg up to three times daily of an extract standardized to contain 3% iridoid glycosides or 50 mg harpagoside total.
Eucalyptus Oil	*Topical—Oil:* Combine 15 ml (½ ounce) of eucalyptus oil with 250 ml (1 cup) of lukewarm water. Or combine 10–20 drops with ½–1 ounce of carrier oil such as jojoba or almond oil. Apply to affected areas as needed.
Glucosamine	*Capsule or Tablet:* Take 500 mg three times a day with meals.
Vitamin E	*Capsule:* Take 400 IU daily of a natural product containing mixed tocopherols.
Willow Bark	*Capsule:* Take an extract standardized to contain 120 to 240 mg of salicylic acids daily. *Caution:* Avoid willow bark if you have an aspirin allergy, bleeding disorder, diabetes, or a peptic ulcer.

STROKE

FEW MEDICAL CONDITIONS ARE AS dangerous as stroke and as widespread among Americans. Stroke is the third leading cause of death and the leading cause of disability among adults in the United States. Every year, 160,000 of the 750,000 stroke victims die a premature death. Many others are left permanently disabled.

WHAT IS IT?

In the simplest of analogies, a stroke is like a heart attack, but it occurs in your brain. It can be of two types. In an *ischemic stroke*—the most common form of stroke—a blood clot blocks blood flow into or within the brain, causing the affected part of the brain to shut down. In the second type of stroke, called a *hemorrhagic stroke*, a blood vessel bursts in the brain and the blood spills out and into the surrounding areas of brain tissue.

Stroke symptoms include sudden weakness, numbness, and paralysis. Speech may become slurred and vision may become blurred. In extreme cases, people experiencing a stroke are seized by a severe headache, which may then be followed by a seizure and/or loss of consciousness. Strokes are a medical emergency, and medical attention for them must be sought immediately, since brain cells begin to die rapidly and in large numbers within minutes after a stroke.

Although strokes are potentially life-threatening conditions, doctors are becoming much better at understanding and treating them, including both minimizing damage during a stroke and rehabilitating people who have experienced strokes. The potential to recover significantly from a stroke has improved tremendously over the past decade.

Just as with the risk of heart attack, lifestyle choices are the keys to preventing strokes: Choosing not to smoke, maintaining a healthy diet and level of physical activity, and reducing stress levels can all help in this regard. Mother Nature also has some friends for helping to prevent strokes and aiding in the recovery from them.

WHAT SHOULD I TAKE?

Make sure to consult your doctor before taking any type of supplement, especially if you have recently suffered from a stroke.

DIETARY DO'S AND DON'TS

Do. Foods rich in important nutrients, including magnesium, potassium, calcium, and fiber, may help to ward off stroke. Try adding avocados, almonds, or oysters to your diet to get more magnesium. Foods packed with potassium include tomatoes, cantaloupe, bananas, and spinach. Foods rich in calcium include green leafy vegetables, broccoli, salmon, and cheese. And increase your intake of carrots, peas, and oats, which are rich in fiber.

Don't. Avoid saturated fats, which may increase cholesterol levels and thereby contribute to blocked arteries, making you more vulnerable to stroke. Substitute monosaturated fats and omega-3 fatty acids, such as those in olive oil and salmon, respectively, for saturated, hydrogenated fats, such as the fats in meat and milk products.

AN APPLE A DAY MAY KEEP STROKE AWAY

A Finnish study investigating the role that the antioxidant quercertin plays in preventing stroke found that eating an apple a day decreases stroke risk in both men and women. By contrast, most other foods containing quercetin did not seem to have stroke-protective effects on the study participants. It remains unclear why apples appear to reduce stroke risk, but researchers suspect that the presence in apples of antioxidants called phenolic acids may play a significant role in this.

While researchers try to pinpoint the exact anti-stroke component of apples, enjoying a daily apple may reduce your stroke risk.

Alpha Lipoic Acid • Coenzyme Q10 (CoQ10)
Garlic • Ginkgo Biloba (Ginkgo) • Magnesium • Melatonin
Omega-3 Fatty Acids • Potassium • Vitamin B Complex

Alpha lipoic acid (ALA) may be good supplement to take in the aftermath of a stroke. Animal studies indicate that ALA may increase the chances of survival and may help the healing process. (For more information on alpha lipoic acid, see page 29.)

CoQ10 is helpful in reducing the risk of stroke because of its blood-pressure lowering effects. Studies have found that supplementation with CoQ10 can significantly decrease blood pressure, especially in people with high blood pressure. Other studies indicate that taking CoQ10 after a stroke may reduce the recurrence of future strokes. (For more information on CoQ10, see page 80.)

Aged **garlic** extract helps regulate blood flow and prevent the formation of blood clots within blood vessels, making it an excellent supplement for helping to prevent ischemic stroke. (For more information on garlic, see page 135.)

Ginkgo, like vitamin E, has mild blood-thinning properties that can help to keep clots from forming on blood vessel walls and obstructing blood flow to or in the brain. In the aftermath of a stroke, ginkgo acts on the brain to help reduce depression and dementia, common consequences from stroke. (For more information on ginkgo, see page 138.)

Preliminary research indicates that **magnesium** may have protective properties against stroke. Drinking water high in magnesium appears to lower stroke risk, and diets lacking sufficient levels of magnesium seem to increase stroke risk. Moreover, magnesium administered intravenously immediately after a stroke is being investigated as a potential stroke treatment. (For more information on magnesium, see page 203.)

Preliminary evidence suggests that **melatonin** may be useful for preventing strokes as well as treating acute strokes. Melatonin is a powerful antioxidant that works to scavenge cell- and tissue-damaging free radical molecules and may have protective effects on the nervous system. However, melatonin should not be taken without first consulting a doctor, especially after a recent stroke or when the risk exists for having one. (For more information on melatonin, see page 208.)

Omega-3 fatty acids are major benefactors for preventing strokes, with some studies indicating that eating two servings of fish rich in omega-3 fatty acids (such as salmon, tuna, and mackerel) reduces the risk of stroke by 50 percent. Omega-3 fatty acids prevent plaque buildup and clotting in the blood vessels, allowing an uninterrupted flow of blood through them. The other advantage of obtaining omega-3 fatty acids from fish is that you can avoid adding more saturated fat to your diet by easily replacing a serving of red meat with a serving of fish (but be aware of the associated risk of mercury toxicity if you do eat large amounts of fish). If you can't get your omega-3 fatty acids from fish, a supplement is still quite helpful for obtaining them. (For more information on omega-3 fatty acids, see page 221.)

Preliminary research suggests there is a correlation between **potassium** intake and decreased risk of stroke, most likely due to its blood pressure–lowering abilities (see page 498). A recent study found that a high intake of potassium—singularly or together with magnesium and fiber—is especially helpful in preventing stroke in men with high blood pressure. (For more information on potassium, see page 233.)

High levels of homocysteine—an amino acid found in the blood—can increase the risk of having a stroke or heart attack. **Vitamin B complex** may be useful in keeping homocystine levels down and providing added insurance against strokes. Folic acid (vitamin B_9) may be especially helpful in reducing the risk of stroke, so be sure your B-complex vitamin contains adequate amounts of this important nutrient. (For more information on vitamin B complex, see pages 277, 279, and 282.)

Several Supplements Don't Mix with Surgery!

Did You Know?

Only a few supplements are recommended for health benefits in preparation for or recovery after surgery. On the other hand, certain supplements may be very dangerous to take immediately before or after surgery. The following supplements should be strictly avoided if you are planning to undergo any kind of surgical procedure:

■ **Echinacea**—Has the potential to adversely interfere with medications often prescribed to surgical patients

■ **Garlic and Ginkgo**—May encourage harmful bleeding because of their blood-thinning capabilities

■ **Ginseng**—May cause hypoglycemia or postoperative bleeding

■ **Kava and Valerian**—May increase the effects of anesthesia, including increased sedation

■ **St. John's Wort**—May interfere with the body's absorption of medications prescribed to surgical patients

The use of all of the above supplements should be discontinued at least 1 week before scheduled surgery, unless otherwise directed by your doctor. If you will be having a surgical procedure, speak with your doctor about any supplements you are taking and find out when you should stop taking them.

MY SUPPLEMENT LIST—STROKE

SUPPLEMENT	RECOMMENDED DOSAGE
Alpha Lipoic Acid	*Capsule:* Take 600–800 mg daily.
CoQ10	*Softgel:* Take 30 to 90 mg daily. While some people may find benefits from taking higher dosages, consult a doctor before exceeding this dosage.
Garlic	*Capsule:* Studies using 2.4 to 7.2 g of aged-garlic extract have yielded positive results. Consult your doctor before taking high dosages of this supplement. *Caution:* People taking anticoagulant medications should consult their doctor before taking garlic supplements. If you are scheduled to have surgery, notify your surgeon if you are taking garlic supplements.
Ginkgo	*Capsule:* Take 120 to 240 mg daily, divided into two or three doses, of an extract standardized to contain 6% terpene lactones and 24% flavone glycosides. *Caution:* People taking anticoagulant medications should consult their doctor before taking ginkgo supplements. If you are scheduled to have surgery, notify your surgeon if you are taking ginkgo supplements.
Magnesium	*Capsule or Tablet:* Take 300 to 400 mg twice daily. *Note:* Ask your doctor before taking magnesium if you have kidney disease. Take magnesium in the form of magnesium glycinate to avoid loose stools. Large amounts of magnesium can cause diarrhea; if this becomes a problem for you, reduce your dosage.
Melatonin	Consult your doctor to determine an appropriate dosage of melatonin for you.
Omega-3 Fatty Acids	*Fish Oil—Capsule:* 2–3 g of omega-3 fatty acids per day, in divided doses, with meals. The amount of omega-3 fatty acid will vary by manufacturer, so be sure to check the product label carefully.
Potassium	*Tablet:* Dosages of 2,400 mg daily are often required to lower blood pressure and achieve stroke protective results; however, dosages this high are not available without a doctor's prescription. Speak with your doctor about taking potassium supplements if you have high blood pressure and are at risk of stroke. *Note:* People taking potassium-sparing diuretics should not take potassium supplements.
Vitamin B Complex	*Tablet:* Take a vitamin B complex in a dose of 50, 75, or 100 mg daily. Read individual product labels for dosage information.

SURGERY PREPARATION

NO MATTER HOW INVASIVE or serious the surgical procedure, preparing for surgery is never easy. Just thinking about having surgery can be daunting, but not addressing the issue can be detrimental to both one's mental health and recovery after surgery.

WHAT IS IT?

To prepare mentally for surgery, ask your doctor as many questions as you need to. There are also supplements you can take before and after surgery to prepare for it and then heal your body. For each of the supplements listed below, you should begin your regimen at least 6 weeks before surgery and continue it for 2 to 3 weeks after the surgery.

WHAT SHOULD I TAKE?

Make sure to consult your doctor before taking any supplements before or after surgery.

*Bromelain · Ginger · Grape Seed Extract
Horse Chestnut · Multivitamin · Peppermint*

Some studies have found that **bromelain** may help in reducing the postoperative pain, bruising, and swelling, especially in people who have undergone nasal surgery, cataract removal, and foot surgery, and in women who have undergone episiotomy. However, since bromelain thins the blood, it may increase the risk of bleeding during or after surgery and should be taken only under the supervision of a doctor. (For more information on bromelain, see page 54.)

Ginger may be especially beneficial for easing nausea associated with surgical anesthesia. Two double-blind studies found that ginger reduced postoperative complaints of nausea. (For more information on ginger, see page 136.)

Studies suggest that **grape seed extract** may be helpful in improving recovery after surgery by reducing leakage from the small blood vessels known as capillaries. One study found that the active ingredient in grape seed extract—known as oligomeric

TMD May Affect Your Dental Health

Did You Know?

A study conducted at the Orofacial Pain Center at the University of Kentucky College of Dentistry found that over 63 percent of patients with TMD reported decreasing their regular visits for professional dental care because of the associated pain. The study matched 40 patients with TMD by age and gender with 40 dentistry patients who did not experience TMD. The results showed that patients with TMD not only avoided dental visits because of the pain caused by TMD, but they also had more difficulty in performing basic daily dental care such as brushing and flossing. People with TMD should take extra precautions to ensure that they do not neglect their teeth. If they do, the consequences can be more detrimental than a pain in the jaw!

proanthocyanidins—decreased the severity of swelling in patients who had recently undergone "face-lift" surgery. **Horse chestnut** may work in a way similar to grape seed extract in reducing inflammation after surgery. (For more information on grape seed extract and horse chestnut, see pages 155 and 169.)

Make sure that your body receives the basic nutrients it requires before and after surgery. Taking a **multivitamin** before and after surgery may be a good way to ensure that your body has a speedy recovery from the physical trauma of surgery. (For more information on multivitamins, see page 9.)

Preliminary research suggests that **peppermint** may be effective in soothing postoperative nausea. (For more information on peppermint, see page 226.)

MY SUPPLEMENT LIST—SURGERY PREPARATION

SUPPLEMENT	RECOMMENDED DOSAGE
Bromelain	*Tablet:* Take 500 milk-clotting units (MCU) or 300 gelatin-dissovling units (GDU) one or two times daily.
Ginger	*Capsule:* Take 1 to 4 g daily, divided into two doses. *Note:* Ginger should only be taken for surgically related nausea under a doctor's supervision.
Grape Seed Extract	*Capsule or Tablet:* Take a supplement containing 300 to 600 mg of oligomeric proanthocyanidins (OPCs) daily.
Horse Chestnut Extract	*Oral—Tablet:* Take 300 mg of an extract standardized to contain 16% to 21% aescin two to three times daily between meals.
Multivitamin	*Tablet:* Take a multivitamin/mineral supplement daily. Read the individual product label for dosage information.
Peppermint	*Tea:* Steep 5 g of dried leaves in 1 cup of boiling water for 5 to 10 minutes. Drink three or four cups daily between meals, as needed.

TEMPOROMANDIBULAR DISORDERS

JUST THINK OF HOW MUCH exercise the average person's jaw gets in a day. Talking, eating, yawning, biting, swallowing, and even chewing gum are all activities we typically take for granted until there is a problem with them. So when the basic act of chewing causes serious pain, it can be a most unpleasant problem.

WHAT IS IT?

The various causes of pain in the jaw and in the muscles that control chewing are known collectively as temporomandibular disorders or TMD. One main symptom of TMD is pain in the temporomandibular joint (or TMJ), which is the hinge joint on each side of the head where the jawbone meets the temporal bone of the skull. Causes of TMD include everything from arthritis, injury, keeping your mouth open for long periods of time in the dentist's chair, and poorly fitting dentures to stress and just plain old wear-and-tear. But the symptoms are typically the same: pain in the jaw, ear, or head, particularly when chewing; tenderness in the jaw muscles; locking of the joint; and sometimes a clicking sound or grating sensation while chewing. TMD can be a very painful condition for some.

Talking to your doctor is the best way to discover your options for dealing with TMD. Everything from anti-inflammatory medications and corrective dental treatment by wearing a splint at night to muscle relaxation techniques can help in reducing symptoms of TMD.

WHAT SHOULD I TAKE?
Boswellia • Bromelain • Glucosamine
Lavender • Lemon Balm • Omega-3 Fatty Acids
St. John's Wort • Valerian

Tenderness in the jaw may result from inflammation in the TMJ. **Boswellia**, **bromelain**, and **glucosamine** may help reduce such inflammation and the jaw pain associated with it. (For more information on boswellia, bromelain, and glucosamine, see pages 52, 54, and 144.)

If the cause of tension in your jaw is stress, **lavender**, **lemon balm**, and **valerian** may be helpful because of their calming effects. Valerian may be especially helpful when taken before bedtime if you find that grinding your teeth in the middle of the night causes jaw pain. (For more information on lavender, lemon balm, and valerian, see pages 184, 190 and 272.)

Omega-3 fatty acids are known to decrease inflammation, which can help ease the pain typically associated with TMD. (For more information on omega-3 fatty acids, see page 221.)

St. John's wort best helps to relieve TMD when the oil is applied directly to the TMJ. St. John's wort also increases levels of serotonin when taken orally, which is often found to be decreased in TMD. (For more information on St. John's wort, see page 262.)

MY SUPPLEMENT LIST—TEMPOROMANDIBULAR DISORDERS

SUPPLEMENT	RECOMMENDED DOSAGE
Boswellia	*Tablet:* Take 300–400 mg three times a day of a standardized extract that contains 37.5% boswellic acids.
Bromelain	Take 300–600 mg three times daily between meals. Look for a product containing 2,400 gelatin-dissolving units (GDU) or 3,600 milk-clotting units (MCU) per gram.
Glucosamine	*Capsule or Tablet:* Take 500 mg three times daily with meals, or 1,500 mg with dinner.
Lavender	*Tea:* Steep 1–2 tsp of lavender flowers in 1 cup of boiling water for 5–10 minutes. Drink up to three cups daily.
Lemon Balm	*Tea:* Steep 1–2 tsp of dried herb in 1 cup of boiling water for 5 to 10 minutes. Drink up to three times daily.
Omega-3 Fatty Acids	*Fish Oil—Capsule:* Take 3–4 g of omega-3 fatty acids per day, in divided doses, with meals. The amount of omega-3 fatty acid will vary by manufacturer, so be sure to check the product label carefully.
St. John's Wort	*Topical—Oil:* Apply an oil made from St. John's wort directly to the skin over the TMJ as needed. *Oral—Capsule:* Take 300 mg up to three times daily of an extract standardized to contain 0.3% hypericin.
Valerian	*Capsule or Tablet:* Take 300 to 500 mg of a standardized extract from 30 to 60 minutes before bedtime. Take 150 to 500 mg daily to decrease anxiety-associated TMJ.
	Note: The strength of valerian products may vary greatly. Be sure to choose a standardized product and carefully follow the instructions on the label.

TINNITUS

WHEN COMPLETE SILENCE SEEMS noisier than it ought to be, you're likely to have tinnitus. For 36 million Americans, the persistent sound of ringing, as well as other buzzes, hisses, roars, and clicks, is an all-too-familiar problem. Focusing on this sound might drive anyone to distraction, especially when it interferes with the enjoyment of silence. Although the noise of tinnitus is, literally, "only in your head," it often seems worse than anything coming from an outside source.

WHAT IS IT?

Tinnitus—from the Latin word *tinnire* meaning "to ring"—can vary from a low roar to a high squeal, and may occur in one or both ears. Sometimes the sound is so loud that it becomes hard to focus on much else, and it may interfere with sleep. Tinnitus can occur for a variety of reasons. One of its most common causes is the gradual deterioration of the auditory cells in the inner ear after the age of 60. Another common cause is that ridiculously loud rock concert you went to as a teenager! Overexposure to loud noise for prolonged periods at any age often "kick-starts" tinnitus. Repeated exposure to loud noises can cause tinnitus and eventually lead to hearing loss. Furthermore, medications, TMJ disorders, head trauma, high blood pressure, and even the accumulation of earwax can also cause tinnitus. And certain factors, such as stress and poor diet, can aggravate existing tinnitus.

In many instances, tinnitus is more of a nuisance than a serious health risk, although in some cases it may be a sign of a more serious health problem. Unfortunately, doctors can do very little to treat tinnitus, and a people with tinnitus can often cope with it only by avoiding irritants (such as loud noises, nicotine, and caffeine), blocking the noise, or managing stress. Even though there is no cure for tinnitus, supplements may provide some relief for ringing ears.

WHAT SHOULD I TAKE?

Ginkgo Biloba (Ginkgo) • Melatonin
Vitamin A • Vitamin B₁₂ • Zinc

Ginkgo, in many clinical research studies, has been shown to markedly improve bloodflow to the brain. This could mean a better

Tips to Temper Tinnitus

Healthy Hints

Although there is no definitive cure for tinnitus, you can adopt certain practices to help assuage its annoying symptoms. Read on for some ideas for living a better quality of life with tinnitus.

■ **Take it without a grain of salt.** Decrease your salt intake. Sodium can slow circulation and aggravate symptoms of tinnitus.

■ **Cut out caffeine.** Stimulants such as caffeine in coffee, soda, or tea (and tobacco) can increase symptoms of tinnitus, especially in excess.

■ **Break the pressure.** If your blood pressure is high, discuss options for reducing it with your doctor, since it may contribute to tinnitus.

■ **Mask it.** When you can't make the ringing of tinnitus go away, try to drown it out with a competing noise such as a ticking clock or a machine that creates "white noise." However, keep in mind that you don't want to make competing noises too loud, since that can also damage your hearing.

blood supply to the cell of the inner ear so that people with tinnitus can improve their daily function, easing ear noise in general. But be patient with ginkgo; it often takes a few weeks to achieve its full effectiveness. (For more information on ginkgo, see page 138.)

Melatonin supplements may be useful in the treatment of tinnitus, especially for people who have trouble sleeping as a result of this disorder. A double-blind, placebo-controlled crossover study of 30 patients with tinnitus showed a decrease in symptoms as well as an improvement in sleep with melatonin supplementation. (For more information on melatonin, see page 208.)

Vitamin A is often linked with inner-ear health, and studies have indicated that individuals with a vitamin A deficiency typically experience auditory problems. A vitamin A supplement may therefore be good insurance for the ears. However, keep in mind that high doses of vitamin A can be dangerous. Consult your doctor to determine the appropriate dosage of this vitamin. (For more information on vitamin A, see page 274.)

Vitamin B$_{12}$ may help to ease tinnitus. Although the way in which it works is not understood, a clinical study showed that vitamin B$_{12}$ benefited people with symptoms of tinnitus. Some studies suggest that people with very low levels of vitamin B$_{12}$ may be prone to developing tinnitus. If you have tinnitus, consult your doctor about checking your levels of vitamin B$_{12}$. (For more information on vitamin B$_{12}$, see page 282.)

Zinc is a mineral present in higher concentrations in the middle ear than anywhere else in the body. Studies have shown that low zinc levels increase the risk of hearing loss, and one study indicated that increasing levels of zinc in the body helped to improve hearing. However, studies also show that zinc may not be helpful for those with normal levels of this vitamin. Ask your doctor to check your zinc level if you have tinnitus. (For more information on zinc, see page 304.)

MY SUPPLEMENT LIST—TINNITUS

SUPPLEMENT	RECOMMENDED DOSAGE
Ginkgo	*Tablet:* Take 120–240 mg daily, divided into three doses, of an extract standardized to contain 6% terpene lactones and 24% flavone glycosides.
Melatonin	*Tablet:* Take 3 to 10 mg before bedtime.

MY SUPPLEMENT LIST—TINNITUS	
SUPPLEMENT	**RECOMMENDED DOSAGE**
Vitamin A	*Capsule:* Take 10,000 IU of daily, with at least 5,000 IU supplied in the form of beta-carotene.
Vitamin B$_{12}$	*Capsule or Tablet:* Take 1,000 mcg per day under the tongue, accompanied by 400 mcg of folic acid taken orally.
	Note: Some people may require injections of vitamin B$_{12}$ if they have problems with its absorption in oral dosage form. Consult your doctor to determine if vitamin B$_{12}$ injections are appropriate for you.
Zinc	*Tablet:* Take 50 mg of zinc each day.
	Note: Be sure to take a copper supplement since large doses of zinc may deplete levels of copper in the body.

TOOTH AND GUM CARE

IF YOU'VE WATCHED ANY television lately, chances are you've been compelled by an overwhelming urge to make your teeth bright, shiny, and healthy. After all, what makes a better impression in life than a gleaming, healthy smile? The good news is that keeping your teeth and gums healthy is a relatively simple matter. All it requires is smart choices about food, sound dental hygiene, and the help of Mother Nature.

WHAT IS IT?

The main cause of tooth and gum disorders is gum disease, which has two major forms: *gingivitis* and *periodontitis*. Gingivitis, which is caused by bacteria, tends to get its start early in life when you're not as diligent about caring for your teeth and gums as you should be. Gingivitis begins when as tiny bacteria, left unchecked, form a sticky substance called *plaque* on the base of the teeth. Gradually, this plaque becomes the cause of gingivitis, resulting in tender, swollen, or bleeding gums. When gingivitis isn't stopped, it gradually becomes periodontitis, which often leads to tooth loss. A diagnosis of periodontitis usually means that gum disease has progressed to the point at which gums are swollen and recessed, and the mouth has an unpleasant taste. Tooth pain, loose teeth, and the presence of pus around teeth are also common symptoms of periodontitis.

About 80 percent of Americans have some form of gum disease. The good news is that its progression to tooth loss can be prevented

CALL YOUR DOCTOR WHEN...

On average, people need to see a dentist twice a year for a tooth cleaning. If you experience any of the following problems between these, you should contact your dentists. Be sure to call your dentist if:

■ You experience dry mouth for an extended period

■ You have difficulty eating because of tooth or mouth pain

■ You notice lesions, sores, or lumps in your mouth

■ You have not had a dental checkup within 2 years

by just a few simple steps. The first is to see your dentist regularly to have problems corrected. Second is to begin brushing and flossing your teeth twice daily, using a soft-bristled brush so that you don't injure your gums. And third is to choose supplements that can help prevent and treat gum disease.

WHAT SHOULD I TAKE?
Calcium • Coenzyme Q10 (CoQ10) • Eucalyptus
Folic Acid • Pycnogenol • Tea Tree Oil
Vitamin C • Vitamin D • Xylitol

Some studies have found that **calcium** may be beneficial to people with periodontal disease. In one study, people who were given 1,000 milligrams daily of calcium experienced an improvement in the symptoms of periodontal disease, including a decrease in bleeding gums and loose teeth. (For more information on calcium, see page 57.)

Some studies suggest that gingivitis may be caused by a deficiency of **CoQ10**. Some experts believe that the body can't repair damaged gum tissue if there is a deficiency in CoQ10. Sometimes, the topical use of CoQ10 is combined with other treatment methods for gingivitis to hasten the healing process. (For more information on CoQ10, see page 80.)

Eucalyptus may protect teeth against plaque-causing bacteria. In one controlled study, 15 participants chewed gum three times daily in place of their regular oral hygiene regimen. The group who chewed gum containing eucalyptus had less plaque buildup at the end of the 4-day study. Eucalyptus is an important ingredient in many mouthwash products, such as Listerine, and mouthwashes containing eucalyptus have been shown in studies to reduce gingivitis and plaque buildup. (For more information on eucalyptus, see page 111.)

A **folic acid** (vitamin B$_9$) mouthwash may provide relief for inflamed gums. A folic acid mouthwash may also be useful for gingivitis associated with pregnancy. Although some studies indicate that folic acid supplements are useful for treating gingivitis, studies have indicated that in pregnancy, a folic acid mouthwash, but not oral supplementation, is effective. (For more information on folic acid, see page 130.)

Pycnogenol may have the ability to reduce gum bleeding and plaque in people with gingivitis. One study of 40 people with gingivitis found that chewing a gum containing pycnogenol significantly reduced bleeding in the gums. This study also indicated that people who chewed pycnogenol gum had less dental plaque buildup that those who did not.

The antiseptic and antifungal properties of **tea tree oil** may be beneficial to oral health. Preliminary research suggests that using mouthwash containing tea tree oil may help reduce plaque and maintain overall good oral hygiene. (For more information on tea tree oil, see page 265.)

People with a deficiency of **vitamin C** are at an increased risk for gum disease. Vitamin C (along with flavonoids) is a powerful antioxidant that can protect gums from cell- and tissue-damaging free radical molecules. In addition, regular doses of vitamin C prevents the proliferation of bacteria that cause plaque. A daily supplement of C will keep your dental defenses up and offer your teeth and gums protection from infection. (For more information on vitamin C, see page 284.)

A study published in the *American Journal of Medicine* found that **vitamin D**, along with calcium (see page 56), may help in reducing tooth loss in the elderly. The study, which was an extension of another trial that tested the effectiveness of vitamin D and calcium for strengthening hips and bones, found that participants who took calcium and vitamin D supplements for 3 years were half as likely to lose teeth as those who did not. People who are not exposed to sunlight and whose dietary intake of vitamin D is low should consider taking vitamin D supplements to make sure that they are getting the adequate amounts of this important vitamin. (For more information on vitamin D, see page 289.)

Xylitol may be helpful in preventing cavities. The World Health Organization has investigated the effect of gum, toothpaste, and candy containing xylitol and found that people who used these xylitol products develop fewer cavities than those who receive no dental treatment. (For more information on xylitol, see page 300.)

MY SUPPLEMENT LIST—TOOTH AND GUM CARE

SUPPLEMENT	RECOMMENDED DOSAGE
Calcium	*Capsule or Tablet:* Take 500 mg twice daily.
CoQ10	*Softgel:* Take 50 mg daily.

(continued)

MY SUPPLEMENT LIST—TOOTH AND GUM CARE (continued)	
SUPPLEMENT	**RECOMMENDED DOSAGE**
Eucalyptus	*Oral:* Eucalyptus can be found in a variety of over-the-counter products such as mouthwash and gum. Be sure to read individual product labels for dosage information. *Note:* Pure eucalyptus oil should not be taken orally unless recommended by a doctor, since even small doses have caused toxic side effects and severe or even fatal reactions.
Folic Acid	*Mouthwash:* Gargle with 5 ml of a 0.1% folic acid solution twice daily for 1 to 2 months. *Tablet:* Take 4 mg of folic acid daily. *Note:* Pregnant women may not benefit from the tablet form of folic acid for gingivitis. The mouthwash form of this vitamin should be used for treating this condition.
Pycnogenol	*Gum:* Chew a gum containing pycnogenol to minimize dental plaque and bleeding gums. Pycnogenol gum may be hard to find; a trained alternative-care specialist may be able to help you find it or offer you a comparable alternative.
Tea Tree Oil	*Oral:* Mouthwash containing 0.5% or less tea tree oil may have oral hygiene benefits. *Caution:* Tea tree oil, even diluted as a mouthwash, should never be swallowed.
Vitamin C	*Capsule or Tablet:* Take 1,000 mg with 500 mg of flavonoids daily, divided into two doses. *Note:* Be sure to use a buffered form of vitamin C. If taking vitamin C causes loose stools, decrease your dosage and then gradually increase the dosage as tolerated.
Vitamin D	*Tablet (Adults age 51 and over):* Take 400 IU daily. *(Adults over age 70):* Take 600 IU daily. Ask your doctor to check your vitamin D level.
Xylitol	*Chewing Gum:* Dosages for cavity prevention range from 4 to 10 g per day, taken in divided dosages after meals. Be sure to read individual product labels for dosage information.

ULCERS

IF YOU'RE OVER THE AGE of 40, you probably remember hearing someone say "If you don't stop stressing me, you're going to give me an ulcer!" But peptic ulcers, once believed to be largely caused by stress, are now known to often result from a bacterial infection in the stomach and upper intestine. Thus, while removing stressful elements from life is always a good idea, you might want to discuss antibiotic therapy with your doctor if you have an ulcer.

WHAT IS IT?

Most ulcers are peptic ulcers, which are open sores that develop in the lining of the stomach, esophagus, and small intestine. Peptic ulcers in the stomach are known as gastric ulcers, while those in the small intestine are called a duodenal ulcer.

In the 1980s, researchers discovered that bacteria called *Helicobater pylori* are the source of about half of all ulcers. Although it is not known how these bacteria enter the body, it is known that once they do enter, they multiply and live on the mucous layer that protects the stomach and small intestine. The bacteria then erode the mucous layer, producing an ulcer. Other causes of ulcer include the regular use of nonsteroidal anti-inflammatory drugs (NSAIDs) such as aspirin or ibuprofen, smoking, and excessive consumption of alcohol.

The primary symptom of a peptic ulcer is pain that can occur anywhere from the navel to the breastbone. The pain can last from 5 minutes to a couple of hours, and typically flares up at night. It also tends to be worse when the stomach is empty.

Ulcers are a fairly common condition in America, and about one out of every 10 people will experience them. Some ways to avoid ulcers include curbing regular use of NSAIDs, cigarettes, and alcohol, and avoiding stress, since it is still a contributing factor even if it's not the primary cause of ulcers.

Fortunately, once an ulcer is diagnosed, treatment only takes a couple of weeks. Some doctors prescribe various medications to reduce the production of acid by the digestive tract. For ulcers caused by *H. pylori*, an antibiotic is often the answer, although Manuka honey may also be effective (see Kitchen Tips, page 602). Adding the following herbs and supplements to the treatment regimen for an ulcer can ease its pain and help prevent its return.

WHAT SHOULD I TAKE?

Chamomile • Garlic • Lactobacillus Acidophilus
Licorice • Mastic • Omega-3 Fatty Acids

Several clinical trials have found that **chamomile** may be helpful in keeping ulcers from developing as well as for encouraging their healing if they have developed. (For more information on chamomile, see page 67.)

CALL YOUR DOCTOR WHEN...

Although having an ulcer is always an unpleasant experience, there are times when immediate medical attention is warranted. Be sure to call your doctor if:
- You vomit blood (the vomit may look like coffee grounds)
- You experience unexplained weight loss
- The ulcer is accompanied by back pain
- You experience nausea or fatigue
- You find blood or what appears like black tar in your stool

Because of **garlic's** antibacterial properties, some experts believe it may be helpful in preventing or treating ulcers by killing the *H. pylori* bacteria that often causes ulcers. (For more information on garlic, see page 135.)

Probiotics, such as **Lactobacillus acidophilus**, may be especially helpful for ulcers caused by *H. pylori* bacteria. Early research suggests that acidophilus may both curb the growth of *H. pylori* and help antibiotic drugs to work more effectively. (For more information on Lactobacillus acidophilus, see page 180.)

Licorice has herbal properties that classify it as a demulcent—a soothing, coating agent for the digestive tract. One form of licorice, known as deglycyrrhizinated licorice extract, is available in chewable wafers that bring pain relief and may accelerate the healing of ulcers. Some studies suggest that deglycyrrhizinated licorice can be as effective as over-the-counter ulcer medications. (For more information on licorice, see page 192.)

Studies show that **mastic** has had overwhelmingly positive effects in reducing stomach secretions and fighting the *H. pylori* bacteria. In one clinical trial of 38 patients with duodenal ulcers, 80 percent had a significant reduction in their ulcer symptoms with mastic, and of these 70 percent also experienced significant tissue healing. (For more information on mastic, see page 206.)

Omega-3 fatty acids may curb the growth of bacteria and thereby protect against duodenal ulcers. (For more information on omega-3 fatty acids, see page 221.)

MY SUPPLEMENT LIST—ULCERS

SUPPLEMENT	RECOMMENDED DOSAGE
Chamomile	*Tea:* Take 1 or 2 tsp or teabags of chamomile with 1 cup of water. Steep for 5 to 10 minutes, and drink three or four times daily.
Garlic	*Fresh:* Eat 1 to 2 cloves of raw garlic daily. *Capsule or Tablet:* Take 600 to 900 mg daily of dried garlic powder, standardized to contain 1.3% allicin.
Lactobacillus Acidophilus	*Capsule:* Take a supplement containing 3 to 5 billion live organisms daily.
Licorice	*Chewable:* Follow the individual product labels for dosage information. *Capsule:* Take two to four 380 mg of deglycyrrhizinated licorice three times a day.
Mastic	*Gum:* Chew 1 to 3 g daily.

MY SUPPLEMENT LIST—ULCERS	
SUPPLEMENT	**RECOMMENDED DOSAGE**
Omega-3 Fatty Acids	*Capsule:* 1–2 g of omega-3 fatty acids per day, in divided doses, with meals. The amount of omega-3 fatty acid will vary by manufacturer, so be sure to check the product label carefully.

URINARY TRACT INFECTION

IF YOU HAVE EVER EXPERIENCED the unpleasant, burning sensation of a urinary tract infection (UTI), you know that the only thing on your mind is getting rid of it, and fast! Urinary tract infections are extremely common, especially in women, who are 10 times more likely to experience UTIs than men, although UTIs in men can be very serious.

WHAT IS IT?

Urinary tract infections occur when bacteria cling to the walls of the tube known as the *urethra*, which carries urine out of the body from the bladder, and begin to multiply. These bacteria can spread up to the urethra to the bladder and, if left untreated, up to the kidneys. Other causes of UTIs are sexually transmitted diseases, such as chlamydial infection, gonorrhea, and mycoplasma infection. Although these latter diseases do not usually spread beyond the urethra, they require treatment of both sexual partners.

UTIs make themselves known by causing pain or burning during urination, a feeling of pressure in the bladder, and/or a constant urge to urinate with only small amounts of urine actually being passed. The pain of a UTI can also occur during sexual intercourse. In some cases, blood or pus can appear in the urine, and cramps and pain may develop in the abdomen. A fever may be an indication that a UTI has spread to the kidneys and requires immediate medical attention.

Some activities can increase the risk of contracting a UTI, including frequent and intense sexual intercourse, pregnancy, or the use of birth control pills. At other times, the infection can strike without apparent cause. Simply drinking more water may help, since water decreases the numbers of bacteria in the urine and aids the body in flushing them out. Luckily, nature can do quite a bit to stop a UTI—and prevent it from coming back again.

FRIENDS AND FOES

If you are taking **uva ursi** to treat a UTI, make sure not to take this herb with **vitamin C** or **cranberry**. Both vitamin C and cranberry acidify the urine, and uva ursi needs an alkaline environment in order to work properly. Separate your doses of uva ursi from those of vitamin C or cranberry by at least 2 hours.

WHAT SHOULD I TAKE?
Bromelain • Cranberry • Garlic
Goldenseal • Lactobacillus Acidophilus • Uva Ursi

Bromelain—an enzyme derived from pineapples—may be a useful accompaniment to the antibiotics often prescribed to treat UTI. Studies suggest that bromelain enhances the effectiveness of antibiotics, ensuring that they eradicate a UTI the first time they are prescribed.

In one study in which people with UTIs were given the combination of bromelain and trypsin (another natural enzyme) along with their prescription antibiotic medication, UTI was eradicated in 100 percent of the group that took bromelain as opposed to only 46 percent of the comparison group that took a placebo. (For more information on bromelain, see page 54.)

Whether you choose to take **cranberry** in capsule or juice form, it is a well-accepted supplement for combating UTI. Cranberry works by acidifying the urine and by making it hard for UTI-causing bacteria to stick to the lining of the urethra. If you opt for cranberry juice, its important to take an unsweetened variety, since sugar makes bacteria flourish. (For more information on cranberry, see page 90.)

Alicin, a sulur-containing compound found in **garlic**, may have antibacterial effects against the bacteria that cause UTIs. Adding a garlic supplement to your UTI-fighting regimen may therefore be another way to kill the bacteria that are causing it. (For more information on garlic, see page 135.)

Tricks for Avoiding UTI

Healthy Hints

You can develop many healthy habits to decrease your chances of developing a UTI. If you experience frequent UTIs, try some of the tips below to stop bacteria in their tracks.

■ Doctors recommend drinking 6 to 8 glasses of water each day to flush any harmful bacteria out of the urinary tract.

■ When you have the urge to urinate, go as soon as possible. Holding in urine can trap bacteria and will increase your chances of developing an infection.

■ Wipe from front to back to prevent bacteria around the anus from entering the vagina or urethra

■ Wear cotton underwear and loose-fitting clothes to keep the genital area dry. Avoid wearing tight-fitting jeans or nylon underwear, which tend to trap moisture, creating a breeding ground for bacteria.

■ When possible, cleanse the genital area with a gentle soap and swab before having sexual intercourse.

■ Urinate shortly after having sexual intercourse. This will help flush away any bacteria that might have entered the urethra during sex.

Goldenseal may have promise in fighting UTIs. Berberine—one of the main alkaloids in goldenseal—is purported to have antibacterial properties. Goldenseal may prevent UTI by preventing bacteria from sticking to the wall of the urinary bladder and urethera, although more research is needed to confirm this. (For more information on goldenseal, see page 151.)

Lactobacillus acidophilus may be helpful for preventing and treating UTIs. Acidophilus inhibits the growth of harmful bacteria and promotes a healthy population of "good" bacteria in the digestive tract. Additionally, if you are taking antibiotics to treat a UTI, be sure to take acidophilus to prevent an accompanying yeast infection. (For more information on Lactobacillus acidophilus, see page 180.)

Uva ursi is an antimicrobial herb that has shown effectiveness like that of vitamin C and cranberry in banishing UTI. Nevertheless, uva ursi should not be taken with vitamin C or cranberry, since they seem to cancel each other's benefits. (For more information on uva ursi, see page 270.)

KITCHEN TIPS

ONIONS MAY HELP PREVENT A UTI

Try eating onions to ward off UTIs. Onions contain allicin, which appears to have antiviral, antifungal, and antibacterial effects. The next time you sense a UTI coming on, add raw onion to your meals to help fight off the invading bacteria!

MY SUPPLEMENT LIST—URINARY TRACT INFECTION

SUPPLEMENT	RECOMMENDED DOSAGE
Bromelain	*Tablet:* Take 250 to 500 mg daily between meals. Look for a product containing 2,400 gelatin-dissolving units (GDU) or 3,600 milk-clotting units (MCU) per gram.
	Note: Be sure to buy an enteric-coated form of bromelain to prevent stomach acid from destroying the enzyme and diminishing its effectiveness.
Cranberry	*Juice:* Drink 16 oz of unsweetened cranberry juice every day (which may be diluted with water). *Capsule:* Cranberry juice extract 500 mg, three times daily, or follow the manufacturer's directions.
Garlic	*Capsule:* Take 600 to 900 mg daily of dried garlic powder, standardized to contain 1.3% allicin.
Goldenseal	*Capsule:* Take 250 to 500 mg daily of an extract standardized to contain 8% to 12% goldenseal alkaloids. *Liquid Extract:* Take 2–4 ml three times daily.
Lactobacillus Acidophilus	*Yogurt:* Consume at least 6 oz of acidophilus-containing yogurt daily. *Capsule:* Take a product containing 1- to 2-billion colony-forming units (CFU) daily.
	Note: Different types of yogurt vary greatly in their potency. Some yogurts—especially frozen yogurts—do not contain any probiotic bacteria and thus do not have any bacteria-fighting effects. Be sure to buy a product that contains a live bacterial culture.

(continued)

SUPPLEMENT	RECOMMENDED DOSAGE

Uva Ursi

Capsule: Take 700–1,000 mg three times per day of an extract standardized to contain 20% arbutin. If symptoms do not improve within 48 hours, consider another method of treatment.

Caution: Uva ursi is not recommended for pregnant or breastfeeding women, or for children. It is not recommended for use beyond 7 days or more than 5 times a year, since it may lead to serious stomach disorders.

VARICOSE VEINS

FOR MANY PEOPLE, spider veins and varicose veins are a medically insignificant but cosmetically unpleasant problem. However, aside from putting a damper on summer, varicose veins can be painful and in rare cases lead to more serious health complications.

WHAT IS IT?

Varicose veins are caused by a "glitch" in the valves inside the veins. Arteries normally help blood to circulate from the heart to the rest of the body, with veins returning the blood to the heart for recirculation. When blood that normally travels to your heart begins to lose the fight against gravity, it flows backward and gets trapped by the valves in your veins. The veins then become enlarged

Simple Steps for Fighting Varicose Veins

Healthy Hints

You can do several things to help prevent varicose veins and to ease their pain and swelling if you already have them. Read on for ideas of how you may be able to ease leg and ankle pain.

■ **Walk it off.** Improve strength and circulation in your legs and veins by exercising regularly. Walking is an ideal aerobic exercise for people with varicose veins.

■ **Shed pounds.** Excess weight can be a stress on your legs, ankles, and feet. If you are overweight, discuss a weight-loss plan with your doctor to help give your veins a break.

■ **Don't cross your legs.** Sitting for prolonged periods, such as in the car or at the office, as well as crossing your legs, can instigate circulatory problems. Elevate your legs when possible, to keep the blood circulating through your veins.

■ **Choose compression stockings.** Special stockings are made to help people with varicose veins. If you experience pain from varicose veins, wear compression stockings. Compression stockings steadily squeeze your legs, helping veins and leg muscles move blood more efficiently. The amount of compression varies by the type and brand of stocking.

■ **Don't just stand there.** Try to avoid standing in the same position for extended periods. Change your position and shift your weight as often as possible to encourage healthy bloodflow.

and appear blue because they are filled with deoxygenated blood. The result? Varicose veins. While varicose veins appear enlarged and gnarled, spider veins, a less apparent, medically insignificant counterpart, have a "crawly" appearance. Women are more likely than men to develop varicose veins, and obesity puts you in the high-risk category for them because of the excess pressure of your body weight on your veins. Heredity is another factor, so chances are if varicose veins run in your family, you will be more likely to get them yourself.

WHAT SHOULD I TAKE?
Gotu Kola • Grape Seed Extract
Horse Chestnut • Vitamin E

Gotu kola is best known for easing symptoms of varicose veins as well as improving overall vein function. Gotu kola helps reduce swelling, tiredness, and discomfort in people with varicose veins. (For more information on gotu kola, see page 153.)

Studies suggest that the bioflavanoids found in **grape seed extract**—called oligomeric proanthocyanidin complexes (OPCs)—may be helpful for treating varicose veins. OPCs may work to improve the strength of collagen, reduce inflammation, and prevent blood vessels from leaking. Although plants such as bilberry, cranberry, green and black tea, and hawthorn contain OPCs, grape seed extract contains exceptionally high levels of these important bioflavanoids. (For more information on grape seed extract, see page 155.)

Research has confirmed the beneficial effects of **horse chestnut** in treating varicose veins. The active compound in horse chestnut—aescin—protects the structure of veins, maintaining the strength of the small vessels known as capillaries during times of stress. (For more information on horse chestnut, see page 169.)

Vitamin E helps blood circulation and may strengthen blood vessels. It has been shown to reduce the risk of blood clots, a dangerous potential side effect of varicose veins. (For more information on vitamin E, see page 292.)

MY SUPPLEMENT LIST—VARICOSE VEINS

SUPPLEMENT	RECOMMENDED DOSAGE
Gotu Kola	*Tablet:* Standardized extracts containing up to 100% total saponins (triterpenoids), 60 mg once or twice per day.

(continued)

MY SUPPLEMENT LIST—VARICOSE VEINS (continued)	
SUPPLEMENT	**RECOMMENDED DOSAGE**
Grape Seed Extract	*Capsule:* Take 200 to 500 mg daily of an extract standardized to contain 92% to 95% oligomeric proanthocyanidins (OPCs) in divided doses between meals.
Horse Chestnut	*Tablet:* Take 300 mg of an extract standardized to contain 16% to 21% aescin two to three times daily between meals.
Vitamin E	*Capsule:* Take 200 to 400 IU once a day of a natural product containing mixed tocopherols.

WARTS

ANYTHING THAT CONJURES UP visions of toads in your mind is probably not a something you want to have. Alas, warts are something that almost all of us have, whether we like it or not. Although usually harmless, they can be quite embarrassing and even disfiguring. Genital warts (spread by sexually transmitted disease) are a problem that merits medical attention.

WHAT IS IT?

There are four major types of warts: *common warts* are small, round and often found on the hands, although they may appear elsewhere; *flat warts* typically grow on the face and backs of the hands; *plantar warts* occur on the soles of the feet; and *genital warts* normally occur externally, though they may appear inside the vagina or anal canal as well. Warts are caused by the viruses known as human papillomaviruses (HPVs) and are contagious. Genital warts are the most contagious and

Protecting Yourself Against Warts

Healthy Hints

Because warts are caused by viruses, they are contagious. Fortunately, you can take steps to decrease your chances of catching contagious viruses. Practice these preventive strategies to protect yourself against warts:

■ **Shoe up.** Don't walk around barefoot in public areas, such as pools and locker rooms. Always wear shoes or sandals in public places, including locker room showers, to avoid coming into contact with HPV.

■ **Groom carefully.** Avoid brushing, clipping, combing or shaving areas where there are warts. If a wart opens,

the virus could spread to other parts of your body.

■ **Don't pick!** Picking at warts is a sure way to encourage the spread of the viruses that cause them. If your child has warts, consider covering them with a bandage.

■ **Pamper your feet.** Warts are more likely to grow on skin that is already damaged than on skin that is smooth and healthy. Keep your feet clean, dry, and healthy to ward off plantar warts.

■ **Don't share.** Towels, socks, and shoes can harbor the HPV that causes warts. To avoid contracting the virus, don't share these items.

serious kind of warts; common, flat, and plantar warts are less likely to spread from one person to another, although they may spread from one part of the body to another.

Common medical treatments for warts include topical drug therapy, cryosurgery (freezing the wart), laser removal of the wart, and surgical removal or cutting out of the wart. Through the use of supplements, you may be able to provide a two-pronged attack on warts and boost your immunity against HPV.

WHAT SHOULD I TAKE?

Genital warts are a serious condition. Make sure to consult your doctor before taking any kind of supplements, especially if you have been diagnosed with genital warts or think you may have genital warts.

Folic Acid · Garlic · Vitamin C · Zinc

Folic acid (vitamin B$_9$) may have immunity-boosting properties that can be useful for treating genital warts. Taken daily, it may reduce the chances of recurring episodes of genital warts. (For more information on folic acid, see page 130.)

When applied topically, **garlic** may help treat warts. In one preliminary study, garlic cloves were placed on the warts of children, and covered with a bandage overnight. In every case, the warts healed after an average of 9 weeks. (For more information on garlic, see page 135.)

Vitamin C may help rid the body of warts indirectly, since it helps to improve immune function, and may therefore help the body destroy the HPV virus more effectively. (For more information on vitamin C, see page 284.)

Zinc may have the ability to inhibit certain viruses in the body, possibly including the HPV virus, thus preventing warts. (For more information on zinc, see page 304.)

MY SUPPLEMENT LIST—WARTS

SUPPLEMENT	RECOMMENDED DOSAGE
Folic Acid	*Tablet:* Take 400 mcg daily.
Garlic	*Topical:* In the study described above, the area around the wart was washed and one half-clove of garlic was applied directly to the wart and covered with a bandage or waterproof tape each night. In the morning, the bandage was removed, and the area was washed thoroughly. This regimen was repeated nightly for about 9 weeks.

(continued)

MY SUPPLEMENT LIST—WARTS (continued)	
SUPPLEMENT	**RECOMMENDED DOSAGE**
Vitamin C	*Capsule or Tablet:* Take 3,000 to 8,000 mg daily. Consult your doctor before taking this dosage of vitamin C, since it is relatively high. *Note:* Be sure to use a buffered form of vitamin C. If taking vitamin C causes loose stools, decrease your dosage and then gradually increase the dosage as tolerated.
Zinc	*Tablet:* Take 15 to 30 mg daily.

WATER RETENTION

THE HUMAN BODY IS 70 percent water. Unfortunately, it sometimes seems as though 69 percent of that water is concentrated in your legs, feet, and ankles. Most women probably remember this feeling from being pregnant. And if you've ever experienced particularly bad premenstrual symptoms (PMS), you're probably familiar with the sensation. Suddenly, your legs, feet, and ankles begin to swell up like balloons, and the accompanying aching, soreness and difficulty moving can make you feel like a prisoner in your own body.

WHAT IS IT?

Water retention, or *edema*, is not a full-fledged medical condition but a symptom of other disorders. It occurs because of an imbalance in the body's transfer of fluids. Swelling from water retention typically affects the limbs, usually the legs and feet. It can occur for a variety of reasons, including standing or sitting for extended periods, exposure to high altitudes or heat, side effects of medication (including hormones, steroids, antidepressant medications, and calcium channel blocker drugs), and occurrence of liver disease or high blood pressure, congestive heart failure, or other circulatory disorders. It may also result from hormonal changes during pregnancy or menstruation.

In some cases, edema can be a serious condition that warrants immediate medical attention. During pregnancy, for example, edema may be caused by a condition known as pre-eclampsia, which is often marked by excessive swelling (see Call Your Doctor When, next page). Other serious diseases of the kidneys, heart, or liver can also cause edema. Pulmonary edema, which occurs when there is a build-up of excess fluid and swelling in the lungs, can be a potentially life-threatening condition. Supplements should not be used to treat edema in these cases.

Although in many cases water retention is not life threatening, it can be a terrible nuisance. The limbs become swollen and unwieldy, and the aching can rise to unbearable pain. But you can take several measures to reduce the occurrence of edema, including eating a low-salt diet, using cold-water compresses, elevating your legs for an hour every day, and swimming. Some supplements may also help relieve the symptoms of edema.

WHAT SHOULD I TAKE?
Bilberry • Dandelion
Horse Chestnut • Quercetin

A number of flavonoids, that are not available in the United States—including coumarin, hydroxyethylrutoside, and diosmin—have been found to reduce various types of edema. As alternatives to these supplements, some experts recommend taking **bilberry** or **quercetin** since they are more readily available in the United States. However, research on these supplements is preliminary, and more study is needed to determine their effectiveness in treating edema. (For more information on bilberry and quercetin, see pages 46 and 236.)

Dandelion has a long history of traditional use as a diuretic and, as a result, the German Commission E (see page 16) has approved its use. One recent animal study found that dandelion when taken in high doses (2 grams per 2.2 pounds of body weight) is equal in effect to furosemide (Lasix), a prescription diuretic. (For more information on dandelion, see page 96.)

Preliminary research suggests that **horse chestnut** may be effective in treating edema, particularly in cases of edema caused by surgery, head injury, or sports injury. This is because the same active compound in horse chestnut that is helpful in preventing and treating varicose veins—aescin—acts as an anti-inflammatory agent, reducing swelling and fluid accumulation. (For more information on horse chestnut, see page 169.)

CALL YOUR DOCTOR WHEN...

During pregnancy, swollen legs, feet, and even hands are normal, albeit uncomfortable symptoms. However, extreme swelling may be the sign of the serious medical condition called pre-eclampsia. This progressive condition occurs in 5 percent of all pregnancies. While bloating is a common accompaniment to pregnancy, be sure to call your doctor if:

■ Your face begins to swell, particularly around the eyes
■ You suspect your blood pressure is high
■ You notice sudden weight gain
■ You experience changes in vision or headaches

MY SUPPLEMENT LIST—WATER RETENTION

SUPPLEMENT	RECOMMENDED DOSAGE
Bilberry	*Capsule or Tablet:* Take 240–1,800 mg once a day of an extract standardized to contain 25% anthocyanidins divided into one to three doses.

(continued)

MY SUPPLEMENT LIST—WATER RETENTION (continued)	
SUPPLEMENT	**RECOMMENDED DOSAGE**
Dandelion	*Tea:* Steep 1 to 2 tsp of dried dandelion root in 1 cup of boiling water for 15–20 minutes; drink twice daily. Higher doses may be required. Consult your doctor to determine an appropriate dose for you.
Horse Chestnut	*Tablet:* Take 300 mg of an extract standardized to contain 16% to 21% aescin two to three times daily between meals.
Quercetin	*Tablet:* Although the optimal dosage is unknown, some experts recommend taking 200 to 500 mg two or three times daily.

WEIGHT LOSS

IN RECENT YEARS, supplements for producing weight loss have received their fair share of bad press. Ephedra in particular, which has been banned by the U.S. Food and Drug Administration (FDA), has proven to be an especially risky weight-loss supplement, resulting in the deaths of some users. However, other supplements have emerged as safe, effective weight-loss aids when used as directed and incorporated into a weight-loss program that includes a lower caloric intake and regular exercise.

WHAT IS IT?

More than 123 million American adults are obese as are 3.1 million people around the world, qualifying obesity as a major epidemic in the United States and as a serious health problem worldwide. With the convenience, ease, and broad availability of food in our country, coupled with our increasingly sedentary lifestyle, the problem has grown continually worse.

People struggling to lose weight—whether they are obese or simply looking to shed a few pounds—often look for "quick-fix" solutions. It's important to remember that conquering obesity will not happen overnight, regardless of what an infomercial might tell you. First and foremost, losing weight comes down to two simple factors: reducing your caloric intake and increasing your level of activity. Of course, eating the right foods (such as fruits and vegetables, whole grains, lean sources of protein, high-fiber foods, and foods with monounsaturated fats) also doesn't hurt. If you have a weight problem, talk to your doctor and a dietitian. Then try some of these safe natural remedies to assist you on the road to a healthy weight.

WHAT SHOULD I TAKE?
Calcium • Cayenne • Chromium
Fiber • 5-Hydroxytryptophan (5-HTP)
Green Tea • Omega-3 Fatty Acids

Although most people associate **calcium** with bone health, numerous studies suggest that it may also help promote weight loss. Data from various studies show that a greater intake of calcium may be associated with a lower body fat content and/or body weight, while a lower intake of calcium may be associated with a higher body fat content and/or body weight. Researchers have speculated that when calcium intake is increased by 300 milligrams, body fat in children may decrease by 2.2 pounds and in adults by 5.5 to 6.6 pounds. More studies are underway to examine the role of calcium in weight loss. (For more information on calcium, see page 57.)

Preliminary research indicates that ingesting **cayenne**—the "hot" in hot peppers—may promote weight loss in at least two ways. The active ingredient, capsaicin, appears to not only curb appetite but also speed the metabolism of dietary fats. (For more information on cayenne, see page 64.)

Chromium, in the form of chromium picolinate, may have promise in the world of weight-loss supplements. Preliminary studies suggest that chromium may reduce fat mass, increase lean body mass, and lead to weight loss, most effectively in women. One study found that supplementation with 200 to 400 micrograms of chromium picolinate daily resulted in an increased body mass and reduced body fat in nondieting, obese people. Another study suggests that chromium may prevent the loss of lean body mass in people on low-calorie diets. (For more information on chromium, see page 77.)

Foods with a high **fiber** content can be useful components of a healthy weight-loss program. Studies show that women who consume more whole-grain foods (as opposed to refined-grain foods) consistently weigh less than those who do not. However, recent studies suggest that fiber may only be useful when it is taken in conjunction with a low-calorie diet. (For more information on fiber, see page 120.)

5-HTP is derived from the seeds of *Griffonia simplicifolia*, an African plant. In studies, it has helped reduce food cravings by boosting the levels of the neurotransmitter serotonin, which typically declines during dieting, precipitating binge urges to eat and

KITCHEN TIPS

OOLONG TEA MAY PROMOTE WEIGHT LOSS

If green tea isn't—well—your "cup of tea," you may opt for the traditional Chinese tea, oolong tea. Long believed to aid in weight loss, this tea was put to the test in a study of 11 Japanese women. Researchers found that the women in the study who consumed oolong tea experienced an increased metabolism and were therefore able to burn more calories. Oolong is a good alternative to green tea, because it contains only about half as much caffeine. However, if you do drink green tea, decaffeinated preparations are available.

carbohydrate cravings. Studies have found that supplementation with 5-HTP in obese people resulted in significant weight loss as well as a lower intake of carbohydrates and in satiety with smaller amounts of food. Another study, of people with type 2 diabetes who were not on restricted diets, found that supplementation with 5-HTP helped to reduce carbohydrate and fat intake. People in this study lost an average of 4.6 pounds in 2 weeks, as compared to a loss of 0.2 pounds in a placebo group. A word of warning, though, people taking antidepressant medications should steer clear of 5-HTP. Be sure to consult your doctor before taking 5-HTP. (For more information on 5-HTP, see page 123.)

Green tea is rich in fat-burning polyphenols, which are present in greatest concentration in extracts of green tea. Studies have indicated green tea to be effective in boosting metabolism and energy expenditure. A study of healthy young men found an increase in energy expenditure and fat oxidation with green tea supplementation. Another study, involving moderately obese people, showed that after 3 months of taking green tea extract, their weight had decreased by 4.6 percent and waist size by 4.48 percent. Preliminary animal studies suggest that

How can I calculate my body mass index?

The body mass index (BMI) is a formula that determines a person's percentage of body fat on the basis of their height and weight. The BMI was established in 1998 by the National Institutes of Health as a way of classifying obesity. Calculating your BMI can be done in five simple steps:

1. Convert your weight from pounds to kilograms. (This is done by dividing your weight by 2.2.)

For example: 135 pounds x 2.2 = 61.36 kg

2. Convert your height from feet to inches. (1 foot = 12 inches)

For example: 5 feet, 5 inches = 65 inches

3. Convert your height to meters. (Multiply your height in inches by 2.54. Then divide your answer by 100.)

For example: 65 inches x 2.54 = 165.1
165.1 divided by 100 = 1.651 meters

4. Multiply your height in meters by itself.

For example: 1.651 x 1.651 = 2.725

5. Divide your weight in kilograms (Step 1) by your height in meters multiplied by itself (Step 4). The answer is your BMI.

For example: 61.36 divided by 2.725 = 22.51.

BMI = 22.51

A BMI of 19 to 24 is within the healthy range for adults; a BMI of 25 to 29 is classified as representing overweight; a BMI of 30 or more is considered to represent obese. BMIs of 25 or more are linked with higher blood pressure, a higher blood fat content, and an increased risk of heart disease and stroke.

Keep in mind that there are some kinks in this calculation: Body builders have more muscle than fat and usually have high BMIs. In the elderly, a BMI of 25 to 27 is often more favorable than a BMI of under 25. *Note:* The BMI is not meant for evaluating children's weight.

green tea may also be helpful as an appetite suppressant. One study, conducted on mice, found that food intake as well as weight gain and fat tissue accumulation decreased after supplementation with green tea. (For more information on green tea, see page 157.)

Omega-3 fatty acids are not weight-loss aids, but they may improve glucose/insulin metabolism and lower cholesterol, thus reducing diabetes and cardiovascular disease, two major health problems typically associated with obesity. It is a wise idea to add omega-3 fatty acids to any weight-loss program. (For more information on omega-3 fatty acids, see page 221.)

MY SUPPLEMENT LIST—WEIGHT LOSS

SUPPLEMENT	RECOMMENDED DOSAGE
Calcium	*Capsule or Tablet:* Take 300 mg in the form of calcium citrate daily.
Cayenne	*Infusion:* Combine 1 cup of boiling water with one-half to 1 tsp of cayenne powder and let it sit for 10 minutes. Mix 1 tsp of this infusion with water and take three or four times a day.
Chromium	*Tablet:* Take 50 to 300 mcg of chromium picolinate up to three times daily.
Fiber	*Capsule:* Take 25 to 35 g daily. *Psyllium:* Take 7 g in 8 oz of liquid up to three times daily. *Methylcellulos (sold as Citrucel):* Take 10.2 g in 8 ounces of liquid, as often as three times per day. *Polycarbophil (sold as Fibercon):* Take 1 g (or 2 caplets) per day. Do not exceed 4 g per day.
5-HTP	*Capsule:* Take 300 to 900 mg daily, divided into three divided doses. *Note:* Do not take 5-HTP without first consulting your doctor.
Green Tea	*Capsule:* Take 100 mg of a decaffeinated extract providing a minimum of 90% total catechins and 70% epigallocatechin gallate.
Omega-3 Fatty Acids	*Oral:* 1–3 g of omega-3 fatty acids per day, in divided doses, with meals. The amount of omega-3 fatty acid will vary by manufacturer, so be sure to check the product label carefully.

YEAST INFECTION

IN THE LIVES OF WOMEN, few health problems are as pesky and irritating as yeast infections. Almost all women get a yeast infection at some point in their lives (before menopause, three of every four women will have at least one yeast infection). It is therefore likely that if you've had a vaginal yeast infection, you're in very good company.

WHAT IS IT?

Despite common misconceptions, vaginal yeast infections are not necessarily caused by poor hygiene or a sexually transmitted microorganism. In fact, the microscopic fungi that cause vaginal yeast infections are quite common, and are everyday residents of the vagina from infancy onward. When the vagina experiences a change in its internal environment—often during menstruation, pregnancy, or during antibiotic therapy—these fungi, named *Candida albicans*, proliferate with the result being persistent itching and sometimes a thick, cottage cheese–like discharge.

You can do several things on a daily basis to prevent vaginal yeast infections. Among the most basic of these measures are to avoid bubble baths, vaginal contraceptives, and damp or tight-fitting clothing. Wearing cotton underwear and removing underwear before bedtime can also help reduce your chances of infection. Medications such as antibiotics and steroids can also often cause yeast infections, especially if taken on a long-term basis. Studies have shown that eating yogurt with active *Lactobacillus acidophilus* cultures can help stave off infection, since this "friendly bacteria" compete with and combat the Candida yeast (see Lactobacillus acidophilus, page 180). And for a first infection, go see your doctor. Then try some of the supplements named below to help fight the infection.

WHAT SHOULD I TAKE?

Boron • Garlic • Lactobacillus Acidophilus
Lavender • Tea Tree Oil

Could my partner be to blame for my recurrent yeast infections?

Q&A

It is often believed that women get recurrent yeast infections because their partners acquire the infection from them and then pass the infections back to them during intercourse. While it's true that men are not immune to yeast infections, new research suggests that their carrying of yeast does not put their partners at a greater risk for recurrent infection.

Researchers at the University of Michigan, who conducted a study of 148 women with recurrent yeast infection and 78 of their male sexual partners, found no link between recurrent yeast infection in women and the presence of yeast in their partners. This is good news for men, who have often received the blame for their partners' yeast infections. Nevertheless, the study did find that women who engaged in sex acts that involve saliva—their partner's or their own—are at a higher risk for recurrent yeast infection.

Several studies have found that boric acid—a chemical compound closely related to **boron**—is beneficial in treating as well as preventing chronic vaginal yeast infections. In a study of 92 women with chronic vaginal infections who were unresponsive to conventional over-the-counter antifungal agents, boric acid was effective in treating 98 percent of the women. Boric acid suppositories are available over-the-counter and may be less expensive than the medications often prescribed to treat chronic yeast infection. (For more information on boron, see page 50.)

Garlic is well known for its antifungal properties. When used in suppository form, garlic may have the ability to combat yeast infection. (For more information on garlic, see page 135.)

Lactobacillus acidophilus is a "friendly" bacteria that, like *Candida albicans*, commonly resides in the vagina. By increasing the levels of *L. acidophilus* in your body, you can fight vaginal yeast infections. Some studies indicate that acidophilus, when used in suppository form, may be almost equal in effect to clotrimazole (Lotrimin), an antifungal medication often prescribed for treating yeast infections. Acidophilus may also be taken as a preventive measure to avoid yeast infection during antibiotic therapy. Antibiotics notoriously increase the chance of developing a yeast infection, as they kill the "good" bacteria as well as the "bad" bacteria. (For more information on Lactobacillus acidophilus, see page 180.)

Lavender, much like its partner tea tree oil (see below), is a useful, nontoxic supplement for stopping fungal infections. To get the best effect against vaginal yeast infection, use essential oil of lavender in a douche once a day. (For more information on lavender, see page 184.)

Tea tree oil is perhaps the most tried-and-true natural remedy for vaginal yeast infections. It is a proven germicide, and in one study it inhibited 11 different bacteria. In treating a yeast infection, it is best to use tea tree oil as a douche. (For more information on tea tree oil, see page 265.)

MY SUPPLEMENT LIST—YEAST INFECTION

SUPPLEMENT	RECOMMENDED DOSAGE
Boron	*Vaginal:* Boric acid suppositories are available in select pharmacies and alternative medicine stores. Follow the individual product labels for application instruction and dosage information.

(continued)

SUPPLEMENT	RECOMMENDED DOSAGE
	Note: Make sure to consult with your doctor before using boric acid over-the-counter suppository treatments.
Garlic	Peel one whole clove of garlic, being careful not to nick the skin. Wrap in sterile gauze and tie with clean, unbleached string or dental floss, then insert. Remove after 12 hours.
Lactobacillus Acidophilus	*Yogurt:* Eat 8 oz of *L. acidophilus*-containing yogurt daily. *Oral—Capsule:* Take 2 to 5 million organisms three times a day. *Vaginal:* Discuss using acidophilus douches and suppositories with your doctor.
Lavender	*Topical:* Apply lavender essential oil 2 or 3 times per day to the vagina.
	Note: Consult your doctor before using lavender to treat yeast infection.
Tea Tree Oil	*Douche:* Tea tree oil may be used in the form of a vaginal douche. Concentrations of up to 40% have been used effectively. Consult your doctor to see whether tea tree oil is appropriate for your individual situation.
	Note: Tea tree oil should be used internally only under a doctor's supervision. Tea tree oil products should first be tested on a small patch of skin in an unobtrusive area of the body to make sure no allergic reaction occurs.

MY SUPPLEMENT LIST—YEAST INFECTION (continued)

INDEX